MARKERS OF NEURONAL INJURY AND DEGENERATION

ANNALS OF THE NEW YORK ACADEMY OF SCIENCES
Volume 679

MARKERS OF NEURONAL INJURY AND DEGENERATION

Edited by Jan N. Johannessen

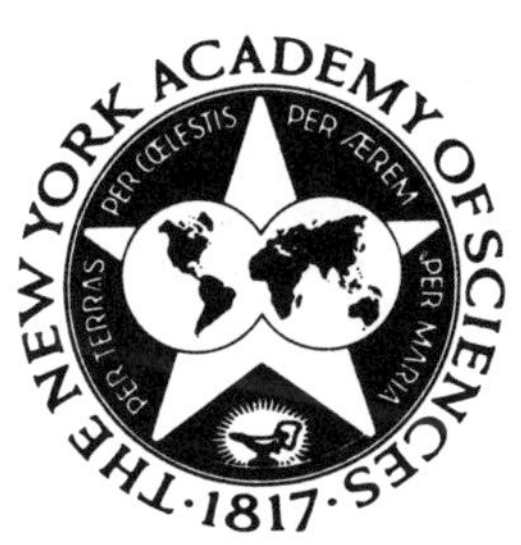

The New York Academy of Sciences
New York, New York
1993

Library of Congress Cataloging-in-Publication Data

Markers of neuronal injury and degeneration / edited by Jan N. Johannessen.

    p.   cm. -- (Annals of the New York Academy of Sciences, ISSN 0077-8923 ; v.679)

    Includes bibliographical references and index.

    ISBN 0-89766-795-6 (cloth : alk. paper). -- ISBN 0-89766-796-4 (pbk. : alk. paper)

    1. Nervous system--Pathophysiology--Congresses. 2. Biochemical markers--Congresses. 3. Nervous system--Degeneration--Congresses. I. Johannessen, Jan N. II. Series.

    [DNLM: 1. Biological Markers--congresses. 2. Nerve Degeneration--congresses. 3. Neurons--physiology--congresses. W1 AN626YL v.679 1993 / WL 102.5 M3456 1993]

Q11.N5 vol. 679

[RC347]

500 s--dc20

[616.8'047]

DNLM/DLC

for Library of Congress

                               93-13753

                                   CIP

Bic/PCP
Printed in the United States of America
ISBN 0-89766-795-6 (cloth)
ISBN 0-89766-796-4 (paper)
ISSN 0077-8923

ANNALS OF THE NEW YORK ACADEMY OF SCIENCES

Volume 679
May 28, 1993

MARKERS OF NEURONAL INJURY AND DEGENERATION[a]

Editor and Conference Organizer
JAN N. JOHANNESSEN

CONTENTS

[a] The papers in this volume were presented at a conference entitled **Markers of Neuronal Injury and Degeneration** held in Bethesda, Maryland on April 22–24, 1992 and sponsored by Sigma Xi, FDA Chapter.

Without the generous financial support of the following agencies of the United States Government this conference would not have been possible.

- ALCOHOL, DRUG ABUSE, AND MENTAL HEALTH
  ADMINISTRATION (ADAMHA)
    —Office of the Administrator
    —Office of Science
- FOOD AND DRUG ADMINISTRATION (FDA)
    —Center for Drug Evaluation and Research—Office of Research
    —Center for Food Safety and Applied Nutrition—Office of
      Toxicological Sciences
    —National Center for Toxicological Research—Division of
      Neurotoxicology
- NATIONAL INSTITUTE FOR OCCUPATIONAL SAFETY AND
  HEALTH (NIOSH)
    —Division of Biomedical and Behavioral Science
- NATIONAL INSTITUTES OF HEALTH (NIH)
    —National Institute on Aging (NIA)—Neuroscience and
      Neuropsychology of Aging Program
    —National Institute of Child Health and Human Development
      (NICHD)—Center for Research for Mothers and Children and
      Mental Retardation and Developmental Disabilities Branch
    —National Institute on Drug Abuse (NIDA)—Neuroscience Research
      Branch
    —National Institute of Environmental Health Sciences
      (NIEHS)—Division of Extramural Research and Training
    —National Institute of Mental Health (NIMH)—Division of Basic Brain
      and Behavioral Sciences
    —National Institute of Neurological Diseases and Stroke
      (NINDS)—Division of Fundamental Neurosciences
- UNITED STATES ENVIRONMENTAL PROTECTION AGENCY (EPA)
    —Division of Neurotoxicology

Preface

JAN N. JOHANNESSEN

Division of Toxicological Research
FDA/CFSAN
8301 Muirkirk Road
Laurel, Maryland 20708

and

M. ANTHONY VERITY

Division of Neuropathology and Brain Research Institute
UCLA Medical Center
Los Angeles, California 90024-1732

During the last decade, numerous studies have identified cellular mechanisms which participate in the initiation and physiological transduction of signaling mechanisms within the central nervous system. A major result of these studies is the recognition that these same pathways, activated abusively, may be transformed into weapons of neuronal destruction. A number of insults are associated with the induction of abnormal cellular processes, resulting in neuronal injury and loss. These include stroke (ischemia), chronic alcoholism, drugs of abuse (amphetamines, "ecstasy"), environmental toxins (*e.g.* heavy metals), food toxins (excitatory amino acids, *e.g.* domoic acid), idiopathic neurodegenerative disease (Parkinson's, Alzheimer's), trauma, and CNS infection.

Biochemical markers used to ascertain the degree of neuronal damage or loss have been those most commonly associated with specific neuronal phenotypes, such as neurotransmitters or their synthetic enzymes and receptors. While these approaches are sensitive, they are highly selective for specific cell types. Furthermore, since loss of a particular transmitter, receptor or enzyme is usually indicative of neuronal loss, these measures do not further our understanding of the degenerative process, but only indicate the magnitude.

Anatomical markers are often useful because specific morphological changes associated with degenerating neurons, including reactive changes in non-neuronal elements, can be visualized. Clearly these morphological changes seen with traditional histological techniques have biochemical correlates. The emphasis of this conference has been on identifying some of the biochemical events which occur during the process of neuronal degeneration rather than those which signal the end result of that process. Furthermore, models of neuronal injury from a wide variety of causes have been included in hopes that certain biochemical events common to injury will emerge.

The expanding list of biomarkers associated with neuronal injury and degeneration should lead to a number of practical benefits. Pursuing the functional roles of these markers in the degenerative process will lead to a more complete understanding of the causes and progression of neuronal injury, point to novel ameliorative strategies. Once current research emphasis in the treatment of neurodegenerative diseases such as parkinsonism, has been on reversal of the disease by neuronal transplant. A more conservative approach is the slowing or halting of the degenerative process by early pharmacological intervention. The success of this strategy will ultimately depend on the ability to detect the earliest stages of the disease. Hence, there is an undisputed need for accurate and sensitive markers of the degenerative process which have predictive diagnostic value.

Accurate and sensitive biomarkers of neuronal injury can also have a practical predictive role in the hazard identification portion of the risk assessment process. The task of identifying neurotoxins which target selective, but unidentified phenotypic targets would be simplified by the availability of markers which denote injury in a number of neuronal subtypes. In addition, prior to overt neuronal loss or irreversible injury, there is often a silent period during which slow degenerative changes are underway. Markers for such damage would be useful for identifying neurotoxins with a slow onset of action.

The wide diversity of approaches for identifying biomarkers of neuronal injury is reflected in this conference proceeding. As the contents readily show, the amount of information on biochemical correlates of neuronal injury is growing rapidly, making it increasingly difficult to cover comprehensively all aspects of this topic within a single conference. However, the diversity of the contributions contained herein will provide an appreciation for the complex integration of events leading to neuronal death, and will serve as a useful source of data and bibliographic information for those interested in the topic.

Altered Calcium Signaling and Neuronal Injury: Stroke and Alzheimer's Disease as Examples[a]

M. P. MATTSON,[b,d] R. E. RYDEL,[c] I. LIEBERBURG,[c] AND
V. L. SMITH-SWINTOSKY[b]

[b]*Sanders-Brown Research Center on Aging and
Department of Anatomy & Neurobiology
University of Kentucky
Lexington, Kentucky 40536-0230*

[c]*Athena Neurosciences Inc.
800F Gateway Blvd.
South San Francisco, California 94080*

INTRODUCTION

Neuronal death, whether "natural" as in development or in different pathological conditions, can result from a variety of causes. At first approximation it would seem that quite different events must be involved in different cases of neuronal death. For example, apoptosis and necrosis, which are morphologically distinct, have generally been related to natural and pathological neuronal death, respectively. Differences in the time course of cell death has also been inferred to indicate the involvement of different mechanisms. Thus, in stroke previously healthy neurons can die within hours to days, while in Alzheimer's disease (AD) neurons may die over periods of weeks to years. Despite these apparent differences in the process of neuronal death, it is reasonable to consider that multiple initiating causes may converge at some point in the cascade of events leading to neuronal injury and death. The present paper considers $[Ca^{2+}]_i$ as a convergence point for multiple initiating causes of neuronal injury ranging from amyloid mismetabolism, to overactivity of glutamatergic systems, to alterations in growth factor signaling. We focus on stroke and AD in this paper because they represent both a disorder that is fairly homogenous in cause (stroke) and another disorder (AD) that is not homogenous in cause, but rather represents a spectrum of alterations that may lead to the similar final result of neurofibrillary degeneration in vulnerable neurons. Therefore, understanding the complexity of cellular signaling mechanisms involved in neuronal survival and death in disorders such as stroke and AD may provide information that can be extrapolated to other neurological disorders, as well as to mechanisms of natural neuronal death.

Ca^{2+} is arguably the most important ion regulating neuronal structure and function.[1] It is therefore not surprising that neurons possess highly elaborate systems for regulating $[Ca^{2+}]_i$ and responding to changes in $[Ca^{2+}]_i$. Regulation of

[a] This work was supported by grants to M.P.M. from the NIH (NS29001 and AG05144), the Alzheimer's Association, and the International Life Sciences Institute.

[d] Address correspondence to Mark P. Mattson, 211 Sanders-Brown Building, University of Kentucky, Lexington, KY 40536-0230; Tel.: (606)257-6040; FAX (606)258-2866.

Ca^{2+} movements across the plasma membrane involves voltage-dependent and ligand-gated Ca^{2+} channels that provide portals through which Ca^{2+} can enter the cytoplasm.[2,3] Moving Ca^{2+} out of the cell against a marked, 10,000-fold, concentration gradient are the plasma membrane Ca^{2+} ATPase and the Na^+/Ca^{2+} exchanger.[4] Within the cytoplasm are a multitude of calcium-binding proteins, some of which may serve to "buffer" calcium and others of which mediate physiological responses to Ca^{2+} (*e.g.*, calmodulin). Proteins responsive to calcium include kinases such as protein kinase C and calcium/calmodulin-dependent protein kinase II,[5] and proteases such as the calpains.[6] Proteins that may sequester calcium include calbindin D-28k and parvalbumin.[7,8] In addition, organelles such as endoplasmic reticulum and mitochondria have efficient mechanisms to remove calcium from the cytoplasm, and can also be induced to release calcium.[9,10]

Calcium mediates adaptive changes in neuronal cytoarchitecture (*e.g.*, neurite outgrowth, synaptic remodeling, and natural cell death) in response to a variety of environmental signals. For example, neurotransmitters,[11] growth factors,[12,13] and cell adhesion molecules[14] can all affect neurite outgrowth and cell survival by modulating $[Ca^{2+}]_i$. A loss of calcium homeostasis resulting in an elevated $[Ca^{2+}]_i$ can cause structural damage to neurons and initiate the process of cell death.[1] Considerable data indicate that excessive elevations of $[Ca^{2+}]_i$ are causally involved in the neuronal degeneration that occurs in: traumatic neuronal injury,[15] stroke,[16,17] AD,[1,18] and Huntington's disease.[19] In each case the excitatory amino acid glutamate may contribute to the calcium influx that is believed to initiate the structural damage and eventual cell death. In theory, alterations in any of the $[Ca^{2+}]_i$-regulating systems described above could lead to a loss of calcium homeostasis. Some of the $[Ca^{2+}]_i$-regulating systems and calcium responsive proteins that are relevant to the problem of neuronal injury and that will be considered in this paper are identified in FIGURE 1. The precise events leading to neuronal damage and death following an aberrant elevation of $[Ca^{2+}]_i$ have not been established. However, accumulating evidence indicates that protein kinases and calcium-dependent proteases are involved. For example, specific activators of protein kinase C can cause neuronal damage and death,[20] and down regulation of protein kinase C can reduce excitotoxic neuronal damage.[21] Similarly, calpain inhibitors have proven effective in protecting neurons against excitotoxic/ischemic insults (see Roberts-Lewis and Siman this volume). Elevations in $[Ca^{2+}]_i$ may also initiate the formation of free radicals which have been implicated in neuronal damage in a variety of conditions.[22]

The present paper illustrates how multiple signaling systems may be involved in neuronal injury and death. The signaling systems discussed here include transduction systems for excitatory amino acids (EAAs), growth factors, and amyloid precursor proteins. The reason we discuss these particular components of neuronal calcium signaling is simply that data exists to support their involvement in the maintenance, plasticity and degeneration of neuronal cytoarchitecture. Although we focus on stroke and AD, we believe that the data considered here are relevant to mechanisms of neuronal damage and death in a variety of pathological conditions, as well as in the proces of "natural" neuronal death.

METHODS

Details of all methods referred to here can be found in previous studies as follows; dissociated cell culture of rat hippocampal and human cortical neurons;[23,24] assessment of neuronal injury;[25] immunocytochemistry and Western blots;[26] fluorescence ratio imaging of intracellular free calcium levels using the calcium indicator dye fura-2;[27,28] adrenalectomy, corticosterone administration and kainic acid injection *in vivo*.[29]

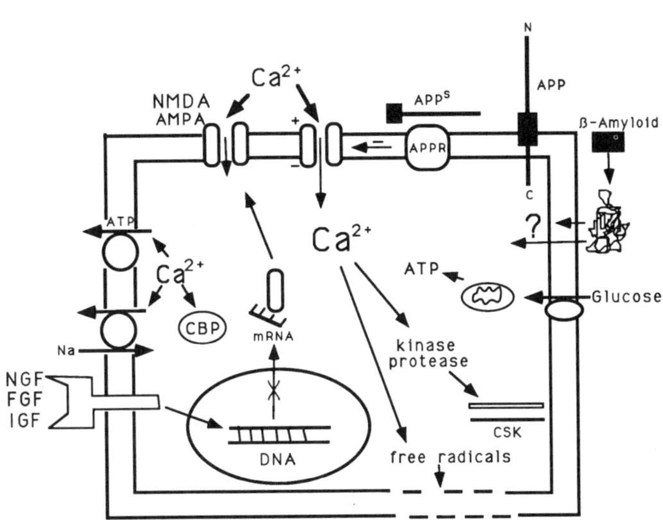

FIGURE 1. Regulation of $[Ca^{2+}]_i$ by excitatory amino acids (EAAs), growth factors, and amyloid precursor protein (APP) products. EAA receptors (NMDA, AMPA) and voltage-dependent calcium channels provide the major sites of Ca^{2+} influx into neurons of brain regions that are vulnerable in stroke and Alzheimer's disease (e.g., hippocampus). Ca^{2+} is normally removed from the cytoplasm by the plasma membrane Na^+/Ca^{2+} exchanger (rapid removal) and Ca^{2+} ATPase (slow removal), organellar sequestration, or Ca^{2+}-binding proteins (CBP). Neurons utilize glucose as an energy source for ATP production. Sustained elevations in $[Ca^{2+}]_i$ result in overactivation of kinases and proteases, and the generation of free radicals all of which contribute to cytoskeletal disruption and membrane damage. Growth factors (*e.g.*, bFGF, NGF and IGFs) stabilize $[Ca^{2+}]_i$ and prevent a loss of $[Ca^{2+}]_i$ homeostasis. For example, bFGF suppresses the expression of a 71 kDa NMDA receptor protein which results in reduced vulnerability to excitotoxicity. Normal proteolytic cleavage of APP results in the liberation of secreted forms of APP (APP^s) which bind to cell surface receptors and cause a reduction in $[Ca^{2+}]_i$. The APP^s can protect neurons against insults such as hypoglycemia. Aberrant APP processing results in both a disruption of the normal neuroprotecive action of APP^s, and the deposition and aggregation of β-amyloid which destablizes $[Ca^{2+}]_i$ and makes neurons vulnerable to excitotoxic/ischemic insults.

DATA AND DISCUSSION

Growth Factors Protect against Ischemic/Excitotoxic Damage by Stabilizing Intracellular Calcium Levels

The vast majority of CNS neurons can be damaged by the excitatory amino acid neurotransmitter glutamate. Neurons are particularly vulnerable to excitotoxicity under conditions of hypoxia and/or hypoglycemia.[30] Data obtained both in neuronal cell culture[25,31,32] and *in vivo*[16,33] indicate that calcium influx caused by glutamate is causally involved in excitotoxic cell damage and death (but see ref. 34, and Dubinsky this volume for further consideration of the mechanism of excitotoxicity). The *N*-methyl-D-aspartate (NMDA) type of glutamate receptor is probably the major site of calcium entry in ischemic/excitotoxic condition,[35] although calcium influx through non-NMDA receptors (see Gibbons *et al.*, this volume) and voltage-dependent calcium channels[36] may also contribute to cell injury. The involvement of calcium in excitotoxic damage is supported by experiments demonstrating that neurons are protected against EAA-induced damage when they are subjected to conditions or agents (*e.g.*, EAA receptor antagonists, removal of extracellular Ca^{2+}, Ca^{2+} channel blockers) that prevent or reduce calcium entry and elevations of $[Ca^{2+}]_i$.[25,35,37]

Several features of calcium-induced neuronal damage in experimental systems are shared with the damage that occurs in neurodegenerative disorders. For example, in rat hippocampal and human cortical cell cultures glutamate and calcium ionophores can elicit changes in the neuronal cytoskeleton similar to those seen in the neurofibrillary tangles of AD and Down syndrome.[26,38] The cytoskeletal alterations include a loss of microtubules, the accumulation of straight filaments, and antigenic changes in the microtubule-associated protein tau and ubiquitin. Tangle-like antigenic changes in tau were also observed in neurons in region CA3 of the hippocampus in rats exposed to kainic acid (FIG. 2). Interestingly, both the neuronal damage and the antigenic changes in tau caused by kainic acid were exacerbated by administration of the glucocorticoid corticosterone,[29] which has been implicated in several neurodegenerative disorders.[39]

Hypoglycemia is a major factor contributing to neuronal damage in stroke, and data also indicate that reduced glucose metablism and reduced glucose transport occur in AD.[40,41] Support for a possible causal role for reduced energy availability/utilization in AD comes from work which showed that hypoglycemia can elicit neurofibrillary tangle-like changes in hippocampal neurons.[42] Glucocorticoids may exacerbate neuronal injury by compromising the function of the neuronal glucose transporter.[39] Reduced glucose availability results in ATP depletion, failure of Ca^{2+} extrusion/buffering systems, membrane depolarization, excess glutamate release, and NMDA receptor activation. All of the preceding alterations would contribute to a neurotoxic increase in $[Ca^{2+}]_i$.

In an initial study we demonstrated that basic fibroblast growth factor (bFGF) can protect cultured rat hippocampal neurons against glutamate neurotoxicity.[43] Subsequently, we found that bFGF can also protect cultured rat hippocampal and human cortical neurons against hypoglycemic damage.[13] The consequences of reduced availability of glucose for neuronal $[Ca^{2+}]_i$ homeostasis and cell survival are illustrated in FIGURE 3. When cultured hippocampal neurons are deprived of glucose they die over a period of 16 to 24 hours. During the first few hours of glucose deprivation there is a reduction in $[Ca^{2+}]_i$ which is associated with a reduction in whole-cell calcium currents.[44] Subsequently, $[Ca^{2+}]_i$ rises slowly through approximately 4–12 hours of hypoglycemia; during this time the neurons appear undamaged. Between 12 and 16 hours of hypoglycemia, $[Ca^{2+}]_i$ rise markedly (3- and 4-fold) and the neurons rapidly degenerate during the next 4 hours. Activation of NMDA receptors is involved in both the elevation in $[Ca^{2+}]_i$ and the cell damage.[35] Thus, neurons are exquisitely sensitive to hypoglycemia since glucose is their sole energy source (neurons do not possess glycogen stores), and because they express excitatory amino acid receptors at high levels.

In addition to bFGF, nerve growth factor (NGF) and insulin-like growth factors

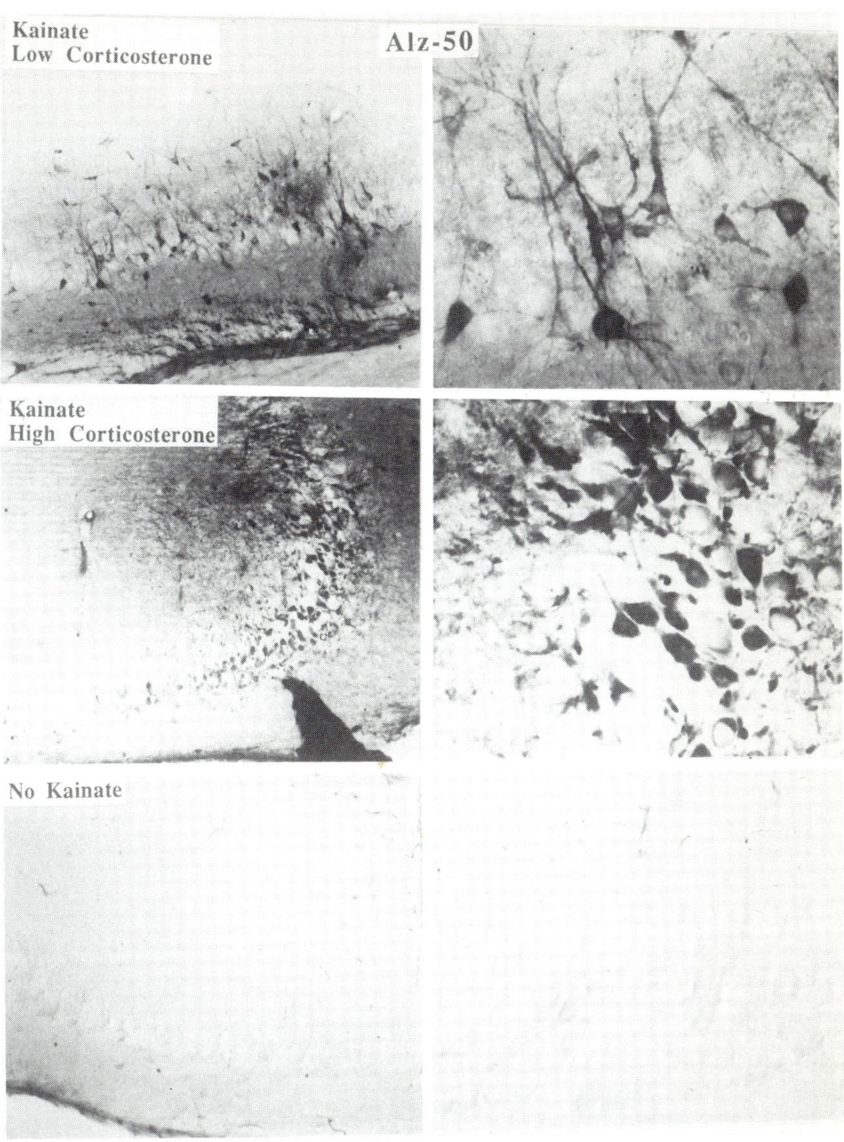

FIGURE 2. Excitotoxic insults *in vivo* can elicit antigenic changes in neurons similar to those seen in Alzheimer neurofibrillary tangles. Shown are coronal sections of rat hippocampus immunostained with antibody Alz-50. Rats were adrenalectomized and administered either a low level (*top panel*) or high level (*middle and bottom panels*) of corticosterone. Kainic acid was then injected unilaterally into region CA1 of the hippocampus and animals were sacrificed 3 hr later. Alz-50 immunoreactivity is seen in neurons of region CA3 of the kainate-injected hippocampus. The cell damage was relatively mild in the animal that received a low level of corticosterone, and neuronal cell bodies and dendrites are immunoreactive, whereas with a high level of corticosterone dendrites deteriorated and only immunoreactive cell bodies remained.

(IGF-1 and IGF-II) protected rat hippocampal and septal neurons against hypogly-cemic damage.[35] All of these growth factors prevented the elevation in $[Ca^{2+}]_i$ that was causally involved in the excitotoxic damage.[13,35,43] Cycloheximide and actinomycin D abolished the neuroprotective effect of bFGF indicating that the

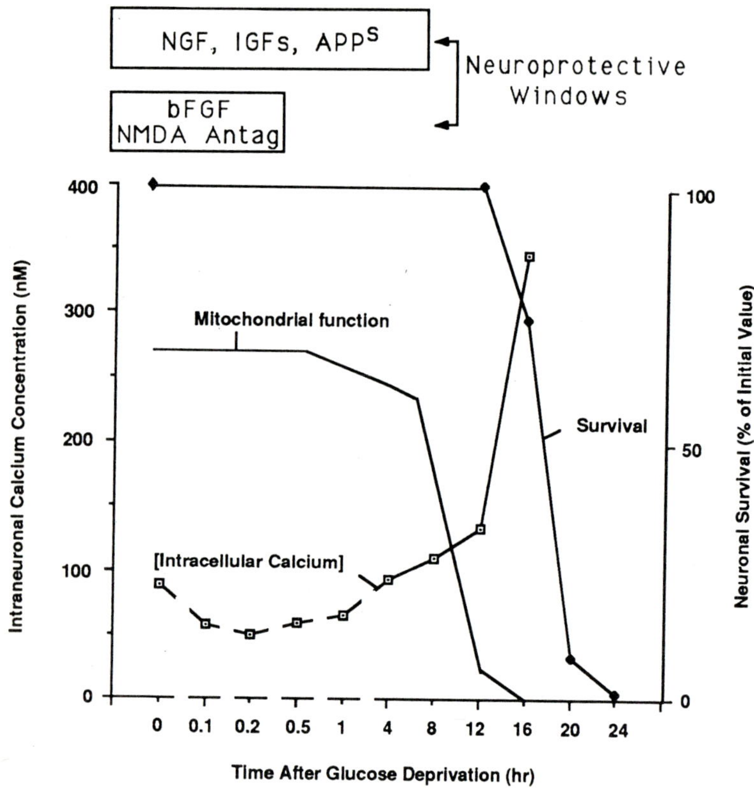

FIGURE 3. Temporal sequence of events occurring in rat hippocampal neurons as the result of glucose deprivation. Following the onset of hypoglycemia (time = 0) the $[Ca^{2+}]_i$ initially falls, then rises modestly between 4 and 12 h, and finally rises rapidly between 12 and 16 h. Neuronal survival is unaffected during the first 12 h of hypoglycemia. After 16 h of glucose deprivation neurons degenerate rapidly. Impairment of mitochondrial function may precede both the late rise of $[Ca^{2+}]_i$ and cell damage. The $[Ca^{2+}]_i$ was measured by fluorescence ratio imaging of the calcium indicator dye fura-2, cell survival was judged by morphological criteria, and mitochondrial function was assessed by their ability to concentrate the dye rhodamine 123. Some of the data used to generate this figure come from a previous study.[44]

mechanism of action of bFGF required protein synthesis.[43] Interestingly, protec-tion from hypoglycemic damage by bFGF required exposure to bFGF prior to or at the time of onset of glucose deprivation, whereas NGF and IGFs were effective in protecting neurons even when added up to 8 hours following the onset of glucose deprivation.[13,35] This difference among growth factors in their "window of opportunity" for neuroprotection suggested that different growth factors have different mechanisms of action.

Growth factors could conceivably protect neurons from glucose deprivation either by preventing ATP depletion or by preventing the consequences of ATP depletion. Two important functions of mitochondria are to generate ATP and to sequester calcium.[10] Damage to mitochondria would therefore be expected to have devastating consequences. We have examined the time course of alteration in mitochondrial function during a hypoglycemic insult. "Healthy" mitochondria accumulate the fluorescent dye rhodamine-123, whereas impaired mitochondria do not accumulate the dye.[46] Within 12 to 14 hours of the onset of hypoglycemia neuronal mitochondria were impaired in their ability to accumulate rhodamine 123 (FIG. 4). The mitochondrial impairment in neurons may precede or accompany both the loss of calcium homeostasis and the cell damage caused by glucose deprivation (FIG. 3). Interestingly, mitochondrial function in astrocytes appeared to be relatively unaffected by hypoglycemia (FIG. 4), probably because astrocytes possess glycogen stores which can be recruited during a period of hypoglycemia. Pretreatment of neurons with bFGF, NGF or IGFs prior to the onset of hypoglycemia prevented the mitochondrial dysfunction. NGF and IGFs were also effective in preventing mitochondrial dysfunction when added at the time of onset of hypoglycemia. These data suggest that growth factors may prevent energy failure in neurons, which may contribute to their ability to "stabilize" $[Ca^{2+}]_i$. In addition, growth factors may prevent the loss of $[Ca^{2+}]_i$ homeostasis resulting from energy failure. Thus, bFGF, NGF and IGFs can protect neurons against the damage normally caused by cyanide or 2,4-dinitrophenol.[17]

Specific Mechanisms of Neuroprotection by Growth Factors

Further insight into the mechanisms whereby growth factors protect neurons against environmental insults has come from recent studies that examined the effects of growth factors on specific neuronal systems involved in $[Ca^{2+}]_i$ regulation (*cf.* FIG. 1). The NMDA type of glutamate receptor[47] is believed to play prominent roles in adaptive processes such as regulation of neurite outgrowth and synaptic plasticity,[11,48] and is almost surely involved in the neuronal damage that occurs in an array of disorders including stroke and AD.[1,16,30] The isolation, purification and cloning of a putative NMDA receptor protein from rat brain[49–51] provided an opportunity to establish the function of this protein and examine its roles in neuronal plasticity and excitotoxicity. The 71 kDa NMDA receptor protein is believed to represent the glutamate binding subunit of a complex of 4 proteins that may comprise a functional NMDA receptor.[51] Using antibodies to the 71 kDa protein we established that: it is expressed in cultured rat hippocampal neurons; the developmental appearance of the protein coincides with appearance of sensitivity of the neurons to NMDA; neurons expressing high levels of the protein are selectively vulnerable to glutamate neurotoxicity; and an antibody to this protein reduces neuronal damage normally caused by glutamate.[52] Additional evidence that the 71 kDa protein is part of a functional NMDA receptor comes from studies in which levels of the 71 kDa protein were selectively reduced using antisense oligonucleotides directed against the mRNA for this protein.[53] Vulnerability to NMDA neurotoxicity was greatly reduced in cultured hippocampal neurons exposed to antisense oligonucleotides for 20 hours (FIG. 5). Furthermore, elevations

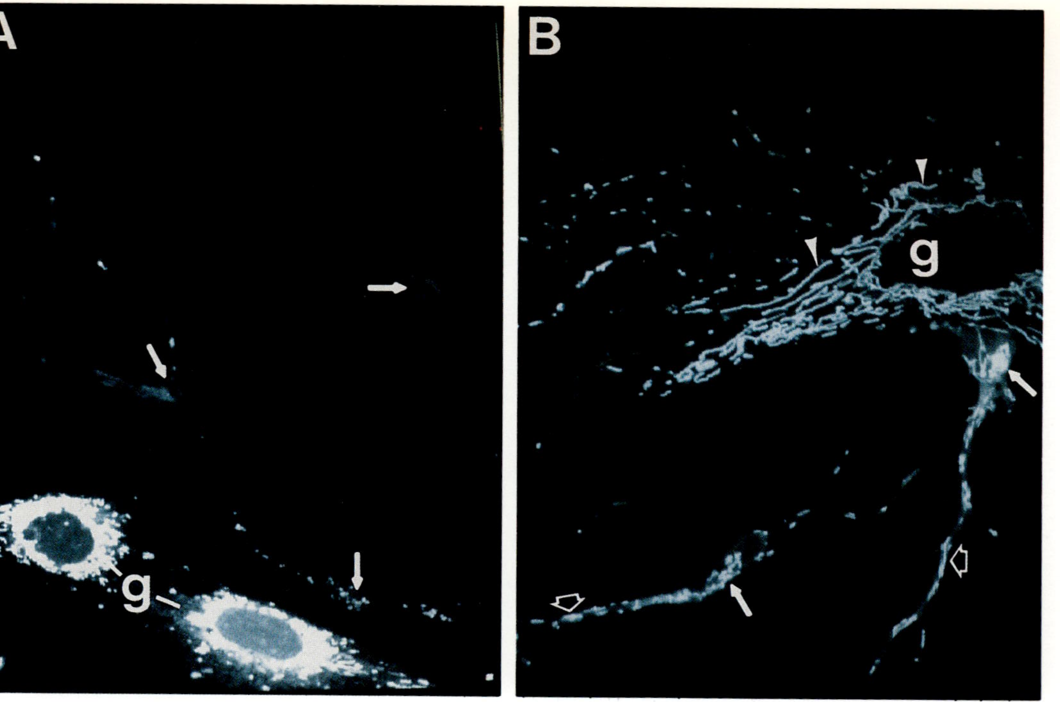

FIGURE 4. Effects of hypoglycemia and growth factors on mitochondrial function. Cultured rat hippocampal cells were deprived of glucose for 14 h, and were then exposed to 10 μM rhodamine 123 for 10 min. Cells were imaged using a confocal laser scanning microscope (Molecular Dynamics), using a Nikon 60× n.a. 1.3 oil immersion lense (0.3 μm optical sections). The cells on the left are from a control glucose-deprived culture, and those in the right panel were from a parallel glucose-deprived culture that had been pretreated for 16 h with 10 ng/ml bFGF. Note that little or no mitochondrial staining is evident in the neurons in the glucose-deprived control culture (*arrows in left panel*), whereas intense staining is present in cell bodies (*arrows*) and axons (*open arrows*) of neurons that had been exposed to bFGF (*arrows in right panel*). Also note that mitochondria in glia (*g*) stain with rhodamine 123 in both cultures (*arrowheads*). These data indicate that bFGF can prevent the loss of mitochondrial function in neurons normally caused by glucose deprivation.

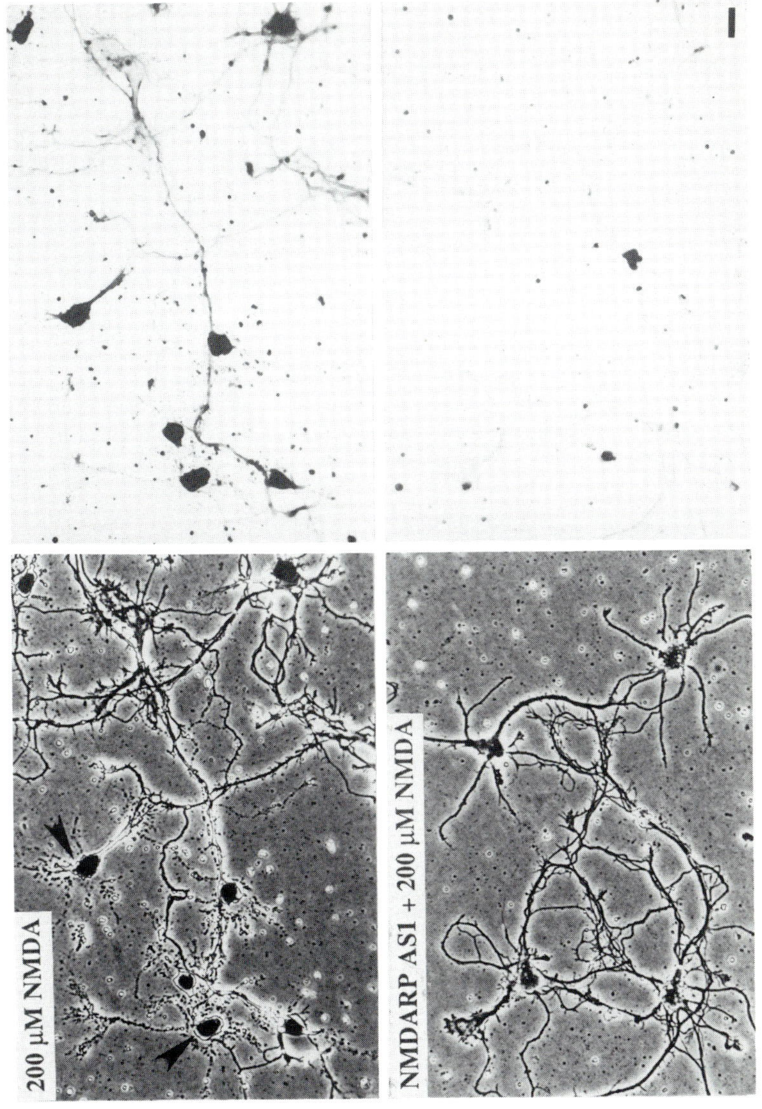

FIGURE 5. An antisense oligonucleotide directed against a 71 kDa NMDA receptor protein can protect cultured hippocampal neurons against excitotoxicity. Phase-contrast (*left*) and bright-field (*right*) light micrographs of cultured rat hippocampal neurons 8 h following exposure to 200 μM NMDA. The cultures were immunostained with a monoclonal antibody to the 71 kDa NMDA receptor protein. The microscope field in the upper panel is from a culture that had not been exposed to antisense oligonucleotide, whereas the cells in the bottom micrographs were pretreated with NMDA receptor protein antisense oligonucleotide (50 μM) for 24 h and then exposed to NMDA. Note that NMDA caused most of the neurons to degenerate in the control culture (*e.g., arrowheads in top panel*), whereas neurons pretreated with NMDA receptor protein antisense were resistant to NMDA toxicity (*bottom*). Scale bar, 10 μm.

of $[Ca^{2+}]_i$ in response to NMDA were greatly attenuated in the antisense-treated cultures.

Western blot and immunocytochemical studies demonstrated that levels of the 71 kDa NMDA receptor protein were markedly reduced in hippocampal neurons after 12 to 48 hours of exposure to bFGF; levels of mRNA for the 71 kDa NMDA receptor protein were also reduced by bFGF.[53] NGF did not affect NMDA receptor protein levels. These data suggest that at least a portion of the neuroprotective effect of bFGF against excitotoxicity can be accounted for by suppression of the expression of an NMDA receptor protein. Since we previously found that the excitoprotective action of bFGF required protein synthesis,[43] it appears that the suppression of NMDA receptor protein expression involves induction of a protein(s) that suppress the expression of the NMDA receptor protein gene. It will certainly be of interest to determine how this regulation occurs and whether regulation of EAA receptors (or other transmitter receptors) by growth factors is a common feature of growth factor actions in the nervous system.

We propose that by regulating the expression of neurotransmitter receptors, growth factors can modulate neuronal plasticity during development and in the adult nervous system. This possibility is consistent with recent reports that growth factors can modify long-term potentiation (LTP), a cellular correlate of learning and memory.[54] Abundant evidence indicates that both neuronal activity (mediated by transmitters) and trophic factors are involved in the regulation of neuronal plasticity in the developing and adult nervous systems.[55] Our data also suggest that neurotransmitter and growth factor systems can be involved in pathological neuronal death. Furthermore, the calcium signaling system appears to be central to both adaptive changes in neuronal structure effected by transmitters and growth factors, and to neuronal degeneration.

Different growth factors are likely to have different mechanisms of action in protecting neurons against environmental insults. This appears to be true for NGF and bFGF since bFGF affects NMDA receptor protein expression whereas NGF does not. In addition, NGF is effective in protecting rat hippocampal neurons against hypoglycemia when added up to 12 hours following the onset of glucose deprivation, whereas bFGF has to be added prior to or at the time of glucose deprivation in order for neuroprotection to be observed.[13] On the other hand a single growth factor may exert multiple influences on calcium homeostasis. Thus, in addition to suppressing NMDA recepor expression bFGF increases the expression of the 28 kDa calcium-binding protein calbindin in hippocampal neurons that normally express lower levels of this protein (M. P. Mattson and S. Christakos, unpublished data).

An important area for future research concerns the mechanism by which neurotransmitters and growth factors affect gene expression. For example, a strong calcium signal is seen in the nucleus following stimulation of neurons by excitatory amino acids (see ref. 56), and excitatory amino acids can turn on immediate early genes.[57] An emerging theme is that activation of growth factor receptors results in the activation of immediate early genes (*e.g.*, *c-fos*, *jun*, *myc*) which are believed to encode transcription factors (see Vendrell *et al.* this volume). Different growth factors can elicit different patterns of immediate early gene expression, which may differ from the immediate early genes turned on by depolarization.[58,59] Although the exact mechanisms by which FGF, NGF, and IGFs exert their protective influences on neurons are unknown, tyrosine kinase activity appears to be a common mechanistic link among receptors for these growth factors.[60–63] Receptors for bFGF[64] and IGF-II[65] are abundant in hippocampus and cerebral cortical neurons, whereas the 75 kDa low affinity NGF receptor and the high affinity NGF receptor (trkA proto-oncogene product) are normally absent or present at very low levels in hippocampal and cortical neurons.[66] However, recent reports indicate that NGF receptors can be induced in hippocampal neurons by environmental insults.[67,68] In fact, recent evidence suggests that both the low affinity NGF receptor (FIG. 6; ref. 13) and trkA (ref. 69; V. L. Smith-Swintosky, D. Clary, F. Lefcort and M. P. Mattson, unpublished data) can be expressed in cultured hippocampal neurons where they may play a neuroprotective role.

Roles for Amyloid Precursor Proteins and β-Amyloid Peptide in Neuronal Degeneration in Alzheimer's Disease

The Alzheimer β-amyloid precursor protein (APP) is a membrane-spanning protein that exists in several forms, including those that either lack (APP695) or contain (APP751, APP770) a protease inhibitor domain.[70–72] APPs have one membrane-spanning segment, a large extracellular N-terminal region, and a shorter intracellular carboxy terminus. The β-peptide consists of a 42 amino acid stretch of APP that lies partially extracellular and partially within the plasma membrane. It is believed that APP is normally processed such that a cleavage occurs within the β-amyloid peptide[73] and that in AD aberrant processing of APP results in the liberation of intact β-peptide.[74,75] It is not yet clear where (*i.e.*, extracellular, intracellular compartments) and how normal and abnormal processing occur. Since the initial descriptions of amyloid accumulations in Alzheimer brains it has been thought that this protein plays a fundamental role in the neuronal damage of AD. Recent evidence suggests that β-amyloid peptide may indeed have either direct neurotoxic actions[76] or may endanger neurons by making them more vulnerable to excitotoxic insults.[28,77]

We recently identified a mechanism whereby β-amyloid peptide may contribute to neuronal degeneration in AD. Exposure of cultured human cortical neurons to β-amyloid peptides resulted in a destabilization of calcium homeostasis such that $[Ca^{2+}]_i$ responses to EAAs, depolarization, and calcium ionophores were greatly potentiated.[28] Neurons pretreated with β-amyloid peptide were more vulnerable to EAA neurotoxicity and neurofibrillary tangle-like changes in the cytoskeleton. The mechanism of action of β-amyloid peptide is unknown but might involve enhancement of calcium influx or disruption of calcium extrusion or buffering. Increased calcium influx could be induced by activation of voltage-dependent calcium channels, EAA receptors or calcium "leak" channels, or β-amyloid peptide might penetrate the membrane and act like a calcium ionophore. It is also conceivable that β-amyloid peptide might compromise the Na^+/Ca^{2+} exchanger or Ca^{2+} ATPase.

Since β-amyloid peptide in senile plaques (which are surrounded by degenerated neurites) in AD consists of fibrillar aggregates, whereas diffuse plaques (which are not associated with degenerated neurons and are believed to represent a precursor to senile plaques) are less aggregated, we have begun studies to determine whether aggregation is required for β-amyloid peptide to destabilize calcium homeostasis. When β-amyloid (aas. 1-38 or 1-40) is added to cell cultures it forms aggregates over a period of several days. In the early stages of aggregation the peptide forms globular accumulations that often accumulate on cell surfaces, and after several days of incubation fibrils form (FIG. 7). Interestingly, there was a strong correlation between the appearance of aggregates and altered $[Ca^{2+}]_i$ responses to glutamate and depolarization (*cf.* 28). In addition, Pike *et al.*,[78] found that "aged" (aggregated) β-amyloid peptides enhanced EAA neurotoxicity in cortical cell cultures. The requirement of aggregation for the effects of β-amyloid peptide on calcium homeostasis therefore seems likely. Although the presence of

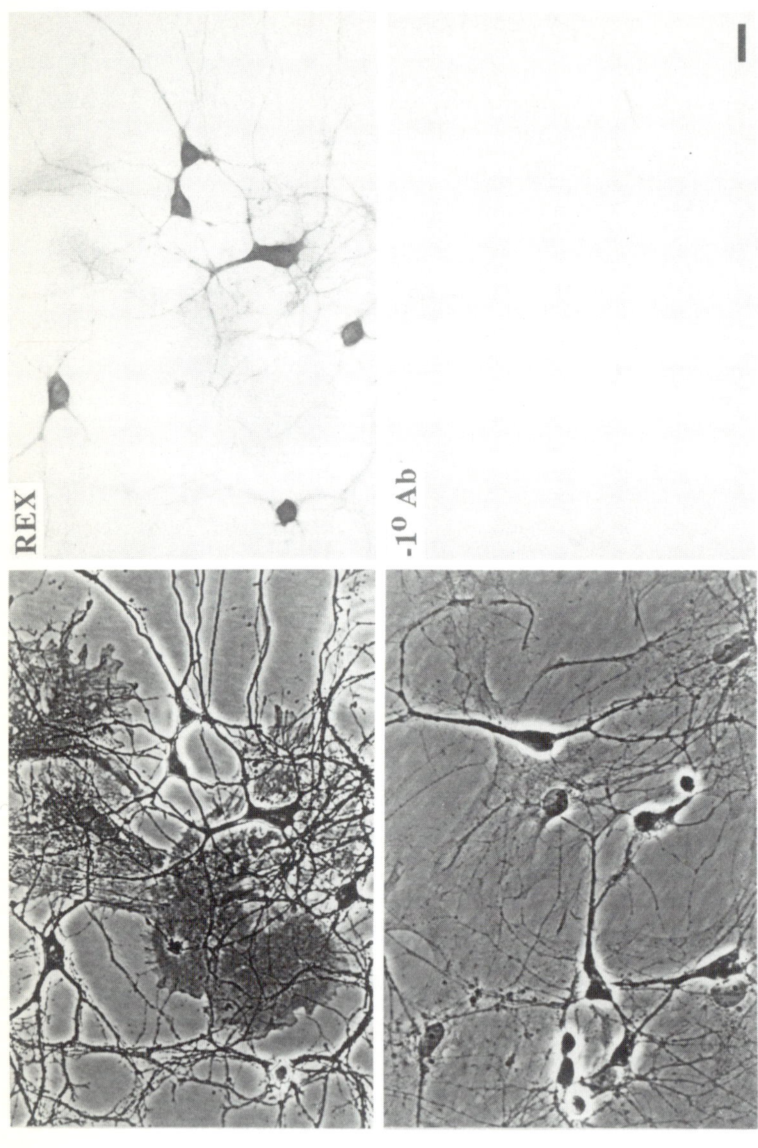

FIGURE 6. NGF receptor immunoreactivity in cultured rat hippocampal neurons. (*Top panels*) Phase-conrast (*left*) and bright-field (*right*) micrographs of fields of embryonic rat hippocampal cells cultured for 11 days and then immunostained with an antibody to the 75 kDa low affinity NGF receptor (antibody REX which was raised against an extracellular domain of the low affinity NGF receptor[91]). Note intense immunoreactivity in neurons and weaker immunoreactivity in astrocytes. (*Bottom panels*) Another 11 day-old culture in which the primary antibody was eliminated from the immunocytochemical staining protocol. Scale bar, 10 μm.

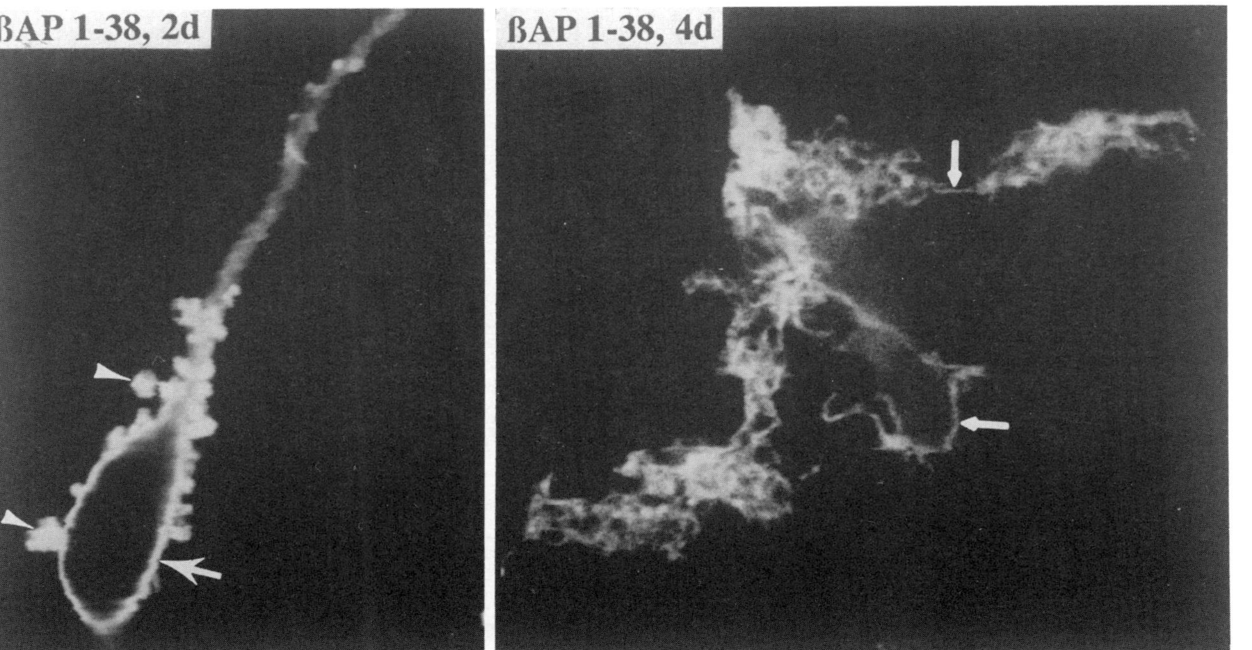

FIGURE 7. Aggregation of β-amyloid peptide. β-amyloid peptide 1-38 (10 μM) was added to cultures of human fetal cortical neurons for either 2 d (*left panel*) or 4 d (*right panel*) at which time cultures were fixed and immunostained with a monoclonal antibody to β-amyloid. Images were acquired using a confocal laser scanning microscope (Molecular Dynamics) with a Nikon 60× n.a. 1.3 oil immersion lense. Note the globular accumulations of β-amyloid immunoreactivity on the neuron after 2 d of exposure (*arrows, left*), and the fiber-like accumulations of β-amyloid immunoreactivity present after 4 d of exposure (*arrows, right*). Also note that the β-peptide immunoreactivity is localized to the plasma membrane and is not present inside the cell. (Modified from Mattson & Rydel.[92])

specific receptors for β-amyloid peptide has been proposed,[76] none has been identified. If aggregation is a prerequisite for the calcium-destabilizing action of β-amyloid peptide, then it seems unlikely that a specific signal transducing receptor is involved.

While β-amyloid deposition resulting from altered APP processing may contribute to neuronal degeneration in AD, an important question that remains to be answered is what is the normal function of secreted forms of β-APP (APP[s])? Since APPs are axonally transported and presumably released at synaptic terminals,[79] it is reasonable to consider that APP[s] play a role in synaptic plasticity. Recent experiments in this laboratory suggest that APP[s] may, in fact, play neuromodulatory and trophic roles. We have found that secreted forms of APP695 and APP751 rapidly lower $[Ca^{2+}]_i$ in cultured rat hippocampal and human cortical neurons.[80] APP[s]695 and APP[s]751 at concentrations from 10 pM to 1 nM cause reductions in $[Ca^{2+}]_i$ within sec to min of exposure. Antibodies to a specific region common to both APP695 and APP751 (aas. 444-592 of APP695) blocked the $[Ca^{2+}]_i$-lowering effects of the APP[s] suggesting that this region was responsible for the $[Ca^{2+}]_i$-lowering effect. These data suggest a possible role for APP[s]s in synaptic plasticity (*i.e.*, LTP). Indeed, LTP apparently requires an elevation in $[Ca^{2+}]_i$ in the postsynaptic cell.[81] More recently we have found that APP[s]695 and APP[s]751 have a neurotrophic effect in hippocampal cell cultures, and can protect neurons against hypoglycemic damage.[82] Hypoglycemic damage is mediated by an elevation in $[Ca^{2+}]_i$,[13] and the APP[s] prevented the loss of calcium homeostasis. Taken together, these data suggest that APP[s] normally play important roles in neuronal plasticity and neuroprotection.

We propose that abnormal processing of APPs in AD disrupts the normal $[Ca^{2+}]_i$-regulating function of APP[s] (FIG. 8). In combination with β-amyloid peptide deposition, APP[s] dysfunction may contribute to a loss of neuronal calcium homeostasis and the neurofibrillary degeneration that occurs in AD.[1] A wide array of data is available that must be taken into account when arriving at a theory for the cause of neuronal degeneration in AD including: information on the genetic and epidemiological aspects of AD; information concerning AD neuropathology at the cellular and molecular levels; age-dependent changes in the brain; and mechanisms of neuronal degeneration and death in experimental systems. Even when each of these areas is considered in isolation, one is led to the conclusion that AD is not a single entity but rather can arise from multiple causes. In some cases, mutations in APP may be of major importance[83] whereas in other cases head trauma[84] or age-associated alterations in brain energy metabolism[40] may be paramount. However, despite the probability of multiple causes leading to AD, it is becoming clearer that altered neuronal calcium homeostasis is involved in the neuronal damage and death that occurs in AD. It is of interest to note that the cellular signaling systems considered above comprise the major hypotheses for the etiology of AD including: the amyloid hypothesis;[85] the EAA hypothesis;[55,86] and the growth factor hypothesis.[55,87] The data described above indicate that a common link between all of these hypotheses is at the level of neuronal calcium homeostasis.

Similarity of "Natural" and Pathological Neuronal Death

Although this paper has focused on mechanisms of pathological neuronal degeneration, it is likely to be the case that there is considerable overlap between these mechanisms of neuronal damage and those operative in "natural" neuronal death. In this regard it is of considerable interest that similarities exist in the events that occur in neurons dying from either NGF deprivation (Deckworth *et al.*, this volume) or glucose deprivation (FIG. 3). In both cases, neurons survive for 12 to 20 hours and then die rapidly during a 4-h time period. In both cases mitochondrial dysfunction apparently precedes morphological signs of cell damage. In both cases

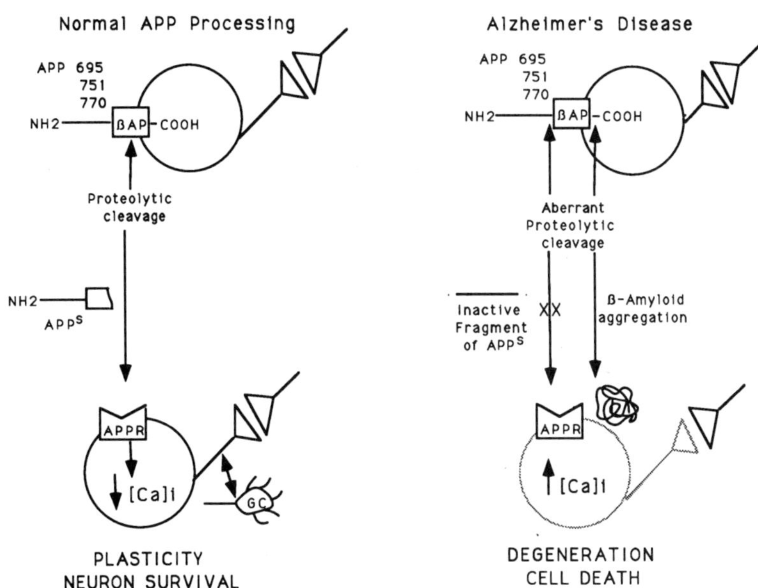

FIGURE 8. The adaptive functions of secreted forms of APP (APP^s), and the consequences of abnormal processing of APP in Alzheimer's disease. APP is a transmembrane protein that exists in at least three forms which either lack (APP695) or contain (APP751 and APP770) a protease inhibitory region. Normal enzymatic processing of APP results in the liberation of APP^s which presumably bind to and activate specific cell surface receptors (APPR) on target cells. Activation of APPR causes a reduction in intracellular calcium levels ($[Ca^{2+}]_i$), and protects against aberrant rises in $[Ca^{2+}]_i$ that can occur when neurons are subjected to adverse conditions (e.g., ischemia, trauma, excitotoxins). By virtue of their ability to regulate and stabilize $[Ca^{2+}]_i$, APP^s play important roles in neuronal plasticity (*e.g.*, regulation of cell survival, neurite outgrowth, LTP). In Alzheimer's disease, APP is aberrantly cleaved. The abnormal processing of APP has two major consequences that endanger neurons. First, the normal $[Ca^{2+}]_i$-stabilizing and neuroprotective function of APP^s is compromised. Second, β-amyloid peptide aggregates and disrupts $[Ca^{2+}]_i$ homeostasis. Thus, aberrant processing of APP renders neurons vulnerable to adverse conditions that accrue with increased age (*e.g.*, reduced glucose uptake and metabolism).

misregulation of $[Ca^{2+}]_i$ seems to play a role in the cell death. Future research efforts should be directed at understanding the signal transduction mechanisms involved in the regulation of natural neuronal survival, and their possible roles in pathological neuron death. The work described above suggests that transduction systems for growth factors, neurotransmitters, and amyloid precursor proteins are among those of considerable prominence with respect to mechanisms of neuronal injury and repair.

Prospects for Preventing and Treating Neurodegenerative Disorders

It is very likely that fundamental knowledge of the cellular signaling mechanisms involved in natural and pathological neuronal injury will lead to effective means of preventing or reducing neuronal damage in disorders such as stroke and Alzheimer's disease. In the case of stroke, clinical trials of excitatory amino acid receptor antagonists and calcium channel blockers are in progress. Moreover, initial cell culture studies demonstrating the effectiveness of growth factors in protecting neurons from excitotoxic/ischemic damage[13,35,43] have led to *in vivo* studies that demonstrated growth factor protection against ischemic injury.[88,89] Clinical trials of NGF administration in Alzheimer's patients are also underway.[90] Our increasing understanding of the normal functions of APP and the mechanisms leading to aberrant processing of APP promise to provide rational treatments for AD. Finally, increasing knowledge of the proteins involved in the regulations of $[Ca^{2+}]_i$ will allow the development of therapeutic agents that, for example, enhance neuronal Ca^{2+} extrusion or buffering.

SUMMARY

Several cellular signaling systems have been implicated in the neuronal death that occurs both in development ("natural" cell death) or in pathological conditions such as stroke and Alzheimer's disease (AD). Here we consider the possibility that neuronal degeneration in an array of disorders including stroke and AD arises from one or more alterations in calcium-regulating systems that result in a loss of cellular calcium homeostasis. A long-standing hypothesis of neuronal injury, the excitatory amino acid (EAA) hypothesis, is revisited in light of new supportive data concerning the roles of EAAs in stroke and the neurofibrillary degeneration in AD. Two quite new concepts concerning mechanisms of neuronal injury and death are presented, namely: 1) growth factors normally "stabilize" intracellular free calcium levels ($[Ca^{2+}]_i$) and protect neurons against ischemic/excitotoxic injury, and 2) aberrant processing of β-amyloid precursor protein (APP) can cause neurodegeneration by impairing a neuroprotective function of secreted forms of APP (APP^s) which normally regulate $[Ca^{2+}]_i$. Altered APP processing also results in the accumulation of β-amyloid peptide which contributes to neuronal damage by destabilizing calcium homeostasis; in AD β-amyloid peptide may render neurons vulnerable to excitotoxic conditions that accrue with increasing age (*e.g.*, altered glucose metabolism, ischemia). Growth factors may normally protect neurons against the potentially damaging effects of calcium influx resulting from energy deprivation and overexcitation. For example, bFGF, NGF and IGFs can protect neurons from several brain regions against excitotoxic/ischemic insults. Growth factors apparently stabilize $[Ca^{2+}]_i$ by several means including: a reduction in calcium influx; enhanced calcium extrusion or buffering; and maintenance or improvement of mitochondrial function. For example, bFGF can suppress the expression of a N-methyl-D-aspartate (NMDA) receptor protein that mediates excitotoxic damage in hippocampal neurons. Growth factors may also prevent the loss of neuronal calcium homeostasis and the increased vulnerability to neuronal injury caused by β-amyloid peptide. Since elevated $[Ca^{2+}]_i$ can elicit cytoskeletal alterations similar to those seen in AD neurofibrillary tangles, we propose that neuronal damage in AD results from a loss of calcium homeostasis. The data indicate that a variety of alterations in $[Ca^{2+}]_i$ regulation may contribute to the neuronal damage in stroke and AD, and suggest possible means of preventing neuronal damage in these disorders.

ACKNOWLEDGMENTS

We greatly appreciate the generous gifts form G. Westkamp and L. Reichardt of antibodies to the low affinity 75 kDa NGF receptor. We thank S. Bose, S. Loughran, J. Mattson and Y. Zhang for technical assistance, and S. Barger, B. Cheng, and J. O'Keefe for critical comments on various aspects of this research. We are particularly grateful to our collaborators: E. K. Michaelis, K. Kumar, E. Elliott, R. M. Sapolsky, and S. Christakos.

REFERENCES

1. MATTSON, M. P. 1992. Calcium as sculptor and destroyer of neural circuitry. Exp. Gerontol. **27:** 29–49.
2. MAYER, M. L. & R. J. MILLER. 1990. Excitatory amino acid receptors, second messengers and regulation of intracellular calcium in mammalian neurons. Trends Pharmacol. Sci. **11:** 254–260.
3. TSIEN, R. W., P. T. ELLINOR & W. A. HORNE. 1991. Molecular diversity of voltage-dependent Ca^{2+} channels. Trends Neurosci. **12:** 349–354.
4. CARAFOLI, E. 1987. Intracellular calcium homeostasis. Ann. Rev. Biochem. **56:** 395–433.
5. KENNEDY, M. B. 1989. Regulation of synaptic transmission in the central nervous system: long-term potentiation. Cell **59:** 777–782.
6. NIXON, R. A. 1989. Calcium-activated neutral proteinases as regulators of cellular function. Ann. N.Y. Acad. Sci. **568:** 198–208.
7. CHRISTAKOS, S., W. B. RHOTEN & S. C. FELDMAN. 1987. Rat calbindin D28k: Purification, quantitation, immunocytochemical localization, and comparative aspects. Meth. Enzymol. **139:** 534–551.
8. MATTSON, M. P., B. RYCHLIK, C. CHU & S. CHRISTAKOS. 1991. Evidence for calcium-reducing and excitoprotective roles for the calcium binding protein calbindin-D_{28k} in cultured hippocampal neurons. Neuron **6:** 41–51.
9. BERRIDGE, M. J. 1984. Inositoltriphosphate and diacylglycerol as second messengers. Biochem. J. **206:** 587–595.
10. ERNSTER, L. & G. SCHATZ. 1981. Mitochondria: A historical review. J. Cell Biol. **91:** 227s–255s.
11. MATTSON, M. P. 1988. Neurotransmitters in the regulation of neuronal cytoarchitecture. Brain Res. Rev. **13:** 179–212.
12. GUNDERSEN, R. W. & J. N. BARRETT. 1980. Characterization of the turning response of dorsal root neurites toward nerve growth factor. J. Cell Biol. **87:** 546–554.
13. CHENG, B. & M. P. MATTSON. 1991. NGF and bFGF protect rat hippocampal and human cortical neurons against hypoglycemic damage by stabilizing calcium homeostasis. Neuron **7:** 1031–1041.
14. JESSELL, T. M. 1988. Adhesion molecules and the hierarchy of neural development. Neuron **1:** 1–13.
15. YOUNG, W. 1992. Role of calcium in central nervous system injuries. J. Neurotrauma **9:** S9–S25.

16. SIESJO, B. K., F. BENGTSSON, W. GRAMPP & S. THEANDER. 1989. Calcium, excitotoxins, and neuronal death in the brain. Ann. N.Y. Acad. Sci. **568:** 234–251.
17. MATTSON, M. P. & B. CHENG. 1992. Growth factors protect neurons against excitotoxic/ischemic damage by stabilizing calcium homeostasis. Stroke. In press.
18. GIBSON, G. E. & C. PETERSON. 1987. Calcium and the aging nervous system. Neurobiol. Aging **8:** 329–343.
19. McDONALD, J. W. & M. V. JOHNSTON. 1990. Physiologial and pathophysiological roles of excitatory amino acids during central nervous system development. Brain Res. Rev. **15:** 41–70.
20. MATTSON, M. P. 1990. Second messengers in neuronal growth and degeneration. *In* Current Aspects of the Neurosciences, Vol. 2: 1–48. (N. Osborne, Ed.) Macmillan, London.
21. FAVARON, M., H. MANEV, R. SIMIAN, M. BERTOLINO, A. M. SZEKELY, G. DeERAUSQUIN, A. GUIDOTTI & E. COSTA. 1990. Down-regulation of protein kinase C protects cerebellar granule neurons in primary culture from glutamate-induced neuronal death. Proc. Natl. Acad. Sci. USA **87:** 1983–1987.
22. JESBERGER, J. A. & J. S. RICHARDSON. 1991. Oxygen free radicals and brain dysfunction. Intern. J. Neurosci. **57:** 1–17.
23. MATTSON, M. P. & S. B. KATER. 1988. Isolated hippocampal neurons in cryopreserved long-term cultures: Development of neuroarchitecture and sensitivity to NMDA. Int. J. Dev. Neurosci. **6:** 439–452.
24. MATTSON, M. P. & B. RYCHLIK. 1990. Cell culture of cryopreserved human fetal cerebral cortical and hippocampal neurons: neuronal development and responses to trophic factors. Brain Res. **522:** 204–214.
25. MATTSON, M. P., P. B. GUTHRIE, B. C. HAYES & S. B. KATER. 1989. Roles for mitotic history in the generation and degeneration of hippocampal neuroarchitecture. J. Neurosci. **9:** 1223–1230.
26. MATTSON, M. P., M. G. ENGLE & B. RYCHLIK. 1991. Effects of elevated intracellular calcium levels on the cytoskeleton and tau in cultured human cortical neurons. Mol. Chem. Neuropathol. **15:** 117–142.
27. MATTSON, M. P., P. B. GUTHRIE & S. B. KATER. 1989. A role for Na^+-dependent Ca^{2+} extrusion in protection against excitotoxicity. FASEB J. **3:** 2519–2526.
28. MATTSON, M. P., B. CHENG, D. DAVIS, K. BRYANT, I. LIEBERBURG & R. E. RYDEL. 1992. β-amyloid peptides destabilize calcium homeostasis and render cultured human cortical neurons vulnerable to excitotoxicity. J. Neurosci. **12:** 376–389.
29. ELLIOTT, E., M. P. MATTSON, P. VANDERKLISH, G. LYNCH, I. CHANG & R. M. SAPOLSKY. 1992. Corticosterone exacerbates kainate-induced alterations in hippocampal tau immunoreactivity and spectrin breakdown in vivo. J. Neurochem, In press.
30. ROTHMAN S. M. & J. W. OLNEY. 1987. Excitotoxicity and the NMDA receptor. Trends Neurosci. **10:** 299–301.
31. CHOI, D. W. 1987. Ionic dependence of glutamate neurotoxicity. J. Neurosci. **7:** 369–379.
32. MATTSON, M. P., P. DOU & S. B. KATER. 1988. Outgrowth-regulating actions of glutamate in isolated hippocampal pyramidal neurons. J. Neurosci. **8:** 2087–2100.
33. SIMON, R. P., J. H. SWAN, T. GRIFFITHS & B. S. MELDRUM. 1984. Blockade of N-methyl-D-aspartate receptors may protect against ischemic damage in the brain. Science **226:** 850–852.
34. DUBINSKY, J. M. & ROTHMAN, S. M. 1991. Intracellular calcium concentration during "chemical hypoxia" and excitotoxic neuronal injury. J. Neurosci. **11:** 2545–2551.
35. CHENG, B. & M. P. MATTSON. 1992. IGF-I and IGF-II protect cultured hippocampal and septal neurons against calcium-mediated hypoglycemic damage. J. Neurosci. **12:** 1558–1566.
36. MATTSON, M. P., P. B. GUTHRIE & S. B. KATER. 1988. Intracellular messengers in the generation and degeneration of hippocampal neuroarchitecture. J. Neurosci. Res. **21:** 447–464.
37. WIELOCH, T. 1985. Neurochemical correlates to selective neuronal vulnerability. Prog. Brain Res. **63:** 69–85.

38. MATTSON, M. P. 1990. Antigenic changes similar to those in neurofibrillary tangles are elicited by glutamate and calcium influx in cultured hippocampal neurons. Neuron **4:** 105–117.
39. SAPOLSKY, R. M. 1987. Glucocorticoids and hippocampal damage. Trends Neurosci. **10:** 346–349.
40. HOYER, S., K. OESTERREICH & O. WAGNER. 1988. Glucose metabolism as the site of the primary abnormality in early-onset dementia of Alzheimer type? J. Neurol. **235:** 143–148.
41. KALARIA, R. N. & S. I. HARIK. 1989. Reduced glucose transporter at the blood-brain barrier and in cerebral cortex in Alzheimer's disease. J. Neurochem. **53:** 1083–1088.
42. CHENG, B. & M. P. MATTSON. 1992. Glucose deprivation elicits neurofibrillary tangle-like antigenic changes in hippocampal neurons: Prevention by NGF and bFGF. Exp. Neurol. **117:** 114–123.
43. MATTSON, M. P., M. MURRAIN, P. B. GUTHRIE & S. B. KATER. 1989. Fibroblast growth factor and glutamate: Opposing roles in the generation and degeneration of hippocampal neuroarchitecture. J. Neurosci. **9:** 3728–3740.
44. CHENG, B., D. MCMAHON & M. P. MATTSON. 1992. Modulation of calcium current, intracellular calcium levels and neuronal survival by hypoglycemia, NGF and bFGF in cultured hippocampal neurons. Brain Res. In press.
45. MATTSON, M. P. & B. RYCHLIK. 1990. Glia protect hippocampal neurons against excitatory amino acid-induced degeneration: Involvement of fibroblast growth factor. Int. J. Dev. Neurosci. **8:** 399–415.
46. LEMASTERS, J. J., J. DIGUISEPPI, A.-L. NIEMINEN & B. HERMAN. 1987. Blebbing, free Ca^{2+} and mitochondrial membrane potential preceding cell death in hepatocytes. Nature **325:** 78–81.
47. ASCHER, P. & L. NOWAK. 1987. Electrophysiological studies of NMDA receptors. Trends Neurosci. **10:** 284–288.
48. COLLINGRIDGE, G. L. & T. V. P. BLISS. 1987. NMDA receptors: Their role in long-term potentiation. Trends Neurosci. **10:** 288–293.
49. CHEN, J.-W., M. D. CUNNINGHAM, N. GALTON & E. K. MICHAELIS. 1988. Immune labeling and purification of a 71-kDa glutamate-binding protein from brain synaptic membranes. J. Biol. Chem. **263:** 417–426.
50. LY, A. M. & E. K. MICHAELIS. 1991. Solubilization, partial purification and reconstitution of glutamate and N-methyl-D-aspartate-activated cation channels from brain synaptic membranes. Biochemistry **30:** 4307–4316.
51. KUMAR, K. N., N. T. TILAKARATNE, P. S. JOHNSON, K. T. EGGERMAN & E. K. MICHAELIS. 1991. Cloning of cDNA for the glutamate-binding subunit of an NMDA receptor complex. Nature **354:** 70–73.
52. MATTSON, M. P., H. WANG & E. K. MICHAELIS. 1991. Developmental expression, compartmentalization, and possible role in excitotoxicity of a putative NMDA receptor protein in cultured hippocampal neurons. Brain Res. **565:** 94–108.
53. MICHAELIS, E. K., H. WANG & M. P. MATTSON. 1991. NMDA receptor protein in cultured hippocampal neurons: developmental expression, relation to excitotoxicity, and regulation by basic FGF. Soc. Neurosci. Abstr. **17:** 74.
54. SASTRY, B. R., S. S. CHIRWA, P. B. Y. MAY & H. MARETIC. 1988. Are nerve growth factors involved in long-term synaptic potentiation in the hippocampus and spatial memory? *In* Synaptic Plasticity and the Hippocampus. G. Buzsaki & H. Haas, Eds.: 101–105. Springer-Verlag. Berlin. pp. 101–105.
55. MATTSON, M. P. 1989. Cellular signalling mechanisms common to the development and degeneration of neuronal cytoarchitecture. Mech. Aging Dev. **50:** 103–157.
56. PRZYWARA, D. A., S. V. BHAVE, A. BHAVE, T. D. WAKADE & A. R. WAKADE. 1991. Stimulated rise in neuronal calcium is faster and greater in the nucleus than the cytosol. FASEB J. **5:** 217–222.
57. SHARP, J. W., S. M. SAGAR, K. HISANAGA, P. JASPER & F. R. SHARP. 1990. The NMDA receptor mediates cortical induction of *fos* and *fos*-related antigens following cortical injury. Exp. Neurol. **109:** 323–332.

58. MORGAN, J. I. & T. CURRAN. 1986. Role of ion flux in the control of c-fos expression. Nature **322:** 552–555.
59. BARTEL, D. P., M. SHENG, L. F. LAU & M. E. GREENBERG. 1989. Growth factors and membrane depolarization activate distinct programs of early response gene expression: dissociation of fos and jun induction. Genes and Development **3:** 304–313.
60. KAPLAN, D. R., B. L. HEMPSTEAD, D. MARTIN-ZANCA, M. V. CHAO & L. F. PARADA. 1991. The trk proto-oncogene product: A signal transducing receptor for nerve growth factor. Science **252:** 554–557.
61. LEE, P. L., D. E. JOHNSON, L. S. COUSENS, V. A. FRIED & L. T. WILLIAMS. 1989. Purification and complementary DNA cloning of a receptor for basic fibroblast growth factor. Science **245:** 57–60.
62. ROBERTS, C. T. & D. LEROITH. 1992. Interactions in the insulin-like growth factor signaling system. News Physiol. Sci. **7:** 69–72.
63. YAYON, A., M. KLAGSBRUN, J. D. ESKO, P. LEDER & D. M. ORNITZ. 1991. Cell surface, heparin-like molecules are required for binding of basic fibroblast growth factor to its high affinity receptor. Cell **64:** 841–848.
64. WANAKA, A., E. M. JOHNSON & J. MILBRANDT. 1990. Localization of FGF receptor mRNA in the adult rat central nervous system by in situ hybridization. Neuron **5:** 267–281.
65. LESNIAK, M. A., J. M. HILL, W. KIESS, M. ROJESKI, C. B. PERT & J. ROTH. 1988. Receptors for insulin-like growth factors I and II: autoradiographic localization in rat brain and comparison to receptors for insulin. Endocrinology **123:** 2089–2099.
66. KOH, S., OYLER, G. A. & HIGGINS, G. A. 1989. Localization of nerve growth factor receptor messenger RNA and protein in the adult rat brain. Exp. Neurol. **106:** 209–221.
67. PIORO, E. P. & A. C. CUELLO. 1990. Distribution of nerve growth factor receptor-like immunoreactivity in the adult rat central nervous system. Effect of colchicine and correlation with the cholinergic system-I. Forebrain. Neuroscience **34:** 57–87.
68. YANKNER, B. A., A. CACERES & L. K. DUFFY. 1990. Nerve growth factor potentiates the neurotoxicity of β amyloid. Proc. Natl. Acad. Sci. USA **87:** 9020–9023.
69. SMITH-SWINTOSKY, V. L. & M. P. MATTSON. 1992. Evidence for the expression of functional low affinity and trkA NGF receptors in cultured hippocampal neurons. Soc. Neurosci. Abstr. **18:** 951.
70. KANG, J., H.-G. LEMAIRE, A. UNTERBECK, J. M. SALBAUM, C. L. MASTERS, K.H. GRZESCKIK, G. MULTHAUP, K. BEYREUTHER & B. MULLER-HILL. 1987. The precursor of Alzheimer's disease amyloid A4 protein resembles a cell-surface receptor. Nature **325:** 733–736.
71. OLTERSDORF, T., L. C. FRITZ, D. B. SCHENK, I. LIEBERBURG, K. L. JOHNSON-WOOD, E. C. BEATTIE, P. J. WARD, R. W. BLACHER, H. F. DOVEY & S. SINHA. 1989. The secreted form of the Alzheimer's amyloid precursor protein with the Kunitz domain is protease nexin-II. Nature **341:** 144–147.
72. DYRKS, T., A. WEIDEMANN, G. MULTHAUP, J. M. SALBAUM, H.-G. LEMAIRE, J. KANG, B. MULLER-HILL, C. L. MASTERS, AND K. BEYREUTHER. 1988. Identification, transmembrane orientation and biogenesis of the amyloid A4 precursor of Alzheimer's disease. EMBO J. **7:** 949–957.
73. ESCH, F. S., P. S. KIEM, E. C. BEATTIE, R. W. BLACHER, A. R. CULWELL, T. OLTERSDORF, D. MCCLURE & P. J. WARD. 1990. Cleavage of amyloid β peptide during constitutive processing of its precursor. Science **248:** 1122–1124.
74. GLENNER, G. G. & C. W. WONG. 1984. Alzheimer's disease: initial report of the purification and characterization of a novel cerebrovascular amyloid protein. Biochem. Biophys. Res. Commun. **120:** 885–890.
75. SISODIA, S. S., E. H. KOO, K. BEYREUTHER & A. UNTERBECK. 1990. Evidence that beta-amyloid protein in Alzheimer's disease is not derived by normal processing. Science **248:** 492–495.
76. YANKNER, B. A., L. K. DUFFY & D. A. KIRSCHNER. 1990. Neurotrophic and neurotoxic effects of amyloid β protein: reversal by tachykinin neuropeptides. Science **250:** 279–282.

77. KOH, J.-Y., L. L. YANG & C. W. COTMAN. 1990. β-amyloid protein increases the vulnerability of cultured cortical neurons to excitotoxic damage. Brain Res. **533:** 315–320.
78. PIKE, C. J., A. J. WALENCEWICZ, C. G. GLABE & C. W. COTMAN. 1991. In vitro aging of β-amyloid protein causes peptide aggregation and neurotoxicity. Brain Res. **563:** 311–314.
79. KOO, E. H., S. S. SISODIA, D. R. ARCHER, L. J. MARTIN, A. WEIDEMANN, K. BEYREUTHER, P. FISCHER, C. L. MASTERS & D. L. PRICE. 1990. Precursor of amyloid protein in Alzheimer disease undergoes fast anterograde axonal transport. Proc. Natl. Acad. Sci. USA **87:** 1561–1565.
80. MATTSON M. P., B. CHENG, A. CULWELL, F. ESCH, I. LIEBERBURG & R. E. RYDEL. 1993. Evidence for excitoprotective and intraneuronal calcium-regulating roles for secreted forms of β-amyloid precursor protein. Neuron. In press.
81. MALENKA, R. C., J. A. KAUER, R. S. ZUCKER & R. A. NICOLL. 1988. Postsynaptic calcium is sufficient for potentiation of hippocampal synaptic transmission. Science **242:** 81–84.
82. CHENG, B. V. L. SMITH-SWINTOSKY, I. LIEBERBURG, R. E. RYDEL & M. P. MATTSON. 1992. Secreted forms of APP increase neuronal survival and protect cultured rat and human CNS neurons against hypoglycemic damage. Soc. Neurosci. Abstr. **18:** 1440.
83. GOATE, A., M. C. CHARTLER-HARLIN, M. MULLAN, J. BROWN, F. CRAWFORD, L. FIDANI, L. GLUFFRA, A. HAYNEST, N. IRVING, L. JAMES, R. MANT, P. NEWTON, K. ROOKE, P. ROQUES, C. TALBOT, R. WILLIAMSON, M. ROSSOR, M. OWEN & J. HARDY. 1991. Segregation of a missense mutation in the amyloid precursor protein gene with familial Alzheimer's disease. Nature **349:** 704–707.
84. ROBERTS, G. W., S. M. GENTLEMAN, A. LYNCH & D. I. GRAHAM. 1991. βA4 amyloid protein deposition in brain after head injury. Lancet **338:** 1422–1423.
85. SELKOE, D. J. 1989. Biochemistry of altered brain proteins in Alzheimer's disease. Ann. Rev. Neurosci. **12:** 463–490.
86. GREENAMYRE, J. T. & A. B. YOUNG. 1989. Excitatory amino acids and Alzheimer's disease. Neurobiol. Aging **10:** 593–602.
87. HEFTI, F., J. HARTIKKA & B. KNUSEL. 1989. Function of neurotrophic factors in the adult and aging brain and their possible use in the treatment of neurodegenerative diseases. Neurobiol. Aging **10:** 515–533.
88. SHIGENO, T., T. MIMA, K. TAKAKURA, K. E. GRAHAM, G. KATO, Y. HASHIMOTO & S. FURUKAWA. 1991. Amelioration of delayed neuronal death in the hippocampus by nerve growth factor. J. Neurosci. **11:** 2914–2919.
89. KNOZAKI K., S. P. FINKLESTEIN & M. F. BEAL. 1993. Basic fibroblast growth factor protects against hypoxia/ischemia and NMDA neurotoxicity in neonatal rats. J Cerebr. Blood Flow Metab. In press.
90. OLSON, L., A. NORDBERG, H. VONHOLST, L. BACKMAN, T. EBENDAL, I. ALAFUZOFF, K. AMBERLA, P. HARWIVIG, A. HERLITZ, A. LILJA, *et al.* 1992. Nerve growth factor affects C-11-nicotine binding, blood flow, EEG, and verbal episodic memory in an Alzheimer patient—case report. J. Neurol. Trans. (Parkinsons) **4:** 79–84.
91. WESTKAMP, G. & L. F. REICHARDT. 1991. Evidence that biological activity of NGF is mediated through a novel class of high affinity receptors. Neuron **6:** 649–663.
92. MATTSON, M. P. & R. E. RYDEL. 1992. β-Amyloid precursor protein and Alzheimer's disease: The peptide plot thickens. Neurobiol. Aging **13:** 617–621.

Calcium Influx and Neurodegeneration[a]

SIMON J. GIBBONS,[b] JAMES R. BRORSON,[b,c]
DAVID BLEAKMAN,[b] PAUL S. CHARD,[b] AND
RICHARD J. MILLER[b]

[b]Department of Pharmacological and Physiological Sciences
[c]Department of Neurology
University of Chicago
947 East 58th Street
Chicago, Illinois 60637

INTRODUCTION

The influx of Ca^{2+} across the plasma membrane of neurons has enormous physiological significance because increases in the free intracellular Ca^{2+} concentration ($[Ca^{2+}]_i$) are linked to a variety of neuronal processes. In addition to being the fundamental messenger as a trigger for neurotransmitter release, Ca^{2+} is a key element in the control of neuronal excitability,[1] integration of electrical signals,[1,2] synaptic plasticity of various types,[3] cellular metabolism,[4] and gene expression.[5] Clearly, control of these processes requires the close regulation of $[Ca^{2+}]_i$. Ultimately all intracellular Ca^{2+} must come from the extracellular medium, although intracellular stores do sequester Ca^{2+} and release it into the cytoplasm which permits rises in $[Ca^{2+}]_i$ when neurons are incubated in the absence of extracellular Ca^{2+}. The entry of Ca^{2+} down its electrochemical gradient is mediated by transiently increasing the permeability of the plasma membrane to Ca^{2+}. This can be achieved by opening Ca^{2+} permeable ion channels of which there are two principal types; voltage gated and ligand gated.[6–8] Voltage gated Ca^{2+} channels are directly activated by changes in the membrane potential whereas ligand gated Ca^{2+} permeable ionophores are opened following neurotransmitter binding to a closely associated receptor.[6] Ca^{2+} influx via both pathways has been implicated in various forms of neurodegeneration; however, it is the possible relevance of receptor operated Ca^{2+} channels to neuronal death which we shall discuss in this paper.

As we have indicated, Ca^{2+} is involved in many fundamental processes relevant to normal cell function, and the $[Ca^{2+}]_i$ is usually closely regulated. Therefore, it is perhaps not surprising that the prolonged elevation of $[Ca^{2+}]_i$ has been directly linked to delayed cell death. A number of endogenous and exogenous compounds including agonists for excitatory amino acid neurotransmitter receptors and capsaicin, the hot flavor of chili peppers, cause delayed cell death in just such a Ca^{2+}-dependent manner. In addition, in several pathological conditions such as ischemia, status epilepticus and trauma, excessive intracellular accumulation of Ca^{2+}

[a] S.J.G. received a long-term fellowship grant from the Human Frontier Science Program, D.B. was supported by a Fulbright Fellowship, P.S.C. by NIH training Grant PHS NR-SA2T32 GMM07151, J.B. by a Howard Hughes Medical Institute Physician Research Fellowship and R.J.M. received funding from the NIH Grants MH-40165, DA-02121, DA-02575 and a Digestive Diseases Core Center Award to Dr. R. Roos (DK-42086).

appears to be the key element in the development of distinct patterns of neurodegeneration.[8,9] An important feature of these forms of neurotoxicity is the time delay between the period of excessively high $[Ca^{2+}]_i$ and the subsequent cell death, this lag time may provide a window of opportunity for therapeutic intervention and seems to offer hope for the development of effective treatments for brain ischemia and stroke.

In ischemia and status epilepticus there is a clear culprit which elicits the Ca^{2+} influx necessary to cause neurodegeneration. Excitatory amino acids, particularly glutamate, mediate excitatory synaptic transmission by acting at neuronal receptors which cause elevated $[Ca^{2+}]_i$. Prolonged stimulation of glutamatergic synapses during epileptiform discharges and the accumulation of glutamate in the extracellular space following ischemia both produce an abnormal spatial and temporal elevation of $[Ca^{2+}]_i$ which ultimately leads to neurotoxicity.[10] This mechanism of action is not limited to endogenous excitatory amino acid agonists; amnesic shellfish poisoning has been directly linked to neurodegeneration caused by the excitatory amino acid receptor agonist domoic acid, an occasional contaminant in mussels.[11]

Ca^{2+}-dependent neurodegeneration is not restricted to the central nervous system; in the peripheral nervous system the effects of Ca^{2+} influx through the capsaicin-activated receptor has been widely used as a tool for studying nociceptive sensory neurons.[12–15] Capsaicin (8-methyl-*N*-vanillyl-6-monemamide) is the pungent ingredient of peppers of the genus capsicum which activates a non-specific conductance permeable to, amongst other cations, Ca^{2+} and Co^{2+}.[12,13,16] In common with excitatory amino acids, capsaicin also causes selective, delayed degeneration of a population of neurons associated with elevated $[Ca^{2+}]_i$. In the case of capsaicin the affected cells are a sub-population of dorsal root ganglion (DRG) neurons of the Aδ and C-fiber type.[17,18] However, there is no clear pathological or physiological correlate of this observation; for example, an endogenous ligand has not been identified for this receptor. Despite this, capsaicin has found some therapeutic use in the alleviation of painful diabetic neuropathies,[19] and the effects of this compound are a useful model of Ca^{2+}-mediated neurodegeneration with particular relevance to the mechanisms controlling Ca^{2+} homeostasis in sensory neurons.

NON-NMDA RECEPTOR–MEDIATED Ca^{2+} INFLUX AND NEURODEGENERATION

The excitatory amino acid receptors can be divided into the ionotropic receptors, which are directly linked to cationic ion channels, and the metabotropic receptors, in which the agonist's action at the receptor leads to the activation of an enzymatic process or modulation of other excitatory amino acid receptors or voltage-sensitive ion channels. An example of the former effect of metabotropic receptors is the G-protein–mediated activation of phospholipase C to produce IP_3.[20] The opening of K^+ conductances and enhanced effectiveness of non-NMDA receptors are examples of the latter.[21,22] The ionotropic receptors are further divided into subclasses identified by the specific synthetic agonist acting at each subclass.[23] The NMDA receptors, activated by *N*-methyl-D-aspartate, are known to be highly permeable to Ca^{2+}, so that they directly contribute to the $[Ca^{2+}]_i$. Thus, they have been considered likely participants in processes of neuronal plasticity and Ca^{2+}-mediated cell death. The non-NMDA receptors, activated by kainate and α-amino-3-hydroxy-5-methyl-4-isoxazolepropionate (AMPA), on the other hand, have conventionally been thought to be Ca^{2+} impermeable,[24] and therefore contributing to the $[Ca^{2+}]_i$ only indirectly, by the Na^+-dependent depolarization of the cell membrane, leading to the opening of voltage-gated Ca^{2+} channels and Ca^{2+} influx by that route.

In part, because of their high Ca^{2+} permeability, the NMDA receptors have received the greatest amount of attention in relation to excitatory amino acid-mediated neuronal death. Work from a number of laboratories has implicated NMDA receptors in *in vitro* models of excitotoxicity,[25,26] and NMDA receptor activation seems to be essential to neuronal damage in several *in vivo* models of ischemia and trauma.[27,28] Yet there is also reason to believe that the NMDA receptor does not account for the whole story of excitotoxic cell death. Kainic acid toxicity is substantially resistant to voltage sensitive Ca^{2+} channel blockers in *in vitro* studies.[29] In certain models of global ischemia, specific antagonists of non-NMDA receptors alone[30] or in combination with NMDA antagonists[31] are neuroprotective. In addition, domoic acid is a selective kainate receptor agonist; therefore activation of non-NMDA receptors is the likely cause of amnesic shellfish poisoning.[10] Recent evidence has also suggested that, in some physiological systems, non-NMDA receptors also share with NMDA receptors the property of a high Ca^{2+} permeability. Murphy and Miller[32] showed that, in cultured striatal neurons, the Ca^{2+} influx induced by kainate could not be entirely blocked by antagonists of voltage gated Ca^{2+} channels. Iino *et al.*[33] showed that a small fraction[34] of cultured hippocampal neurons expressed receptors activated by kainate which were Ca^{2+} permeable, giving rise to an inwardly rectifying current-voltage (I-V) relationship. They denoted these Ca^{2+}-permeable 'type II' kainate receptors, in distinction from the typical 'type I' kainate receptors, which are Na^+ permeable, Ca^{2+} impermeable, and have an I-V relationship that is approximately linear. Other authors have also reported evidence for Ca^{2+}-permeable non-NMDA receptors in various types of cultured neurons.[35-37] Additionally, the cloning of several non-NMDA receptor subunits has revealed that these subunits, when expressed in various combinations in oocytes or cell lines, can give rise to receptors which are either Ca^{2+}-permeable or Ca^{2+}-impermeable.[38,39]

Thus non-NMDA receptor–activated Ca^{2+} channels may contribute to excitotoxicity and in order to study this, we sought a suitable *in vitro* system. The first system that we chose to study were cerebellar Purkinje neurons because several of their features indicate that Ca^{2+}-mediated processes may be particularly important in these cells.[40] They are known to have profuse glutamatergic synaptic inputs and to be extremely sensitive to hypoxic and ischemic neuronal injury.[41] In addition, most studies have found that in adult tissues, Purkinje neurons lack NMDA receptors.[42] Thus it would seem that excitotoxicity mediated by pathways other than the NMDA receptor might be particularly important to the vulnerability of Purkinje cells. In our culture system the majority of neurons were identified as Purkinje cells by immunocytochemistry; less than one-third expressed NMDA receptors but all viable neurons responded to kainate.[40]

As mentioned earlier, the standard model of excitatory amino acid receptors would hold that the Ca^{2+} influx upon activation of non-NMDA receptors is due to Na^+ influx through the receptor ionophore, causing depolarization and Ca^{2+} influx through voltage-gated Ca^{2+} channels. If this were the explanation for the kainate-induced rise in $[Ca^{2+}]_i$ in the cultured cerebellar neurons, it should not occur if the external Na^+ were replaced by an impermeant cation such as *N*-methyl-D-glucamine (NMDG). In some cells, this indeed seemed to the case, in that there was little or no Ca^{2+} influx in Na^+ free solutions, despite large $[Ca^{2+}]_i$ rises in response to kainate in Na^+-containing solutions. However, in most of the cells studied, a substantial Ca^{2+} influx was observed even in Na^+-free conditions.[43] Some 77% of cells responded in a 2 mM Ca^{2+}, 140 mM NMDG (2 CaNMDG) solution to 30 μM kainate, with increases in the $[Ca^{2+}]_i$ of up to 1 μM. In cells exposed to kainate in both Na^+-containing and Na^+-free solutions, the $[Ca^{2+}]_i$ increases in Na^+-free solutions were about 60% of those in Na^+-containing solutions. The concentration dependence of this kainate-induced Ca^{2+} influx showed a threshold concentration of between 3 μM and 10 μM kainate; AMPA also could induce a Na^+-independent Ca^{2+} influx. The effects of kainate in either Na^+-containing or Na^+-free media were not reduced by the NMDA receptor antagonist 2-amino-5-phosphonopentanoate (AP5) (50 μM), but could be completely blocked by the non-NMDA antagonist 6-cyano-7-nitroquinoxaline-2,3-dione (CNQX) (10 μM).[43] These data suggested that the non-NMDA receptors might be directly Ca^{2+}-permeable.

In order to confirm the conclusion that kainate causes Ca^{2+} influx in these cerebellar neurons that does not involve voltage-sensitive Ca^{2+} channels, we made use of both pharmacological and physiological approaches. We attempted to block Ca^{2+} influx using the nonselective organic voltage-gated Ca^{2+} channel antagonist TA-3090 (clentiazem).[44] TA-3090 effectively inhibited both depolarization-induced whole cell Ca^{2+} currents and 50 mM K^+-induced Ca^{2+} influxes. In contrast, when kainate-induced Ca^{2+} influxes were examined in 2 CaNMDG-containing solutions, TA-3090 was ineffective at blocking the $[Ca^{2+}]_i$ rise. Similarly, under voltage clamp conditions in 2 CaNMDG solutions, kainate-induced inward currents were unaffected by TA-3090, nor were they inhibited by 100 μM Cd^{2+}, an inorganic blocker of voltage-gated Ca^{2+} channels.

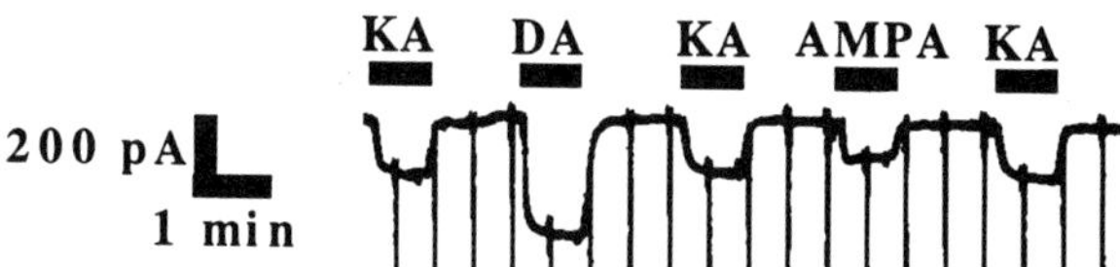

FIGURE 1. Non-NMDA receptor agonist–induced Ca^{2+} currents in voltage clamped cerebellar neurons. Under whole-cell voltage clamp conditions, which prevented activation of voltage gated Ca^{2+} channels, kainate (KA) (100 μM), AMPA (30 μM), and domoate (DA) (100 μM) all induced inward currents in a cerebellar neuron under ionic conditions isolating inward Ca^{2+} currents. Agonist-induced currents were recorded at the holding potential of -100 mV, with depolarization to 0 mV every 30 seconds. (Intracellular solution: 140 mM NMDG fluoride, 10 mM BAPTA; extracellular solution: 2 mM Ca^{2+}, 140 mM NMDG, 0.5 μm tetrodotoxin, 20 μM bicuculline.)

Another way to eliminate contributions of voltage-gated Ca^{2+} currents to Ca^{2+} influx is to prevent depolarization of the cell membrane by whole-cell voltage clamping. Kainate also produced clear Ca^{2+} influx in Na^+-free medium into the majority of neurons that were voltage clamped at -80 mV, a potential at which high threshold Ca^{2+} currents are not activated in these cells.[43] This Ca^{2+} influx, activated by AMPA, kainate and domoate, could be measured as an inward current (FIG. 1). However, there were also cells that did not respond in this way. In these cells showing neither a Ca^{2+} influx nor an inward current in Na^+-free medium, large kainate-induced currents could still be observed in Na^+-containing medium, without concomitant increases in $[Ca^{2+}]_i$.[43]

Current-voltage relationships for kainate-induced currents were measured both in Na^+-containing and Na^+-free media, using 100 μM Cd^{2+} to block voltage gated Ca^{2+} currents. In Na^+-containing media, the kainate-induced large inward currents had approximately linear I-V relationships, similar to results previously reported for kainate-induced currents.[24] In contrast, the kainate-induced currents recorded in Na^+-free external solutions were much smaller in magnitude, and displayed inward rectification[43] as was described for the type II kainate receptors in hippocampal neurons[33] and for the Ca^{2+} permeable non-NMDA receptors in oocytes injected with the glutamate subunit messenger RNA.[38] The I-V curves for the kainate-induced currents recorded in NMDG shifted in the positive direction when the external Ca^{2+} was raised for 2 mM to 10 mM, again indicating the opening of a Ca^{2+}-permeable channel.[43]

Given that in these cerebellar neurons the Ca^{2+} permeable non-NMDA receptors were always coexpressed with a substantially larger kainate-induced Na^+ conductance (unlike in the subset of hippocampal neurons where Iino *et al.*[33] apparently found only the type II kainate receptors), it could be argued that this relatively small kainate-induced Ca^{2+} current matters little to the Ca^{2+} homeostasis of these neurons. We therefore also wished to obtain an indication of the relative contributions in the cultured neurons of voltage gated Ca^{2+} channels and Ca^{2+} permeable non-NMDA receptors to Ca^{2+} influx in a more physiological medium containing Na^+. In "responding" cells (those with a Ca^{2+} influx when stimulated with kainate in Na^+-free solutions), TA-3090, while substantially reducing the 50 mM K^+-induced increase in $[Ca^{2+}]_i$, produced only about 13% inhibition of the kainate-induced peak $[Ca^{2+}]_i$ responses in Na^+-containing solutions. These data are consistent with the idea that when neurons possess Ca^{2+}-permeable non-NMDA receptors, kainate-stimulated Ca^{2+} influx occurs substantially via this pathway even in the presence of Na^+.

Ca^{2+}-permeable non-NMDA receptors constructed in oocytes are very nonselective with respect to cation permeability and are quite permeable to Co^{2+},[45] which does not significantly permeate voltage sensitive Ca^{2+} channels, NMDA receptors or Ca^{2+}-impermeable non-NMDA receptors. Using a histochemical silver staining method to identify Co^{2+}-uptake, Pruss *et al.*[37] have shown that stimulation with kainate causes Co^{2+} influx through Ca^{2+}-permeable non-NMDA receptors in neurons. Following this method, we found that 65% of the cerebellar neurons in culture showed Co^{2+}-uptake staining following incubation with 100 μM kainate. This effect was blocked by 20 μM CNQX, but not by 50 μM AP5. The morphology of neurons stained for Co^{2+}-uptake included both those with Purkinje cell morphology and also some non-Purkinje cells.[43]

These data clearly demonstrated that kainate can activate a substantial Ca^{2+} influx in Purkinje cells and other cerebellar neurons which does not require cell depolarization and influx via voltage sensitive Ca^{2+} channels. What seems particularly significant is that this phenomenon does not only occur in a minority of neurons, but in the majority of cultured cerebellar cells where these receptors seem to coexist with traditional types of non-Ca^{2+}–permeable non-NMDA receptors. Moreover, judging by Co^{2+}-uptake staining data,[37] these results are not just confined to cell culture but are also observed in the mature rat brain. This implies non-NMDA as well as NMDA receptors can produce damagingly large and prolonged elevations of neuronal $[Ca^{2+}]_i$. We have begun to investigate whether such Ca^{2+}-permeable kainate receptors might be responsible for excitotoxicity in these cultured cerebellar neurons. Preliminary evidence suggests that kainate can indeed induce delayed excitotoxic cell death through Na^+-independent pathways in these neurons, and that this is fully blocked by CNQX and partially by removal of extracellular Ca^{2+}.[46] These results suggest that in these neurons, Ca^{2+} permeation through the kainate receptor plays an important role in excitotoxicity. Thus the role played by excitatory amino acid receptors in clinical situations might well include Ca^{2+} influx through non-NMDA receptors as well as NMDA receptors, with different pathways having different relative importance in various neuronal cell types.

Another situation in which non-NMDA receptor mediated excitotoxicity has been proposed to contribute to a disease state is the degeneration of a subpopulation of interneurons in the dentate hilus following ischemia and status epilepticus[47] as well as in animal models of these diseases.[48] These cells express a distinct set

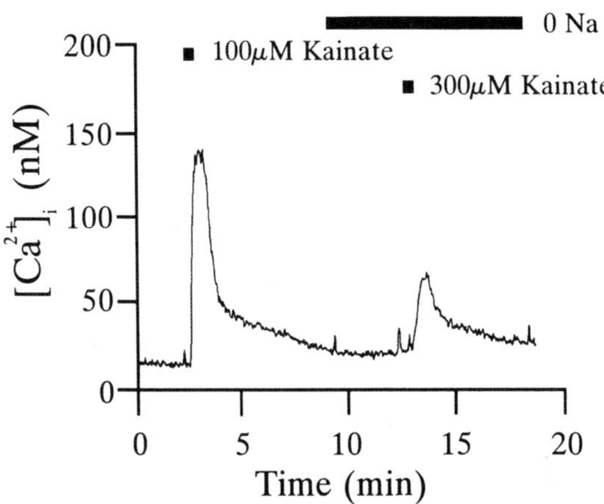

FIGURE 2. Direct Ca^{2+} entry through kainate receptor-activated channels in dentate hilar neurons. Fura-2-based $[Ca^{2+}]_i$ microfluorimetry was used to assess responses to kainate in cultured neurons from the rat dentate gyrus. Tetrodotoxin (0.5 μM) was used throughout to block synaptic transmission that may have contributed to responses. Exposure of a neuron to 100 μM kainate in normal HEPES buffered Hank's balanced salt solution produced a rapid rise in somatic $[Ca^{2+}]_i$ which returned to basal levels within 8 minutes. In the absence of extracellular sodium (replaced by an equimolar quantity of N-methyl-D-glucamine), a smaller but reproducible rise in $[Ca^{2+}]_i$ is observed. In this cell, a higher concentration (300 μM) of kainate was tested in the absence of sodium.

of neuromodulators, in particular somatostatin and GABA, which together with the absence of the Ca^{2+}-binding proteins, calbindin D28K and parvalbumin, and their morphological appearance sets them apart from other populations of hilar interneurons.[49] By dissociating cells from 5-day-old rats and using particular culture conditions we can obtain an enriched population of such hilar interneurons for studying their excitatory amino acid pharmacology.[50] Using single cell $[Ca^{2+}]_i$ microfluorimetry, we observe kainate-induced rises in $[Ca^{2+}]_i$ in the majority of cells which are also observed in the absence of extracellular Na^+, albeit with a reduced effect (FIG. 2). We concluded that Ca^{2+}-permeable non-NMDA receptors are also present on these cells and confirmed this by using the Co^{2+} uptake assay described previously for Purkinje cells. The majority of neurons take up Co^{2+}

following incubation with 100 μM kainate (FIG. 3a), an effect which is substantially reduced by 10 μM CNQX (FIG. 3b).

Thus somatostatin containing hilar neurons do express Ca^{2+} permeable non-NMDA receptors. However, it is not clear whether this is only true for this subpopulation of hilar interneurons or whether all hilar interneurons express type II non-NMDA receptors. The hilar region certainly took up Co^{2+} to a greater degree than other hippocampal regions in the intact slice[51] but it was not apparent that there is a difference between different neuronal types in the hilus. There are several other factors which probably contribute to hilar cell vulnerability such as the absence of Ca^{2+}-binding proteins[52] and the likely presence of dual excitatory synaptic inputs from the mossy fibers and perforant path. Indeed studies in the intact hippocampal slice indicate that hilar interneurons are notably more excitable than other hippocampal neurons.[53] However, there is a precedent for type II non-NMDA receptors being associated with vulnerability of a subgroup of neurons in a mixed population in studies on cortical cell cultures.[54] It remains to be seen whether *in vivo* degeneration of hilar interneurons can be mediated by non-NMDA receptors alone or whether Ca^{2+} entry through NMDA receptors inevitably contributes to excitotoxicity where both non-NMDA and NMDA Ca^{2+}-permeable receptors are present.

CAPSAICIN-INDUCED DEGENERATION OF DORSAL ROOT GANGLION NEURONS

Although it can be demonstrated that Ca^{2+} influx, particularly through receptor-operated channels, is a key element in the forms of neurodegeneration described thus far, the sequelae which ultimately result in cell death are less clear. We have used the capsaicin-induced degeneration of DRG neurons to study the processes which may underlie this particular case of Ca^{2+}-induced delayed cell death. In the CNS, NMDA receptor-mediated neurodegeneration has been associated with the activation of the thiol-dependent protease calpain (ref. 55 and Roberts-Lewis and Siman, this volume). We have therefore examined the ability of calpain inhibitors to prevent capsaicin-induced cell death because of the coincident feature of capsaicin and NMDA-induced cell death, namely Ca^{2+} influx.

Twenty-four hours after a 20-min treatment with 100 μM capsaicin in 10 mM extracellular Ca^{2+}, 35% of the DRG neurons were killed. To determine whether Ca^{2+} entry was the trigger for cell death, we removed extracellular Ca^{2+} during incubation with capsaicin. Under these conditions, and when the neurons were loaded with the Ca^{2+} chelator BAPTA (1,2-bis(2-aminophenoxy)ethane N,N,N',N'-tetraacetic acid), cell survival was normal. Cell death was also prevented by incubation with the capsaicin receptor antagonist ruthenium red (1 μM).

The effect of two calpain inhibitors was studied on capsaicin-induced cell death. One compound was the naturally occurring cysteine protease inhibitor, E64[56] and the other was a synthetic calpain inhibitor Cbz-Val-Phe-H (MDL 28,170).[57] Incubation of the cells with both inhibitors significantly increased cell survival when assessed 24 hours after capsaicin application (FIG. 4). These compounds did not affect either capsaicin evoked whole cell inward currents or more specifically, capsaicin-induced Ca^{2+} influx.

Western blot analysis indicated that capsaicin application also increased the degradation of the calpain preferred substrate, α-spectrin (240 Kda) and that this increase could be significantly reduced by treatment with either of the calpain

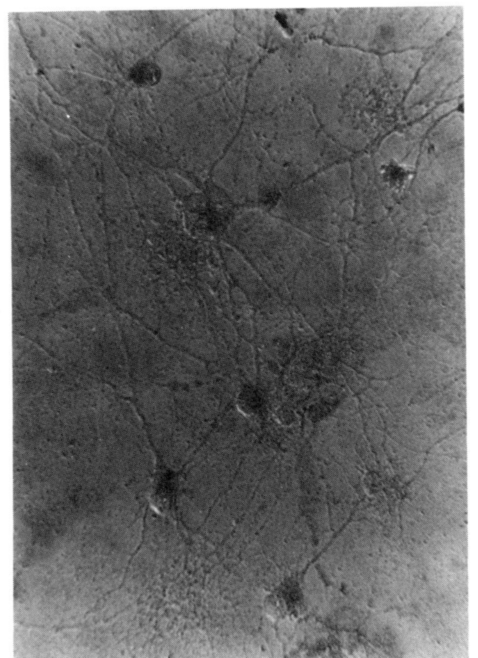
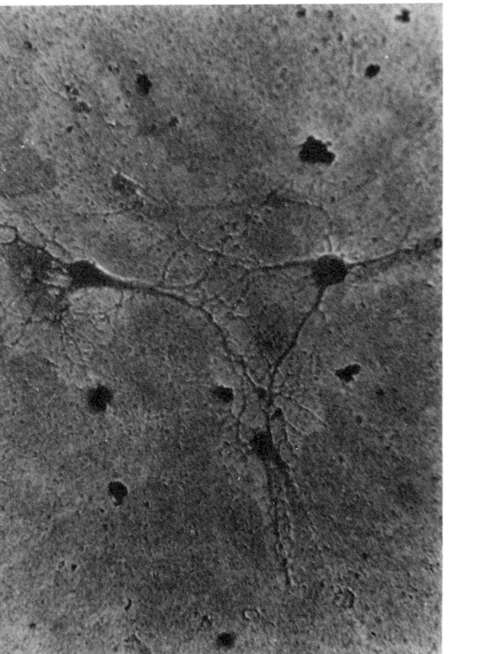

FIGURE 3. Silver staining of Co^{2+} uptake following kainate application. **A.** 100 μM kainate caused uptake of Co^{2+} into a majority of neurons cultured from the dentate gyrus as indicated by the dark staining of both the soma and neurites with silver grains. Co^{2+} does not permeate voltage-sensitive Ca^{2+} channels or NMDA receptors therefore this technique showed the cells which allowed direct influx of divalent cations through the kainate receptor. **B.** Under the same incubation conditions, considerably reduced silver staining was observed when kainate was incubated with the selective kainate receptor antagonist CNQX (10 μM) therefore the effect is specifically due to kainate receptor activation.

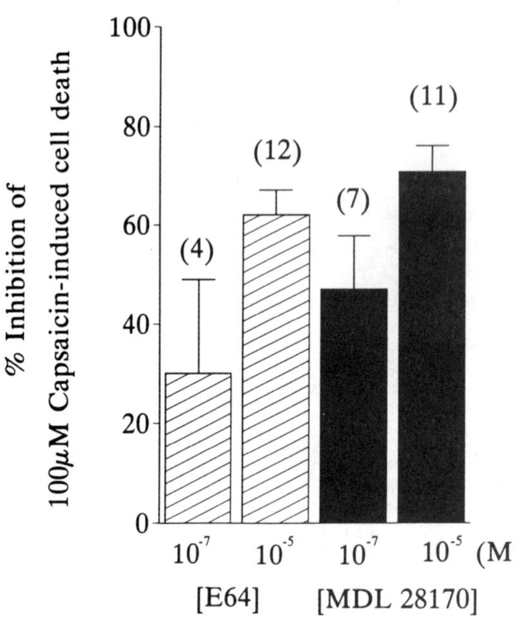

FIGURE 4. Concentration-dependent inhibition of the capsaicin-induced (100 μM) death of cultured dorsal root ganglion neurons by the Ca^{2+}-activated protease inhibitors E64 and MDL-28,170. Cells were incubated in a medium containing capsaicin for 20 min and then allowed to recover for 24 h at which point cell death was assessed using the vital stain fluorescein diacetate and DNA intercalating agent propidium iodide. Protease inhibitors were added 20 min before incubation with capsaicin and were present in all media until the cell death assay. Percentage inhibitions were calculated from the corresponding control coverslips. The data are plotted as mean ± the standard error of the mean. The numbers in parentheses indicate the number of separate experiments.

inhibitors. The increased formation of breakdown products was not observed when capsaicin was applied in the absence of extracellular Ca^{2+}.

These data imply that capsaicin mediated neurotoxicity is a consequence of Ca^{2+} influx and increased calpain activity is the mechanism by which elevated $[Ca^{2+}]_i$ initiates the processes leading to cell death. The importance of calpain in this form of Ca^{2+} influx-induced neurotoxicity is not unique, as we mentioned earlier NMDA receptor–mediated cell death in the CNS can be substantially ameliorated by the use of calpain inhibitors[55] implying that calpain activity may be a significant contributor to Ca^{2+} mediated neurotoxicity in general.

Ca^{2+} INFLUX THROUGH RECEPTOR OPERATED CHANNELS DOES NOT KILL ALL CELL-TYPES

Ca^{2+} influx through receptor operated channels does appear to contribute to Ca^{2+}-dependent delayed neurodegeneration and this Ca^{2+}-induced cell death is mediated in part by induction of calpain activity in both DRG neurons following capsaicin application and in the hippocampus following application of NMDA. However, this does not mean that compounds such as glutamate and capsaicin are only toxic to cells which express Ca^{2+} permeable receptors nor that Ca^{2+} permeable receptors always make a cell particularly vulnerable to excitotoxins. For example, we have observed type II non-NMDA receptor responses in cultured astroglia and, in the studies of Williams and colleagues[51] CA3 pyramidal cells, which are selectively killed by kainate but not NMDA, do not express Co^{2+}-permeable non-NMDA receptors. In our studies, large increases in $[Ca^{2+}]_i$ can be measured following application of kainate, AMPA and domoate to a population of cultured rat cortical astroglia. A majority of these cells do not have voltage sensitive Ca^{2+} currents therefore depolarizing agents do not cause elevated $[Ca^{2+}]_i$ unless a Ca^{2+} permeable ionophore is activated. Confirmation that the observed rise in Ca^{2+} was due to divalent cation conductance was obtained using fura-2 based microfluorimetry with Co^{2+} as the principal extracellular divalent. Co^{2+} quenches emitted fluorescence from fura-2 at both 340 and 380 nm excitation wavelengths therefore any Co^{2+} entry into fura-2 loaded cells can be monitored. In FIGURE 5, no significant change in fluorescence is measured when a normal

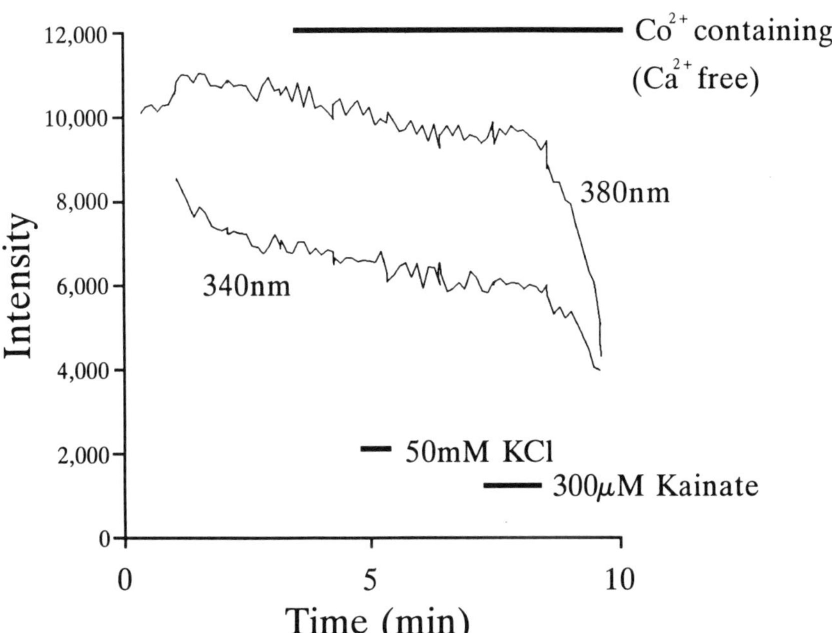

FIGURE 5. Divalent cation permeable kainate receptors are present in cultured cortical astroglia. Using Fura-2-based microfluorimetry, we measured the emission of light at a wavelength of 510 nm following excitation of the Fura-2-loaded astroglia with light at the dual wavelengths of 380 and 340 nm. In normal extracellular solution (containing 2 mM Ca^{2+}) and when the Ca^{2+} ions were completely replaced with equimolar amounts of Co^{2+}, no change in emitted fluorescence was observed. As expected, a depolarizing solution of 50 mM K^+ (equimolar replacement for Na^+) had no effect. This indicates that either no voltage-sensitive Ca^{2+} channels were present of that any channels present were not permeable to or were blocked by Co^{2+}. However, application of 300 μM kainate did cause a rapid decrease in emitted light due to excitation by light at both 340 or 380 nm wavelengths. We conclude that Co^{2+} entered the cell through the kainate-activated conductance and bound intracellular Fura-2, quenching the fluorescence.

medium containing 2 mM Ca^{2+} is exchanged with a medium containing 2 mM Co^{2+} in place of the Ca^{2+}. As expected, 50 mM K^+ has no effect on the fluorescence but application of 300 μM kainate causes a rapid quenching of the light intensity indicating the opening of a divalent permeable conductance. Kainate also causes dose-dependent increases in intracellular Ca^{2+} in 2 CaNMDG media so we believe that Ca^{2+} permeable kainate receptors are present in these cells. Work on cerebellar fusiform glial cells[58] and Bergmann glia in the intact cerebellar slice[59] indicates that cultured cortical astroglia are not unique in expressing type II non-NMDA receptors which serves to emphasize the point that receptor operated Ca^{2+} channels can be expressed in cells such as glia which are resistant to excitotoxicity and it is not the receptor-operated Ca^{2+} channel which makes a neuron vulnerable *per se*.

IN CONCLUSION

Delayed neurodegeneration depends upon distinct temporally and spatially defined rises in $[Ca^{2+}]_i$ and the presence or absence of particular Ca^{2+}-activated proteins including enzymes, buffers and transporters. However, certain pathologies are clearly the consequence of excessive Ca^{2+} influx and understanding the means of Ca^{2+} influx and the effectors of subsequent cell death could provide useful new therapeutic strategies in the treatment of these diseases.

ACKNOWLEDGMENTS

We wish to thank James A. Holzwarth, Dr. Ning-Sheng Wang, Patricia Manzolillo, Hawke H. Yoon, Jonathan R. Savidge, and Ursulla Matke for invaluable assistance with the experiments described in this paper.

REFERENCES

1. MARTY, A. 1989. Trends Neurosci. **12:** 420–424.
2. LLINAS, R. R. 1988. Science. **242:** 1654–1664.
3. MALENKA, R. C., J. C. KAUER, D. J. PERKEL & R. A. NICOLL. 1989. Trends Neurosci. **12:** 444–450.
4. SZEKELY, A. M., E. COSTA & D. R. GAYSON. 1990. Molec. Pharmacol. **38:** 624–633.
5. MCCORMACK, J. G., A. P. HALESTRAP & R. M. DENTON. 1990. Physiol. Rev. **70:** 391–425.
6. MILLER, R. J. 1990. FASEB J. **4:** 3291–3299.
7. MAYER, M. L. & R. J. MILLER. 1990. Trends Pharmacol. Sci. **11:** 254–260.
8. CHOI, D. W. 1987. J. Neurosci. **7:** 369–379.
9. SIESJO, B. & F. BENGTSSON. 1989. J. Blood Flow Metab. **9:** 127.
10. MILLER, R. J. 1992. Trends Neurosci. **15:** 317–319.
11. NOVELLI, A., J. KISPERT, M. T. FERNANDEZ-SANCHEZ, A. TORREBLANCA & V. ZITKO. 1992. Brain Res. **577:** 41–48.
12. WOOD, J. N., J. WINTER, I. F. JAMES, H. P. RANG, J. YEATS & S. BEVAN. 1988. J. Neurosci. **8:** 3208–3220.
13. BLEAKMAN, D., J. R. BRORSON & R. J. MILLER. 1990. Br. J. Pharmacol. **101:** 423–431.
14. HOLZER, P. 1991. Pharmacol. Rev. **43:** 143–201.
15. MAGGI, C. A. 1991. J. Autonomic Nervous System **33:** 1–14.
16. WINTER, J. 1987. Neurosci. Lett. **80:** 134–140.
17. JANCSO, G., E. KIRALY & A. JANCSO-GABOR. 1977. Nature. **270:** 741–743.

18. MARSH, S. J., C. E. STANSFIELD, D. A. BROWN, R. DAVEY & D. MCCARTHY. 1987. Neurosci. **23:** 275–289.
19. BERNSTEIN, J. E., N. J. KORMAN, D. R. BICKERS, M. V. DAHL & L. E. MILLIKAN. 1989. J. Am. Acad. Dermatol. **21:** 265–270.
20. SLADECZEK, F., M. RECASENS & J. BOCKAERT. 1988. Trends Neurosci. **11:** 545–549.
21. BLEAKMAN, D., K. I. RUSIN, P. S. CHARD, S. R. GLAUM & R. J. MILLER. 1992. Mol. Pharmacol. **42:** 192–196.
22. CONSTANTI, A. & V. LIBRI. 1992. Eur. J. Pharmacol. **214:** 105–106.
23. WATKINS, J. C., P. KROGSGAARD-LARSEN & T. HONORE. 1990. Trends Pharmacol. Sci. **11:** 25–33.
24. MAYER, M. L. & G. L. WESTBROOK. 1987. Physiol. Rev. **394:** 501–527.
25. ROTHMAN, S. M. & J. W. OLNEY. 1987. Trends Neurosci. **10:** 299–302.
26. REGAN, F. G. & D. W. CHOI. 1991. Neurosci. **43:** 585–591.
27. PARK, C. K., D. G. NEHLS, D. I. GRAHAM, G. M. TEASDALE & J. MCCULLOCH. 1988. Ann. Neurol. **24:** 543–551.
28. FADEN, A. I. & R. P. SIMON. 1988. Ann. Neurol. **23:** 623–626.
29. WEISS, J. H., D. M. HARTLEY, J. KOH & D. W. CHOI. 1990. Science **247:** 1474–1477.
30. SHEARDOWN, M. J., E. O. NIELSEN, A. J. HANSEN, P. JACOBSEN & T. HONORE. 1990. Science **247:** 571–574.
31. KAKU, D. A., M. P. GOLDBERG & D. W. CHOI. 1991. Brain Research. **554:** 344–347.
32. MURPHY, S. N. & R. J. MILLER. 1989. J. Pharm. Exp. Ther. **249:** 184–193.
33. IINO, M. S., S. OZAWA & K. TSUZUKI. 1990. J. Physiol. **424:** 151–165.
34. OZAWA, S., M. IINO & K. TSUZUKI. 1991. J. Neurophysiol. **66:** 2–11.
35. HOLOPAINEN, I., M. O. K. ENKVIST & K. E. O. AKERMAN. 1989. Neurosci. Lett. **98:** 57–62.
36. OGURA, A., K. AKITA & Y. KUDO. 1990. Neurosci. Res. **9:** 103–113.
37. PRUSS, R. M., R. C. AKESON, M. M. RACKE & J. L. WILBURN. 1991. Neuron. **7:** 509–518.
38. HOLLMAN, M., M. HARTLEY & S. HEINEMANN. 1991. Science **252:** 851–853.
39. BARNES, J. M. & J. M. HENLEY. 1992. Prog. Neurobiol. **39:** 113–133.
40. BRORSON, J. R., D. BLEAKMAN, S. J. GIBBONS & R. J. MILLER. 1991. J. Neurosci. **11:** 4024–4043.
41. LLINAS, R. & M. SUGIMORI. 1980. J. Physiol. (Lond.) **305:** 171–195.
42. AUDINAT, E., T. KNOPFEL & B. H. GAHWILER. 1990. J. Physiol. (Lond.) **430:** 297–313.
43. BRORSON, J. R., D. BLEAKMAN, P. S. CHARD & R. J. MILLER. 1992. Mol. Pharmacol. **41:** 603–608.
44. BLEAKMAN, D., P. S. CHARD, S. FOUCART & R. J. MILLER. 1991. J. Pharm. Exp. Ther. **259:** 430–438.
45. MCGURK, J. F., R. S. ROGINSKI, R. S. ZUKIN & M. V. L. BENNETT. 1991. Soc. Neurosci. Abstr. **17:** 335.
46. BRORSON, J. R., P. A. MANZOLILLO & R. J. MILLER. 1992. Neurology (Abstracts). **42:** 196.
47. MELDRUM, B. & J. GARTHWAITE. 1990. Trends Pharmacol. Sci. **11:** 379–387.
48. SLOVITER, R. S. 1987. Science **235:** 73–76.
49. KOSAKA, T., J.-Y. WU & R. BENOIT. 1988. Exp. Brain Res. **71:** 388–398.
50. GIBBONS, S. J. & R. J. MILLER. 1992. Soc. Neurosci. Abstr. **18:** 613.11.
51. WILLIAMS, L. R., R. F. PREGENZER & J. A. OOSTVEEN. 1992. Brain Res. **581:** 181–189.
52. MATTSON, M. P., B. RYCHLIK, C. CHU & S. CHRISTAKOS. 1991. Neuron. **6:** 41–51.
53. SCHARFMAN, H. E. 1991. J. Neurosci. **11:** 1660–1673.
54. TURETSKY, D. M., M. P. GOLDBERG & D. W. CHOI. 1992. Soc. Neurosci. Abst. **18:** 43.2.
55. SIMAN, R., J. C. NOSZEK & C. KEGERISE. 1989. J. Neurosci. **9:** 1579–1590.
56. MEHDI, S. 1991. Trends Pharmacol. Sci. **16:** 150–153.
57. ARLINGHAUS, L., S. MEHDI & K. S. LEE. 1991. Eur. J. Pharm. **209:** 123–125.
58. BURNASHEV, N., A. KHODOROVA, P. JONAS, P. J. HELM, W. WISDEN, H. MONYER, P. H. SEEBURG & B. SAKMANN. 1992. Science **256:** 1566–1570.
59. MULLER, T., T. MOLLER, T. BERGER, J. SCHNITZER & H. KETTENMANN. 1992. Science **256:** 1563–1566.

Examination of the Role of Calcium in
Neuronal Death

JANET M. DUBINSKY

Department of Physiology
University of Texas Health Science Center
7703 Floyd Curl Drive
San Antonio, Texas 78284-7756

Perhaps the most popular hypothesis regarding mechanisms which contribute to neuronal death involves elevations in intracellular calcium ($[Ca^{2+}]_i$). From a wide variety of experiments focusing on cerebral hypoglycemia and ischemia, Siesjo originally formulated that elevations of cytosolic calcium consequent to energy failure initiate a number of calcium-activated intracellular processes causing cell death.[1] This view was later expanded to include calcium entry through the *N*-methyl-D-aspartate (NMDA) subtype of GLU receptor as well as calcium entry through voltage dependent calcium channels (VDCC).[2] Regardless of the origin of this $[Ca^{2+}]_i$ rise, it has been generalized that elevated levels of $[Ca^{2+}]_i$ are toxic to neurons.[2,3] As with all generalizations, abundant experimental evidence exists that is consistent with the hypothesis. Alterations in $[Ca^{2+}]_i$ are closely linked with the process of cell death following ischemic or excitotoxic injury. However, small perturbations may be sufficient to trigger the loss of viability rather than large calcium overloads. Furthermore, neurons may die from other causes, independent of changes in $[Ca^{2+}]_i$. The purpose of this discussion is to focus on the *limitations* of the *generalized* calcium hypothesis regarding differing forms of neuronal death.

In the nervous system, neuronal death occurs developmentally during normal synaptogenesis and perhaps with advanced aging, and abnormally as a consequence of ischemia, trauma or disease processes. For normally occurring cell death and hypoxia or hypoglycemia-induced neuronal death, experimental approaches manipulating the known causes, availability of growth factors, blood supply, oxygen or glucose, in both *in vivo* and *in vitro* models provide good experimental systems in which to study the steps involved in the mechanisms of neuronal death. Cell death associated with epilepsy may result from excitotoxicity consequent to overstimulation.[4] The direct causes of cell death associated with aging processes, Huntington's disease, Parkinson's disease, and other neurodegenerative diseases remain speculative. Manipulations of experimental models for these diseases are less informative since these models only mimic the still unknown causes. Therefore, this discussion is limited to cell death in those systems with known causative agents.

This article is not intended to challenge the involvement of calcium in the process of neuronal cell death associated with excitotoxicity, ischemia or hypoglycemia. Rather, the experiments presented here are discussed in an effort to delimit more clearly the conditions, both temporal and spatial, in which calcium influx, following GLU receptor activation, participates in eventual toxicity. Global measurements of $[Ca^{2+}]_i$ from neuronal somas may not reflect the relevant compartment in which calcium-associated changes may be occurring. Local alterations in $[Ca^{2+}]_i$ and its homeostasis within postsynaptic structures may disrupt normal functioning to a sufficient extent to produce degeneration initially in dendrites and subsequently in cell bodies.[5] Furthermore, the absence of any rises in $[Ca^{2+}]_i$ associated with growth-factor deprivation-induced neuronal death illustrates the point that not every form of cell death is associated with $[Ca^{2+}]_i$ increases.

Glutamate-induced toxicity, hypothesized to contribute to ischemia-induced necrosis,[6] has been extensively studied in *in vitro* models[7-9] where $[Ca^{2+}]_i$ can be directly observed with indicator dyes.[10] In tissue culture models of excitotoxicity, application of GLU or agonists at NMDA receptors produce two independently measurable events: 1) rapid elevations in $[Ca^{2+}]_i$ on a time scale of minutes,[11-22] and 2) eventual neuronal death on a time scale of many hours.[15,16,18,19,21,22] Neuronal death can occur rapidly as a result of osmotic imbalance following a large ionic influx[23] or on a delayed time scale over the course of a day.[8,24] The delayed neuronal death appears to be dependent upon the presence of extracellular calcium and its presumed influx through NMDA channels.[8,24,25] The extent and duration of the rise in $[Ca^{2+}]_i$ appear variable and depend largely on the way individual experiments have been conducted (TABLE 1). A few laboratories have reported massive increases in $[Ca^{2+}]_i$ in response to excitatory amino acid stimulation (≥ 1 μM).[18,26,27] Many other laboratories have reported only modest rises from similarly prepared tissues (≤ 500 nM).[12-15,20,22,28] Thus the toxic effects of calcium influx may result from moderate displacements of intracellular levels.

Modest elevations in $[Ca^{2+}]_i$ are also reported following prolonged hypoglycemia.[29,30] More recent experiments demonstrated that this rise does not occur immediately upon removal of glucose, but after 16 hours, coincident with observable neuronal death (Mattson, this volume). A more rapid response in alterations in $[Ca^{2+}]_i$ was observed after the combined insult of both hypoglycemia and hypoxia.[31]

Several laboratories have convincingly shown that the rises in $[Ca^{2+}]_i$ correlated with the eventual fate of the cell.[15,16,18,19,27] Manev and colleagues correlated the peak level of $[Ca^{2+}]_i$ immediately after an excitotoxic insult with eventual cell death 24 hours later.[15,19] Kudo and colleagues, on the other hand, reported that death correlated with the length of time that $[Ca^{2+}]_i$ remained above basal levels rather than with the absolute level of calcium reached.[18] In the most recent study to examine this correlation, Randall and Thayer[27] monitored $[Ca^{2+}]_i$ in cultured hippocampal neurons continuously over a 3-h period with the dye Indo-1. They reported two rises in $[Ca^{2+}]_i$: 1) an initially very high response reaching micromolar levels, which recovered and 2) a secondary increase 1–3 hours later. Only the secondary $[Ca^{2+}]_i$ increase correlated with cell death. It should be noted that the secondary rise was only observed in neurons that had previously undergone the initial calcium disequilibrium. The variability in these correlations echoes the uncertainty about how elevations in $[Ca^{2+}]_i$ mediate the subsequent cell death.

However, correlations may not necessarily imply causation. Both alterations in $[Ca^{2+}]_i$ and eventual cell death may be caused by the same initial triggering events. The early rises in $[Ca^{2+}]_i$ may not be the mediator of the cell death process. Elevations in $[Ca^{2+}]_i$ may be parallel events[32] that trigger other processes contributing to or amplifying the initial toxic event.[33] The strongest evidence for causation is provided by the prevention of cell death upon removal of extracellular calcium for as little as 30 minutes immediately after exposure to toxic levels of GLU.[8,24,25] In separate experiments monitoring $[Ca^{2+}]_i$, external solution with no added calcium greatly attenuated but did not totally block GLU-induced rises in $[Ca^{2+}]_i$.[22] Hypoglycemia-induced death among cultured neurons was also successfully prevented in nominally calcium-free external solution.[29]

Yet, other experimental manipulations which prevented the GLU receptor-associated rises in $[Ca^{2+}]_i$ did not fully protect against excitotoxic damage. Among

TABLE 1. Comparison of *in Vitro* Experiments Examining GLU-induced Intracellular Ca^{2+} Changes

Preparation	Insult	Max Level of $[Ca^{2+}]_i$ Attained	Toxicity	Recovery of Basal $[Ca^{2+}]_i$	Methodological Notes	Reference
Cultured embryonic mouse striatum, 11–21 div	≥5 min of GLU, NMDA, KA	~400 nM	n.e.[a]	yes	fura-2-AM, bath perfusion, 37°C	12
Isolated adult guinea pig CA1 neurons	several seconds of GLU	300 nM	n.e.	no	fura-2-AM, GLU iontophoresis, 30–32°C	13
Cultured embryonic mouse cortex, 8 div	≥5 min 100 μM GLU	400 nM	n.e.	only with rinses in 2 div cultures	fluo-3-AM, direct dilute addition, 37°C	14
Cultured postnatal rat cerebellar granule cells, 7–8 div	50–500 μM GLU	~260 nM	correlate $[Ca^{2+}]_i$ after GLU removal with eventual toxicity	only with 5 μM GLU	fura-2-AM simultaneous with PI uptake, RT	15
Cultured postnatal rat cerebellum, 7 div	56 mM K^+ → 100 μM GLU →	~550 nM ~275 nM	n.e.	slow	fura-2-AM, direct addition, perfusion rinses, 32°C	20
Cultured postnatal rat hippocampus, 14–18 div	45 min 500 μM GLU	400 nM	not correlated with $[Ca^{2+}]_i$ when using GLU, GLU + antagonists or high K^+	no	fura-2-AM, direct addition, trypan blue uptake or exclusion, RT	21
Cultured postnatal rat hippocampus, 14–18 div	5 min 300 μM GLU →	~350 nM	toxic	no	fura-2-AM, bath perfusion, trypan blue uptake or exclusion, 33–35°C	22
	5 min 3 mM NaCN →	~1.1 μM	not toxic	yes		

Cultured postnatal rat hippocampus, 14–18 div	5 min, 500 μM GLU	~450 nM	toxic	yes	fura-2-AM, direct addition and discrete rinses, trypan blue uptake or exclusion, 33–35°C	42
Cultured embryonic rat hippocampus, 7–17 div	1 min 500 μM GLU	~450 nM	n.e.	yes	fura-2-AM, bath perfusion, ?RT	28
Cultured postnatal rat cerebellar granule cells, 10–13 div	500 μM GLU	~550 nM	parallel dose response curves for increases in $[Ca^{2+}]_i$ ($ED_{50} = 6\ \mu$M) and toxicity ($LD_{50} = 10\ \mu$M)	n.e.	fura-2-AM, discrete solution changes, MTT assay, 35–36°C	19
Cultured embryonic rat hippocampus, 4–14 div	5–15 min 1 mM GLU	1–2 μM	correlated with rate of recovery from $[Ca^{2+}]_i$ elevation	yes	fura-2-AM, discrete solution changes, count phase bright neurons, 37°C	18
Cultured embryonic mouse cortex, 9 div	10 μM GLU $\rightarrow$ 50 mM KCl $\rightarrow$	1 μM $\rightarrow$ 700 nM $\rightarrow$	increased LDH no change LDH	n.e.	fluo-3-AM, LDH release, ?RT	26
Cultured embryonic rat hippocampus, $\geq$10 div	5 min 100 μM GLU	2.8 μM	correlated with secondary increase $[Ca^{2+}]_i$	yes, followed by secondary increase in $[Ca^{2+}]_i$	indo-1-AM, stop-flow perfusion, assess death by loss of indo-1 fluorescence, RT	27

[a] n.e., not examined.

cultured hippocampal neurons, GLU receptor antagonists, CNQX or APV in combination with toxic levels of GLU, completely prevented increases in $[Ca^{2+}]_i$ but only partially attenuated toxicity.[21] MK-801 also blocked the GLU-induced rise in $[Ca^{2+}]_i$ as well as the associated toxicity.[21] Thus, some components of excitotoxic death may not be mediated by calcium. In a model of hypoxia, rapid neuronal death among cultured cortical neurons induced by continuous exposure to the glycolytic inhibitor iodoacetate and the electron transport inhibitor rotenone correlated with early rises in $[Ca^{2+}]_i$.[34] Removal of extracellular calcium prevented the increase in $[Ca^{2+}]_i$ but did not alter cell fate as a consequence of this energy depleting treatment.[34] Thus, some manipulations which prevent globally detectable alterations in $[Ca^{2+}]_i$ are not protective.

In addition to observations of hypoxic and excitotoxic cell death without alterations in $[Ca^{2+}]_i$, other instances involving large elevations in $[Ca^{2+}]_i$ have not produced any toxic consequences. High concentrations of extracellular potassium produce increases in $[Ca^{2+}]_i$ to a micromolar or more,[11,22,26,35] presumably from influx through VDCC, which are not toxic to cultured neurons.[21,26] On the contrary, protracted exposure to high potassium promotes survival of many different kinds of neurons in tissue culture.[36-38] Elevations of $[Ca^{2+}]_i$ to micromolar levels, much higher than those generally reported for GLU or NMDA stimulation (see above), have also been observed following sodium cyanide exposure as a model of "chemical hypoxia" without any deleterious consequences.[22] These experiments argue against the notion that every general increase in $[Ca^{2+}]_i$ is toxic to neurons. Indeed, gradual increases in $[Ca^{2+}]_i$ may be part of the normal developmental processes of neurite extension, neuronal differentiation and growth factor independent survival.[38-41]

It should also be noted that calcium homeostasis is not permanently shifted to higher levels after excitotoxic exposure. When monitoring indicator dye fluorescence for an hour or more following a brief toxic insult, $[Ca^{2+}]_i$ recovered to basal levels.[27,42] Indeed, loading the indicator dye into hippocampal neurons in the hours following an excitotoxic insult revealed that $[Ca^{2+}]_i$ did not remain elevated, but returned to resting levels and remained so for up to 13 hours.[42] So if alterations in $[Ca^{2+}]_i$ are involved in triggering or amplifying the process of cell death, only short periods of elevation may be necessary. The absence of $[Ca^{2+}]_i$ elevation during the hours following GLU exposure also argues that any toxicity attributable to prolonged, low level activation of non-NMDA type GLU receptors is probably not acting through a global increase in $[Ca^{2+}]_i$. These experiments emphasize the importance of delimiting the temporal sequence and spatial locations at which calcium elevations may contribute to the lethal consequences of excitotoxicity.

Other types of experiments are supportive of a role of calcium involvement but do not directly demonstrate that calcium is required for the eventual death to occur. Calcium ionophores, which artifically increase membrane permeability to calcium and therefore promote large, abnormal increases in $[Ca^{2+}]_i$, also cause a delayed neuronal death.[8,43] This is not surprising since ionophores were purified from bacterial toxins with cytolytic activity.[44] These manipulations produce massive calcium overload and may mimic the process of calcium influx and subsequent cell demise in excitotoxicity. Yet these experiments do not necessarily show that every elevation of $[Ca^{2+}]_i$ is toxic.

The best studied example among neuronal populations where death occurs in the absence of alterations in $[Ca^{2+}]_i$ concerns the naturally occurring cell death among peripheral neurons. This apoptotic type of death occurs in the absence of sustaining levels of trophic growth factor usually provided by the synaptic target. *In vitro,* sympathetic and dorsal root ganglion cells are dependent upon exogenous nerve growth factor (NGF) for survival during the first several weeks.[38,45–48] Over the course of the first 3 weeks *in vitro,* these neurons became increasingly independent of NGF, surviving for increasingly longer time periods after NGF withdrawal, eventually becoming totally independent.[47,48] In parallel with the increasing NGF independence, the basal $[Ca^{2+}]_i$ rose from initial values just under 100 nM to levels between 200–240 nM.[41,47] High potassium, which elevated $[Ca^{2+}]_i$, substituted for NGF to promote survival among peripheral neurons less than 3 weeks *in vitro.*[38,41] Depletion of extracellular calcium lowered $[Ca^{2+}]_i$ and prevented attainment of NGF independence.[47] Additionally, during the 2 days of survival following NGF withdrawal, $[Ca^{2+}]_i$ remained constant or decreased slightly. No increases were observed 24 hours after NGF withdrawal, even though these neurons were committed to die.[41] Thus it appears that moderate increases in basal $[Ca^{2+}]_i$ promote survival among these peripheral neurons and that death by growth factor-deprivation is not accompanied by initial, large deviations of $[Ca^{2+}]_i$ from basal levels.

Neuronal cell death can occur by any number of mechanisms, many of which might be associated with an early calcium-dependent event. Elevation of $[Ca^{2+}]_i$ will undoubtedly activate calcium-dependent proteases, protein kinases, phospholipases, and possibly endonucleases in different compartments of different neuronal populations.[49] These processes could contribute to eventual toxicity. Several points are to be emphasized concerning calcium's contribution. 1) Ca may not be the sole agent responsible for neurodegeneration. Increases in $[Ca^{2+}]_i$, in association with disruption of other homeostatic events may participate in the induction and amplification of a toxic insult.[33] 2) All elevations of $[Ca^{2+}]_i$ may not lead to toxic consequences. The neuronal soma may not be the appropriate site to monitor relevant changes in calcium homeostasis. 3) The extent to which $[Ca^{2+}]_i$ is elevated may not determine the severity of the toxic insult. Local transients or sustained low level augmentations may be equally effective threshold events. 4) Some forms of neuronal cell death may not involve early elevations in $[Ca^{2+}]_i$. Massive influx of $[Ca^{2+}]_i$ coincident with membrane breakdown occurs in the later stages of cellular demise.

Disturbances of intracellular calcium are most certainly invovled in neuronal cell death triggered by overstimulation of GLU receptors. However, the extent to which $[Ca^{2+}]_i$ must rise to initiate lethal consequences may be limited depending upon intracellular location and previous cellular activity. The duration of the disruption in calcium homeostasis may be a more important parameter than the absolute level of $[Ca^{2+}]_i$ reached. In neuronal cell death consequent to metabolic compromise or energy deprivation, alterations in $[Ca^{2+}]_i$ may not be essential for subsequent death. Finally, in other forms of neuronal degeneration, *e.g.* after growth factor deprivation, alterations in $[Ca^{2+}]_i$ may not be involved until after neurons are committed to die. Since intracellular calcium homeostasis is so tightly regulated, potentially lethal insults may produce disturbances of resting calcium levels. In some cases, these calcium fluctuations may amplify a toxic insult and result in cell death. Alternatively, homeostasis may be restored and death may be averted. In other cases, cell death may ensue from other causes, despite the perturbations, and perhaps even restoration, of calcium homeostasis.

REFERENCES

1. SIESJO, B. K. 1981. Cell damage in the brain: A speculative synthesis. J. Cereb. Blood Flow Metab. **1:** 155–185.
2. SIESJO, B. K. & F. BENGTSSON. 1989. Calcium fluxes, calcium antagonists, and calcium-

related pathology in brain ischemia, hypoglycemia, and spreading depression: A unifying hypothesis. J. Cereb. Blood Flow Metab. **9:** 127–140.

3. ORRENIUS, S., D. J. MCCONKEY, G. BELLOMO & P. NICOTERA. 1989. Role of Ca^{2+} in toxic cell killing. Trends Pharmacol. Sci. **10:** 281–285.

4. SLOVITER, R. S. 1991. Permanently altered hippocampal structure, excitability, and inhibition after experimental status epilepticus in the rat: The "dormant basket cell" hypothesis and its possible relevance to temporal lobe epilepsy. Hippocampus **1:** 41–66.

5. MATTSON, M. P., P. DOU & S. B. KATER. 1988. Outgrowth-regulating actions of glutamate in isolated hippocampal pyramidal neurons. J. Neurosci. **8:** 2087–2100.

6. CHOI, D. W. & S. M. ROTHMAN. 1990. The role of glutamate neurotoxicity in hypoxic-ischemic neuronal death. Ann. Rev. Neurosci. **13:** 171–182.

7. CHOI, D. W., M. MAULUCCI-GEDDE & A. R. KRIEGSTEIN. 1987. Glutamate neurotoxicity in cortical cell culture. J. Neurosci. **7:** 357–368.

8. CHOI, D. W. 1987. Ionic dependence of glutamate neurotoxicity. J. Neurosci. **7:** 369–379.

9. ROTHMAN, S. M. 1984. Synaptic release of excitatory amino acid neurotransmitter mediates anoxic neuronal death. J. Neurosci. **4:** 1884–1891.

10. GRYNKIEWICZ, G., M. POENIE & R. Y. TSIEN. 1985. A new generation of Ca^{2+} indicators with greatly improved fluorescence properties. J. Biol. Chem. **260:** 3440–3450.

11. MURPHY, S. N. & R. J. MILLER. 1989. Regulation of Ca^{++} influx into striatal neurons by kainic acid. J. Pharm. Exp. Therap. **249:** 184–193.

12. MURPHY, S. N., S. A. THAYER & R. J. MILLER. 1987. The effects of excitatory amino acids on intracellular calcium in single mouse striatal neurons in vitro. J. Neurosci. **7:** 4145–4158.

13. CONNOR, J. A., W. J. WADMAN, PHILLIP E. HOCKBERGER & R. K. S. WONG. 1988. Sustained dendritic gradients of Ca^{2+} induced by excitatory amino acids in CA1 hippocampal neurons. Science **240:** 649–653.

14. WAHL, P., A. SCHOUSBOE, TAGE HONORE & J. DREJER. 1989. Glutamate-induced increase in intracellular Ca^{2+} in cerebral cortex neurons is transient in immature cells but permanent in mature cells. J. Neurochem. **53:** 1316–1319.

15. DE ERAUSQUIN, G. A., H. MANEV, A. GUIDOTTI, E. COSTA & G. BROOKER. 1990. Gangliosides normalize distorted single-cell intracellular free Ca^{2+} dynamics after toxic doses of glutamate in cerebellar granule cells. Proc. Natl. Acad. Sci. USA **87:** 8017–8021.

16. MANEV, H., M. FAVARON, A. GUIDOTTI & E. COSTA. 1989. Delayed increase of Ca^{2+} influx elicited by glutamate: Role in neuronal death. Mol. Pharmacol. **36:** 106–112.

17. FURUYA, S., H. OHMORI, T. SHIGEMOTO & H. SUGIYAMA. 1989. Intracellular calcium mobilization triggered by a glutamate receptor in rat cultured hippocampal cells. J. Physiol. **414:** 539–548.

18. OGURA, A., M. MIYAMATO & Y. KUDO. 1988. Neuronal death in vitro: Parallelism between survivability of hippocampal neurons and sustained elevation of cytosolic Ca^{2+} after exposure to glutamate receptor agonist. Exp. Brain Res. **73:** 447–458.

19. MILANI, D., D. GUIDOLIN, L. FACCI, T. POZZAN, M. BUSO, A. LEON & S. D. SKAPER. 1991. Excitatory amino acid-induced alterations of cytoplasmic free Ca^{2+} in individual cerebellar granule neurons: Role in neurotoxicity. J. Neurosci. Res. **28:** 434–441.

20. CIARDO, A. & J. MELDOLESI. 1991. Regulation of intracellular calcium in cerebellar granule neurons: Effects of depolarization and of glutamatergic and cholinergic stimulation. J. Neurochem. **56:** 184–191.

21. MICHAELS, R. L. & S. M. ROTHMAN. 1990. Glutamate neurotoxicity in vitro: Antagonist pharmacology and intracellular calcium concentrations. J. Neurosci. **10:** 283–292.

22. DUBINSKY, J. M. & S. M. ROTHMAN. 1991. Intracellular calcium concentrations during "chemical hypoxia" and excitotoxic neuronal injury. J. Neurosci. **11:** 2545–2551.

23. ROTHMAN, S. M. 1985. The neurotoxicity of Excitatory Amino Acids is Produced by Passive Chloride Influx. J. Neurosci. **5:** 1483–1489.

24. ROTHMAN, S. M., J. H. THURSTON & R. E. HAUHART. 1987. Delayed neurotoxicity of excitatory amino acids in vitro. Neurosci. **22:** 471–480.

25. HARTLEY, M. & D. W. CHOI. 1989. Delayed rescue of N-methyl-D-aspartate receptor-mediated neuronal injury in cortical culture. J. Pharm. Exp. Therap. **250:** 752–758.
26. FRANDSEN, A. & A. SCHOUSBOE. 1991. Dantrolene prevents glutamate cytotoxicity and Ca^{2+} release from intracellular stores in cultured cerebral cortical neurons. J. Neurochem. **56:** 1075–1078.
27. RANDALL, R. D. & S. A. THAYER. 1992. Glutamate-induced calcium transient triggers delayed calcium overload and neurotoxicity in rat hippocampal neurons. J. Neurosci. **12:** 1882–1895.
28. GLAUM, S. R., W. K. SCHOLZ & R. J. MILLER. 1990. Acute- and long-term glutamate-mediated regulation of $[Ca^{++}]_i$ in rat hippocampal pyramidal neurons in vitro. J. Pharm. Exp. Therap. **253:** 1293–1302.
29. CHENG, B. & M. P. MATTSON. 1991. NGF and bFGF protect rat hippocampal and human cortical neurons against hypoglycemic damage by stabilizing calcium homeostasis. Neuron **7:** 1031–1041.
30. CHENG, B. & M. P. MATTSON. 1992. IGF-I and IGF-II protect cultured hippocampal and septal neurons against calcium-mediated hypoglycemic damage. J. Neurosci. **12:** 1558–1566.
31. GOLDBERG, M. P. & D. W. CHOI. 1990. Intracellular free calcium increases in cultured cortical neurons deprived of oxygen and glucose. Stroke **21** (Suppl. III): 75–77.
32. HOSSMANN, K. A., B. G. OPHOFF, R. SCHMIDT-KASTNER & U. OSCHLIES. 1985. Mitochondrial calcium sequestration in cortical and hippocampal neurons after prolonged ischemia of the cat brain. Acta Neuropathol. (Berl.) **68:** 230–238.
33. CHOI, D. W. 1990. Cerebral Hypoxia: Some new approaches and unanswered questions. J. Neurosci. **10:** 2493–2501.
34. NEDERGAARD, M. 1991. Energy depletion kills neurons independently of cytosolic calcium. J. Cereb. Blood Flow Metab. **11** (Suppl. 2): S421. (Abstract)
35. MURPHY, S. N. & R. J. MILLER. 1989. Two distinct quisqualate receptors regulate Ca^{2+} homeostasis in hippocampal neurons in vitro. Mol. Pharmacol. **35:** 671–680.
36. SCOTT, B. S. 1977. The effect of elevated potassium on the time course of neuron survival in cultures of dissociated dorsal root ganglia. J. Cell Physiol. **91:** 305–316.
37. COLLINS, F. & J. D. LILE. 1989. The role of dihydropyridine-sensitive voltage-gated calcium channels in potassium-mediated neuronal survival. Brain Res. **502:** 99–108.
38. KOIKE, T., D. P. MARTIN & E. M. JOHNSON, JR. 1992. Role of Ca^{2+} channels in the ability of membrane depolarization to prevent neuronal death induced by trophic-factor deprivation: Evidence that levels of internal Ca^{2+} determine nerve growth factor dependence of sympathetic ganglion cells. Proc. Natl. Acad. Sci. USA **86:** 6421–6425.
39. COHAN, C. S., J. A. CONNOR & S. B. KATER. 1987. Electrically and chemically mediated increases in intracellular calcium in neuronal growth cones. J. Neurosci. **7:** 3588–3599.
40. MATTSON, M. P. & S. B. KATER. 1987. Calcium regulation of neurite elongation and growth cone motility. J. Neurosci. **7:** 4034–4043.
41. EICHLER, M. E., J. M. DUBINSKY & K. M. RICH. 1992. Relationship of intracellular calcium to dependence on nerve growth factor in dorsal root ganglion neurons in cell culture. J. Neurochem. **583:** 263–269.
42. DUBINSKY, J. M. 1992. Intracellular calcium levels during the period of delayed excitotoxicity. J. Neurosci. In press.
43. MATTSON, M. P., B. RYCHLIK, J. S. YOU & J. E. SISKEN. 1991. Sensitivity of cultured human embryonic cerebral cortical neurons to excitatory amino acid-induced calcium influx and neurotoxicity. Brain Res. **542:** 97–106.
44. PRESSMAN, B. C. 1976. Biological applications of ionophores. Ann. Rev. Biochem. **45:** 501–530.
45. GREENE, L. A. 1977. Quantitative in vitro studies on the Nerve Growth Factor (NGF) requirement of neurons. I. Sympathetic neurons. Dev. Biol. **58:** 96–105.
46. GREENE, L. A. 1977. Quantitative in vivo studies on the nerve growth factor (NGF) requirements of neurons II. Sensory neurons. Dev. Biol. **58:** 106–113.
47. KOIKE, T. & S. TANAKA. 1991. Evidence that nerve growth factor dependence of

sympathetic neurons for survival in vitro may be determined by levels of cytoplasmic free Ca^{2+}. Proc. Natl. Acad. Sci. USA **88:** 3892–3896.

48. EICHLER, M. E. & K. M. RICH. 1989. Death of sensory ganglion neurons after acute withdrawal of nerve growth factor in dissociated cell culture. Brain Res. **482:** 340–346.

49. ORRENIUS, S., D. J. McCONKEY, D. P. JONES & P. NICOTERA. 1988. Ca^{2+}-activated mechanisms in toxicity and programmed cell death. ISI Atlas of Science 319–324.

Cellular Responses of Identified Lamprey Central Neurons to Axonal and Dendritic Injury

An *in Situ* Model for Studying Cellular Injury on the Single Cell Level in the Vertebrate CNS

GARTH F. HALL

Department of Neurology (Neuroscience)
Harvard Medical School
Center for Neurologic Diseases
Department of Neurology
Children's Hospital
Boston, Massachusetts 02115

The spectrum of degenerative and regenerative changes seen in neurons following mechanical injury shares important features with both the cellular pathology resulting from chemical, excitotoxic and ischemic injury and that induced by neurodegenerative diseases such as Alzheimer's Disease (AD) and amyotrophic lateral sclerosis (ALS). Neurons affected by these conditions exhibit early changes in second messenger levels (particularly intracellular Ca++ and protein kinase C), followed by major cytoskeletal reorganizations, changes in protein synthesis, phosphorylation, transport and degradation and often a loss of cellular polarity. The ultimate effects of these changes range from cellular degeneration and death to successful recovery of normal function. In this article, I will describe the responses of giant identified neurons in the hindbrain of the larval sea lamprey to axonal and dendritic amputation and will present this system as a model with major technical advantages for studying the effects of cellular injury on a single cell level in a vertebrate central nervous system (CNS) *in situ*. The effects of axotomy on lamprey central neurons will then be discussed in the context of the degenerative neuronal pathology following the various types of cellular injury outlined above which forms the common focus of these proceedings.

THE LAMPREY CNS AS A MODEL SYSTEM FOR STUDYING THE RESPONSE TO NEURONAL INJURY IN SINGLE CELLS *IN SITU*

The giant Muller and Mauthner neurons in the brain and spinal cord of the larval sea lamprey (*Petromyzon marinus*) has been a longstanding subject for studies of spinal cord injury that have focused on the cellular correlates of behavioral recovery following spinal transection.[1-7] During the last few years, these cells have also been used to examine the cell biology underlying the neuronal response to injury.[8-18] In this paper, I will present the lamprey CNS as an experimental system with a number of technical advantages over other lower vertebrate systems as well as over mammalian preparations for the study of CNS injury in vertebrates. Some of these advantages are: 1) Muller and Mauthner cells are unusual among mature vertebrate central neurons in that they sprout vigorously following axotomy and recognize at least some appropriate targets in the spinal cord.[6] Behavioral recovery from spinal transection occurs within several weeks, and because of the simplicity of spinally mediated behaviors in the lamprey, can be readily analyzed in detail using sophisticated computer techniques. 2) Muller and Mauthner cells are individually identifiable and have highly stereotyped locations and dendritic and axonal morphology[19] (see FIGS. 1 and 2). This permits one to make precise lesions (such as amputation of parts of dendritic trees) in living animals and to work with single, morphologically sterotyped cells in different animals. 3) Muller and Mauthner somata are extremely accessible; they are large (60–100 microns across) and can be easily seen and injected intracellularly in the living animal (FIG. 1), allowing pharmacological perturbation experiments that directly affect only the injected cell. 4) The larval lamprey CNS has little or no intrinsic vasculature, making neurons resistant to lesions that in higher vertebrates might cause widespread ischemic effects. The lamprey CNS thus provides many of the technical advantages of cell cultures while allowing one to ask questions that are best answered in the context of single neurons *in situ*.

Effects of "Distant" Axotomy in the Spinal Cord on Muller and Mauthner Cells

Localized degenerative changes begin occurring in the transected axons of Muller and Mauthner neurons near the lesion site within minutes of "distant" axotomy in the spinal cord at a distance of 1 cm or more from their somata in the hindbrain (FIG. 1). One of the first effects of axotomy is the induction of a large flux of $Ca++$ and other cations into the axon stump from the extracellular fluid at the site of axotomy.[11] A recent Fura-2 study[18] has demonstrated that this flux is transient, persisting for 1 day or less following axotomy and is localized to the area within several hundred microns of the lesion. Within a few hours of axotomy, both the proximal and distal stumps of the cut axons retract from the lesion site and often form large bulbs;[12] this is accompanied by partial proteolysis[20] and spatial rearrangements[21] of neurofilaments at the lesion site. Studies have shown that the influx of extracellular cations is opposed by an imposed electrical field when the local degeneration and retraction of the axon stumps is inhibited and axonal regeneration is promoted, whereas amplification of the inflowing current accelerates local degeneration and retards regeneration.[12,22] It is thus likely that the mechanism by which axotomy induces these initial degenerative changes involves an increase in the level of intracellular Ca^{++} and the activation of $Ca++$ dependent proteases[23] either as a consequence of the influx of extracellular $Ca++$ at the lesion site mentioned above, or the release of bound $Ca++$ from intracellular stores due to local depolarization.[24]

Changes begin to appear in the somata and dendrites of these cells by several days following distant axotomy, with chromatolysis evident by 8 days post axotomy in some cases[25] and phosphorylation of somatodendritic neurofilaments (NFs) appearing by 14 days.[14] The first signs of axonal regeneration appear as neurofilamentous branches from the axon stump within 45 μm of the lesion in some neurons by 7 days post axotomy,[21] by which time changes in the electrophysiological properties of the axon stump membrane (notably an increase in $Ca++$ conductance) have become established.[13] Regeneration into and across the spinal lesion is clearly established in some cells by 2 weeks post axotomy.[1–3,6–7] Sprouts make synaptic contacts onto other elements in the cord,[3] some of which are appropriate (*i.e.* onto motoneurons).[6] The cytoskeleton of the regenerating sprouts

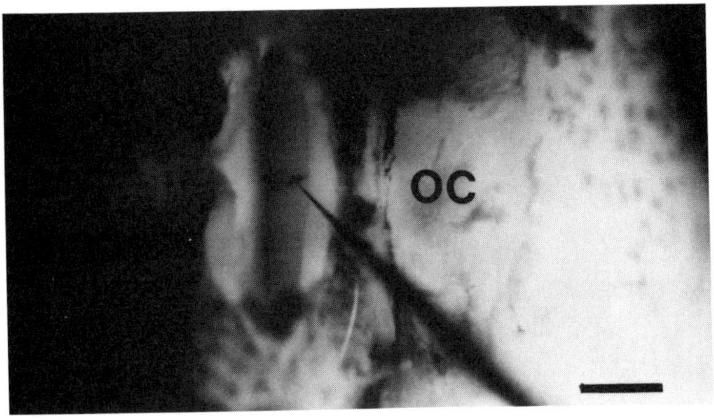

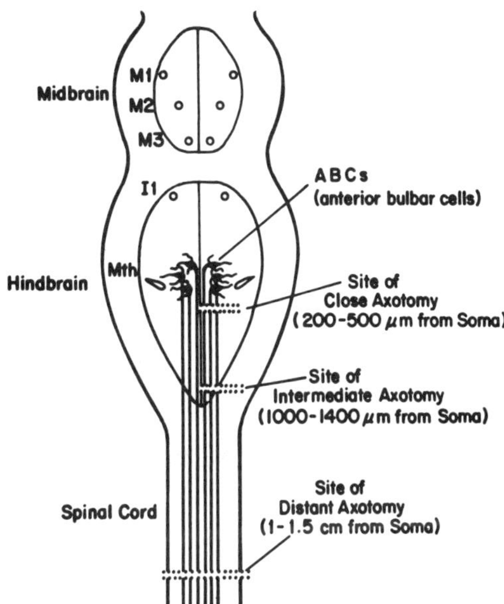

FIGURE 1. *Top:* Dorsal view of a lamprey head showing the hindbrain exposed and illuminated as it would be for microinjection. The somata of two Anterior Bulbar Cells (ABCs) and the Mauthner Cell (MC) on the right side of the brain have been filled with 0.5% Fast Green via a microelectrode (shown pointing at the MC soma). OC = otic capsule. Scale Bar = 500 μm.

Bottom: Schematic diagram of the brain and spinal cord of the lamprey (dorsal view) showing the locations of the three most anterior pairs of bulbar reticulospinal cells (ABCs). The locations of other Muller (M1-3, I1) and Mauthner (Mth) somata are also shown.

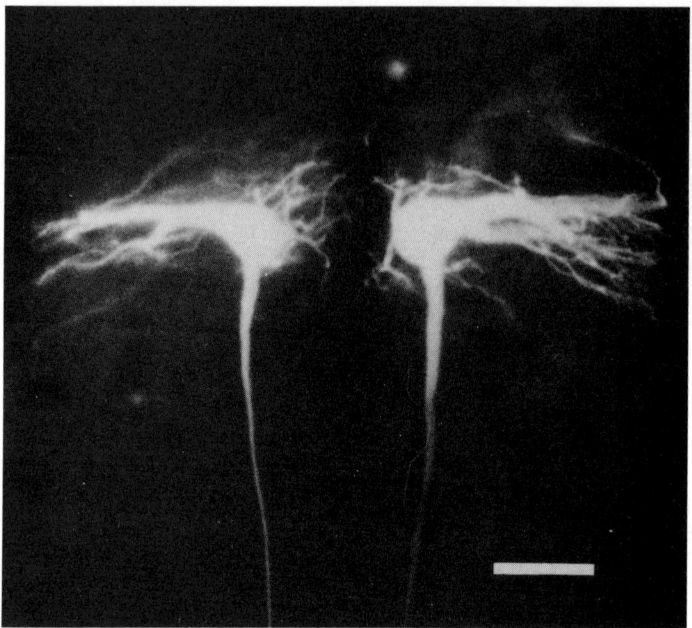

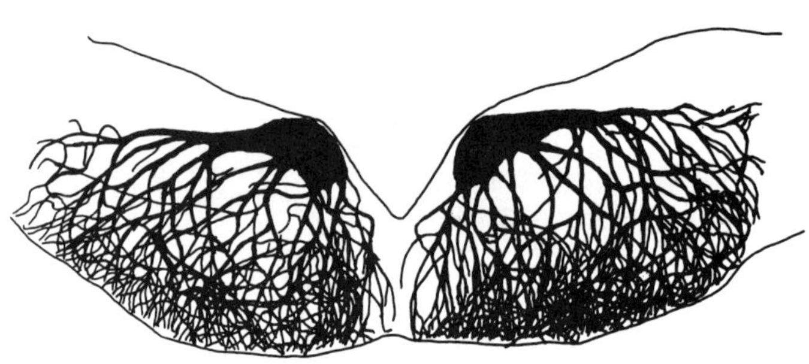

FIGURE 2. Normal ABC morphology. **A:** Dorsal view of a pair of ABCs that have been injected with Lucifer Yellow showing the normal morphology of ABC dendrites and the proximal region of the axon. Most dendrites extend ventrally or ventrolaterally from either the some or the lateral dendrite out of the plane of view. The dendritic tree is relatively flattened in the rostrocaudal dimension, with most dendrites remaining within 100 μm of the plane of the soma. By contrast, the axon is linear and unbranched, extending caudally for nearly the entire length of the spinal cord. **B:** Cross sectional reconstruction of the same cells shown in A. Note that ABC dendrites taper steadily from base to tip without varicosities and branch at regular intervals, with the finest dendrites being evenly distributed along the ventral margin of the brain. ABC dendrites do not cross the central sulcus. Scale Bar = 100 μm.

resembles that of the parent axons, consisting mainly of NFs with very few microtubules (MTs). This is true even in the sprout tips, which also contain a large number of electronlucent vesicles.[3,14,21] The trajectories followed by regenerating Muller and Mauthner axons also resemble those of the parent axons; sprouts tend to be linear, unbranched and follow axial guidance cues in both the brain and spinal cord. In addition, sprouts show a preference for caudal growth in the spinal cord, but not in the brain.[7,9]

By 2 to 3 months or more post axotomy, degenerative changes begin to appear in most Muller and Mauthner cells. The somata of the affected cells begin to swell and the resting membrane potential recorded in the soma is often reduced by 30–40 mV.[9,25,26] This is accompanied by dendritic retraction in which the primary dendritic trunks are narrowed and many higher order dendrites are lost outright (FIGS. 3 and 4). The overall extent of the dendritic field is also reduced, and electrophysiological and ultrastructural evidence suggests that many or most of the synapses onto the dendrites of the axotomized cells are lost.[14,26] There is some evidence to suggest that many of the regenerating axonal sprouts also begin to retract at late times post axotomy;[4] however it is unclear whether this occurs to all sprouts or only to those that have failed to form appropriate synaptic connections.

Degenerative changes accompanying dendritic retraction can also be seen in the cytoskeleton. By 50–60 days post axotomy, there is a clear loss of immunocyto-chemical staining for tubulin in the region around the nucleus and near the plasma membrane, suggesting that there is a loss of MTs in the cell body and dendrites by this time post axotomy (FIGS. 5 and 6). This is particularly marked in the case of staining for acetylated tubulin, a marker for stable microtubules. Phosphoryla-tion of somatodendritic neurofilaments first appears at relatively early times post axotomy (FIG. 6), before the onset of overt degenerative changes. However, NF phosphorylation becomes more marked with time, and by late times post axotomy, phosphorylated NFs appear to displace MTs in the perinuclear region (FIG. 5). Some cells also exhibit a marked staining with antibodies specific for ubiquitin, further suggesting that degenerative changes are underway.

Virtually all Muller and Mauthner cells appear to survive for at least 6 months following axotomy, although by this time the degenerative changes described above become quite marked in most cells.[26] In a few preparations examined more than 1 year post axotomy, a minority of cells were missing, suggesting that some or perhaps all Muller and Mauthner cells eventually die following axotomy. Whether this is due to the failure of the moribund cells to reestablish their original postsynaptic contacts (as might be expected in light of results from many other systems) is presently unknown.

Effects of "Close" Axotomy and "Dendrotomy" on Neuronal Polarity

Over the past few years I have focused my research in this system on the cellular effects of "close" axotomy in the hindbrain (FIG. 1) at a point within 500 μm the somata of Mauthner neurons and a subset of Muller cells (anterior bulbar cells or ABCs, see FIGS. 1 and 2). Many of the effects of distant axotomy described above also occur following close axotomy in ABCs, often at an accelerated rate. As with distant axotomy, close axotomy induces chromatolysis, cytoskeletal changes and the onset of axonal regeneration within the first two weeks post axotomy, followed by dendritic retraction accompanied by further progressive cytoskeletal changes and synapse loss. However, one major difference between the effects of the two types of lesion is that close axotomy causes the affected

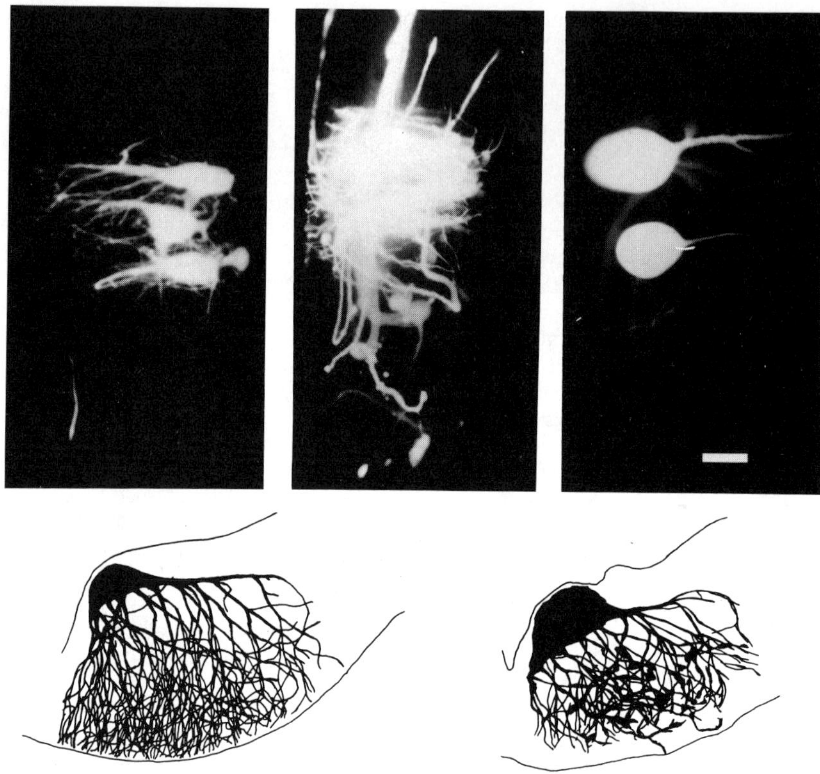

FIGURE 3. Dendritic sprouting and retraction following close axotomy. *Top left:* ABCs 27 days after axotomy of the caudalmost cell. In this animal, the main lesion was on the contralateral side of the brain (not shown). The lesion crossed the midline to cut the axon of the caudalmost cell, leaving the other 2 intact. The intact cells do not sprout, whereas 2 sprouts can be seen emerging from the dendrites of the axotomized cell, one of which extends caudally from the dendritic field following a trajectory parallel to the axons of the intact cells. *Top center:* Two ABCs 50 days following close axotomy showing profuse ectopic axonal regeneration from the dendrites. *Top right:* Two ABCs 181 days following close axotomy showing severe retraction of the dendritic tree. Note the swollen soma and the reduced diameter of the lateral dendrite when compared to intact ABCs. *Bottom:* Cross sectional reconstructions of an intact ABC (left) and on 220 days following close axotomy (right). Note the reduced complexity and extent of the dendritic tree and the presence of swollen dendritic tips. Scale Bar = 50 μm.

neuron to lose its normal cellular polarity. Normally, axotomy induces a neuron to regenerate its axon specifically from the cut end of the axon stump, bypassing other sites within the cell. Following close axotomy, axonal regeneration is redistributed to the dendritic tips from the axon stump, with the total amount of sprouting (measured by summing the lengths of all sprouts from a given cell) remaining the same as that caused by a more distant axotomy[8,9] (FIG. 3). Thus close axotomy causes the neuron to lose its ability to funnel new growth specifically into the appropriate cellular location, and thus to lose an important aspect of its normal cellular polarity. The ectopically regenerating "dendritic" sprouts closely resemble axons in their gross morphology, ultrastructure and the paths that they follow within the brain[9,14] (FIG. 4), and orthotopic and ectopic sprouts cannot be distinguished form one another by these criteria. The phenomenon of axonal regeneration from the dendrites is accompanied by major cytoskeletal changes in the soma and dendrites, with elecron microscopy of the neurons giving rise to ectopic sprouts showing a dramatic loss of somatodendritic microtubules and corresponding increase in neurofilaments[14] (FIG. 7).

One advantage of using ectopic axonal regeneration from the dendrites as a model for axonal regeneration is that sprouting is occurring from uninjured processes, so that there is no confusion between local degenerative changes at the

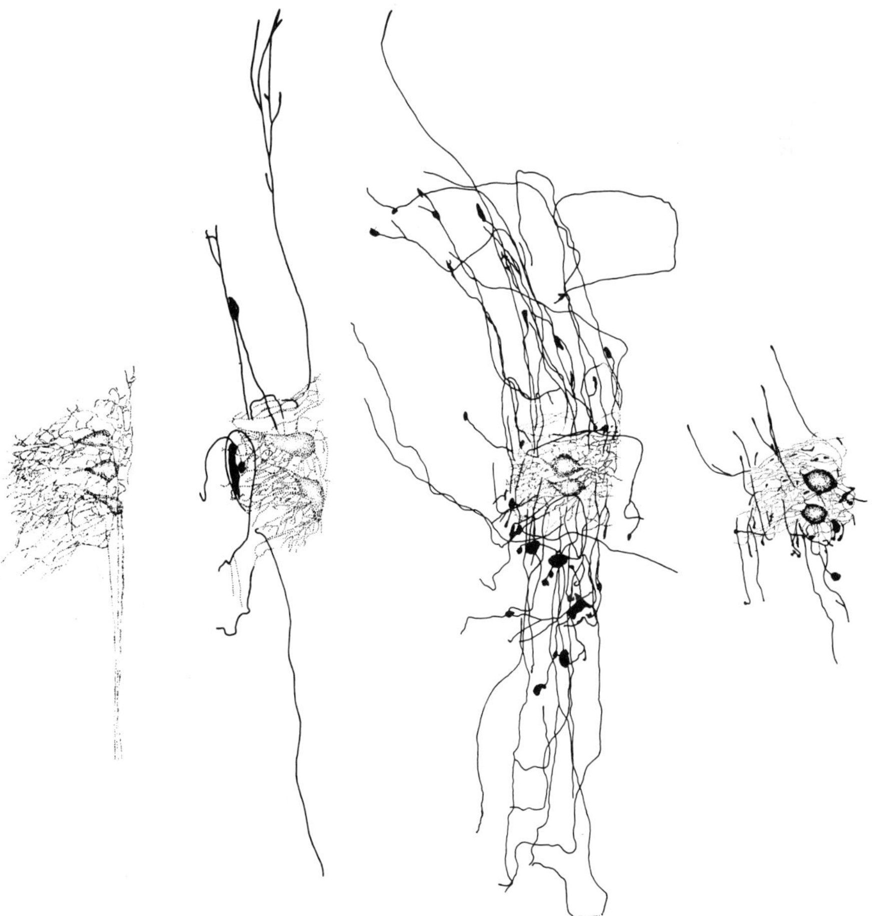

FIGURE 4. Tracings showing the time course of dendritic sprouting and retraction following close axotomy. Intact (*extreme left*) and axotomized ABCs at successively longer times after close axotomy (*left center*, 62 days; *right center*, 113 days; *extreme right*, 181 days). Processes in solid black are sprouts; stipple denotes dendritic tree and soma.

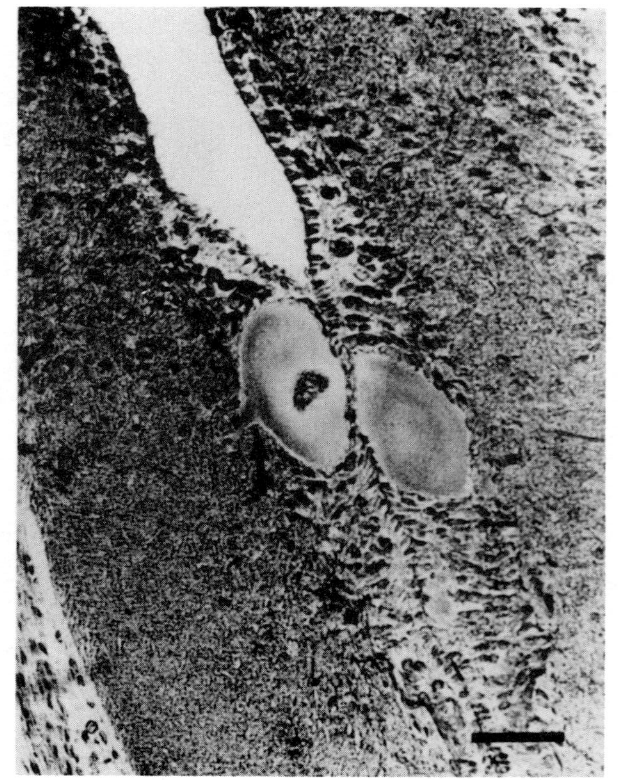

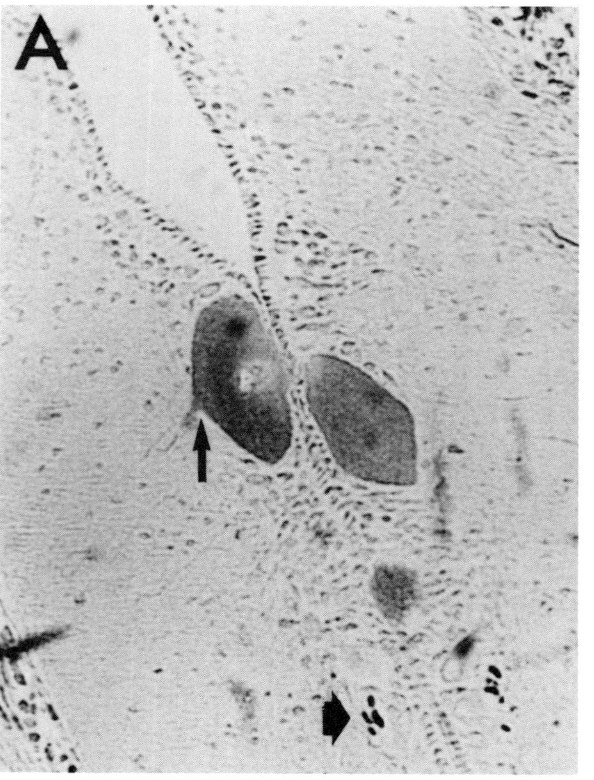

FIGURE 5. Somatodendritic cytoskeletal changes following distant axotomy. Adjacent sections through the soma and dendrites of a pair of ABCs 92 days following axotomy in the spinal cord at the level of the 5th gill (distant axotomy, see FIG. 1). **A** is stained for phosphorylated NFs with mAb RMO34, **B** is stained with mAb 6-11b (courtesy of Dr. Gianni Piperno), which recognized acetylated (stably polymerized) α tubulin. Note that while there has been a clear loss of MT staining and an invsion of phosphorylated NFs into the soma, especially in the perinuclear region, the proximal dendrite (*arrows,* both sections) retains stable MTs. Scale Bar = 100 μm.

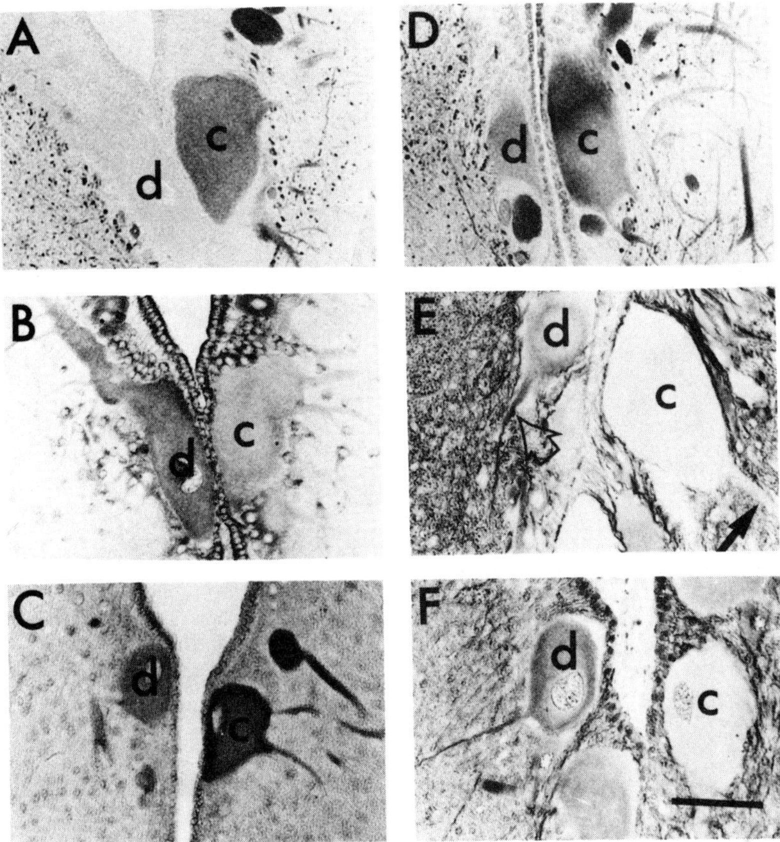

FIGURE 6. Comparison of the effects of close and distant axotomy. Sections through ABCs at various times following close axotomy of the ABC at right (marked c) and distant axotomy of the cell at left (marked d). **A, B:** adjacent sections through ABCs 14 days following lesioning, at the same time as the onset of dendritic sprouting following close axotomy. Section A is stained with the mAb RMO34, specific for highly phosphorylated NFs. Note that the soma of the distantly axotomized cell does not yet show staining while the ABC subjected to close axotomy is heavily stained. Section B is stained with RMd015, a mAb specific for nonphosphorylated NFs. Note the inverse pattern of staining when compared with RMO34. Panel **C** shows a section taken from a different lamprey 14 days post lesion and stained with RMO308, which recognizes a phosphorylation independent epitope on NFs. Note that by this time there is also more NF protein present in the soma and dendrites following close axotomy than there is following distant axotomy. **D:** Section taken 22 days post lesion and stained with the mAB RMO62, specific for phosphorylated NFs. Note that some staining has begun to appear in the distantly axotomized cell, but that it is not as intensively stained as following close axotomy. **E, F:** Sections taken from a brain 50 days post lesion, at a time when extensive dendritic sprouting is found following close axotomy. Section E is stained for acetylated (stably polymerized) tubulin, while F is stained for total alpha tubulin. Note that the loss of MTs following close axotomy is greater than the following distant axotomy, and that this loss extends into the dendrites (**E,** *solid arrow*) following close axotomy, but not following distant axotomy (**E,** *hollow arrow*). Scale Bar = 50 μm.

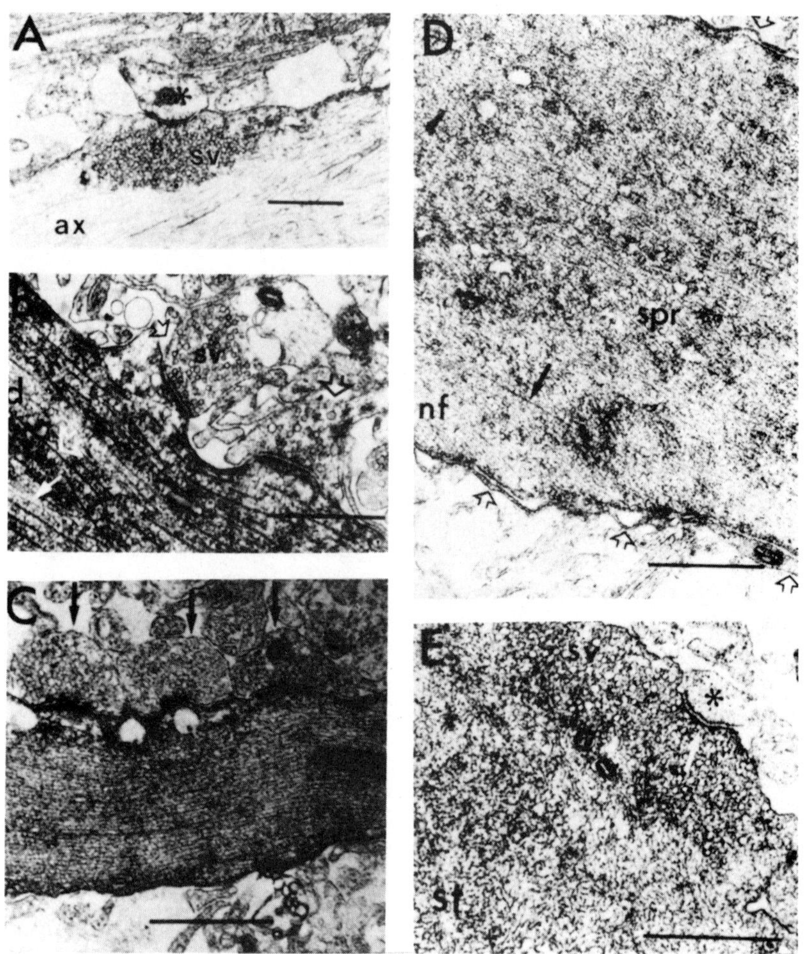

FIGURE 7. Effect of close axotomy on ABC ultrastructure. **A:** Normal axonal ultrastructure showing a cytoskeleton consisting mainly of NFs with relatively few MTs. The axon makes an *en passant* synapse onto an unidentified postsynaptic element in the caudal hindbrain. **B:** Normal dendritic ultrastructure of an intact ABC filled with horseradish peroxidase. The dendritic cytoskeleton consists mainly of MTs (open white arrow) and has relatively few NFs (solid white arrow). ABC dendrites are invariably postsynaptic to other cells. Open black arrows denote presynaptic terminals, SV: synaptic vesicles. **C:** Longitudinal section through an ABC dendrite (d) 57 days after close axotomy. Note that the cytoskeleton consists almost entirely of NFs aligned along the axis of the dendrite, while MTs are rare. Dendrites of axotomized ABCs remain postsynaptic to other neurons (*arrows*). **D:** Section taken from the shaft of a dendritic sprout. Note the NF dominated cytoskeleton and the presence of cellular elements wrapping the sprout. (*hollow arrows*). Occasional MTs (*solid arrow*) can also be seen. **E:** Section through a swollen sprout tip (st) showing a synapse in which the sprout contains synaptic vesicles (sv) and is the presynaptic element. The postsynaptic element (*asterisk*) is unidentified. Note that the NFs appear swirled and disorganized when compared to those in the sprout shaft (**D**). All Scale Bars = 1 μm.

lesion site and the first signs of regeneration. Consequently, the time at which regeneration begins is better defined for ectopic sprouting than it is for orthotopic regeneration in this system. That said, the times of onset of axonal sprouting following close and distant axotomy appear to be roughly similar; the very first signs of both orthotopic and ectopic sprouting are seen in a few cells by one week or so post axotomy and most cells exhibit regenerating sprouts by 2 to 3 weeks.[8,9,21] However, if ABCs are first subjected to distant axotomy in the spinal cord 30 days prior to close axotomy, the onset of ectopic sprouting is accelerated, with dendritic sprouts seen in most cells within the first few days of close axotomy.[9] This suggests that while the cellular mechanisms underlying axonal regeneration require 1 to 2 weeks to be activated following axotomy, the loss of normal polarity is much more rapid and can occur within a few days of close axotomy.

The effect of dendritic amputation (dendrotomy) on the pattern of ectopic axonal regeneration in axotomized ABCs gives some further hints as to the nature of the factors that control the polarity of regeneration following axotomy. If the lateral dendrites of otherwise intact ABCs are amputated by a longitudinal scalpel lesion in the hindbrain, no obvious gross morphological changes occur in the dendrites between 20 and 120 days post lesion. However, if ABCs that have previously been subjected to distant axotomy are subjected to dendrotomy, some sprouting occurs from the site of the dendritic lesion by 20 days post dendrotomy.[10] Furthermore, the distribution of sprouting following close axotomy can also be altered by dendrotomy, which again results in sprouting occurring preferentially from lesioned dendrites. These results emphasize the importance of the proximity of the lesion site as a determinant of the cellular location of axonal regeneration, and are consistent with a major role for localized Ca++ influx in initiating sprouting.

Cytoskeletal Changes Preceding Dendritic Sprouting following Close Axotomy

The mechanism of polarity loss following close axotomy in ABCs has been the focus of a series of experiments that I have recently undertaken in collaboration with Dr. Ken Kosik. We have focused our attention on the nature and time course of cytoskeletal changes that occur before and during the onset of ectopic axonal regeneration following close axotomy. Our rationale has been that since ectopic axonal regeneration is accompanied by major cytoskeletal rearrangements in the dendrites of affected cells by 8 to 10 weeks after the onset of sprouting[14] (FIG. 7), such changes might be intimately related to a loss of dendritic identity following close axotomy and thus might precede sprouting and play a causal role in the loss of normal polarity.

We used immunocytochemical analysis of Bouins fixed serial sections through the somata and dendrites of ABCs at early times following unilateral close axotomy to assess the effects of close axotomy on the distribution and modifications of MTs and NFs in axotomized ABCs in comparison to contralateral controls[16] (FIG. 8). A panel of monoclonal antibodies that recognize total alpha tubulin, stably polymerized (acetylated) tubulin and labile microtubules or unpolymerized (tyrosinated) tubulin were used to assess the effects of close axotomy on the distribution and polymerization state of microtubules. We also used four mABs recognizing various phosphorylation states of lamprey neurofilament protein which were provided by Dr. Virginia Lee, who was also a collaborator on the project. Lampreys have only one NF subunit, as opposed to the three found in most mammalian NFs, and the lamprey NF protein possesses characteristics of all three mammalian

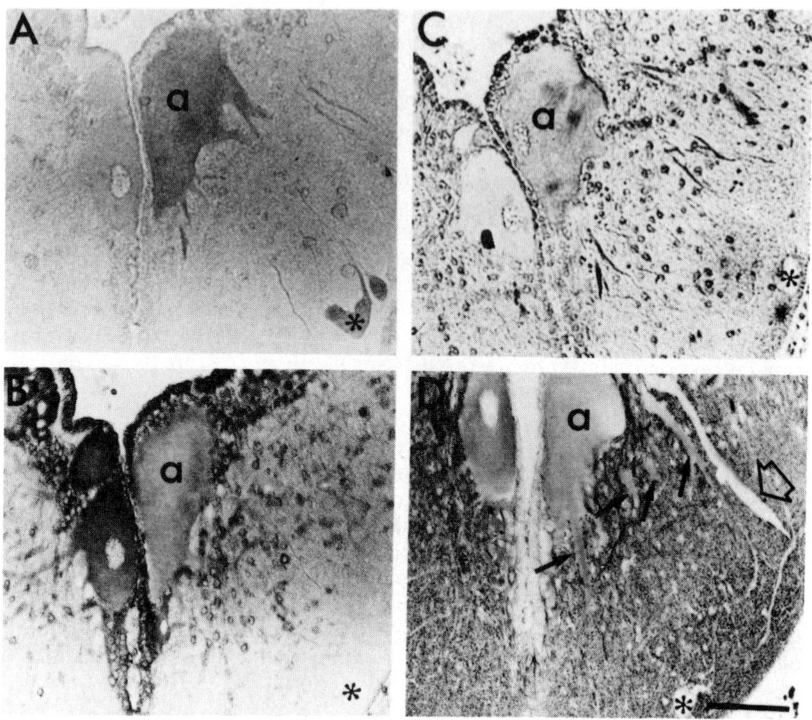

FIGURE 8. Cytoskeletal changes accompanying dendritic sprouting following close axotomy (**A–D**) Sections showing ABC somata and dendrites following close axotomy of cells on the right (a) 16 days previously. The cells on the left (c) were left intact to serve as controls. Axotomized ABCs give rise to dendritic sprouts (asterisks). Sections were stained for (**A**) highly phosphorylated NFs (RMO34), (**B**) non-phosphorylated NFs (RMd015), (**C**) tyrosinated (labile) MTs (TUB-1) and (**D**) acetylated (stably polymerized) tubulin (6-11b). Sections A–C are adjacent sections taken of a single pair of ABCs, section D is from a different lamprey. All of the sprouts indicated by asterisks arise from the dendrites of the cells shown (*arrows*); in D the course of the dendrite is traced (*long, narrow arrows*) with the missing portions of its trajectory present in adjacent sections. The sprout stains more intensely for phosphorylated NFs and less intensely for non-phosphorylated NFs and tyrosinated tubulin than the soma and dendrites of the parent ABC. (**D**) Overall staining for stably polymerized MTs in the axotomized cell is slightly reduced relative to control levels, and a swollen dendrite (*broad arrow*) is nearly devoid of MT staining along its entire length. Other primary dendrites (*arrows*) of the axotomized cell resemble the control cell. A dendritic sprout tip (*asterisk*) arising from an adjacent dendrite (*long narrow arrows*) is also devoid of staining. The dendrite lacking staining (*hollow arrow*) does not taper normally as do nearby dendrites (*solid arrows*), but shows a pronounced swelling, a preliminary to dendritic sprouting. Scale bars = 50 μm.

NF subunits.[27] The anti-NF antibodies (RMO34, RMO62, RMdO15 and RMO308) have all been extensively characterized by Dr. Lee and her colleagues in both lamprey and mammals, and have been shown to specifically recognize heavily phosphorylated, moderately phosphorylated, dephosphorylated and phosphorylation independent sites respectively on the carboxyl terminus sidearm domains of mammalian NF-H[28] and the lamprey NF protein.[27]

We found that close axotomy results in rapid changes from the normal staining patterns of each of these mAbs in the somata and dendrites of ABCs and Mauthner cells. Close axotomy induces a dramatic increase in staining for phosphorylated NFs and a decrease in staining for nonphosphorylated NFs by 6 days post axotomy in virtually all cells examined. This is accompanied by an increase in staining for tyrosinated tubulin. By the time ectopic axonal regeneration from the dendrites begins, the staining for total NF protein in the soma and dendrites is increased and staining for acetylated (stably polymerized) tubulin has decreased somewhat in most ABCs, with the most dramatic decreases seen in those dendrites that are giving rise to ectopic sprouts (FIG. 8). These observations suggest that close axotomy results in two events that might be mechanistically linked to the loss of normal polarity following close axotomy: 1) the destabilization of dendritic MTs and 2) the phosphorylation of dendritic NFs. Furthermore, a comparison of the effects of close and distant axotomy shows that while both NF phosphorylation and MT destabilization in ABC dendrites precede ectopic sprouting following close axotomy, neither appears to occur before the onset of orthotopic regeneration following distant axotomy, and extensive MT destabilization (as measured by a complete loss of staining for acetylated tubulin) does not occur in the dendrites even at late times (92 days) post axotomy[15] (FIGS. 5 and 6).

We then chose to utilize the unusual experimental accessibility of the lamprey CNS to manipulate NF phosphorylation directly by microinjecting individual ABCs and MCs *in situ* with specifically acting agents. We found that specific inhibitors and activators of Protein Kinase C (PKC) were able to block somatodendritic NF phosphorylation induced by close axotomy and artificially induce NF phosphorylation in intact cells respectively (FIG. 9, TABLES 1 and 2). The phosphatase inhibitor okadaic acid also proved to be an effective inducer of NF phosphorylation in intact cells. An interesting feature of these results is that the effects of these agents took several days to develop and were long lasting, with a time course mimicking that of NF phosphorylation following close axotomy.[17] This suggests an indirect "triggering" role for PKC in the mechanism of NF phosphorylation following axotomy, especially as the agents used to induce NF phosphorylation in this study (di(octanoyl)glycerol and okadaic acid) are known to leave cells within minutes or hours of administration in other systems.[29]

In summary, giant reticulospinal neurons in the lamprey CNS respond to axotomy with a variety of morphological and physiological changes beginning with a localized (and possibly general) increase in intracellular Ca++, up-regulation of a PKC-like activity in the soma and dendrites resulting in NF phosphorylation, chromatolysis and axonal regeneration. If the site of axotomy is sufficiently close to the soma, these responses are accompanied by an invasion of the soma and dendrites by phosphorylated NFs, a destabilization of dendritic MTs and ectopic axonal regeneration from the dendrites. Beginning at 2 to 3 months following either close or distant axotomy, degenerative changes begin to occur in most cells; these include a retraction and thinning of the dendritic tree with the outright loss of many higher order dendrites, a partial loss of presynaptic contacts, and the eventual reteraction of both ectopic and orthotopically regenerating axonal sprouts. Some loss of microtubules and increase in NFs in the soma and dendrites appear to be permanent consequences of axotomy even after distant axotomy; these changes are far more marked following close axotomy, which eventually causes the loss of most somatodendritic microtubules and their replacement with phosphorylated NFs.

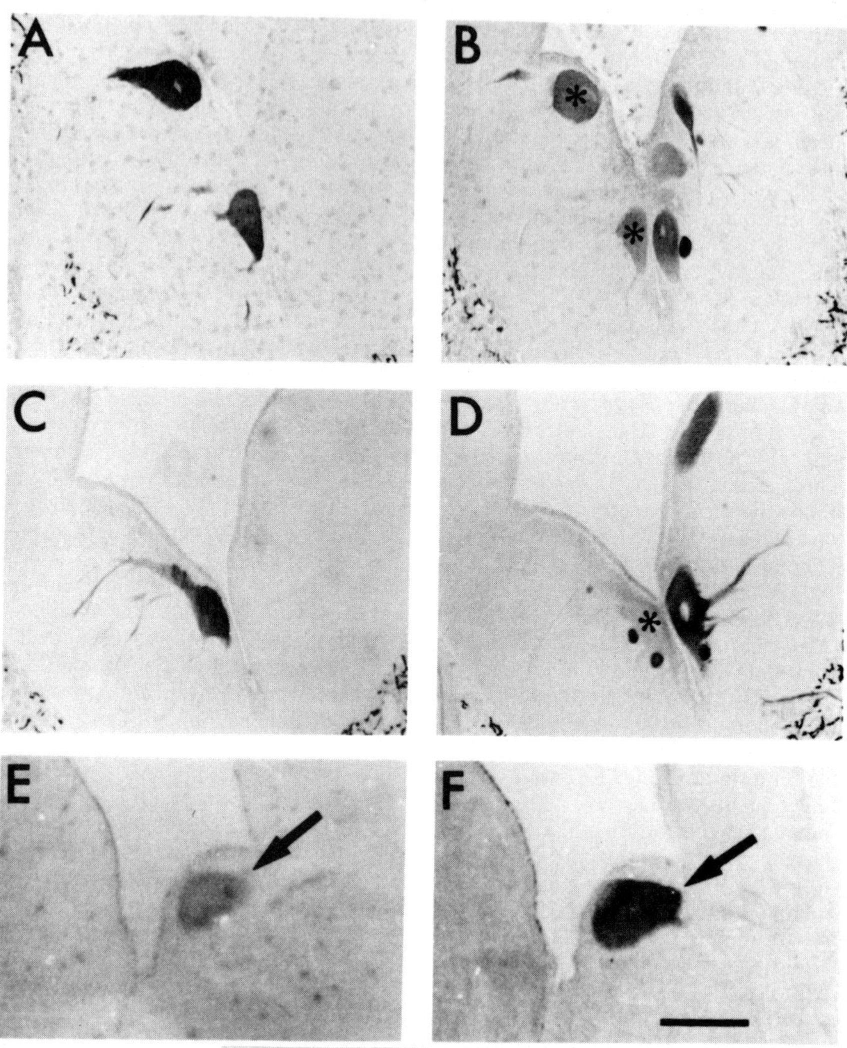

FIGURE 9. Effects of microinjecting PKC specific inhibitory peptides, control peptides, and okadaic acid into ABCs and MCs. **A–D:** ABCs and MCs were injected with 0.5 mM protein kinase C pseudosubstrate inhibitory peptide (panels C and D), or an inactive analog of this peptide at the same concentration (panels A and B) and subjected to close axotomy. Serial transverse sections through the hindbrain were taken 6 days post axotomy. Sections in panels A and C were stained for rabbit IgG (coinjected with the peptides) to identify the injected cells. Adjacent sections (panels B and D) were stained with the antiphosphorylated NF mAbs RMO62 (B) or RMO34 (D). Note that in D, the injected cell (asterisk) stain much more lightly for somadendritic phosphorylated NFs than do uninjected cells in the same sections, while the inactive analogue has no effect (B). **E–F:** Intact ABCs and MCs were injected with the serine/threonine phosphatase inhibitor okadaic acid at 150 μM in the electrode tip and examined 6 days later. Panel E was stained for rabbit IgG to identify the injected cell (*arrow*). An adjacent section (F) was stained with RMO34. Note that staining for phosphorylated NFs is prominent by 6 days post injection. Scale bar = 100 μm.

TABLE 1. Effects of PKC Inhibitors on Axotomy-induced Somatodendritic NF Phosphorylation

		Days Post Axotomy	Injected Cell[a] Clearly Weaker than Uninjected Cells	Injected Cell within Range of Uninjected Cells	Injected Cell Clearly Stronger than Uninjected Cells	Statistical Significance (Chi-square Test)
Agents Injected at Time of Close Axotomy			$-$	$\pm$	$+$	
Second messenger–activated kinase inhibitors	Sphingosine (1 mM)	6	6	3	0	$p < 0.05$
	K252a (10 μM)	6	8	6	1	$p \approx 0.1$
PKC-specific inhibitory peptides	19-36 peptide (500 μM)	6	17	8	0	$p < 0.005$
	19-36 peptide (500 μM)	15	8	3	0	$p < 0.05$
	EGF peptide (1 mM)	6	9	1	0	$p < 0.005$
Controls	IgG alone	6	5	15	2	All $p > 0.95$[b]
	19-36 control (500 μM)	6	12	26	3	vs. other
	19-36 control (500 μM)	15	4	12	1	controls
Unbiased distribution (vs. controls)[c]			13	53	13	$0.8 > p > 0.2$

PKC, protein kinase C; 19-36 peptide, PKC pseudosubstrate peptide inhibitor; 19-36 control; inactivated pseudosubstrate peptide analog, EGF peptide, epidermal growth factor receptor substrate sequence for PKC (another specific PKC inhibitor). Concentrations in parentheses are concentrations in the electrode tip. a: cell/cell comparisons are within the same brain section; b: compared in a 3 × 3 chi square analysis; c: expected distribution if no artifacts induced by injection of control substances are present.

TABLE 2. Effects of DiC8 and Okadaic Acid on Intact Neurons

		Days Post Injection	No Staining Above Background Staining of Uninjected Cells	Clear Staining Above Background	Statistical Significance (Chi-square Test)[b]
			±	+	
Agents Injected into Intact Neurons					
Diacylglycerol (DiC8)	1 mM	3	17	4	$0.8 > p > 0.2$
		6	12	6	$p < 0.05$
		15	6	5	$p < 0.01$
Okadaic Acid	10 μM	6	6	4	$p < 0.05$
	50 μM		3	5	$p < 0.005$
	150 μM		0	6	$p < 0.005$
	150 μM	3	5	5	All $p < 0.005$ vs.
		6	0	6	controls, $p < 0.005$
		9	1	6	3 days vs. 6–9 days[c]
Controls	IgG alone	6	15	1	All $p \approx 0.9$
	DMSO		7	0	vs. other
	Racemized DiC8[a]		5	1	controls

DMSO, dimethylsulfoxide; DiC8, di(octoyl)glycerol; a: stock solution allowed to stand at 4 degrees C for 24 h before use; b: compared in a 2×3 chi square analysis; c: compared in a 2×3 chi square anlaysis after 6 and 9 day data were combined.

DISCUSSION OF THE RESPONSE OF LAMPREY
CENTRAL NEURONS TO INJURY IN THE CONTEXT
OF THE INJURY AND DISEASE LITERATURE
OF THE MAMMALIAN CNS

The array of responses of lamprey central neurons to mechanical injury described above demonstrates that axotomy activates or alters fundamental cellular mechanisms vital for axonal regeneration and the maintenance of normal cellular polarity and perhaps (ultimately) cellular viability. These findings suggest that the lamprey CNS, with its multiple technical advantages, might be a suitable system for the investigation of the cellular mechanisms underlying the response to various types of injury in identified vertebrate central neurons *in situ*. However, before one can adopt the lamprey CNS as an *in situ* model for neuronal injury and neurotoxic disease states as they occur in less accessible mammalian systems, one must ask whether the responses to injury seen in lamprey neurons are comparable to and congruent with those seen in other vertebrate systems. The degree to which such a congruence exists is discussed below.

Axotomy of mammalian central neurons initially results in many cellular changes similar to those seen in the lamprey. As in the lamprey, axotomy typically induces localized changes in intracellular Ca++ levels,[30] phosphorylation of somatodendritic NFs[31] and chromatolysis[32] during the first few days post axotomy. These similarities are particularly evident in large neurons[31] and are more pronounced and occur sooner if the site of axotomy is close to the soma. Furthermore, many of the degenerative changes that occur at late times post axotomy in lamprey ABCs and MCs have also been well studied and documented in various vertebrate systems. Axotomy of frog spinal[33] and rat hypoglossal[34] motoneurons results in dendritic retraction by several weeks post axotomy which is characterized by a shrinkage of the dendritic field and the thinning and loss of higher order dendrites very similar to that seen in lamprey ABCs. In many cases[35] this retraction is accompanied by a loss of presynaptic contacts, again similar to the lamprey. It has also been shown that many of these "retrograde" degenerative effects of axotomy can be reversed by reestablishing postsynaptic contacts;[34] whether this is also true in lamprey is not yet known.

One major point of difference between the response of lamprey and mammalian central neurons to axotomy is the ability (lacking in mammals) of lamprey neurons to sprout vigorously and at least partially regenerate their axons. However, in the last few years it has been shown that mature mammalian central neurons do have an intrinsic ability to regenerate their axons when environmental factors hostile to axonal regeneration that are normally present in the mammalian CNS are either neutralized[36] or replaced with a favorable environment.[37] Thus the intrinsic regenerative abilities of mammalian central neurons appear to be no different from those of mammalian peripheral neurons and peripheral and central neurons in lower vertebrates.

Another (apparently) distinctive feature of axonal regeneration in the lamprey is the predominance of phosphorylated NFs and the paucity of other cytoskeletal elements in the growing axonal tips[14] (FIGS. 7 and 8). This cytoskeletal structure is quite unlike that seen in "classic" growth cones found on growing neurites in cell culture and in developing nervous systems, which consist primarily of actin filaments, microtubules and their associated proteins. It has been traditionally assumed that NFs play a relatively minor role in neurite outgrowth during development, although some recent studies have indicated that NFs are essential for process outgrowth under certian circumstances.[38,39] It should be noted that little is known about the ultrastructure of the growing tips of regenerating axons in the CNS (as distinct from developing axons or regenerating axons in the PNS) in the mammalian CNS owing to the lack of most central regeneration in mammals discussed above and the difficulty of unambiguously identifying actively growing tips from cut axons. An ultrastructural study of regenerating axons in the optic tract of the goldfish[40] has suggested that NFs are prominent in regenerating sprouts even at the earliest times post axotomy, and reported that they have a "swirled" appearance that closely resembled that seen in lesioned ABC axons at the lesion site.[21] However, it still cannot be definitively established whether this observation, like those in many previous studies reflects axotomy-induced alterations to the cytoskeleton existing prior to the lesion, the presence of new growth, or a mixture of the two. The phenomenon of ectopic axonal regeneration in lamprey ABCs allows one to see that phosphorylated NFs play a prominent role in the first new growth of regenerating large axons; it remains to be seen whether they are functionally important to sprout growth in the lamprey, and if so, if they play similar roles in the regenerating CNS of other vertebrate systems. The paths followed by both orthotopically and ectopically regenerating sprouts in the lamprey do resemble those seen in the development and regeneration of other vertebrate central neurons; they follow general axial guidance cues in both the brain and spinal cord[6,41] similar to those thought to guide developing spinal axons in a variety of other lower vertebrates.[42,43]

Finally, one must consider whether the loss of polarity that accompanies axotomy close to the soma in the giant neurons of the lamprey CNS is an idiosyncratic quirk of this system or if it reflects some general principle of process regeneration in vertebrates. There have been a number of reports of ectopic axonal regeneration following axotomy in various invertebrate systems over the past 15 years.[44–46] In each of these cases, either the distance of the lesion site from the soma or the presence or length of a proximal axon stump determined if a loss of polarity would occur. One instance of ectopic axonal regeneration following close axotomy has been reported in mammals,[47] where multiple myelinated sprouts were observed emerging from the dendrites of cat spinal motoneurons following ventral rhizotomy. The tendency of many vertebrate central neurons to die following axotomy close to the soma and the general inability of mammalian central neurons to regenerate their axons at all following axotomy may have prevented the widespread observation of polarity loss following close axotomy in the mammalian CNS. In addition, since axotomy generally must occur very close to the soma (within several hundred microns) to elicit the loss of neuronal polarity, most neurons in the mammalian CNS are relatively inaccessible to experimental lesions that might provoke ectopic axonal regeneration. However, it has been shown that traumatic injury to the head frequently results in the axotomy of central neurons in humans;[48] head trauma has also been implicated in the development of neurofibrillary tangles (NFTs) and the loss of polarity in some neurons similar to that seen in AD.[49] It is thus possible that the loss of polarity following close axotomy is fairly widespread among vertebrates and that the cellular mechanisms underlying this phenomenon have general significance in establishing and maintaining dendritic and axonal identity.

In summary, although a great deal remains to be learned about the cellular response to axotomy and axonal development and regeneration in the lamprey, what is known suggests that the cellular response of giant lamprey central neurons to axotomy is probably fairly typical of vertebrates in general.

The Response to Axotomy of Lamprey Central Neurons as a Model for Other Types of Neuronal Injury and the Cellular Pathology of Neurodegenerative Diseases

One of the main themes of this meeting has been the commonality of many of the cellular mechanisms underlying the effects of injury and various degenerative diseases on vertebrate neurons. Although each of these pathological conditions has some distinctive features, the broad overlap between the various cellular events that follow the onset of these conditions is striking. Ischemia, excitotoxic and mechanical injury (*i.e.* axotomy) all result in an initial perturbation of intracellular Ca++ levels and a consequent activation of protein kinases, as does administration of beta amyloid.[30,50–51] Recent evidence also suggests that a cellular inability to control CNS glutamate levels (presumably resulting in excitotoxic neuronal injury) may underlie the neurodegenerative pathology of ALS.[52] The phosphorylation of cytoskeletal proteins (particularly neurofilament and tau proteins) is a prominent feature in all of these conditions and is probably a consequence of this initial Ca++ perturbation. The phosphorylation of these proteins in turn appears to have major functional effects, influencing their intracellular distribution, transport and binding characteristic vis-à-vis other proteins.[53–55] Aspects of normal cellular polarity are also lost in most neurodegenerative conditions, with changes in the distribution of tau and/or NFs being hallmarks of ALS, AD and neurodegeneration following ischemic and traumatic injuries.[52,56–58] These changes are often manifested by the accumulation of neurofibrillary tangles (consisting of abnormally phosphorylated tau and (possibly) NFs in the somata and dendrites of affected cells),[59,60] In AD and in some cases of traumatic injury,[49,59] this is accompanied by a loss of somatodendritic MTs and aberrant sprouting of axonlike processes from the dendrites that resembles the dendritic sprouting of lamprey giant neurons following close axotomy.

The common features of neuronal responses to various types of injury and the cellular pathology of neurodegenerative diseases suggest the tantalizing possibility that they are all manifestations of a generalized cellular mechanism set in motion by various types of injury or stress. One of the most challenging aspects of elucidating the roles that these common pathological elements might play in such a mechanism is the difficulty of determining whether causal relationships exist between them as they occur *in situ*. This is exacerbated by the variability and widespread nature of these pathological features, which suggests that they may be induced or influenced by a complex interplay of both cell intrinsic and environmental changes caused by injury and/or disease. It seems to me that the technical advantages of the lamprey CNS afford a unique opportunity to directly test *in situ* the nature of relationships between apparently important cellular events (increases in intracellular Ca++, phosphorylation of somatodendritic NFs, loss of neuronal polarity, etc.) on a single cell basis, and thus determine whether, to what extent and how the pathological mechanisms of neurodegenerative conditions and the effects of neuronal injury are interrelated.

REFERENCES

1. ROVAINEN, C. M. 1976. Regeneration of Muller and Mauthner axons after spinal transection in larval lampreys. J. Comp. Neurol. **168:** 545–554.
2. SELZER, M. E. 1978. Mechanism of functional recovery and regeneration after spinal cord transection in the larval sea lamprey. J. Physiol. (Lond.) **277:** 395–408.

3. WOOD, M. R. & M. J. COHEN. 1981. Synaptic regeneration and glial reactions in the transected spinal cord of the lamprey. J. Neurocytol. **10:** 57–79.
4. YIN, H-S. & M. E. SELZER. 1983. Axonal regeneration in the lamprey spinal cord. J. Neurosci. **3:** 1135–1144.
5. YIN, H.-S., S. A. MACKLER & M. E. SELZER. 1984. Directional specificity in the regeneration of lamprey spinal axons. Science **224:** 894–896.
6. MACKLER, S. A. & M. E. SELZER. 1985. Regeneration of functional synapses between individual recognizable neurons in the lamprey spinal cord. Science **229:** 774–776.
7. MACKLER, S. A., H-S. YIN & M. E. SELZER. 1986. Determinants of directional specificity in the regeneration of lamprey central neurons. J. Neurosci. **6:** 1814–1821.
8. HALL, G. F. & M. J. COHEN. 1983. Extensive dendritic sprouting induced by close axotomy of central neurons in the lamprey. Science **222:** 518–521.
9. HALL, G. F. & M. J. COHEN. 1988a. The pattern of dendritic sprouting and retraction induced by axotomy of lamprey central neurons. J. Neurosci. **8**(10): 3584–3597.
10. HALL, G. F. & M. J. COHEN. 1988b. Dendritic amputation redistributes sprouting evoked by axotomy in lamprey central neurons. J. Neurosci. **8**(10): 3598–3606.
11. BORGENS, R. B., L. F. JAFFE & M. J. COHEN. 1980. Large and persistent electrical currents enter the transected lamprey spinal cord. Proc. Natl. Acad. Sci. USA **77:** 1209–1213.
12. ROEDERER, E. N. H. GOLDBERG & M. J. COHEN. 1983. Modification of retrograde degeneration in transected spinal axons of the lamprey by applied DC current. J. Neurosci. **3:** 153–160.
13. MacVICAR, B. A. & R. R. LLINAS. 1985. Barium action potentials in regenerating axons of the lamprey spinal cord. J. Neurosci. Res. **13:** 323–335.
14. HALL, G. F., A. POULOS & M. J. COHEN. 1989. Sprouts emerging from the dendrites of axotomized lamprey central neurons have axonlike ultrastructure. J. Neurosci. **9:** 588–599.
15. HALL, G. F., V. M-Y. LEE & K. S. KOSIK. 1990. Major cytoskeletal changes precede dendritic sprouting following close axotomy of lamprey giant central neurons. Soc. Neurosci. Abst. Vol. 10.
16. HALL, G. F., V. M-Y. LEE & K. S. KOSIK. 1991. Microtubule destabilization and neurofilament phosphorylation precede dendritic sprouting after close axotomy of lamprey central neurons. Proc. Natl. Acad. Sci. USA **88:** 5016–5020.
17. HALL, G. F. & K. S. KOSIK. 1993. Axotomy induced neurofilament phosphorylation can be blocked in situ by microinjection of protein kinase A and C inhibitors into identified lamprey neurons. Neuron. In press.
18. STRAUTMAN, A. F., R. J. CORK & K. R. ROBINSON. 1990. The distribution of free calcium in transected spinal axons and its modulation by applied electric fields. J. Neurosci. **10:** 3564–3575.
19. SCHULTZ, R., E. C. BERKOWITZ & D. C. PEARSE. 1956. The electron microscopy of the lamprey spinal cord. J. Morphol. **98:** 251–273.
20. HALL, G. F. & V. M-Y. LEE. 1992. High neurofilament packing density in lesioned giant lamprey axons is correlated with neurofilament sidearm proteolysis. Soc. Neurosci. Abst. Vol. 12.
21. McHALE, M. K. & M. J. COHEN. 1983. Ultrastructure of regenerating giant axons in the lamprey CNS. Soc. Neurosci.
22. BORGENS, R. B. E. ROEDERER & M. J. COHEN. 1981. Enhanced spinal cord regeneration in lamprey by applied electric fields. J. Neurosci. **213:** 611–617.
23. SCHLAEPFER, W. W. 1987. Neurofilaments: Structure, Metabolism and implications in disease. J. Neuropathol. Exp. Neurol. **46:** 117–129.
24. HOLLIDAY, J., R. J. ADAMS, T. J. SEJNOWSKI & N. C. SPITZER. 1991. Calcium induced release of calcium regulates differentiation of cultured spinal neurons. Neuron **7:** 787–796.
25. FISHMAN, P. S. 1975. A study of dendritic form in identified lamprey neurons. PhD dissertation, Yale University.
26. HALL, G. F. 1985. Morphological plasticity of lamprey central neurons evoked by axonal and dendritic injury. PhD dissertation, Yale University.

27. PLEASURE, S. J., M. E. SELZER & V. M-Y. LEE. 1988. Lamprey neurofilaments combine in one subunit the features of each mammalian neurofilament protein, but are highly phosphorylated only in large axons. J. Neurosci. 9(2): 698–709.

28. LEE, V. M-Y., M. J. CARDEN & J. Q. TROJANOWSKI. 1986. Novel monoclonal antibodies provide evidence for the in situ existence of a nonphosphorylated form of the largest neurofilament subunit. J. Neurosci. 6: 850–858.

29. KLUMPP, S., P. COHEN & J. SCHULTZ. 1990. Okadaic acid, an inhibitor of protein phosphatase 1 in *Paramecium*, causes sustained Ca++ dependent backward swimming in response to depolarizing stimuli. EMBO J. 9: 685–689.

30. MATTSON, M. P., M. MURAIN & P. B. GUTHRIE. 1990. Localized calcium influx orients axon formation in embryonic hippocampal pyramidal neurons. Dev. Brain Res. 52 201–209.

31. GOLDSTEIN, M. E., H. S. COOPER, J. BRUCE, M. J. CARDEN, V. M-Y. LEE & W. W. SCHLAEPFER. 1987. Phosphorylation of neurofilament proteins and chromatolysis following transection of rat sciatic nerve. J. Neurosci. 7(5): 1586–1594.

32. LIEBERMAN, A. R. 1971. The axon reaction: A review of the principal features of perikaryal responses to axon injury. Int. Rev. Neurobiol. 14: 49–124.

33. CERF, J. A. & L. W. CHACKO. 1958. Retrograde reaction in motoneuron dendrites following ventral root section in the frog. J. Comp. Neurol. 109: 205–216.

34. SUMNER, B. E. H. & W. E. WATSON. 1971. Retraction and expansion of the dendritic tree of motor neurons of adult rat induced in vivo. Nature 233: 273–275.

35. KERNS, J. M. & E. J. HINSMAN. 1973. Neuroglial response to sciatic neurectomy. 2: electron microscopy. J. Comp. Neurol. 151:255–280.

37. DAVID, S. & A. J. AGUAYO. 1981. Axonal elongation into peripheral nervous system bridges after central nervous system injury in adult rats. Science 214: 931–933.

36. SCHNELL, L. & M. E. SCHWAB. 1990. Axonal regeneration in the rat spinal cord produced by an antibody against myelin-associated neurite growth inhibitors. Nature 343: 269–272.

38. SZARO, B. G., P. GRANT, V. M-Y. LEE & H. GAINER. 1991. Inhibition of axonal development after injection of neurofilament antibodies into a *Xenopus laevis* embryo. J. Comp. Neurol. 308: 576–585.

39. SHEA, T. B., M. L. BEERMAN & R. A. NIXON. 1991. Sequential requirement for cytoskeletal constituents during axonal initiation, elongation and stabilization. J. Cell Biol. 115 3(2): 163a.

40. LANNERS, H. N. & B. GRAFSTEIN. 1980. Early stages of axonal regeneration in the goldfish optic tract: An electron microscopic study. J. Neurocytol. 9: 733–751.

41. COHEN, M. J. & G. F. HALL. 1986. The control of neuron shape during development and regeneration. Neurochem. Pathol. 5: 331–343.

42. CONSTANTINE-PATON, M. & R. CAPRANICA. 1976. Axonal guidance of developing optic nerves in the frog. J. Comp. Neurol. 170: 17–32.

43. NORDLANDER, R. H. & M. SINGER. 1982. Morphology and position of growth cones in the developing *Xenopus* spinal cord. Dev. Brain Res. 4: 181–193.

44. MURPHY, A. D. & S. B. KATER. 1980. Sprouting and functional regeneration of an identified neuron in Helisoma. Brain Res. 186: 251–272.

45. ROEDERER, E. & M. J. COHEN. 1983. Regeneration of an identified neuron in the cricket: Control of sprouting from dendrites, soma and axon. J. Neurosci. 3: 1835–1847.

46. SCHACHER, S. & E. PROSHANSKY. 1983. Neurite regeneration by aplysia neurons in dissociated tissue culture: Modulation by hemolymph and the presence of the initial axon segment. J. Neurosci. 3: 2403–2413.

47. LINDA, H., M. RISLING & S. CULLHEIM. 1985. "Dendraxons" in regenerating motoneurons in the cat: Do dendrites grow new axons after central axotomy? Brain Res. 358: 329–333.

48. STRICH, S. B. 1961. Shearing of nerve fibres as a cause of brain damage due to head injury. The Lancet (26 Aug): 443–448.

49. TOKUDA, T., S. IKEDA, N. YANAGISAWA, Y. IHARA & G. G. GLENNER. 1991. Re-examination of ex-boxers brains using immunohistochemistry with antibodies to amyloid beta-protein and tau protein. Acta Neuropathol. 82; 280–285.

50. MATTSON, M. P. 1991. Evidence for the involvement of protein kinase C in neurodegenerative changes in cultured human cortical neurons. Exp. Neurol. **112:** 95–103.
51. KOWALL, N. W., M. F. BEAL, J. BUSCIGLIO, L. K. DUFFY & B. A. YANKNER. 1991. An in vivo model for the neurodegenerative effect of beta amyloid and protection by substance P. Proc. Natl. Acad. Sci. USA **88:** 7247–7251.
52. ROTHSTEIN, J. D., L. J. MARTIN & R. W. KUNCL. 1992. Decreased glutamate transport by the brain and spinal cord in amyotrophic lateral sclerosis. N. Engl. J. Med. **326:** 1464–1468.
53. NIXON, R. A. & R. K. SIHAG. 1991. Neurofilament phosphorylation: A new look at regulation and function. TINS **14**(11): 501–505.
54. OLMSTED, J. B. 1986. Microtubule associated proteins. Ann. Rev. Cell Biol. **2:** 421–457.
55. LETERRIER, J.-F., J. WONG, R. K. H. LIEM & M. L. SHELANSKI. 1984. Promotion of microtubule assembly by neurofilament associated microtubule associated proteins. J. Neurochem. **43:** 1385–1391.
56. CORSELLIS, J. C. J. BRUTON & D. FREEMAN-BROWNE. 1973. The aftermath of boxing. Psychol. Med. **3:** 270–303.
57. KATO, T., A. HIRANO, T. KATAGIRI, H. SASAKI & S. YAMADA. 1988. Neurofibrillary tangle formation in the nucleus basillis of Meynert ipsilateral to a massive cerebral infarct. Ann. Neurol. **23:** 620–623.
58. GREENMAYRE, J. T. & A. YOUNG. 1989. Excitatory amino acids and Alzheimer's disease. Neurobiol. Aging **10:** 593–602.
59. KOWALL, N. W. & K. S. KOSIK. 1987. Axonal disruption and aberrant localization of tau protein characterize the neuropil pathology of Alzheimer's disease. Ann Neurol. **22:** 639–643.
60. CORK, L. C., N. H. STERNBERGER, L. A. STERNBERGER, M. F. CASANOVA, R. G. STRUBLE & D. L. PRICE. 1986. Phosphorylated neurofilament antigens in neurofibrillary tangles in Alzheimer's Disease. J. Neuropathol. Exp. Neurol. **45:** 56–64.

Changes in Protein Phosphorylation in Cultured Neurons after Exposure to Methyl Mercury

THEODORE A. SARAFIAN AND M. ANTHONY VERITY

Department of Pathology (Neuropathology)
UCLA Center for Health Sciences
Los Angeles, California 90024

INTRODUCTION

The ubiquity and diversity of protein kinase enzymes underscores their fundamental role as metabolic regulators in biological systems.[1] All cell types depend heavily on the action of protein kinases for the control of homeostatic modulatory processes. In the nervous system, however, protein phosphorylation takes on uniquely specialized roles.[2-4] The phosphorylation of proteins represents an important component of intercellular communication which is the primary function of the nerve cell.

TABLE 1 lists a variety of examples of key neuronal functions mediated by protein phosphorylation. Membrane potential and excitability, neurotransmitter synthesis and release and post-synaptic receptor-mediated responses must all be carefully regulated by the interplay between the unusually abundant protein kinases and the diverse substrate proteins found in the nervous system.

PROTEIN PHOSPHORYLATION AND NEUROTOXICITY

Considering the central role of these specialized reactions it is not surprising that agents or conditions which result in abnormal protein phosphorylation may cause profound and selective neuroinjury. A striking example is provided by the Dunce mutant of *Drosophila melanogaster*.[5] The "learning" defect in this otherwise normal fly is the result of a specific abnormality in cAMP metabolism with consequent perturbation of protein phosphorylation. The locus of the mutation resides in one of the three genes encoding cAMP phosphodiesterase enzymes.[6] This specific subclass of enzyme is calmodulin-insensitive and functions in the molecular pathway for mermory formation in the adult fly.

Other examples indicate the involvement of protein kinase C in mechanisms of neurotoxic injury. For instance the phorbol ester, phorbol-12-myristate 13-acetate (PMA) has been shown to be toxic to cultured hippocampal neurons after 24-h exposure to 10–100 nM.[7] These studies revealed that disruption of a variety of second messenger signaling pathways results in neuritic degeneration and/or cell death. Phorbol ester is also neurotoxic to retinal neurons of the retinal degeneration (rdg) mutant of Drosophila, a fly which is rendered blind by exposure to light.[8] Both light and PMA produce the same pattern of degeneration of retinal neurons in this mutant. Thus it was concluded that either PKC is an integral component of

TABLE 1. Protein Phosphorylation and Neuronal Function

Function	Proteins Phosphorylated
1. Neurotransmitter synthesis	Neurotransmitter enzymes
2. Neurotransmitter release	Synaptic vesicle proteins
3. Membrane/action potential	Ion channel proteins
4. Neuritogenesis	Cytoskeletal proteins

the stimulus-response pathway leading to degeneration or that PKC modulates a critical element of this pathway. The discovery of a double mutant of rdg which lacks a form of PKC called eye PKC lends further support for the central role of this enzyme in the neurodegenerative process of the rdg mutant.[9] This double mutant retains functional neurons following light exposure and identifies the specific enzyme mediating this unusual neurodegenerative paradigm.

An association between PKC and glutamate-mediated excitotoxicity has been described in cultures of cerebellar granule neurons.[10] In these cultures 24-h exposure to 50 μM glutamate results in prolonged elevation of Ca_i^{2+} and activation of phosphatidyl inositol turnover causing abnormally sustained activation of PKC.[11,12] These events culminate in the death of 85–90% of the neurons after 24 hours. This toxicity, however, is largely prevented if the PKC inhibitor, ganglioside GT1b, is included in the incubation medium with glutamate.[13] Moreover, cells depleted of both soluble and membrane-bound PKC by 24-h PMA-induced down-regulation were resistant to glutamate.[14] The degree of resistance correlated directly with extent of clearance of PKC activity from the cells. A key observation was that PKC-depleted cells did not manifest sustained elevation of Ca_i^{2+} during glutamate exposure suggesting the involvement of PKC in loss of Ca_i^{2+} homeostasis during excitotoxic injury.

Thus evidence is mounting for the involvement of protein phosphorylation, particularly by PKC, as a key component of neurotoxic pathways.

METHYL MERCURY AND THE CEREBELLAR GRANULE NEURON

The insidious and disastrous outbreak of mercury poisoning which spread through the cities of Minimata and Nigata in the 1950s and 1960s served to alert the world to the growing threat of anthropogenic mercury in the environment.[15] Sources of mercury include air, water and food, particularly sea food.[16] Currently there is increasing concern over dental amalgam fillings as a source of chronic mercury exposure.[17–19] Grinding teeth and/or chewing food produce intraoral levels of mercury vapor which can be twofold above permissible exposure levels established by OSHA (50 μg/m^3).[20] Once inhaled or ingested mercury has a low turnover rate and requires up to a year for elimination from the body.

Methyl mercury (MeHg) is one of the most neurotoxic chemical forms of mercury, causing a variety of maladies ranging from tremor and sensory disturbance to gross incoordination, limb deformity and deterioration of intellect.[21] One area of the brain which is especially sensitive to MeHg is the granule layer of the cerebellum which manifests extensive neuronal destruction and accounts for the pervasive loss of coordination in chronic MeHg toxicity.[22] These cells provide a convenient experimental model since they can be studied in relative isolation using cell suspension preparations or cell cultures.[23,24]

METHYL MERCURY STIMULATES PROTEIN PHOSPHORYLATION

Exposure of cultured cerebellar granule neurons to MeHg for 24 hours produced a surprising dose-dependent stimulation of protein phosphorylation which was not observed in cultured glial cells (FIG. 1).[24] Phosphorylation was measured by labeling cells for 2–4 hours with 1.0 mCi/ml [^{32}P]orthophosphate in phosphate-free DMEM, followed by extraction of cells with 2% NP 40 in buffer and determination of TCA-insoluble cpm. The observed neuron-specific stimulation by MeHg was not due to changes in intracellular [^{32}P]ATP specific activity, increased ^{32}P incorporation into TCA-insoluble lipid fractions or changes in rate of ^{32}P turnover in labeled proteins (data not shown).

Analysis of individual phosphoproteins by 2D polyacrylamide gel electrophoresis (2D PAGE) revealed that proteins did not increase their ^{32}P content uniformly. Some displayed MeHg-induced increases of >300% while others displayed no change or a slight decrease in labeling.[25] This variability in phosphorylation suggested that one or more protein kinase activities were stimulated by MeHg.

MECHANISM OF METHYL MERCURY–INDUCED STIMULATION

Could MeHg stimulate protein kinase activity by direct interaction with enzyme in a manner analogous to the effect of lead acetate on PKC?[26] Studies using cell-free protein kinase assays for cAMP-dependent, Ca^{2+}/calmodulin-dependent, tyrosine kinases and PKC failed to disclose stimulation at any concentration of

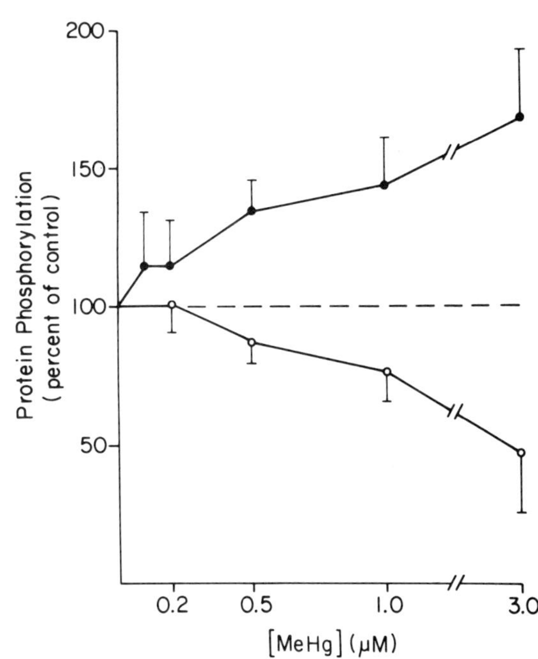

FIGURE 1. Effect of MeHg on phosphorylation in cerebellar neuronal (●) and glial (○) cultures. Cells treated 24 h with MeHg were labeled 4 hours with 0.5 mC$_i$/ml [^{32}P]orthophosphate and extracted with 2% NP40 in 0.01 M Tris HCl buffer pH 7.4. Aliquots were precipitated and washed with cold 10% TCA and dpm determined in protein pellets. Protein content was determined in a parallel series of MeHg-treated wells extracted with 1 N NaOH. Values calculated as dpm ^{32}P/mg protein are expressed as % of control and represent means of 6 determinations ± SEM. $p < 0.05$ for 1 and 3 µM MeHg compared with control using paired t-test.

MeHg tested (10^{-7}-10^{-4} M) (FIG. 2). Thus direct stimulatory interaction with kinase enzyme seems unlikely. A more plausible explanation would be activation of second messenger pathways and our studies have indicated that the levels of two second messengers, Ca^{2+} and inositol phosphate, can be elevated by MeHg under appropriate conditions. Studies with $^{45}Ca^{2+}$ revealed two MeHg-induced

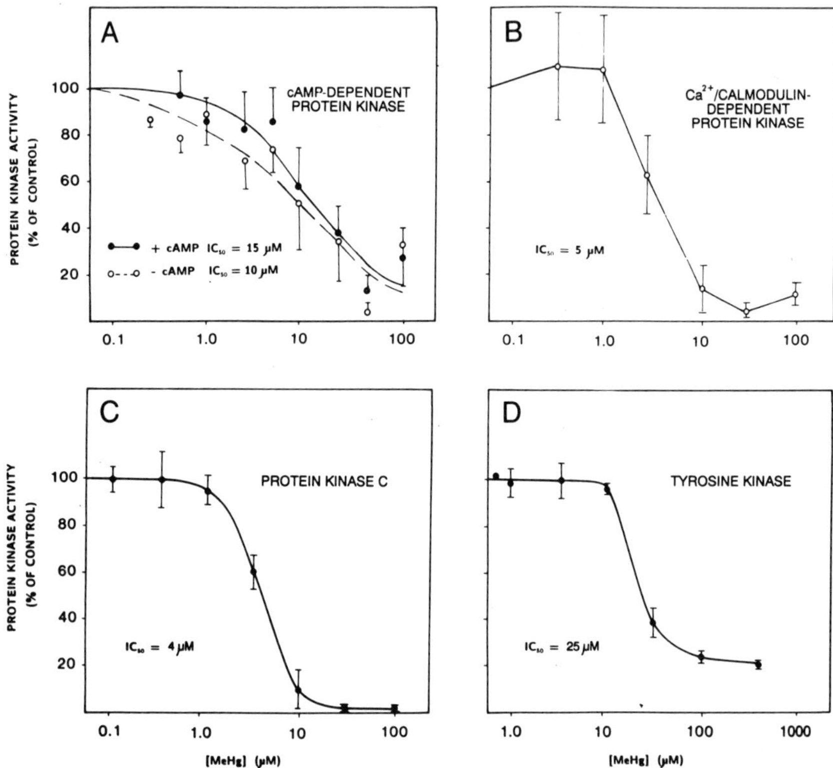

FIGURE 2. MeHg inhibition curves for proteins kinase activities. Values are means ± SEM (N = 3–8). Protein kinase C was partially purified form adult rat brain by DEAE-cellulose and Phenyl-Sepharose (Pharmacia-LKB) chromatography. All other enzyme activities were derived directly from cultured cerebellar granule neurons.

changes in Ca^{2+} metabolism: 1) Increased rate of $^{45}Ca^{2+}$ uptake in neuronal cultures (TABLE 2) and 2) Increased total and ionophore A23187-releasable $^{45}Ca^{2+}$ following 24 h exposures to 3 and 5 μM MeHg (TABLE 3). These changes in Ca^{2+} content were not observed in glial cell cultures, nor were they produced by triethyl lead or mercuric chloride (Data not shown). Disturbance of Ca^{2+} homeostasis by MeHg has been described previously and could well contribute to changes in

TABLE 2. Effect of 24-Hour MeHg on ^{45}Ca Uptake Rate

[MeHg] (μM)	cpm / μg Protein	% of Control
0	10.4 $\pm$ 0.78	(100)
1	13.0 $\pm$ 0.81	125
3	13.6 $\pm$ 1.5	131
5	37.2 $\pm$ 8.5	358

All cells used had been in culture 1–3 weeks. Uptake assays were performed by incubating MeHg-treated cells 5 min with 5 μC$_i$ ^{45}Ca (35°C) and washing with 5 mM EGTA in modified Krebs-Ringer buffer. Cells were then extracted with 1 N NaOH and cpm and protein content was determined in appropriate aliquots. Values represent means of 6 determinations $\pm$ SEM. $p < .025$ for 1 μM and 5 μM MeHg compared with control using Bonferroni-corrected Students t-test with paired data.

protein phosphorylation patterns.[27] Changes in inositol phospholipid turnover were observed at both 30 min and 24 hours following MeHg exposure (TABLE 4). Cells prelabeled with [^{3}H]myo-inositol were treated with MeHg in the presence of 10 mM LiCl. Formic acid extracts of these cells contained higher levels of labeled total inositol phosphate eluted from AG 1-X8 anion ion exchange columns. Again the response was specific for neuronal cultures and MeHg.

These observations imply the activation of phospholipase C by MeHg which would also mean protein kinase C stimulation since diacylglycerol is a requisite coproduct of phospholipase C activity.

TABLE 3. Effect of 24-Hour MeHg Exposure on A23187-Releasable ^{45}Ca Levels

[MeHg] (μM)	Neuronal Injury Index	Neuronal cpm / μg Protein	Neuronal % of Control	Glial Injury Index	Glial cpm / μg Protein	Glial % of Control
0	0	7.8 $\pm$ 0.9	(100)	0	4.9 $\pm$ 1.0	(100)
0.5	0	7.9 $\pm$ 1.1	101			
1	0	8.3 $\pm$ 0.9	106	0	4.5 $\pm$ 1.6	92
3	1	12.2 $\pm$ 1.9^a	156	0	6.1 $\pm$ 0.7	124
5	2	17.2 $\pm$ 2.4^a	220	2	5.8 $\pm$ 2.2	118

Cells were treated 24-hours with MeHg and ^{45}CaCl$_2$, washed and then incubated 30 min at room temperature in Krebs-Ringer buffer containing 50 μM calcium ionophore A23187. A23187-releasable cpm was determined by subtracting cpm released in the absence of A23187 from that in the presence in parallel culture wells. Values for injury index represent visual estimations of the degree of cellular injury incurred after 24-h exposures using a scale 0–5. Based on experiments using trypan blue as an indicator of cell mortality, the injury index corresponded approximately to the following percent viabilities: 0 = 85 to 100, 1 = 70 to 85, 2 = 50 to 70, 3 = 25 to 50, 4 = 10 to 25, 5 = 0 to 10. Values for cpm/μg protein represent means of 6 to 12 determinations $\pm$ SEM.

^{a} $p < .05$ compared with control using Bonferroni-corrected Student's t-test with unpaired data.

WHICH PROTEIN KINASE IS ACTIVATED?

In order to characterize effects of MeHg on intracellular protein kinase activities 2D PAGE patterns of ^{32}P-labeled proteins were analyzed following short-term (1 h) exposure of cells to specific kinase-modulatory agents. The phorbol ester, PMA, a specific activator of PKC, dramatically alters protein phosphorylation patterns in cerebellar granule cell culture with the appearance of several new spots, and enhanced labeling of 10–15 other proteins (FIG. 3). Select changes are indicated by arrows in FIGURE 3 with notable increases at M_r 27,000, pI 6.4 and 7.5, M_r 65,000, pI 6.4–6.5 and M_r 43,000, pI 5.1–5.4. The group of proteins at M_r 65,000 stain positively for tau factor by Western blot analysis. Forskolin, which activates adenylcylase and consequently cAMP-dependent protein kinase, produced a distinct pattern of changes with increases in a protein of M_r 60,000, pI 5.5 which stains with anti-tubulin antibody by Western blot analysis and an M_r 55,000, pI 5.7

TABLE 4. Effect of 30-Minute MeHg Exposure on Inositol Phosphate Level in Neuronal and Glial Culture

[MeHg] (μM)	Neuronal $\dfrac{\text{cpm}}{\mu\text{g Protein}}$	% of Control	Glial $\dfrac{\text{cpm}}{\mu\text{g Protein}}$	% of Control
0	49.3 ± 5.6(9)	(100)	19.8 ± 5.6(4)	(100)
1	51.6 ± 5.6(6)	105	22.8 ± 4.4(4)	115
3	77.6 ± 10.2(6)	157[a]	24.7 ± 6.7(4)	125
5	96.1 ± 14.0(9)	195[b]	19.6 ± 8.4(4)	99
10	107.1 ± 20.2(6)	217[b]		

Cells prelabeled overnight with [³H] myo-inositol were washed twice with modified Krebs-Ringer buffer containing 10 mM LiCl and then incubated 30 min at 36°C with balanced salt solution (25 mM Tris HCl, pH 7.4, 15 mM glucose, 120 mM NaCl, 5.5 mM KCl, 0.8 mM $MgCl_2$ 1.8 mM $CaCl_2$) containing MeHg (0–20 μM) and 10 mM LiCl. Following a wash with modified Krebs-Ringer buffer, cells were extracted and analyzed for total inositol phosphate using formate AG 1-X8 anion exchange columns.

Values from cpm/μg protein represent means ± SEM (number of determinations).

[a] $p < 0.025$ using Bonferroni-corrected t-test.

[b] $p < 0.01$.

protein (FIG. 4). The only change which was similar to that induced by PMA was an acidic shift in pI of the group of microheteromers at M_r 43,000, pI 5.0–5.4. The Ca^{2+} ionophore A23187 (5 μM) had virtually no effect on protein phosphorylation during the 1-h analysis (Data not shown).

One hour exposure to MeHg at 5 and 10 μM produced changes which were almost identical to that of PMA (FIG. 5). New spots of M_r 27,000, pI 6.4 and pI 7.5 and M_r 35,000, pI 6.4 appeared and increased phosphorylation was observed for proteins of M_r 65,000, pI 6.4–6.5 and M_r 43–45,000, pI 4.9–5.4. The latter group of proteins had a greater abundance of more acidic forms than that produced by PMA treatment, suggesting phosphorylation of multiple alternative sites in MeHg-trated cells.

The effects of MeHg on protein phosphorylation were completely blocked by 25 μM staurosporine and 200 μM H7 suggesting that PKC mediates the MeHg effects (data not shown).

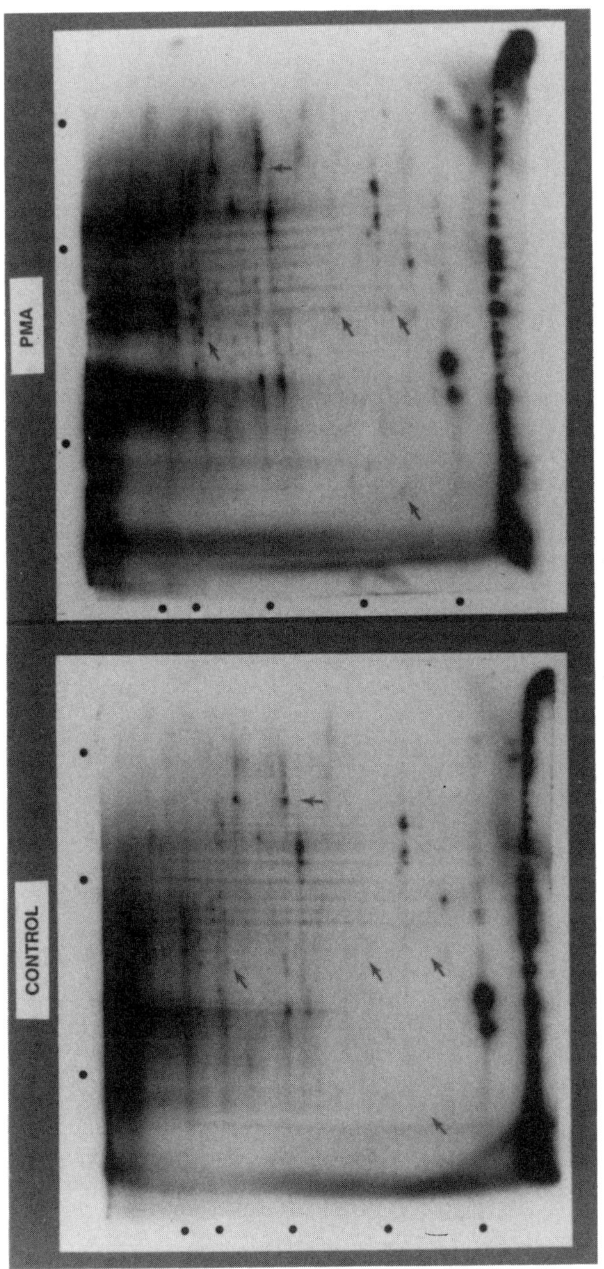

FIGURE 3. 2D PAGE profiles for phosphoproteins from control and 0.1 μM PMA-treated cultured granule neurons. Cells were treated 1 hour with PMA during labeling with [32P]orthophosphate. Electrophoresis was performed essentially by the method of O'Farrell (J. Biol. Chem. **250:** 4007–4021). Dots on left side represent M_r markers (top to bottom): 97,000, 66,000, 43,000, 31,000, 21,000. Dots above gels represent pH (left to right): 7, 6, 5. Arrows identify select proteins demonstrating altered phosphorylation with treatment.

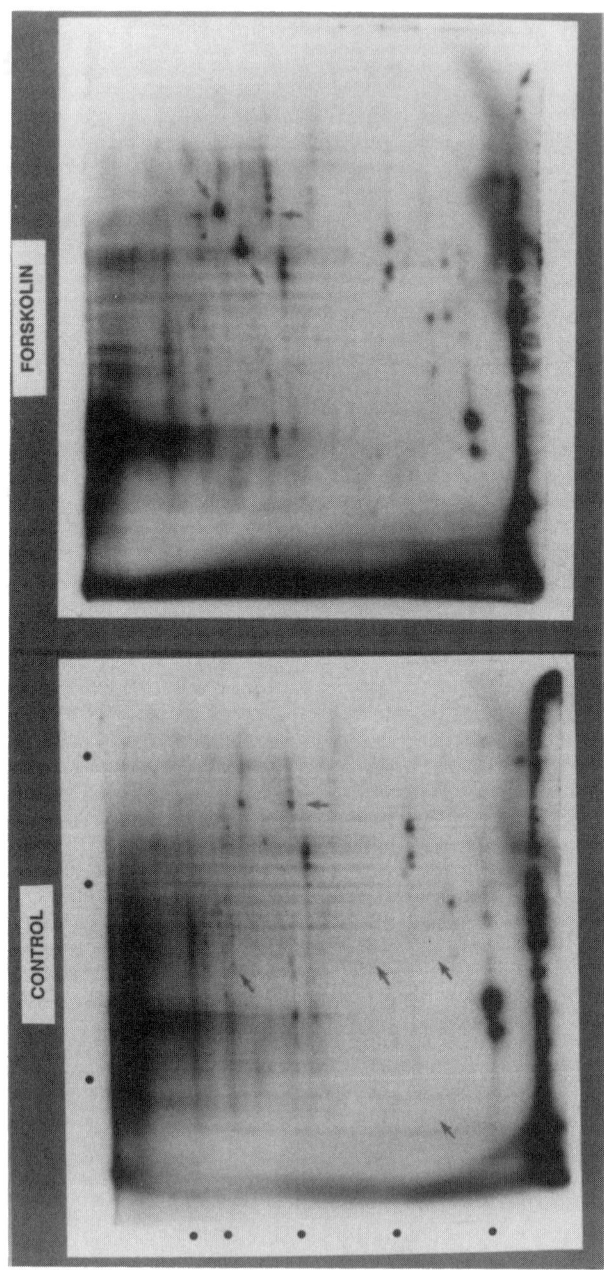

FIGURE 4. 2D PAGE profiles for control and 25 μM forskolin-treated granule neuron phosphoproteins.

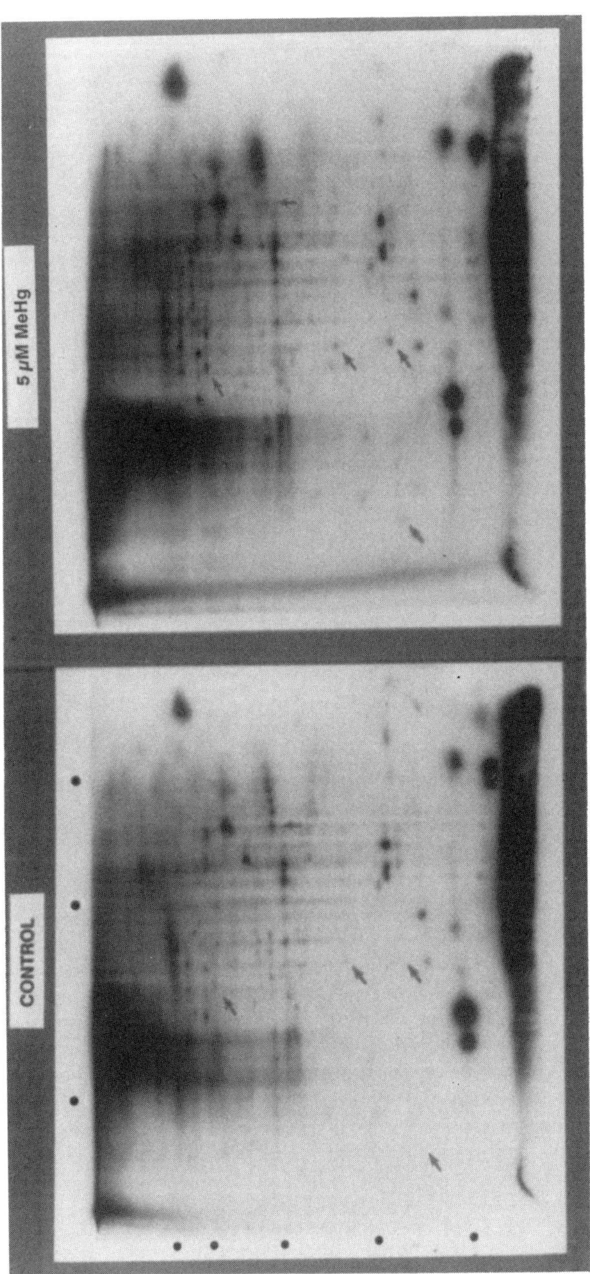

FIGURE 5. 2D PAGE profiles for control and 5 μM MeHg-treated granule neuron phosphoproteins.

CAN MeHg CAUSE DOWN-REGULATION OF PKC?

Complete loss of responsiveness to 100 nM PMA results from 24-h pretreatment with 10 μM PMA implying depletion of PKC from all cells by the process known as down-regulation (FIG. 6A). However, 24 h exposure to 3 or 5 μM MeHg, sufficient to produce overt toxicity, did not eliminate or substantially diminish stimulation of phosphorylation by 100 nM PMA (FIG. 6B). These results indicate that the PKC enzyme remains active throughout the degenerative period following MeHg exposure and suggests the possibility of concurrent activation of PKC and inhibition of the proteolytic enzyme, calpain, believed to be responsible for the down-regulation phenomenon.

CONCLUSION

Disturbance in the regulation and specificity of protein phosphorylation would be expected to have profound disruptive effects on neuronal function.[28] It is not presently clear whether or not such functional disruption can, by itself, lead to neuronal death. However, several reports have been published wherein such a scenario seems likely.[7,10] In addition to the previously mentioned connections between protein kinase C and neurotoxicity there is the well-known abnormality of cytoskeletal fibrillar proteins characteristic of Alzheimer's disease. Degenerating neurons in this disorder manifest gross accumulation of tau factor, neurofilament, and amyloid plaques.[29] Abnormal and excessive phosphorylation of each of these components has been characterized suggesting that altered protein kinase activity may be the primary event in the pathogenesis of neuritic lesions.[28,30] Our present observations of increased phosphorylation of numerous proteins, including cytoskeletal proteins, by low concentrations of MeHg provides another intriguing circumstance wherein abnormalities of protein phosphorylation are associated with neurotoxic injury.

It is well known that, in addition to energy sources and basic nutrients, neurons require trophic or survival factors in order to maintain viability.[31,32] Teleologially this requirement arises from the developmental neurobiologic process of neuronal elimination which serves to assure that only those neurons which have achieved appropriate functional synaptic connections are destined to survive. This competitive selection process, which can be modeled by NGF deprivation of sympathetic neurons in culture, has been hypothesized to involve the induction of an endogenous "death program."[33] Numerous studies have shown that NGF and other trophic factors alter protein phosphorylation and that these phosphorylation reactions are required to produce the various morphologic and biochemical effects of these factors.[34–36] It is conceivable that the "death program" associated with factor deprivation can be activated by specific changes in the state of neuronal protein phosphorylation and it may be speculated that some neurotoxins may act by activating the phosphorylation pathways required for expression of the death program. The present data provides evidence that MeHg may represent such a neurotoxin.

ACKNOWLEDGMENTS

The authors would like to thank Steve Kaufman, Sharon Belkin and Carol Gray for contributed artwork, and Luiza Vartavarian and Dr. Sylvia Aguiar for technical

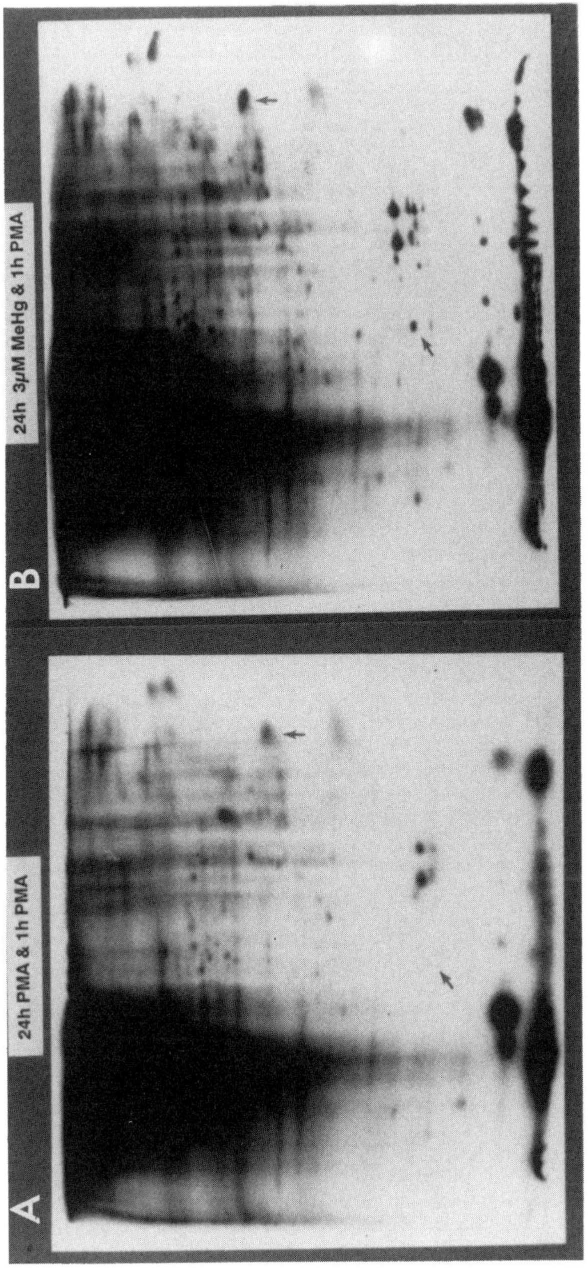

FIGURE 6. Effect of 24-h pretreatment with 10 μM PMA (**A**) or 3 μM MeHg (**B**) on ^{32}P phosphoprotein pattern produced by 1-h 0.1 μM PMA. Arrows identify select protein kinase C substrates.

assistance. We are also indebted to Dr. Dale Bredesen for insightful comments and suggestions.

REFERENCES

1. HANKS, S. K., A. M. QUINN & T. HUNTER. 1988. The protein kinase family: Conserved features and deduced phylogeny of the catalytic domains. Science **241:** 42–52.
2. NAIRN, A. C., H. C. HEMMINGS & P. GREENGARD. 1985. Protein kinases in the brain. Ann. Rev. Biochem. **54:** 931–976.
3. NESTLER, E. J. & P. GREENGARD. 1984. Protein phosphorylation in the nervous system. John Wiley and Sons. New York.
4. WALAAS, S. I. & P. GREENGARD. 1991. Protein phosphorylation and neuronal function. Pharmacol. Rev. **43:** 299–349.
5. DUDAI, Y., Y-N. YAN, D. BYERS, W. G. QUINN & S. BENZER. 1976. *Dunce,* a mutant of Drosophila deficient in learning. Proc. Natl. Acad. Sci. USA **73:** 1684–1688.
6. SHOTWELL, S. L. 1983. Cyclic adenosine 3′:5′-monophosphate phosphodiesterase and its role in learning in Drosophilia. J. Neurosci. **3:** 739–747.
7. MATTSON, M. P., P. B. GUTHRIE & S. B. KATER. 1988. Intracellular messengers in the generation and degeneration of hippocampal neuroarchitecture. J. Neurosci. Res. **21:** 447–464.
8. MINKE, B., C. T. RUBINSTEIN, I. SAHLY, S. BAR-NACHUM, R. TIMBERG & Z. SELINGER. 1990. Phorbol ester induces photoreceptor-specific degeneration in a Drosophilia mutant. Proc. Natl. Acad. Sci. USA **87:** 113–117.
9. SMITH, D. P., R. RANGANATHAN, R. W. HARDY, J. MARX, T. TSUCHIDA & C. S. ZUKER. 1991. Photoreceptor deactivation and retinal degeneration mediated by a photoreceptor-specific protein kinase C. Science **254:** 1478–1484.
10. MANEV, H., E. COSTA, J. T. WROBLEWSKI & A. GUIDOTTI. 1990. Abusive stimulation of excitatory amino acid receptors: A strategy to limit neurotoxicity. FASEB J. **4:** 2789–2797.
11. MANEV, H., M. FAVARON, A. GUIDOTTI & E. COSTA. 1989. Delayed increase in Ca^{2+} influx elicited by glutamate: Role in neuronal death. Mol. Pharmacol. **36:** 106–112.
12. NICOLETTI, F., J. T. WROBLEWSKI, A. NORELLI, H. ALHO, A. GUIDOTTI & E. COSTA. 1986. The activation of phospholipid metabolism as a signals transducing system for excitatory amino acids in primary cultures of cerebellar granule cells. J. Neurosci. **6:** 1905–1911.
13. FAVARON, M., H. MANEV, H. ALHO, M. BERTOLINO, B. FERRET, A. GUIDOTTI & E. COSTA. 1988. Gangliosides prevent glutamate and kainate neurotoxicity in primary neuronal cultures of neonatal rat cerebellum and cortex. Proc. Natl. Acad. Sci. USA **85:** 7351–7355.
14. FAVARON, M., H. MANEV, R. SIMAN, M. BERTOLINO, A. M. SZEKELY, G. DEERAUSQUIN, A. GUIDOTTI & E. COSTA. 1990. Down regulation of protein kinase C protects cerebellar granule neurons in primary culture from glutamate-induced neuronal death. Proc. Natl. Acad. Sci. USA **87:** 1983–1987.
15. SMITH, W. E. & A. M. SMITH. 1975. Minimata. Holt Rinehart and Winston. New York.
16. NRIAGU, J. O., Ed. 1979. The Biogeochemistry of Mercury in the Environment. Elsevier/North Holland. New York.
17. CLARKSON, T. W., J. B. HURSCH, P. R. SAGER & T. L. M. SYVRESEN. 1988. Mercury. *In* Biological Monitoring of Toxic Metals. T. W. Clarkson, L. Friberg, G. F. Nordberg & P. R. Sager, Eds.: 199–246. Plenum Press. New York.
18. MOLIN, M., B. BERGMAN, S. L. MARKLUND, A. SCHUTZ & S. SKERFING. 1990. Mercury, selenium and gluathione peroxidase before and after amalgam removal in man. Acta Odontol. Scand. **48:** 189–202.
19. DANSCHER, G., P. HORSTED-BINDSLEV & J. RUNGBY. 1990. Traces of mercury in organs from primates with amalgam fillings. Exp. Mol. Pathol. **52:** 291–299.
20. LEWIS, R. J. 1991. Hazardous Chemicals Desk Reference, Second Ed.: 750. Van Nostrand Reinhold. New York.

21. SUZUKI, T., N. IMURA & T. W. CLARKSON, Eds. 1991. Advances in mercury toxicology. Plenum Press. New York.

22. REUHL, K. R., L. W. CHANG & J. W. TOWNSEND. 1981. Pathological effects of in utero methyl mercury exposure on the cerebellum of the golden hamster. I. Early effects upon the neonatal cerebellar cortex. Environ. Res. **26:** 281–306.

23. SARAFIAN, T. A., J. HAGLER, L. VARTAVARIAN & M. A. VERITY. 1989. Rapid cell death induced by methyl mercury in suspensions of cerebellar granule neurons. J. Neuropathol. Exp. Neurol. **48:** 1–10.

24. SARAFIAN, T. A. & M. A. VERITY. 1990. Methyl mercury stimulates protein ^{32}P-phospholabelling in cerebellar granule cell culture. J. Neurochem. **55:** 913–921.

25. SARAFIAN, T. A. & M. A. VERITY. 1990. Altered patterns of protein phosphorylation and synthesis caused by methyl mercury in cerebellar cell culture. J. Neurochem. **55:** 922–929.

26. MARKOVAC, J. & G. W. GOLDSTEIN. 1988. Picomolar concentrations of lead stimulate brain protein kinase C. Nature **334:** 71–73.

27. KOMULAININ, H. & S. C. BONDY. 1987. Increased free intrasynaptic Ca^{2+} in chemical toxicity. Toxicol. Appl. Pharmacol. **88:** 77–86.

28. SAITOH, T., E. MASLIAH, L-W. JIN, G. M. COLE, T. WIELOCH & I. P. SHAPIRO. 1991. Protein kinases and phosphorylation in neurologic disorders and cell death. Lab. Invest. **64:** 596–616.

29. KATZMAN, R. & T. Saitoh. 1991. Advances in Alzheimer's disease. FASEB J. **5:** 278–286.

30. ZHANG, H., N. H. STERNBERGER, L. J. RUBINSTEIN, M. M. HERMAN, L. I. BINDER & L. A. STERNBERGER. 1989. Abnormal processing of multiple proteins in Alzheimer disease. Proc. Natl. Acad. Sci. USA **86:** 8045–8049.

31. CUNNINGHAM, T. J. 1982. Naturally occurring neuron death and its regulation by developing neural pathways. Int. Rev. Cytol. **74:** 163–186.

32. CLARKE, P. G. H. 1985. Neuronal death in the development of the vertebrate nervous system. Trends. Neurosci. **8:** 345–349.

33. MARTIN, D. P., T. L. WALLACE, & E. M. JOHNSON. 1990. Cytorine arabinoside kills post-mitotic neurons in a fashion resembling trophic factor deprivation: Evidence that a deoxychytidine-dependent process may be required for nerve growth factor signal transduction. J. Neurosci. **10:** 184–193.

34. ALETTA, J. M., S. A. LEWIS, N. J. COWAN & L. A. GREENE. 1988. Nerve growth factor regulates both the phosphorylation and steady-state levels of microtubule-associated protein 1.2(MAP 1.2). J. Cell Biol. **106:** 1573–1581.

35. GLOWACKA, D. & J. A. WAGNER. 1990. Role of cAMP-dependent protein kinase and protein kinase C in regulating the morphological differentiation of PC12 cells. J. Neurosci. Res. **25:** 453–462.

36. KALMAN, D., B. WONG, A. HORVAI, M. J. CLINE & P. H. O'LAQUE. 1990. Nerve growth factor acts through cAMP-dependent protein kinase to increase the number of sodium channels in PC12 cells. Neuron **2:**355–366.

Spectrin Proteolysis in the Hippocampus: A Biochemical Marker for Neuronal Injury and Neuroprotection

JILL M. ROBERTS-LEWIS AND ROBERT SIMAN

Departments of Pharmacology and Biochemistry
Cephalon, Inc.
145 Brandywine Parkway
West Chester, Pennsylvania 19380

INTRODUCTION

It is well established that a precipitous or sustained rise in intracellular calcium levels can lead to neuronal death.[1] This state can result from excessive release of the endogenous excitatory amino acids (EAAs) glutamate and aspartate, or by administration of agonist analogs of these "excitotoxins." EAA-induced perturbations in calcium homeostasis have clearly been implicated in the neuronal death related to ischemia, and may be involved in other neurodegenerative diseases or traumatic injuries, as well.[2-4]

For a number of years, attention has been focused on the pharmacological blockade of EAA receptors or calcium channels as a strategy for designing neuroprotective agents. However, an interest in identifying relevant intracellular "downstream" targets has emerged more recently. A few of the calcium-sensitive intracellular events that have been associated with neuronal death include the activation of proteases, protein kinases, phospholipases (leading to formation of free radicals and lipid peroxidation), and a calcium-dependent endonuclease activity leading to DNA fragmentation (apoptosis).[3-7] Defining the role of these intracellular mechanisms in the processes of neuronal death will provide relevant new biochemical markers of neuronal injury and degeneration, as well as novel therapeutic targets for drug discovery efforts.

The calcium-activated neutral cysteine protease, calpain I (μ-calpain), has many characteristics which suggest that it may play a key role in the mechanisms underlying EAA-induced neuronal death.[2,3] Calpain I is localized in neurons that are selectively vulnerable to excitotoxin- or ischemia-induced degeneration,[8] and is activated by the low micromolar calcium concentrations that are thought to be achieved intracellularly during pathological conditions such as ischemia or following excitotoxin administration.[9,10] Preferred substrates of calpain I include major neuronal structural proteins, such as neurofilament polypeptides, microtubule-associated proteins, tubulin, and spectrin.[11] The large scale proteolysis of any or all of these structural components could lead to a global and lethal failure of the structural integrity of the neuron. In fact, activation of calpain I has been linked to cellular degeneration associated with a number of diseases and neuropathologies, including spinal and head trauma, peripheral nerve injury, demyelinating disease, muscular atrophy, lens cataract formation, and cerebral ischemia.[12-19]

Measurement of spectrin proteolysis provides a relevant, easily detectable biochemical marker of calpain activation.[11,19,20] A number of studies have suggested that the pathological induction of spectrin proteolysis is directly related to subsequent neuronal death. For example, Siman et al.[20] have shown that spectrin is degraded in vulnerable regions of the hippocampus within 3 hours following intracerebral infusion of the EAA analogs, kainic acid or N-methyl D-aspartate (NMDA). The appearance of spectrin proteolytic fragments is maximal at 24 hours and persists for several days following EAA administration. The magnitude of this excitotoxin-induced proteolysis of spectrin is also dose-dependent and positively correlated with the magnitude of structural damage, as well as the specific regions of the hippocampus sustaining damage, after EAA administration.[20] TABLE 1 summarizes the correspondence between the induction of neuronal damage ("neurotoxicity") and calpain I-mediated spectrin proteolysis ("calpain activation"). In addition to serving as a biochemical index of neuronal damage, the calpain

TABLE 1. Correspondence between Excitotoxin-induced Neuronal Damage and Calpain I-mediated Spectrin Proteolysis

Condition	Neurotoxicity	Calpain Activation
Kainate, 0.25 μg	+	+
Kainate, 1 μg	+ +	+ +
	Area CA3	Area CA3
Kainate, 1 μg (6 h)	+	+
NMDA, 40 μg	+	+
NMDA, 80 μg	+ +	+ +
Kainate, 1 μg + CPP, 2 μg	+ +	+ +
NMDA, 80 μg + CPP, 2 μg	−	−

Excitatory amino acid (EAA) activation of calpain I and induction of hippocampal damage in vivo show a tight correspondence. Neurotoxicity was evaluated by silver impregnation histochemistry, while calpain activation was assessed by Western blot analysis with spectrin antibodies. CPP = carboxypiperazin-4-yl-propylphosphonate, a selective and potent NMDA receptor antagonist which has little or no affinity for kainate receptors. + + = maximal effect; + = moderate effect; − = no effect. In all cases, each EAA treatment had parallel effects on neuronal damage and calpain I activation.

I-mediated spectrin degradation may be an important contributor to neuronal disintegration. Spectrin is an actin-binding protein and it links actin-based microfilaments to the plasma membrane, but calpain I digestion of spectrin may lead to membrane detachment of the spectrin-actin network.[21,22]

We have also measured spectrin breakdown products in the vulnerable CA1 region of the hippocampus 24 hours following 5 minutes of global cerebral ischemia in the gerbil (data not shown). The degradation of spectrin in the hippocampus is maximal at 3 to 4 days, and absent by one week following ischemia, consistent with the evolution of secondary or delayed deterioration that occurs at 3–4 days in this model. In fact, Seubert et al.[19] have shown a measurable induction of spectrin proteolytic fragments in the hippocampus as early as 15 minutes after global cerebral ischemia. Clearly, calpain activation is an early event associated with this neuropathological insult which precedes and may actually be causally related to subsequent neuronal death. Lee et al.[23] have also shown that in vivo administration of the protease inhibitor, leupeptin, attenuated both spectrin proteolysis and neuronal degeneration of the hippocampus following global ischemia in the gerbil. Furthermore, they have demonstrated that the hippocampus from leupeptin-treated gerbils subjected to ischemia retained normal physiological responsiveness up to two weeks following the ischemic insult.

In the present report, we will further demonstrate that the *ex vivo* analysis of spectrin proteolysis can provide a useful index of neuronal injury, and that this analysis can be profitably used to rapidly evaluate the *in vivo* efficacy of potential neuroprotective compounds.

METHODS

Kainic Acid (KA)-induced Hippocampal Damage

For the histological analysis male and female Sprague-Dawley rats (200–350 g) were anesthetized with Nembutal (50 mg/kg i.p.) and administered 0.4 μg of K-252a, or vehicle (DMSO) in a total of 5 μl intracerebroventricularly (ICV), 30 minutes prior to and about 3 and 24 hours following delivery of 0.6 μg KA in 5 μl ICV. Sham-operated animals received vehicle infusions instead of KA and K-252a. ICV infusions were delivered through a cannula permanently implanted about one week earlier at stereotaxic coordinates: anterior-posterior at bregma, 1.5 mm lateral to bregma, and 4.4 mm ventral from the top of the skull.

For the biochemical analysis, anesthetized female Sprague-Dawley rats (200–250 g) received an ICV infusion of 0.4 μg K-252a, or vehicle, simultaneously with 0.6 μg of KA in a total of 5 μl through a 10 μl Hamilton syringe positioned at the stereotaxic coordinates described above.

N-Methyl-D-Aspartate (NMDA)-induced Hippocampal Damage

Female Sprague-Dawley rats (200–250 g) were anesthetized with Nembutal (50 mg/kg i.p.) and received 7 μg of aurintricarboxylic acid (ATA) or vehicle simultaneously with 3 μg NMDA in a total of 1 μl into the dorsal hippocampus at sterotaxic coordinates −3.3 mm posterior from bregma, lateral 2.3 mm from the midline and ventral 4.3 mm from the top of the skull. Animals treated with MK-801 were administered an NMDA infusion as described above, and MK-801 (1 mg/kg i.p.) or vehicle immediately following the NMDA infusion. Sham-operated animals received an intrahippocampal infusion of vehicle instead of NMDA or drug.

Biochemical Analysis

Calpain I-sensitive proteolysis of spectrin was evaluated in homogenates of the hippocampus using an immunoblot analysis described by Siman *et al.*[20] Briefly, rats were sacrificed by decapitation 24 hours following NMDA or kainate treatment, and the dorsal hippocampus was dissected out of the brain and homogenized in 20 mM Tris-HCl (pH 7.4) containing 0.1 mM phenylmethylsulfonyl-fluoride. Proteins from aliquots of each homogenate were separated by SDS-PAGE, and an immunoblot analysis was used to quantitate the amount of NMDA- or kainate-induced spectrin proteolysis in each sample. The amount of spectrin proteolysis in each sample was measured by digitizing the breakdown product bands with computerized image analysis (R & M Biometrics, Nashville, TN).

Histological Analysis

Rats were sacrificed by decapitation 2 weeks following kainic acid treatment, and the brains were rapidly removed and frozen on dry ice. A series of slide-mounted coronal sections from each brain was stained with thionin and examined microscopically by an observer who was unaware of the group identity of the sections. Damage to the hippocampus was quantitated by summing the total number of subfields of the hippocampus (CA 1-4) on both left and right sides of the brain, that suffered a loss of pyramidal cells.

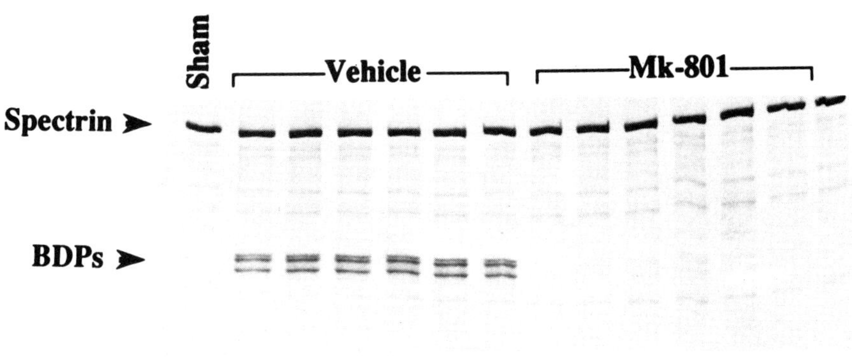

FIGURE 1. Western blot of NMDA-induced spectrin proteolysis following systemic treatment with MK-801. Each lane represents the hippocampus from one animal. All animals except shams received an intrahippocampal infusion of NMDA followed immediately by an i.p. injection of vehicle or MK-801. Shams (shown in the first and last lanes) received an intrahippocampal infusion of vehicle, but no NMDA or MK-801. The NMDA-induced increase in hippocampal spectrin breakdown products (BDPs) is significantly reduced in the hippocampus from animals receiving MK-801 compared to vehicle-treated controls.

RESULTS

Effect of an NMDA Antagonist on NMDA-induced Spectrin Proteolysis

Hippocampal pyramidal cell death induced by NMDA can be largely prevented by administration of the non-competitive NMDA antagonist, MK-801.[24] In order to evaluate whether this treatment would also prevent NMDA-induced spectrin proteolysis in the hippocampus, rats were injected with MK-801, or vehicle, immediately following an infusion of NMDA into the dorsal hippocampus. The hippocampus from MK-801-treated rats showed significantly less spectrin proteolysis than that from vehicle-treated rats (FIG. 1), consistent with the neuroprotective effects seen with histological methods of analysis after MK-801 treatment.[24]

Effect of a Protein Kinase Inhibitor on KA-induced Cell Death and Spectrin Proteolysis

There is some evidence to suggest that protein kinases may be involved in the cascade of events that contribute to cell death under various conditions. For example, gangliosides (GM$_1$), which block the translocation of protein kinase C to the membrane and its sustained activation following persistent EAA receptor stimulation, have been shown to be neuroprotective against EAA-mediated cell death.[25] The protein kinase inhibitor, K-252a, also prevents cultured chick dorsal root ganglion neurons from dying in the absence of requisite growth factors.[26] Furthermore, intracerebral pretreatment of rodents with K-252a or staurosporine (an analog of K-252a) may reduce hippocampal cell death induced by transient global ischemia *in vivo*.[27,28] To examine the possibility that inhibition of protein kinases might also prevent EAA-induced neuronal death *in vivo*, rats were treated with K-252a (ICV), or vehicle, in conjunction with administration of a neurotoxic dose of the EAA analog, kainic acid. As shown in FIGURE 2, K-252a treatment significantly reduced the extent of hippocampal damage sustained 2 weeks following infusion of kainic acid. Furthermore, the same treatment also resulted in a significant attenuation of hippocampal spectrin proteolysis 24 hours following kainic-acid infusion (FIGS. 3 and 4).

Effect of an Endonuclease Inhibitor on NMDA-induced Spectrin Proteolysis

Apoptosis, or programmed cell death, is believed to be the process by which the size of a neuronal population is regulated during development. This is thought to be an active process requiring gene expression and protein synthesis in order to be successfully executed.[29,30] Apoptotic cell death is characterized by inter-nucleosomal DNA cleavage mediated by a calcium-dependent endonuclease activity.[29,30] A few reports have suggested that there may be some commonalties between apoptosis and certain forms of neuronal death. For example, DNA degra-

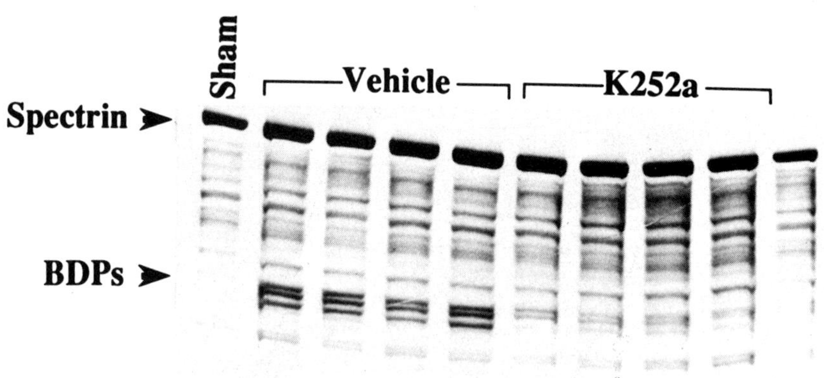

FIGURE 2. Western blot of kainic acid-induced spectrin proteolysis following central administration of K-252a. Each lane represents the hippocampus from one animal. All animals except shams received an ICV infusion of kainic acid together with vehicle or K-252a. Shams (shown in the first and last lanes) received an ICV infusion of vehicle, but no kainic acid or K-252a. The kainic acid-induced increase in hippocampal spectrin breakdown products (BDPs) is significantly reduced in the hippocampus from animals receiving K-252a treatment compared to vehicle-treated controls.

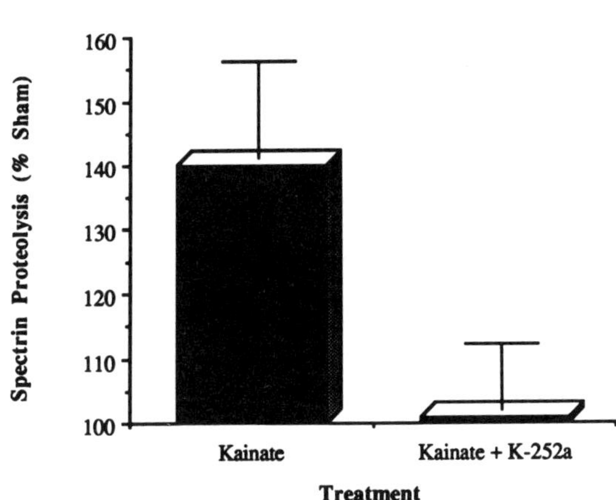

FIGURE 3. Analysis of kainic acid-induced spectrin proteolysis following central administration of K-252a. Rats received an ICV infusion of kainic acid (kainate) together with vehicle or K-252a. Sham control animals received an ICV infusion of vehicle, but no kainic acid or K-252a. All animals were sacrificed 24 h later, and homogenates of the hippocampus were analyzed for spectrin breakdown products using the immunoblot methods described in the text and shown in FIGURE 2. The magnitude of spectrin proteolysis is expressed as a percent increase in spectrin breakdown products over sham control values. Data shown are the mean percent increase in spectrin breakdown products from vehicle (kainate) or K-252a (kainate + K-252a) treated samples ± SEM. Sham = 100%.

dation is elicited by glutamate agonists,[31] and the endonuclease inhibitor, aurintricarboxylic acid (ATA) prevents PC12 cell death induced by NGF deprivation *in vitro*.[32] To begin to explore the possibility of a common mechanism underlying EAA-induced neuronal death and apoptosis *in vivo*, rats were treated with ATA, or vehicle, simultaneously with an infusion of NMDA directly into the dorsal hippocampus. ATA treatment resulted in a profound reduction of NMDA-induced spectrin proteolysis in the hippocampus, as illustrated in FIGURE 5.

CONCLUSIONS

Activation of the calcium-dependent neutral cysteine protease, calpain I, is an early feature of excitotoxin- and ischemia-induced neuronal injury. The cytoskeletal protein, spectrin, is a preferred substrate of calpain I, and spectrin proteolysis occurs within minutes to hours following calcium-mediated neuronal injury. The extent of neuronal damage is correlated with the magnitude of spectrin proteolysis.

Measurement of injury-induced spectrin breakdown products can also provide a useful means of assessing the neuroprotective activity of agents acting through diverse mechanisms. We have shown that three structurally and functionally dissimilar compounds attenuated spectrin proteolysis induced by administration of the excitotoxins kainic acid or NMDA. Treatment of rats with the known neuroprotective NMDA antagonist, MK-801, resulted in a significant inhibition of spectrin proteolysis in the hippocampus 24 hours following an intrahippocampal NMDA infusion. A protein kinase inhibitor, K-252a, similarly attenuated spectrin

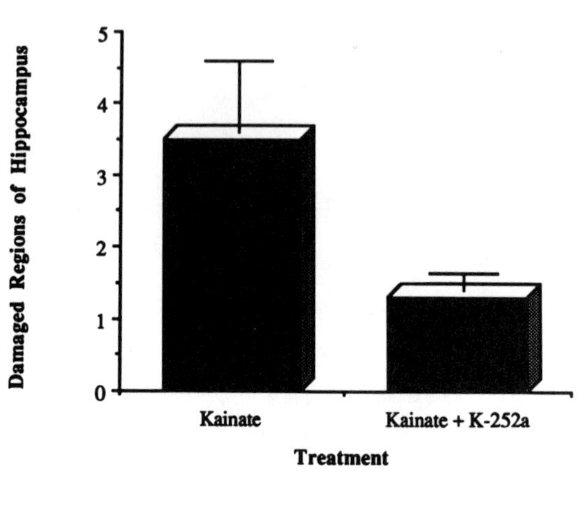

FIGURE 4. Histological analysis of kainic acid-induced hippocampal damage following central administration of K-252a. Rats received an ICV infusion of kainic acid together with vehicle or K-252a. All animals were sacrificed two weeks later, and damage to the hippocampus was evaluated using histological methods described in the text. Data shown are the mean number of CA-regions of the hippocampus damaged from vehicle (kainate) or K-252a (kainate + K-252a) treated animals ± SEM. K-252a treatment significantly reduced the extent of hippocampal damage sustained following an infusion of kainic acid compared to vehicle-treated controls.

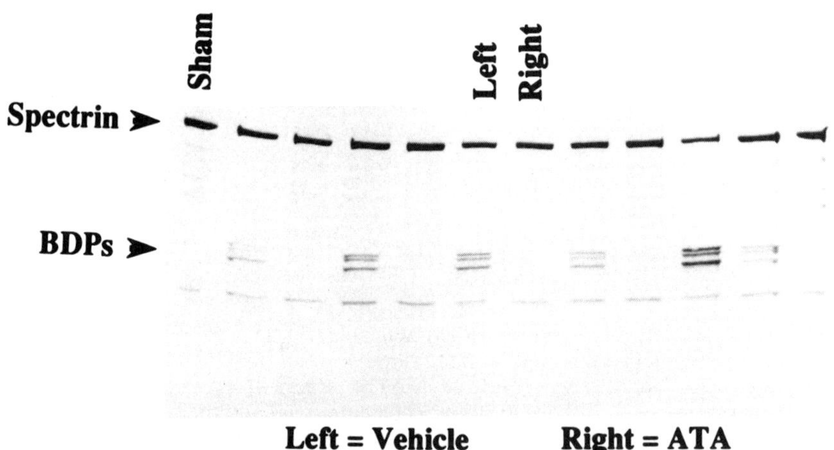

FIGURE 5. Western blot of NMDA-induced spectrin proteolysis following central administration of aurintricarboxylic acid (ATA). Each pair of lanes represents the left and right hippocampus from one animal. All animals except shams received intrahippocampal infusions of NMDA into both left and right sides together with vehicle (left hippocampus), or ATA (right hippocampus). Shams (shown in the first and last lanes) received an intrahippocampal infusion of vehicle, but no NMDA or ATA. The NMDA-induced increase in hippocampal spectrin breakdown products (BDPs) is significantly reduced in the hippocampus receiving ATA treatment compared to the vehicle-treated control side.

breakdown as well as pyramidal cell damage in the hippocampus following intraventricular infusion of kainic acid. Finally, an endonuclease inhibitor, aurintricarboxylic acid, which has been reported to reduce apoptotic cell death,[29] almost completely eliminated hippocampal spectrin breakdown 24 hours following an intrahippocampal infusion of NMDA. These results indicate that the neuroprotective activity of mechanistically dissimilar compounds is associated with an attenuation of excitotoxin-induced spectrin proteolysis. Thus, spectrin proteolysis appears to be a good marker for neuronal injury and assessing the neuroprotective activity of potential therapeutic compounds, as well as a tool for evaluating the role of different biochemical pathways in the intracellular cascades leading to neuronal death in pathological states.

ACKNOWLEDGMENTS

The authors would like to thank V. R. Marcy and Y. Zhao for their expert technical contributions, and Dr. M. E. Lewis for many insightful suggestions and a critical reading of the manuscript.

REFERENCES

1. SIESJO, B. K. 1981. J. Cereb. Blood Flow Metab. **1:** 155–185.
2. SIMAN, R. 1990. *In* Neurotoxicity of Excitatory Amino Acids. A. Guidotti, Ed.: 145–161. Raven Press. New York.
3. SEUBERT, P. & G. LYNCH. 1990. *In* Intracellular Calcium-Dependent Proteolysis. R. L. Mellgren & T. Murachi, Eds.: 251–263. CRC Press. Boca Raton, FL.
4. FAROOQUI, A. A. & L. A. HORROCKS. 1991. Brain Res. Rev. **16:** 171–191.
5. BAZAN, N. G. 1989. Ann. N.Y. Acad. Sci. **559:** 1–16.
6. MANEV, H., E. COSTA, J. T. WROBLEWSKI & A. GUIDOTTI. 1990. FASEB J. **4:** 2789–2797.
7. SERVER, A. C. & W. C. MOBLEY. 1991. *In* Apoptosis. The Molecular Basis of Cell Death. L. D. Tomei & F. O. Cope, Eds.: 263–278. Cold Spring Harbor Laboratory Press. Plainview, NY.
8. SIMAN, R., C. GALL, L. S. PERLMUTTER, C. CHRISTIAN, M. BAUDRY & G. LYNCH. 1985. Brain Res. **347:** 399–403.
9. REGEHR, W. G., J. A. CONNOR & D. W. TANK. 1989. Nature. **341:** 533–536.
10. PUMAIN, R. & U. HEINEMANN. 1985. J. Neurophysiol. **53:** 1–16.
11. SIMAN, R. & J. C. NOSZEK. 1988. Neuron **1:** 279–287.
12. BADALAMENTE, M. A., L. C. HURST & A. STRACHER. 1989. Proc. Natl. Acad. Sci. USA **86:** 5983–5987.
13. AZUMA, M., T. R. SHEARER, T. MATSUMOTO, L. L. DAVID & T. MURACHI. 1990. Exp. Eye Res. **51:** 393–401.
14. LIBBY, P. & A. L. GOLDBERG. 1978. Science. **199:** 534–536.
15. SINGH, I. & A. K. SINGH. 1983. Neurosci. Lett. **39:** 77–82.
16. SATO, A., R. H. QUARLES, R. O. BRADY & W. W. TOURELOTTE. 1984. Ann. Neurol. **15:** 264–267.
17. SCHLAEPFER, W. W. & M. B. HASLER. 1979. Brain Res. **168:** 299–309.
18. IWASKI, Y. H. EZUKA, T. YAMAMOTO, H. KONNO & S. KADOYA. 1985. Brain Res. **347:** 124–126.
19. SEUBERT, P., K. LEE & G. LYNCH. 1989. Brain Res. **492:** 366–370.
20. SIMAN, R., J. C. NOSZEK & C. KEGERISE. 1989. J. Neurosci. **9:** 1579–1590.
21. HU, R.-J. & V. BENNETT. 1991. J. Biol. Chem. **266:** 18200–18205.
22. HARRIS, A. S. & J. S. MORROW. 1990. Proc. Natl. Acad. Sci. USA **87:** 3009–3013.

23. LEE, K. S., S. FRANK, P. VANDERKLISH, A. ARAI & G. LYNCH. 1991. Proc. Natl. Acad. Sci. USA **88:** 7233–7237.
24. FOSTER, A. C., R. GILL, J. A. KEMP & G. N. WOODRUFF. 1987. Neurosci. Lett. **76:** 307–311.
25. FAVARON, M., H. MANEV, H. ALHO, M. BERTOLINO, B. FERRET, A. GUIDOTTI & E. COSTA. 1988. Proc. Natl. Acad. Sci. USA **85:** 7351–7355.
26. BORASIO, G. D. 1990. Neurosci. Lett. **108:** 207–212.
27. ABE, K., M. YOSHIDOMI & K. KOGURE. 1989. Ann. N.Y. Acad. Sci. **559:** 259–268.
28. HARA, H., H. ONODERA, M. YOSHIDOMI, Y. MATSUDA & K. KOGURE. 1990. J. Cereb. Blood Flow Metab. **10:** 646–653.
29. KERR, J. F. R. & B. V. HARMON. 1991. *In* Apoptosis. The Molecular Basis of Cell Death. L. D. Tomei & F. O. Cope, Eds. 5–29. Cold Spring Harbor Laboratory Press. Plainview, NY.
30. LOCKSHIN, R. A. & Z. ZAKERI. 1991. *In* Apoptosis. The Molecular Basis of Cell Death. L. D. Tomei & F. O. Cope, Eds.: 47–60. Cold Spring Harbor Laboratory Press. Plainview, NY.
31. KURE, S., T. TOMINAGA, T. YOSHIMOTO, K. TADA & K. NARISAWA. 1991. Biochem. Biophys. Res. Commun. **179:** 39–45.
32. BATISTATOU, A. & L. A. GREENE. 1991. J. Cell Biol. **115:** 461–471.

The Lysosomal System in Neuronal Cell Death: A Review[a]

RALPH A. NIXON[b–e] AND ANNE M. CATALDO[b,c]

[b]Laboratories for Molecular Neuroscience
Mailman Research Center, McLean Hospital
Belmont, Massachusetts 02178

[c]Department of Psychiatry
[d]Program in Neuroscience
Harvard Medical School
Boston, Massachusetts 02115

INTRODUCTION

The destructive potential of proteases on cells may have been apparent to Salkowski in 1891 when, investigating intracellular proteolysis for the first time, he discovered the phenomenon of autolysis, which includes the self-digestion of tissue proteins.[1] Further studies of the autolytic process in brain in the 1920s[1–3] and the identification of a group of proteolytic enzymes known as cathepsins[1] were followed three decades later by deDuve's discovery of specialized membrane-limited organelles that contain the cathepsins and the many other acid hydrolases of the cell.[4,5] The concept of the lysosome as a physical barrier that prevents highly lytic enzymes from digesting the cells' own cytoplasm presaged not only the role of lysosomes in normal intracellular protein turnover but also their participation in other physiologic and pathologic autolytic phenomena. Among these proposed physiologic functions were the elimination of foreign material introduced into cells by phagocytosis and the digestion of parts or the whole of cells during normal development, involution, metamorphosis, and secretion.[5,6] The possibility that, in pathologic states, damaged lysosomes might release into the cytoplasm hydrolytic enzymes that injure or even kill the cell also became appreciated as soon as the protective role of the lysosomal membrane was realized.[7] The notion of lysosomes as "suicide bags" stimulated experimentation on lysosomes in injured cells, including work by deDuve on ischemic hepatocytes which appeared to support the concept, at least as a late degenerative event.[8] Evidence for intracellular rupture of lysosomes as a common early event in cell injury, however, is still controversial.[9] A close association between lysosomal alterations and the phenomenon of cell death has nevertheless remained a popular and intuitively appealing notion that continues to influence the interpretation of pathologic mechanisms.

[a] The research leading to the data presented from these laboratories was supported by grants from the National Institute on Aging AG08208, AG05134 and AG10916. The McLean Hospital Brain Tissue Research Center is supported by Public Health Service Grant R01-MH/NS31862 and an award from the Seidel Research Fund.

[e] Address correspondence to: Dr. Ralph A. Nixon at the Laboratories for Molecular Neuroscience, Mailman Research Center, McLean Hospital, Belmont, MA 02178.

In this review, we evaluate the behavior of the lysosomal system in relation to various forms of neuronal cell death. Properties of the lysosomal system and problems encountered in its investigation are briefly considered before discussing the relative importance of lysosomes at early and late stages of the cell death process. The developmental state and metabolic individuality of the neurons being studied, as well as the nature of the etiologic event and its chronicity are discussed as factors influencing if, when and how the lysosomal system is called into play as part of the neurodegenerative process. Although the role of lysosomes in neurodegeneration has not been previously considered in detail, reviews on the lysosomal system in neurons,[10–12] and on the general biology[13–15] and pathobiology[6,16] of the lysosomal system have appeared.

THE LYSOSOMAL SYSTEM

Lysosomes are ubiquitous acidic vacuoles containing over 40 hydrolytic enzymes that have acid pH optima and are capable of breaking down most biological polymers to monomers.[7,11] The lysosome originates within a system of intracellular membrane compartments known as the cytoplasmic vacuolar system,[13–15] the main components of which include the nuclear envelope, endoplasmic reticulum, and Golgi complex. The lysosome is the centerpiece of a polymorphic family of acidic vesicular organelles known as the endosomal-lysosomal system (FIG. 1), which includes Golgi-derived vesicles containing newly synthesized hydrolases (primary lysosomes), secondary lysosomes which contain engulfed material and hydrolytic enzymes, and residual bodies containing accumulated indigestible material (FIG. 2). These various lysosomal compartments rapidly and extensively communicate with each other by receptor-targeted membrane fusion,[13] thereby creating an efficient mechanism for protein and membrane trafficking between the Golgi apparatus and the plasma membrane.

As the terminal degradative compartment of the cell,[7,15] lysosomes are the final destination for a broad array of intracellular and endocytosed materials. When the lysosomal system is activated, pre-lysosomal compartments are formed either by the endocytosis of extracellular material (heterophagosomes) or by the engulfment of intracellular organelles or cytoplasm (autophagosomes) (FIG. 1). These compartments eventually fuse with primary lysosomes to form various types of secondary lysosomes (FIG. 3), including autophagic vacuoles, multilamellar bodies (MLB), multivesicular bodies (MVB), and dense bodies, which reflect the nature of the internalized material and represent various transitional states in the digestion process. A rise in their numbers is considered one type of evidence for increased activity of the lysosomal system.[17] Successful lysosomal function calls for the conversion of most complex cellular constituents to monomers (*e.g.*, proteins to amino acids) which may then be reutilized in biosynthesis.

Complete digestion of the material within secondary lysosomes, in principle, should leave little or no residual substrate within the lysosome. Incomplete or unsuccessful digestion, on the other hand, causes undigested material to accumulate and to generate a family of residual bodies (tertiary lysosomes) distinguished in some instances by the nature of the undegraded material that accumulates.[12] An autofluorescent matrix or pigment portion and varying amounts of lipid collect in lipofuscin granules, one of the most common types of residual bodies[12,18–20] (FIGS. 2 and 4). Hydrolases similar to those found in primary and secondary

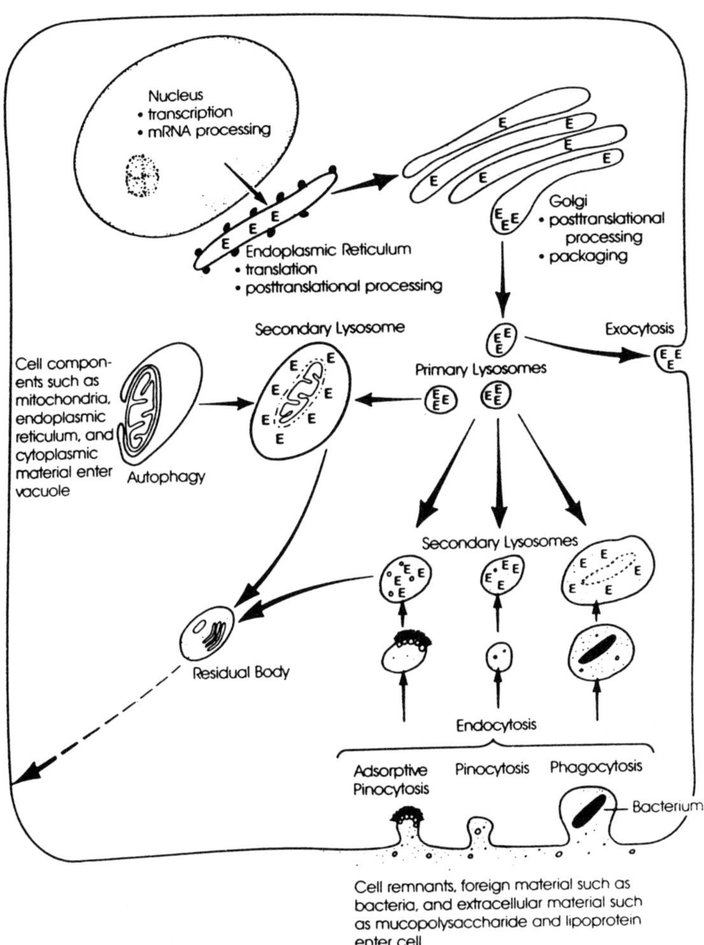

FIGURE 1. The biological life of a lysosome. Acid hydrolases, including precursor forms (represented by E) are synthesized in the ER and undergo posttranslational processing and packaging within the Golgi apparatus. This schematic representation outlines several alternative fates for a newly formed primary lysosome. These include direct export from the cell, fusion with intracellular constituents (autophagy) or internalized material (hetero-phagy) to form secondary lysosomes, and development of residual bodies containing the undigested remnants of heterophagic/autophagic processing. (Reproduced from ref. 87 with permission.)

lysosomes (FIG. 4) may also be present but in widely varying levels in tertiary lysosomes such as lipofuscin granules.[12] Lipofuscin granules (FIG. 4), bounded by a single layer of membrane, have a complex polymorphic structure which is characterized by various combinations of electron lucent lipoid material, electron opaque bodies, and spherical, laminated structures of alternating dense and light bands (myelin figures).[20] In brain, six varieties of lipofuscin have been distinguished ultrastructurally in terms of shape, and relative amount and structure of pigment and content of lipid.[21] Nearly a century of investigation supports claims for lipofuscin accumulation as being among the most prominent and reliable mor-

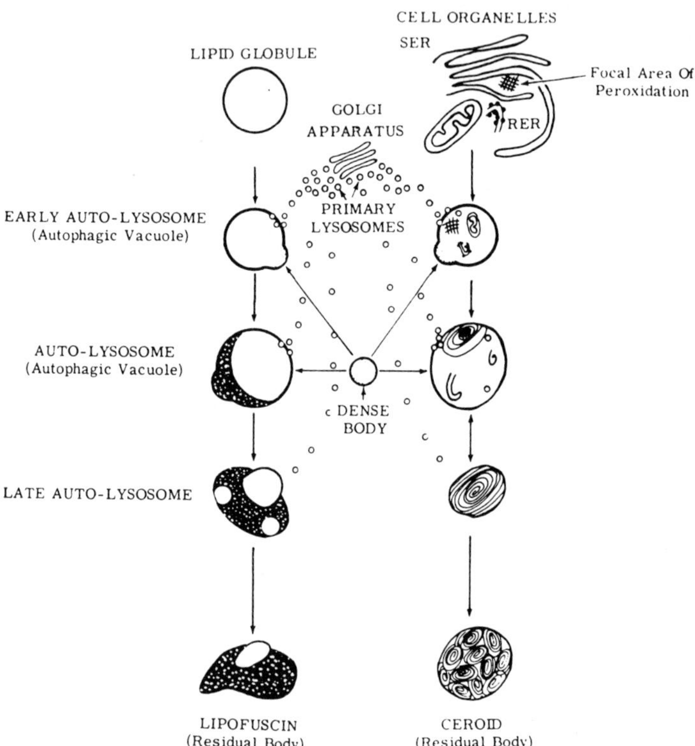

FIGURE 2. Biogenesis of lipopigments. Formation of lipopigment granules begins with the production of acid hydrolases in the smooth endoplasmic reticulum (SER) followed by subsequent packaging in the Golgi apparatus, sorting, and receptor-mediated translocation of newly synthesized acid hydrolases to primary lysosomes. Autophagocytosis of intracellular lipid and/or cell organelles enclosed by membrane donated by the ER fuse with primary lysosomes, resulting in the formation of organelles defined as secondary lysosomes, autosomes or autophagic vacuoles. The incomplete digestion of the material within the autophagic vacuole yields residual material that accumulates (especially within non-dividing cells) in complex organelles called residual bodies. In brain, the lipopigments, lipofuscin and ceroid, are two types of residual bodies that autofluoresce with ultraviolet light. (Reproduced from ref. 12 with permission.)

pologic correlates of cellular aging in some postmitotic cells such as brain (FIG. 5) and muscle (reviews in refs. 12 and 19). This relationship and the observations that lipofuscin accumulation is accelerated in certain pathologic conditions (FIG. 6) have fueled the notion that lipofuscin is a harbinger of metabolic compromise

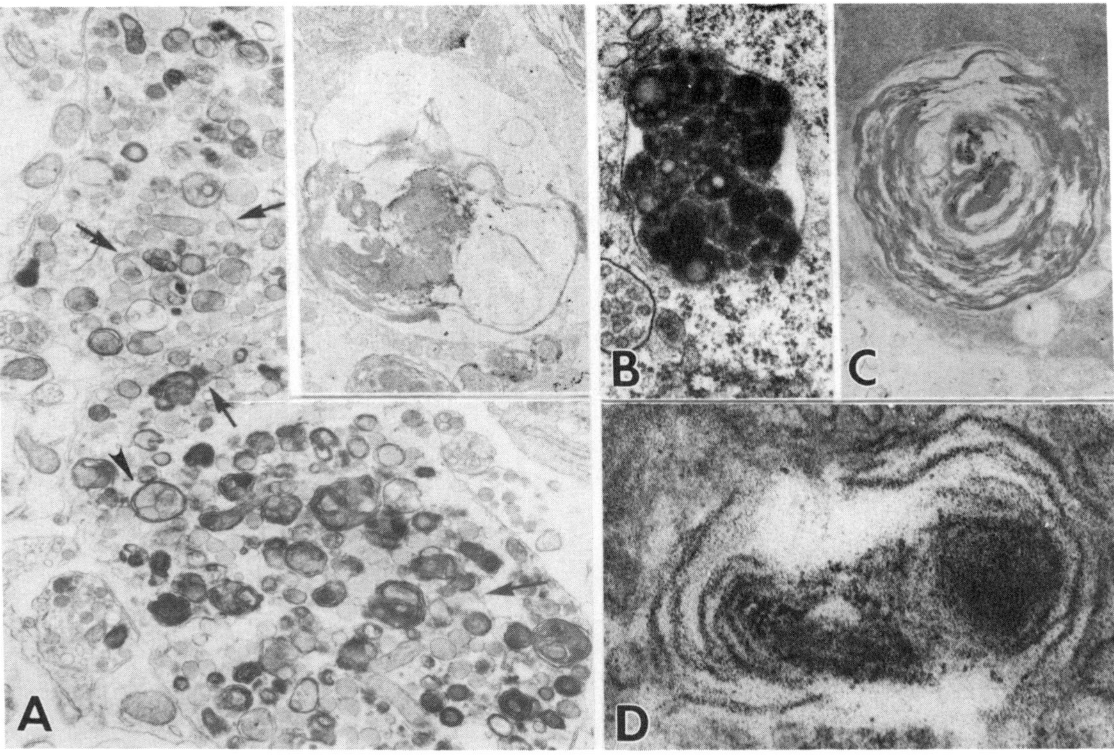

FIGURE 3. In the neurohypophysis of a salt-stressed mouse, some preterminal swellings contain numerous secondary lysosomes in the form of multilamellar bodies (**A**, *arrowhead and inset*). Segments of ER (**A**, *arrows*) appear to wrap around some of these structures. Other types of secondary lysosomes commonly seen in neural and non-neural tissues include multivesicular bodies (**B**), myelin whorls (**C**), and autophagic vacuoles (**D**).

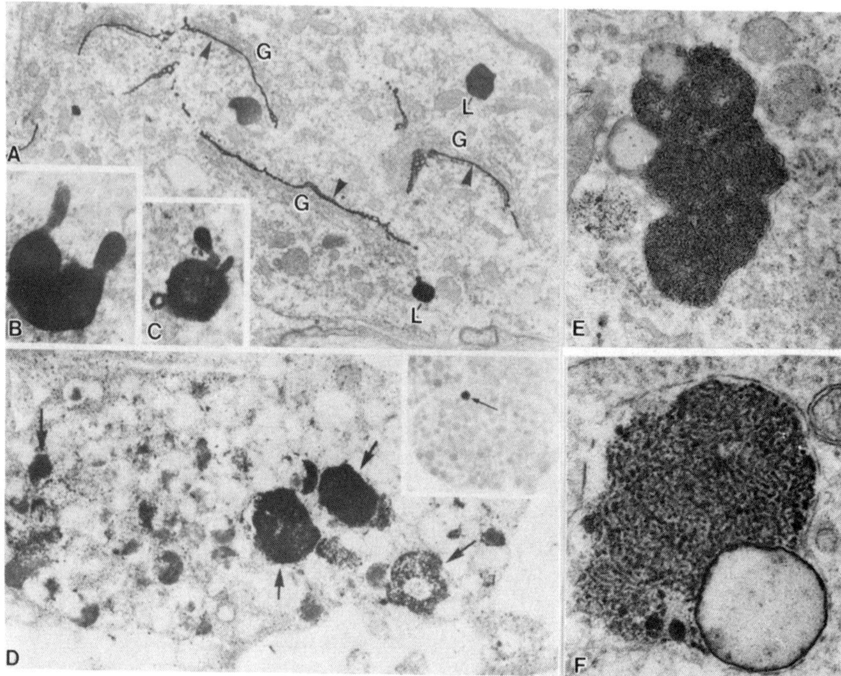

FIGURE 4. In the cell body of a mouse supraoptic neuron (**A**), acid phosphatase activity is localized in some secondary lysosomes (L) and in the transmost Golgi saccule (G, *arrowheads*) which corresponds to GERL. In a supraoptic neuron of a salt-stressed mouse, acid phosphatase-positive tubules measuring 100–200 nm wide are confluent with perikaryal secondary lysosomes (**B** and **C**). Acid hydrolase-positive lysosomes similar in size to autophagic/crinophagic vacuoles and 100–300 nm wide secretory granules (**D**, *arrows*) are prevalent in a preterminal swelling from a salt-stressed mouse, but are rare in preterminals of the neurohypophysis from a control mouse (**D**, *inset, arrow*). Residual structures such as lipofuscin granules (**E** and **F**) are types of tertiary lysosomes that are common in postmitotic cells such as neurons. These structures commonly contain some hydrolase activity.

or functional decline,[152,153] although the case for this idea is not unequivocal[19,22,23] as discussed later.

LYSOSOMAL SYSTEM ANALYSIS: PROBLEMS AND LIMITATIONS

Assessing the relative importance of particular metabolic events to the mechanisms of neuronal cell death is difficult, and the relationship of the lysosome system to neurodegeneration is no exception. In evaluating past studies, we applied several criteria that, if satisfied, might indicate an important contribution of the lysosomal system to neuronal cell death. These include: 1) a lysosomal response that precedes the typical morphologic changes of cellular necrosis or apoptosis; 2) a lysosomal response of sufficient magnitude to distinguish it from normal physiologic responses; and 3) a reasonably direct biologic link between the lysosomal response and the cell death process. Unfortunately, these criteria are not always easily applied to the existing data. Information about changes in specific organelles of the lysosomal system is often not quantitative or available from control and experimental cell populations of adequate size for statistical analysis. When the neurodegenerative condition is examined at a single stage in

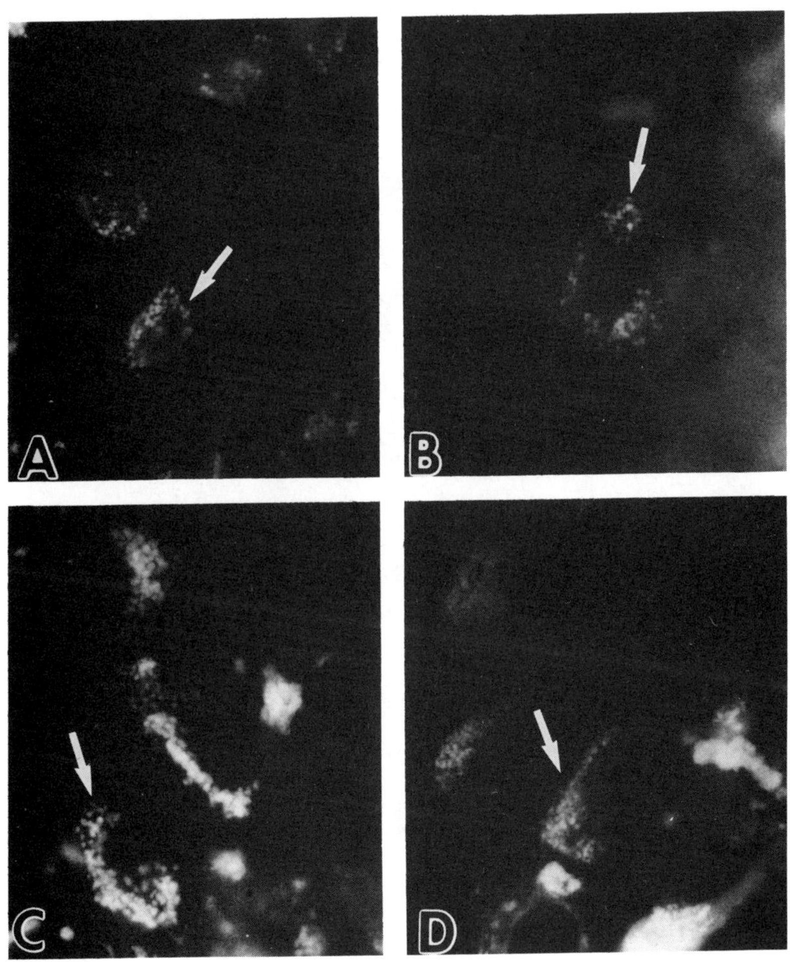

FIGURE 5. Lipofuscin granules are one of the most common types of residual bodies. An increase in the numbers of these autofluorescent granules is a common feature of aging in some neuronal cell types. Random neurons within cortical laminae III and V of a young individual (**A** and **B**) contain minimal autofluorescent lipofuscin (*arrows*). Neurons from the same region of the brain from an aged control individual (**C** and **D**) show increased numbers of lipofuscin granules (*arrows*).

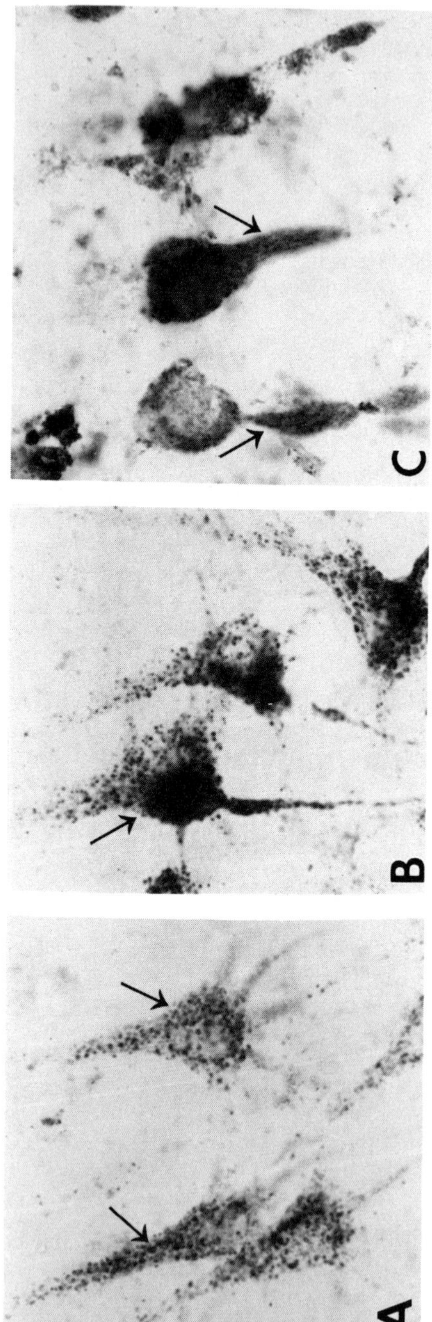

FIGURE 6. In neurons from an aged control brain (**A**), cathepsin-D reactive lysosomes (*arrows*) are abundant in the cell soma and proximal dendrites and scarce in the axon. In brains from individuals with Alzheimer disease (**B**) and Batten's disease (**C**), distinctive alterations are seen in the content and distribution of hydrolase-positive lysosomes (*arrows*), predominantly in the form of lipofuscin granules and ceroid, respectively.

disease progression, the timing of lysosomal changes relative to other structural alterations may not be apparent. As discussed later, metabolic and structural differences among neurons that vary in type or developmental stage or that come from different species may also influence the lysosomal response and limit the ability to compare studies of different neuronal systems.

Even a minimal evaluation of the lysosomal response and its physiological significance requires that secondary lysosomes be distinguished from residual bodies, because these organelles may provide different information about the functional state of the system. Measurements of intracellular autofluorescence, for example, only report on lipofuscin accumulation and give relatively little information about secondary lysosomes and lysosomal system activity. Enzyme cytochemical markers may label individual components of the lysosomal compartment selectively but, by light microscopy, do not necessarily discriminate between them. Even at the electron microscope level, the morphologic appearance of the lysosomal system represents only a static image of the system at a single instant. Whether, for example, lipofuscin has accumulated because of more rapid production, impaired removal, or redistribution from other parts of the neuron may not be easily discerned without applying methods that can monitor the dynamics of lysosome biogenesis and trafficking at various stages of the pathologic process. Finally, some lysosomal disturbances that might be highly relevant to cell death mechanisms, such as a change in lysosomal membrane stability or permeability, are not easily monitored, especially in postmortem tissue. Despite these limitations, the available data yield several potentially useful impressions about the participation of the lysosomal system in neuronal cell injury and cell death.

RESPONSES OF THE LYSOSOMAL SYSTEM IN NEURODEGENERATIVE STATES

Several general morphological patterns of lysosomal system response to neurodegeneration can be identified from a survey of the neuropathological literature (TABLES 1–3). It is important to emphasize that in many of these studies we could not exclude the possibility that changes have occurred in the dynamics or biochemistry of the neuronal lysosomal system that might be highly relevant to cell death but were not evident morphologically. For example, disruption of a population of lysosomes, as might be induced by lysosomotrophic agents,[24] may be highly cytotoxic but may not be easily detected without special techniques. On the other hand, certain aspects of lysosomal behavior, such as lysosomal system activation and increased lysosomal proteolysis, seem usually to be reflected morphologically.[17]

Neuronal cell death in some pathologic states proceeds in the apparent absence of a lysosome response detectable by standard ultrastructural analyses (TABLE 1). The long list of conditions in TABLE 1, which includes examples of necrotic or apoptotic cell death,[43] suggests that activation of the lysosomal system, at least as evidenced morphologically, is not a universal concomitant of neuronal cell death. Because cells eventually lyse in all forms of cell death, however, the rupture of lysosomes and leakage of hydrolytic enzymes are inevitable consequences of end-stage cell death. At this late stage of the process, lysosomal rupture may be less of a critical factor in the mechanism of cell death than in the process of breaking down and removing cellular debris.

In another heterogeneous group of neuropathologic states (TABLE 2), lysosomal

TABLE 1. Neurodegenerative States Associated with Minimal Morphologic Response of the Neuronal Lysosomal System

Natural neuronal cell death—development[25–28]
Peripheral deprivation—development[26–30]
Purkinje cell degeneration (Pcd mutation)[31,32]
Werdnig Hoffman disease[33]
Ischemia[34,35]
Experimental hypertensive injury[36]
Radiation (acute)[37]
Acrylamide neurotoxicity[38]
Triortho cresylphosphate neurotoxicity[39]
Aluminum neurotoxicity[40]
Amyotrophic lateral sclerosis[41]
Creutzfeldt-Jakob disease[42]

system activation, reflected by modest increases in secondary lysosomes (autophagic vacuoles, dense bodies or MLBs), takes place in association with ultrastructural changes typical of either necrosis or apoptosis (TABLE 2). In some cases, the lysosomal changes were known to occur after degeneration was well under way, suggesting that lysosomal system activation was probably not causal but rather a secondary response to the degenerative process. Although such a response may contribute to cell injury, it is equally possible that these lysosomal activities are compensatory and reflect the cell's attempt to survive the insult by breaking down non-essential components and using these materials for repair. The variables that distinguish the lysosomal system response in the conditions listed in TABLE 2 from the minimal response seen in the TABLE 1 group are not clear, though several possibilities are discussed in a later section.

Several types of lysosomal responses may clearly precede most other alterations of cytoplasmic or membranous ultrastructure in certain neurodegenerative states (TABLE 3). In a few of these conditions, the predominant response is autophagic—an activation of the lysosomal system as evidenced by prominent increases in secondary lysosomes. The autophagic response is often accompanied by an increased accumulation of residual bodies, as in Alzheimer's disease[64–71] and chloroquine toxicity.[57,60] As considered further below, increased autophagy is not necessarily a pathologic response in these conditions. In a wide variety of physiologic states, cells greatly increase the rate of autophagy as one step in the restructuring process that accompanies major morphogenetic events or changes in availability of nutrients.[7,17] These autophagic responses are reversible and, rather than having lethal consequences, represent one important way that cells adapt successfully to changing conditions. Early autophagic responses in some pathologic states may, therefore, reflect regenerative attempts that ultimately fail to sustain the neuron.

TABLE 2. Neurodegenerative States Associated with Late Morphologic Responses of the Neuronal Lysosomal System

Axotomy[44–47]	Radiation[53]
Chromatolysis[44,46,48]	Guanethidine[54]
Malnutrition[49]	n-Hexane[55]
Wobbler mutation[50–52]	

In some forms of neurodegeneration, residual bodies or abnormal lysosomes containing storage material accumulate as a predominant early feature of the degenerative process (TABLE 3). Though seemingly quite diverse in etiology, most of these degenerative states seem to share one of two general molecular features that may help to explain the early lysosomal involvement, namely a direct impairment of the lysosome's degradative machinery or an enhanced generation of modified substrates that resist digestion.

More than 25 lysosomal storage diseases have now been discovered in which genetic defects in one of the many acid hydrolases or other proteins of the lysosome are associated with progressive neurodegeneration.[87,88] In these diseases, sub-

TABLE 3. Neurodegenerative Conditions Associated with Prominent Early Responses of the Neuronal Lysosomal System

Secondary Lysosome Alterations
  Chloroquine[57,60]
  Nutritional deprivation—Anuran[61]
  Natural cell ceath—Anuran[62,63]
  Alzheimer's disease[64-71]
Lipofuscin
  Chloroquine[57]
  Leupeptin[57-60]
  Vitamin E deficiency[72,73]
  Irradiation (chronic)[37]
  Parkinson's disease[74]
  Motor neuron degeneration—late-onset mouse mutation[75]
  Progressive supranuclear palsy[76]
  Medial frontal epilepsy[77]
  Alzheimer's disease[64-71,78,79]
Ceroid[80-84]
  Neuronal ceroid lipofuscinoses (*e.g.*, Batten's, Kuf's)[80-84]
  Hermansky-Pudlak syndrome[85]
  Myoclonus epilepsy[86]
Storage Bodies[16,84,87-89]
  Sphingolipidoses (*e.g.*, Niemann, Pick, Gaucher, Tay-Sachs)[90,91]
  Mucopolysaccharidoses (*e.g.*, Hurler)[90]
  Glycoproteinoses (*e.g.*, mannosidoses)[92]
  Acid lipase deficiency (*e.g.*, Wolman)[93]
  Glycogenoses type II (*e.g.*, Pompe)[94,95]
  Mucolipidoses (*e.g.*, Type I)[84]

strates that are normally degraded by the defective enzyme accumulate and generate abnormal lysosomes with distinctive light microscopic and ultrastructural features that may be diagnostic for the particular disease. The lysosomal system may also be involved directly in other hereditary diseases where the precise molecular defect is still unknown. For example, ceroid lipofuscinosis or Batten's disease and related disorders including Kuf's disease[80-84] and myoclonus epilepsy with Lafora bodies[86] result in the accumulation of ceroid lipopigment, which is morphologically similar but biochemically distinct from lipofuscin.[12] Defective lysosomal proteolysis has been suggested as the molecular basis for certain types of this disorder.[96-98] Unquestionably, in these storage disorders, defective functioning of lysosomes results in neuronal cell death, but it is far from clear whether the defective lysosome is the direct cause of cell death in any of these conditions. The functional impairment of any organelle essential to neuron function might be expected to lead indirectly to cell death even though the organelle is not part of a specific cell death mechanism.

Lysosomal function may also be directly impaired by chemical toxins, leading to residual body accumulation and neurodegeneration. Leupeptin, an inhibitor of the lysosomal protease cathepsins and other cysteine proteases, causes ceroid lipofuscin and dense bodies to form rapidly[57–60] and induces Purkinje cell degeneration.[57] Interestingly, neocortical pyramidal cells also accumulate lipofuscin but do not degenerate, indicating that, as in normal aging, abundant lipofuscin accumulation does not necessarily signal the demise of the cell. Chloroquine, one of a family of lysosomotropic agents,[60,99,100] poisons the lysosome system in another way. After diffusing into lysosomes as a neutral species, it becomes protonated and trapped because of the impermeability of the lysosomal membrane to cations. Lysosomal proteolysis is inhibited as the pH of the lysosome rises above the optimum for most proteolytic enzymes. Under these conditions, abundant multilamellar bodies appear together with accumulations of lipofuscin,[57] Purkinje cells degenerate, and axonal dystrophy may occur in other neuronal populations.[57–60]

Many of the other neuropathologic states in TABLE 3, though quite diverse in etiology, share in common metabolic disturbances that may result in the chemical modification of cellular constituents, thereby rendering them less digestible by lysosomal hydrolases. The target of the modification is most often the membrane. Considerable support exists for the theory that lipopigment accumulation arises largely from abnormal peroxidation of lipids due to free radical injury to membranes.[101,102] In vitamin E deficiency, the classical example of experimentally induced lipofuscinosis, cells are partly deprived of one of the most effective antioxidant agents for removing peroxides and blocking free radical formation.[103] Oxidation of membrane lipids and proteins by free radicals is considered a major toxic effect of chronic radiation.[47,104,105] Lipid peroxidation is also selectively increased in the substantia nigra in Parkinson's disease.[106,114] Mesencephalic dopaminergic neurons, which degenerate in this disease, are at particular risk for generating free radicals during the synthesis of neuromelanin[107,108] as well as the oxidative degradation of dopamine by monoamine oxidase B, an enzyme enriched in the substantia nigra.[109] Abnormalities of iron handling in Parkinson's disease may also predispose neurons to form toxic hydroxyl and superoxide radicals.[110–115] Although the case for excessive lipid peroxidation in Alzheimer's disease is not as well developed, injury or dysfunction of membranes is suggested by changes in membrane lipid composition,[116,117] altered activities and properties of integral membrane proteins,[118] marked increases in lipolytic enzymes,[119] and altered iron homeostasis.[120,121]

FACTORS INFLUENCING LYSOSOMAL SYSTEM RESPONSES IN NEURONAL CELL DEATH

The foregoing discussion suggests that etiologic factors, particularly those targeting specific organelles, greatly influence the nature and timing of lysosomal responses during neurodegeneration. The importance of the inciting stimulus to cell death is further illustrated by the responses of chick isthmo optic neurons induced to die by different treatments. If only afferent connections to the neuron are removed, cell death is accompanied by a robust autophagic response and increased hydrolase expression.[30] If deefferentation is combined with deafferentation, however, these cells exhibit a much more modest autophagic response even though they degenerate at the same rate.[30] In other studies of the same neuron population, deefferentation alone resulted in a nuclear pattern of degeneration with little evidence of a significant lysosomal response.[28] These and other observations show that varying lysosomal system responses can be elicited within the same neuron depending on the pathologic insult that initiates cell death. The degeneration of Purkinje cells, for example, may be associated with little apparent lysosomal response in genetic disorders[31,32] or after axotomy[45] but is accompanied by greatly increased autophagy in chloroquine neurotoxicity or accumulation of ceroid lipofuscin in leupeptin toxicity.[57]

Other variables that may influence the cell's responses to a metabolic insult include species differences, stage of neuronal development, duration of the insult, and pace of cell death. Earlier studies providing the strongest evidence linking the lysosomal system with mechanisms of neuronal cell death have tended to involve lower vertebrates and invertebrates. Robust accumulations of dense bodies and autophagic vacuoles accompany the programmed cell death of lateral motor column neurons in *Rana pipiens*[62] and of neuron populations in the crab.[63] Large lipofuscin accumulations are also seen after chronic irradiation in neurons of *Torpedo*.[37] These prominent lysosomal responses contrast with those exhibited by neurons undergoing developmentally regulated cell death in different mammalian and avian species (TABLE 1). Variability in the extent of lipofuscin accumulation within the same neurons (*e.g.*, Purkinje cells) from different species during normal aging[122] also point to possible species-dependent influences on lysosomal function.

The stage of development of neurons is believed to influence their vulnerability and patterns of degeneration. For example, a neuron that dies before it reaches its normal target may exhibit a quite different degenerative pattern (*e.g.*, "nuclear") than the one observed when death occurs after these targets are reached (*e.g.*, "cytoplasmic").[19] Developmental factors may also be relevant to the lysosomal response in neurodegeneration. Lysosomes concentrate within dendrites in early development, but, with maturity, the lysosomal density decreases in these processes and increases in the perikaryon.[123] Residual bodies are infrequent in immature neurons but accumulate markedly with age.[23] What these developmental differences imply about the efficiency of the lysosome is unclear; nevertheless, they may relate to observations that morphological lysosomal responses tend to be less striking in immature *mammalian* neurons that die in various conditions including naturally occurring cell death[25-28] or cell death induced either by peripheral deprivation[26-30] or as a result of various mutations.[31,32,50-52] Developmentally regulated cell death in some lower vertebrates and invertebrates may be exceptions,[62,63] as previously discussed. The lysosomal response in dying anterior horn cells of young mice expressing the Wobbler mutation[50-51] is minimal compared to the massive lipofuscinosis that accompanies loss of the same cell population in the motor neuron degeneration (Mnd) mouse, a mutant strain in which motor neurons degenerate only in late adulthood (FIG. 7). Obviously, factors other than maturational state could also explain these differences.

Other variables likely affect the kind of lysosomal changes that a neuron will display before it degenerates, but information is not sufficient to isolate these variables and evaluate them independently of the overriding influence of etiologic factors. The metabolic individuality of different cell populations may account for the 10-fold higher lipofuscin accumulation in inferior olivary neurons compared to Purkinje cells during aging[124,141] and may explain some regional differences in lysosomal response in some pathologic states. The tendency of conditions with more protracted disease courses (*e.g.*, vitamin E deficiency, Parkinson's disease, Alzheimer's disease, motor neuron degeneration mutation) (TABLE 3) to display prominent accumulation of residual bodies (FIGS. 7–9) may suggest that the pace

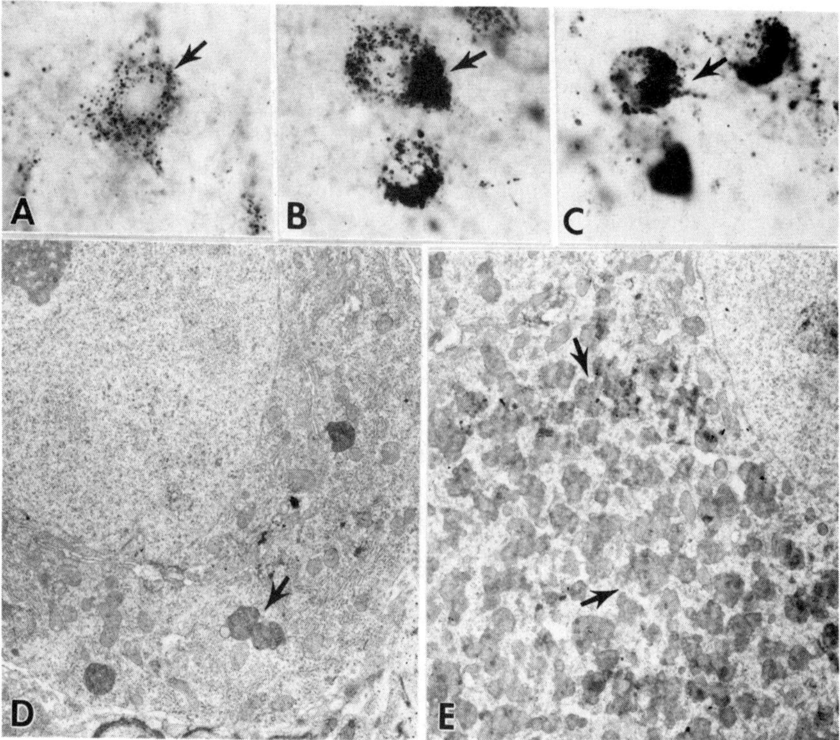

FIGURE 7. The immunolabeling pattern in anterior horn cells of control mice decorated with an antibody to cathepsin D (**A**) contrasts with that in motor neurons of mice harboring the Mnd (motor neuron degeneration) mutation which causes a late-age-onset degenerative state. Increased levels of cathepsin D (*arrows*) are detected at the presymptomatic (**B**) and mild to moderate (**C**) stages of the disorder. Lipofuscin granules were dramatically increased and structurally altered in affected Mnd neurons when compared with cells from age-matched control animals (**D** and **E**, arrows).

of cell death may affect the extent to which the lysosomal system can respond and the nature of this response. For example, the accumulation of residual bodies in degenerating neurons of Torpedo after chronic low-dose radiation, but not in neurons induced to die more quickly by high-dose radiation,[37] is consistent with this idea, although these observations can also be explained in other ways.

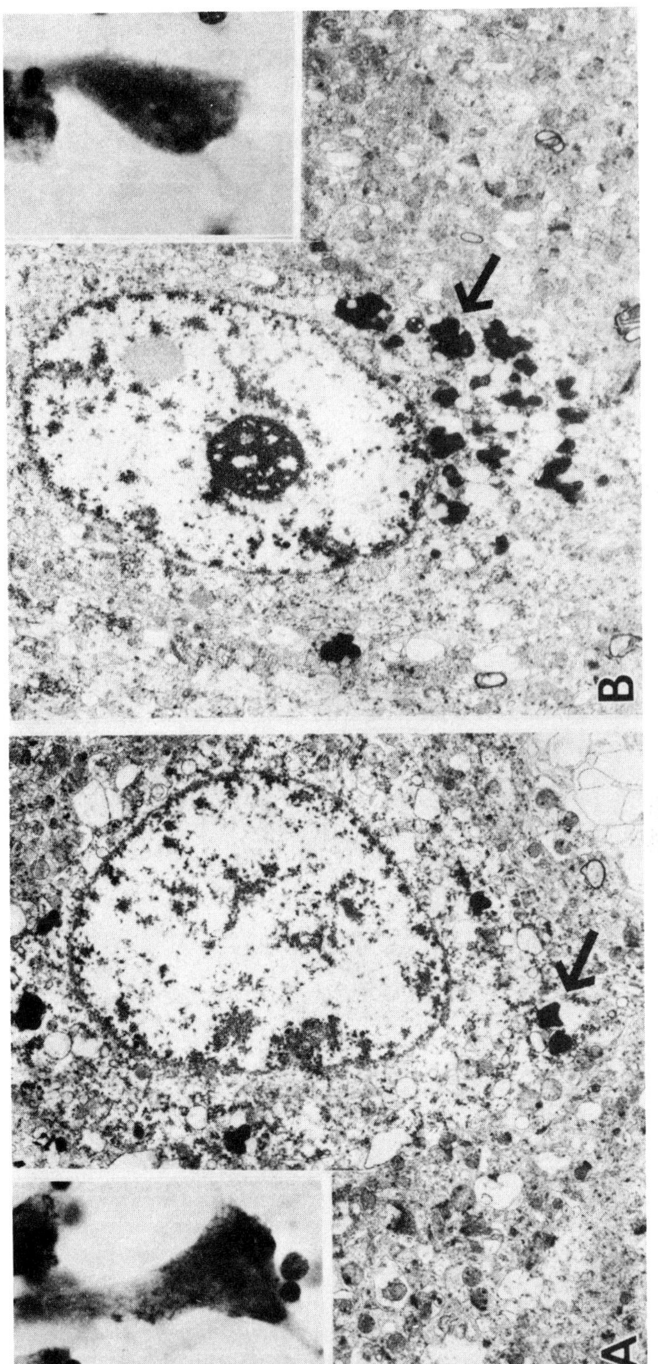

FIGURE 8. Immunoelectron labeling studies show residual bodies/lipofuscin granules (*arrows*) stained by an antibody to the lysosomal hydrolase, cathepsin D, in neurons from a control (**A**) and Alzheimer's (**B**) brain. This increase in immunoreactive organelles precedes chromatolytic changes that are detectable by Nissl staining in the same cells at lower magnification (**A** and **B**, *insets*).

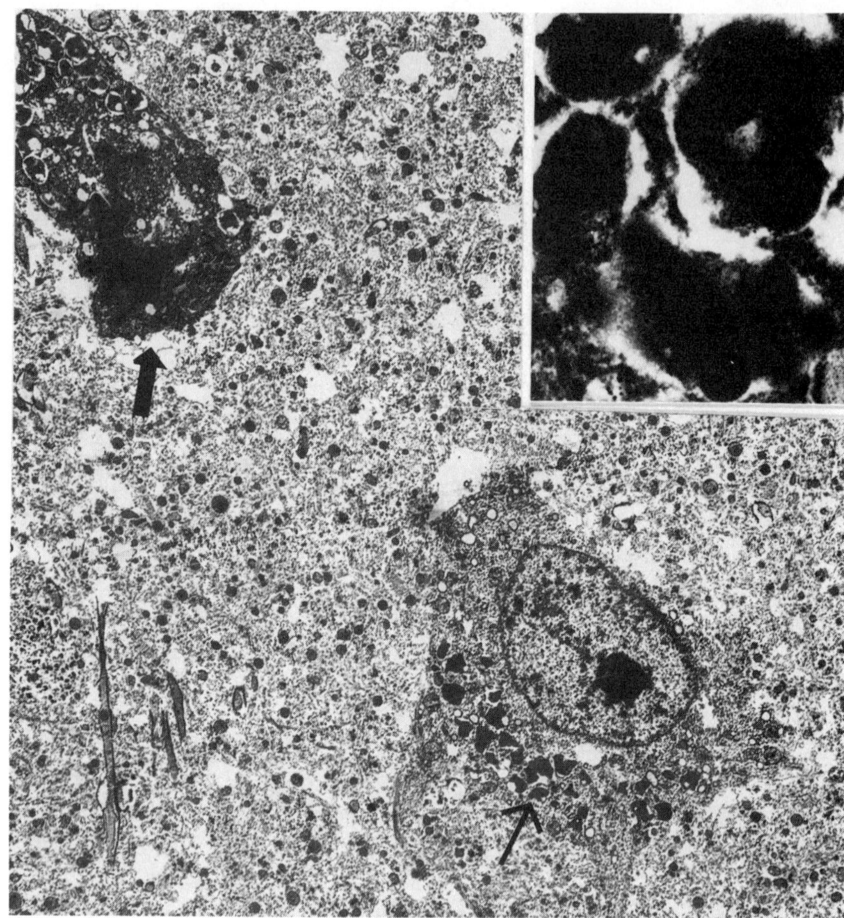

FIGURE 9. Two neurons from an Alzheimer's disease brain are decorated by an antibody to the lysosomal hydrolase, hexosaminidase A (HEX). One relatively normal-appearing neuron (*lower right*) contains abundant immunoreactive lipofuscin (*thin arrow*). A second degenerating neuron contains individual reactive lipofuscin granules as well as large HEX-positive lipofuscin aggregates (*thick arrow*). A higher magnification of this material is shown in the inset. From ref. 68, used with permission.)

RELATIONSHIP OF LYSOSOMAL CHANGES TO NEURONAL CELL DEATH

Given that various lysosomal system responses can be elicited during neurodegeneration, what is the evidence that these lysosomal changes contribute directly to the demise of the cell and are not a compensatory response or a metabolic disturbance separate from the neurodegenerative mechanism? Few studies in neurons address this question definitively. Conceivably, the lysosomal system could contribute to cell death in several ways: 1) rupture of the lysosome and intracellular release of lytic enzymes might cause the uncontrolled digestion of cellular constituents; 2) autophagy may exceed the rate of replacement of essential cellular constituents; 3) accumulation of secondary lysosomes or residual bodies might sterically interfere with transport mechanisms, metabolic pathways, and structural integrity of the cell, and 4) lysosome dysfunction might disrupt processes critical to cellular vitality including protein synthesis, gluconeogenesis, *etc.*

Lysosomal rupture or intracellular leakage of lysosomal hydrolases has perhaps the greatest potential as a mechanism for directly killing cells. Cellular self-digestion would be expected from the uncontrolled actions of some proteases and other hydrolases including, RNAse and DNAse, which retain partial activity at neutral pH. Under conditions of hypoxia, the solubilization and activation of these enzymes may be accelerated due to metabolic acidosis.[125] Several degenerative states involving non-neural cells are known where lethal injury has been shown to be initiated by lysosomal rupture.[9] The inciting toxic agent in these cases accumulates in the lysosome and damages the lysosomal membrane. Silica[126] or sodium urate crystals[127] phagocytosed by macrophages or leukocytes interact with, and eventually rupture, the lysosomal membrane as evidenced by the intracellular dispersal of lysosomal hydrolases and the liberation of the crystals themselves into the cytoplasm. A variant of this form of lethal cell injury results from the accumulation in lysosomes of certain photosensitive dyes which then damage the lysosomal membrane if a peroxidation reaction is induced by exposing the cells to appropriate wavelengths of light in the presence of oxygen.[9,128] Finally, certain weakly basic amines designed to have detergent activity concentrate several hundred-fold in lysosomes and appear to increase the intracytoplasmic leakage of one or a few lysosomal hydrolases.[99] In the case of one such agent, cysteine cathepsins were the major cytotoxic factors released from the lysosome.[24] In sublethal stages of certain forms of cell injury, particularly those initiated by calcium overload, mitochondrial changes are among the earliest subcellular alterations. It has been proposed that lysosomes catalyze the disruption of mitochondrial oxidative phosphorylation through the coupled action of a lipolytic (phospholipid-hydrolyzing) enzyme within the lysosomal membrane and phospholipase A.[129] Subsequent mitochondrial swelling in later stages of cell injury are thought to be due to membrane-lytic lipids generated by lysosomal lipases.[130] In the nervous system, membrane stability of neuronal lysosomes is reported to be reduced as a result of normal aging[131] and Alzheimer's disease,[132] but the possibility of lysosome rupture as a killing mechanism has not been investigated in any detail.

As discussed earlier, stimulation of autophagy is a common response to many physiological stimuli, and massive increases in autophagic vacuoles may increase massively and reversibly in cells that do not degenerate.[17] For example, chlorpromazine induces in cultured rat dorsal root ganglion neurons a rapid and robust increase in autophagic vacuoles and MLBs associated with increases in acid phosphatase activity.[56] Chromatolytic changes are uncommon, mitochondria are normal and the endoplasmic reticulum and Golgi apparatus are minimally affected. Although the actions of chlorpromazine are not fully understood, some of its main effects are believed to be exerted mainly on membranes, especially those of lysosomes within which the drug is thought to concentrate.[56,133–135]

Lipofuscin may accumulate in some neurons in aging brain to levels that seem to distend the perikaryon[70,136] (FIG. 6). These accumulations may be associated with cell death within some neuronal populations[137,138] but not in others.[139] Moreover, aging-related cell death may take place in some cell populations that do not accumulate lipofuscin,[140] suggesting that these two phenomena are not directly linked. It has been proposed that very large accumulations of lipofuscin in some neurons represent at least a physical impediment to cell function;[152,153] however, evidence for this has been equivocal.[19,22,23,142] For example, the accumulation of lipofuscin in large amounts during aging has little effect on cellular function as reflected in alterations of RNA levels and nucleolar volume.[124] On the other hand, an aging-related decrease in mitral cells of the rat olfactory bulb strongly correlated with an increase in the volume of dense bodies, which preceded a sharp decrease in rough ER and mitochondrial volume.[138] These results and the earlier discussion suggest that lipofuscinosis may well reflect particular states of altered metabolism, but its role as an effector of cell dysfunction or cell death is still questioned.

Lysosomal degradation serves several critical regulatory functions in the cell besides the normal turnover of intracellular organelles and internalized extracellular components. Amino acid and glucose homeostasis both depend on the proper catabolism of proteins and carbohydrates.[143–146] Lysosomes influence vitamin B12 metabolism by degrading a cobalamin binding protein important in the uptake of the vitamin.[147,148] Cholesterol biosynthesis is also regulated in part by the endocytosis and degradation of circulating low-density lipoprotein particles.[149–151] Primary defects in the lysosomal system are likely to impact negatively on the viability of neurons especially in the face of other superimposed metabolic insults or normal age-related impairments. Although it is difficult to assess their contribution in any given degenerative condition, such effects could be a significant factor in the neuronal cell death associated with many of the neuropathologic states in TABLE 3.

SUMMARY AND CONCLUSIONS

The lysosomal system has often been considered a prominent morphologic marker of distressed or dying neurons. Lysosomes or their constituent hydrolases have been viewed in different neuropathologic states as either initiators and direct agents of cell death, agents of cellular repair and recompensation, effectors of end-stage cellular dissolution, or autolytic scavengers of cellular debris. Limited data and limitations of methodology often do not allow these potential roles to be discriminated. In all forms of neurodegeneration, it may be presumed that lysosomes ultimately rupture and release various hydrolases that promote cell autolysis during the final stages of cellular disintegration. Beyond this perhaps universal contribution to cell death, the degree to which the lysosomal system may be involved in neurodegenerative states varies considerably. In many conditions, morphologic evidence for activation of the lysosomal system is minimal or undetectable. In other cases, lysosomal activation is evident only when other morphologic signs of cell injury are also present. This level of participation may be viewed as either an attempt by the neuron to compensate for or repair the injury or a late-stage event leading to cell dissolution. The early involvement of the lysosomal system in neurodegeneration occurs most commonly in the form of intraneuronal accumulations of abnormal storage profiles or residual bodies (tertiary lysosomes). Very often the lysosomal involvement can be traced to a primary defect or dysfunction of lysosomal components or to accelerated or abnormal membrane breakdown that leads to the buildup of modified digestion-resistant substrates within lysosomes. Because they are often striking, changes in the lysosomal system are a sensitive morphologic indicator of certain types of metabolic distress; however, whether they reflect a salutary response of a compromised neuron or a mechanism to promote cell death and removal of debris from the brain remains to be established for most conditions. Factors that may influence the lysosomal response during lethal neuronal injury include species differences, stage of neuronal development, duration of injury and pace of cell death. The lysosomal system may be more closely coupled to certain forms of neuronal cell death in lower vertebrate or invertebrate systems than in mammalian systems.

ACKNOWLEDGMENTS

The authors wish to thank Drs. Peter Hollenbeck, Stephen Berman and Sherry Bursztajn for helpful comments on the manuscript, and Mrs. Johanne Khan for assistance with manuscript preparation.

REFERENCES

1. NEUBERGER, A. 1981. Trends Biochem. Sci. **6:** 139–141.
2. GIBSON, C. A., F. UMBREIT & H. C. BRADLEY. 1921. J. Biol. Chem. **47:** 333–339.
3. POPE, A. & R. A. NIXON. 1984. Neurochem. Res. **9:** 291–323.
4. DE DUVE, C., B. C. PRESSMAN, R. GIANETTI, R. WATTIAUX & F. APPELMAN. 1955. Biochem. J. **60:** 604–617.
5. DE DUVE, C. 1959. *In* Subcellular Particles. T. Hayashi, Ed.: 128–159. The Ronald Press. New York.
6. YU, Q.-C. & L. MARZELLA. 1990. *In* Cell Death Mechanisms of Acute and Lethal Cell Injury. W. J. Mergner, R. T. Jones & B. F. Trump, Eds. Vol. **1:** 143–178. Medical Publishers, Inc., New York.
7. DE DUVE, C. & R. WATTIAUX. 1966. Annu. Rev. Physiol. **28:** 435–492.
8. DE DUVE, C. & H. BEAUFAY. 1959. Biochem. J. **73:** 610–616.
9. HAWKINS, H. K. 1980. *In* Pathobiology of Cell Membranes. Vol. II: 251–285. Academic Press, Inc. New York.
10. NOVIKOFF, A. B. 1967. *In* The Neuron. H. Hyder, Ed.: 319–377. Elsevier. New York.
11. KOENIG, H. 1984. *In* Structural Elements of the Nervous System, Handbook of Neurochemistry, 2nd Ed. A. Lajtha, Ed. Vol. **7:** 177–204. Plenum Press. New York.
12. SIAKOTOS, A. N. & D. ARMSTRONG. 1975. *In* Neurobiology of Aging: An Interdisciplinary Life-Span Approach. J. M. Ordy & K. R. Brizzee, Eds. Advances in Behavioral Biology, Vol. **16:** 369–399. Plenum Press. New York.
13. STEINMAN, R. M., I. S. MELLMAN, W. A. MULLER & Z. A. COHN. 1983. J. Cell Biol. **96:** 1–27.
14. ANDERSON, R. G. W. & L. ORCI. 1988. J. Cell Biol. **106:** 539–543.
15. KORNFELD, S. & I. MELLMAN. 1989. Annu. Rev. Cell Biol. **5:** 483–525.
16. IANCU, T. C. 1992. Ultrastruc. Pathol. **16:** 231–244.
17. PFEIFER, U. 1987. *In* Lysosomes; Their Role in Protein Breakdown. H. Glaumann & F. J. Gallard, Eds.: 3–60. Academic Press. New York.
18. BRIZZEE, K. R. & J. M. ORDY. 1981. *In* Age Pigments. R. S. Sohal, Ed.: 101–154. Elsevier/North-Holland Biomedical Press. Amsterdam.
19. BRIZZEE, K. R. & J. M. ORDY. 1981. *In* Age Pigments. R. S. Sohal, Ed.: 317–334. Elsevier/North-Holland Biomedical Press. Amsterdam.
20. KENT, S. 1976. Geriatrics **31:** 128–137.
21. BOELLAARD, J. W. & W. SCHLOTE. 1986. Acta Neuropathol. (Berl.) **71:** 285–294.
22. SWAAB, D. F. 1991. Neurobiol. Aging **12:** 317–324.
23. SOHAL, R. S. 1981. *In* Age Pigments. R. S. Sohal, Ed.: 303–316. Elsevier/North-Holland Biomedical Press. Amsterdam.
24. WILSON, P. D., R. A. FIRESTONE & J. LENARD. 1987. J. Cell Biol. **104:** 1223–1229.

25. PANNESE, E., L. LUCIANO, S. IURATO & E. REALE. 1976. Acta Neuropathol. (Berl.) **36:** 209–220.
26. SOHAL, G. S. & T. A. WEIDMAN. 1978. Exp. Neurol. **61:** 53–64.
27. CHU-WANG, I.-W. & R. W. OPPENHEIM. 1978. J. Comp. Neur. **177:** 33–58.
28. PILAR, G. & L. LANDMESSER. 1976. J. Cell Biol. **68:** 339–356.
29. WRIGHT, L. L., T. J. CUNNINGHAM & A. J. SMOLEN. 1983. J. Neurocytol. **12:** 727–738.
30. CLARKE, P. G. H. & M. EGLOFF. 1988. Anat. Embryol. (Berl.) **179**(2): 103–108.
31. LANDIS, S. C. & R. J. MULLEN. 1978. J. Comp. Neurol. **177:** 125–133.
32. O'GORMAN, S. 1985. J. Comp. Neurol. **234:** 298–316.
33. MURAYAMA, S., T. W. BOULDIN & K. SUZUKI. 1991. Acta Neuropathol. **81:** 408–417.
34. MARCOUX, F. W., M. L. WEBER, A. W. PROBERT, JR. & M. A. DOMINICK. 1992. Ann. N.Y. Acad. Sci. **648:** 303–305.
35. DESHPANDE, J., K. BERGSTEDT, T. LINDÉN, H. KALIMO & T. WIELOCH. 1992. Exp. Brain Res. **88:** 91–105.
36. Z.-NAGY, I, V. Z.-NAGY, T. CASOLI & G. LUSTYIK. 1989. Adv. Exp. Med. Biol. **266:** 93–106; discussion 106–107.
37. PISANTI, F. A., L. LUCADAMO & E. A. TOTARO. 1989. Adv. Exp. Med. Biol. **266:** 135–141; discussion 141–142.
38. STERMAN, A. B. 1983. J. Neuropathol. Exp. Neurol. **42**(2): 166–176.
39. PRINEAS, J. 1969. J. Neuropathol. Exp. Neurol. **28**(4): 598–621.
40. TERRY, R. D. & A. PEÑA. 1965. J. Neuropathol. Exp. Neurol. **24:** 200–210.
41. HIRANO, A. 1991. Adv. Neurol. **56:** 91–101.
42. GONATAS, N. K., R. D. TERRY & M. WEISS. 1965. J. Neuropathol. Exp. Neurol. **24**(4): 575–598.
43. KERR, J. F. R. & B. V. HARMON. 1991. *In* Apoptosis: The Molecular Basis of Cell Death.: 5–29. Cold Spring Harbor Laboratory Press. Cold Spring Harbor, NY.
44. DIXON, J. S. 1967. Nature **215:** 657–658.
45. BRAND, S. & E. MUGNAINI. 1976. Exp. Brain Res. **26:** 105–119.
46. HOLTZMAN, E., A. B. NOVIKOFF & H. VILLAVERDE. 1967. J. Cell Biol. **33:** 419–435.
47. HOLTZMAN, E. & E. R. PETERSON. 1969. J. Cell Biol. **43:** 55a.
48. BARRON, K. D., E. D. MEANS & E. LARSEN. 1974. J. Neuropathol. Exp. Neurol. **20**(3): 344–362.
49. LODIN, Z., J. FALTIN, J. BOOHER & J. HARTMAN. 1974. Acta Histochem. **48**(Suppl.): 262–285.
50. HIRSCH, H. E., J. M. ANDREWS & M. E. PARKS. 1974. J. Neurochem. **23:** 935–941.
51. MITSUMOTO, H. & W. G. BRADLEY. 1982. Brain **105:** 811–834.
52. ANDREWS, J. M. 1974. J. Neuropathol. Exp. Neurol. **33**(2): 285–307.
53. PICK, J. 1965. J. Cell Biol. **26:** 335–351.
54. KOISTINAHO, J. & A. HERVONEN. 1989. Neurosci. Lett. **102:** 349–354.
55. SELKOE, D. J., L. LUCKENBILL-EDDS, M. L. SHELANSKI. 1978. J. Neuropathol. Exp. Neurol. **37**(6): 768–789.
56. BROSNAN, C. F., M. B. BUNGE & M. R. MURRAY. 1970. J. Neuropathol. Exp. Neurol. **29**(3): 337–353.
57. IVY, G. O., F. SCHOTTLER, J. WENZEL, M. BAUDRY & G. LYNCH. 1984. Science **226:** 985–987.
58. IVY, G. O., S. KANAI, M. OHTA, G. SMITH, Y. SATO, M. KOBAYASHI & K. KITANI. 1990. *In* Lipofuscin and Ceroid Pigments. E. A. Porta, Ed.: 31–47. Plenum Press. New York.
59. TAKAUCHI, S. & K. MIYOSHI. 1989. Acta Neuropathol. **78:** 380–387.
60. KLINGHARDT, G. W. 1978. Int. J. Neurol. **11**(4): 331–341.
61. SREBRO, Z. 1966. J. Comp. Neurol. **126**(1): 65–73.
62. DECKER, R. S. 1974. J. Cell Biol. **61:** 599–612.
63. TRUMAN, J. W. 1984. Ann. Rev. Neurosci. **7:** 171–188.
64. GONATAS, N. K., W. ANDERSON & I. EVANGELISTA. 1967. J. Neuropathol. Exp. Neurol. **26**(1): 25–39.
65. KRIGMAN, M. R., R. G., FELDMAN & K. BENSCH. 1965. Lab. Invest. **14:** 381–396.
66. SUZUKI, K. & R. D. TERRY. 1967. Acta Neuropathol. **8:** 278–284.

67. CATALDO, A. M. & R. A. NIXON. 1990. Proc. Natl. Acad. Sci. USA **87:** 3861–3865.
68. CATALDO, A. M., P. A. PASKEVICH, E. KOMINAMI & R. A. NIXON. 1991. Proc. Natl. Acad. Sci. USA **88:** 10998–11002.
69. CATALDO, A. M., C. Y. THAYER, E. D. BIRD, T. R. WHEELOCK & R. A. NIXON. 1990. Brain Res. **513:** 181–192.
70. NIXON, R. A., A. M. CATALDO, P. A. PASKEVICH, D. J. HAMILTON, T. R. WHEELOCK, L. KANALEY-ANDREWS. 1992. Ann. N.Y. Acad. Sci. **674:** 65–88.
71. NAKAMURA, Y. M. TAKEDA, H. SUZUKI, H. HATTORI, K. TADA, S. HARIGUCHI, S. HASHIMOTO & T. NISHIMURA. 1991. Neurosci. Lett. **130:** 195–198.
72. SAITO, K., T. YOKOYAMA, M. OKANIWA & S. KAMOSHITA. 1982. Acta Neuropathol. (Berl.) **58:** 187–192.
73. NELSON, J. S., C. D. FITCH, V. W. FISCHER, G. O. BROUN, JR. & A. C. CHOU. 1981. J. Neuropathol. Exp. Neurol. **40**(2): 166–186.
74. ULFIG, N. 1989. Neurosci. Res. **6:** 456–462.
75. CATALDO, A. & R. A. NIXON. Unpublished.
76. TELLEZ-NAGEL, I. & H. M. WISNIEWSKI. 1973. Arch. Neurol. **29:** 324–327.
77. VAQUERO, J., S. OYA, M. MANRIQUE, J. BUJÁN, A. P. LOZANO & G. BRAVO. 1979. Acta Neurochirurgica **46:** 233–241.
78. DOWSON, J. H. 1982. Br. J. Psychiat. **140:** 142–184.
79. DOWSON, J. H., C. Q. MOUNTJOY, M. R. CAIRNS & H. WILTON-COX. 1992. Neurobiol. Aging **13:** 493–500.
80. ZEMAN, W. & A. N. SIAKOTOS. 1973. *In* Lysosomes and Storage Diseases. H. G. Hers & F. Van Hoof, Eds.: 519–550. Academic Press. New York.
81. MARTIN, J.-J. 1991. Dev. Neurosci. **13:** 331–338.
82. NADKARNI, S., D. H. DESHPANDE, V. P. MONDKAR & E. P. BHARUCHA. 1979. J. Neurol. Sci. **43:** 395–404.
83. ZEMAN, W. 1976. *In* Progress in Neuropathology. H. M. Zimmerman, Ed. Vol. III: 203–223. Grune & Stratton. New York.
84. LAKE, B. D. 1984. *In* Greenfields Neuropathology. J. Hume-Adams, J. A. N. Corsellis & L. W. Duchen, Eds., 4th edit.: 491–572. Arnold. London.
85. WITKOP, C. J., JR., L. S. WOLFE, S. X. CAL, J. G. WHITE, D. TOWNSEND & K. M. KEENAN. 1987. Am. J. Med. **82:** 463–469.
86. COLLINS, G. H., R. R. COWDEN & A. H. NEVIS. 1968. Arch. Pathol. **86:** 239–254.
87. BEAUDET, A. L. 1991. *In* Harrison's Principles of Internal Medicine, 12th edit. J. D. Wilson *et al.*, Eds.: 1845–1854. McGraw Hill. New York.
88. HERS, H. G. & F. VANHOOF, Eds. 1973. Lysosomes and Storage Disorders. Academic Press. New York.
89. NEUFELD, E. G., T. W. LIM & L. J. SHAPIRO. 1975. Ann. Rev. Biochem. **44:** 357–376.
90. WALLACE, B. J., B. W. VOLK, L. SCHNECK & H. KAPLAN. 1965. Arch. Pathol. **80**(5): 466–486.
91. GONATAS, N. K., R. D. TERRY, R. WINKLER, S. R. KOREY, C. J. GOMEZ & A. STEIN. 1964. J. Neuropathol. Exp. Neurol. **22**(4): 557–580.
92. SUNG, J. H., M. HAYANO & R. J. DESNICK. 1977. J. Neuropathol. Exp. Neurol. **36:** 807–820.
93. KAMOSHITA, S. & B. H. LANDING. 1968. Am. J. Clin. Pathol. **49:** 312–318.
94. IVY, G. O. & J. W. GURD. 1988. *In* Lipofuscin-1987: State of the Art. I. Zs.-Nagy, Ed.: 83–108. Proc. of Intl. Symposium held in Debrecen, Hungary. Elsevier. Amsterdam.
95. MANCALL, E. L., G. E. APONTE & R. G. BERRY. 1965. J. Neuropathol. Exp. Neurol. **24:** 85–96.
96. IVY, G. O. 1992. Ann. N.Y. Acad. Sci. **674:** 89–102.
97. GRACY, R. W., K. YUKSEL, M. L. CHARMAN, J. K. CINI, M. JAHANI, H. S. LU, B. ORAY & J. M. TAIENT. 1985. *In* Modification of Proteins During Aging: 1–18. Alan R. Liss. New York.
98. KATZ, M. L. 1990. *In* Lipofuscin and Ceroid Pigments. E. A. Porta, Eds.: 109–119. Plenum Press. New York.
99. DE DUVE, C., T. DE BARSY, B. POOLE, A. TROUET, P. TULKENS & F. VANHOFF. 1974. Biochem. Pharmacol. **23:** 2495–2531.

100. BHACHATARRYA, T. K., T. K. CHATTERJEE & J. J. GHOSH. 1983. Biochem. Pharmacol. **32:** 2965–2968.
101. TAPPEL, A. L. 1973. Fed. Proc. **32**(8): 1870–1874.
102. CLAUSEN, J. 1984. Acta Neurol. Scand. **70:** 345–355.
103. TAPPEL, A. L. 1975. *In* Pathobiology of Cell Membranes. B. F. Trump & A. U. Arstilla, Eds. Vol. 1: 145–170. Academic Press. New York.
104. DE, A. K., S. CHIPALKATTI & A. S. AIYAR. 1983. Radiation Res. **98:** 637–645.
105. DE, A. K. & A. S. AIYAR. 1978. Strahlentherapie **154:** 134–138.
106. DEXTER, D. T., C. J. CARTER & F. R. WELLS. 1989. J. Neurochem. **52:** 381–89.
107. KASTNER, A., E. C. HIRSCH, O. LEJEUNE, F. JAVOY-AGID, O. RASCOL & Y. AGID. 1992. J. Neurochem. **59:** 1080–1089.
108. MANN, D. M. A. & P. O. YATES. 1983. Mech. Aging Dev. **21:** 193–203.
109. KONRADI, C., J. KORNHUBER & L. FROELICH. 1989. Neuroscience **33:** 383–400.
110. JENNER, P. 1989. J. Neurol. Neurosurg. Psychiatry Spec. Suppl.: 22–28.
111. SAGGU, H., J. COOKSEY & D. DEXTER. 1989. J. Neurochem. **53:** 692–96.
112. PERRY, T. L., D. V. GODIN & S. HANSEN. 1982. Neurosci. Lett. **33:** 305–310.
113. CALNE, D. B. 1992. Ann. Neurol. **32:** 799–803.
114. FAHN, F. & G. COHEN. 1992. Ann. Neurol. **32:** 804–812.
115. AGID, Y. 1991. Lancet **337:** 1321–1327.
116. PETTEGREW, J. W. 1989. Ann. N.Y. Acad. Sci. **568:** 5–28.
117. NITSCH, R. M., J. K. BLUSZTAJN, A. G. PITTAS, B. E. SLACK, J. W. GROWDEN & R. J. WURTMAN. 1992. Proc. Natl. Acad. Sci. USA **89**(5): 1671–1675.
118. BOSMAN, G. J., I. G. P. BARTHOLOMEAU & W. J. DE GRIP. 1991. Gerontology **37:** 95–112.
119. FAROOQUI, A. A., L. LISS & L. A. HORROCKS. 1988. Ann. Neurol. **23:** 306–308.
120. KVIETYS, P. R. 1989. Am. J. Physiol. **257:** H1640–1646.
121. DESVERGNE, B. 1989. Eur. J. Cell Biol. **49:** 162–170.
122. BRIZZEE, K. R., B. KAACK & P. KLARA. 1975. *In* Neurobiology of Aging: An Interdisciplinary Life-Span Approach. J. M. Ordy & K. R. Brizzee, Eds. Advances in Behavioral Biology, Vol. 16: 463–484. Plenum Press. New York.
123. CARR, V. M. & S. G. SIMPSON. 1978. J. Comp. Neurol. **182:** 727–740.
124. MANN, D. M. A., P. O. YATES & J. E. STAMP. 1978. J. Neurol. Sci. **378:** 83–93.
125. GOLDSTEIN, I. M. 1974. *In* Symposium on the Cell in Shock, sponsored by the Upjohn Company, April 25–27, 1974. pp. 30–34.
126. KANE, A. B., R. P. STANTON, E. G. RAYMOND, M. E. DOBSON, M. G. KNAFELC & J. L. FARBER. 1980. J. Cell Biol. **87:** 643–651.
127. WEISSMAN, G. & G. A. RITA. 1972. Nature (Lond.) New Biol. **240NB:** 167.
128. ALLISON, A. C., J. A. MAGNUS & M. R. YOUNG. 1966. Nature (Lond.) **209:** 874–878.
129. VAZQUEZ-COLON, L., F. D. ZIEGLER & W. B. ELLIOTT. 1966. Biochemistry **5**(4): 1134–1139.
130. MELLORS, A., A. L. TAPPEL, P. L. SAWANT & I. D. DESAI. 1967. Biochim. Biophys. Acta 143: 299–309.
131. NAKAMURA, Y., M. TAKEDA, H. SUZUKI, H. MORITA, K. TADA, S. HARIGUCHI & T. NISHIMURA. 1989. Neurosci. Lett. **97:** 215–220.
132. BOWEN, D. M., C. B. SMITH & A. N. DAVISON. 1973. Brain **96:** 849–856.
133. ROY, D., PATHAK, D. N. & R. SINGH. 1984. J. Neurochem. **42**(3): 628–633.
134. SAMORAJSKI, T. & C. ROLSTEN. 1976. Exp. Gerontol. **11:** 141–147.
135. POPOV, C. S. 1974. *In* Advances in Biochemical Psychopharmacology. I. S. Forrest, C. J. Cann & E. Usdin, Eds. Vol. 9: 229–244. Raven Press. New York.
136. BRAAK, H. 1979. Acta Neuropathol. (Berl.) **46:** 197–202.
137. BRIZZEE, K. R., J. M. ORDY, J. HANSCHE & B. KAACK. 1976. *In* Neurobiology of Aging. R. D. Terry & S. Gershon, Eds.: 229–244. Raven Press. New York.
138. HINDS, J. W. & N. A. MCNELLY. 1979. J. Comp. Neurol. **184:** 811–820.
139. BRODY, H. 1970. Interdisc. Top. Gerontol. **7:** 9–21.
140. BRAAK, H. & E. BRAAK. 1987. Anat. Embryol. (Berl.) **176:** 315–330.
141. MANN, D. M. A. & P. O. YATES. 1974. Brain **97:** 481–488.
142. DAVIES, J. D. & A. P. FOTHERINGHAM. 1981. Exp. Gerontol. **16**(2): 119–125.

143. PFEIFFER, U. 1973. Virchows Arch. (Cell Pathol.) **12:** 195–206.
144. NEELY, A. N., J. R. COX, J. A. FORTNEY, L. M. SCHWORER & G. E. MORTIMORE. 1977. J. Biol. Chem. **252:** 6948–6954.
145. MORTIMORE, G. E. 1982. Nutri. Rev. **40:** 1–25.
146. MORTIMORE, G. E., N. J. HUTSON & C. A. SURMACZ. 1983. Proc. Natl. Acad. Sci. USA **80:** 2179–2183.
147. YOUNGDAHL-TURNER, P. & L. E. ROSENBERG. 1978. J. Clin. Invest. **61:** 133–141.
148. YOUNGDAHL-TURNER, P., I. S. MELLMAN, R. H. ALLEN & L. E. ROSENBERG. 1979. Exp. Cell Res. **118:** 127–134.
149. BROWN, M. S. & J. L. GOLDSTEIN. 1976. Science **191:** 150–154.
150. BROWN, M. S., P. T. KOVANEN & J. L. GOLDSTEIN. 1981. Science **212:** 628–635.
151. BROWN, M. S. & J. L. GOLDSTEIN. 1986. Science **232:** 34–47.
152. STREHLER, L., D. MARK & A. S. MIDVAN. 1959. J. Gerontol. **14:** 430–441.
153. LOCKSHIN, R. A. 1985. *In* CRC Handbook of Aging. V. J. Cristofalo, Ed.: 137–148. CRC Press, Inc. Boca Raton, FL.

Mechanisms of Phospholipase A$_2$ Activation and Neuronal Injury

M. ANTHONY VERITY[a]

Division of Neuropathology and Brain Research Institute
UCLA Medical Center
Los Angeles, California 90024-1732

The phospholipases catalyze the deacylation of phosphoglycerides to produce free fatty acids and lysophosphoglyceride. The phospholipase A$_2$ (PLA$_2$) enzymes share a common catalytic property: the hydrolysis of the sn-2 fatty acyl position of phosphatides. Prolonged, abusive or unmodulated PLA$_2$ activation will lead to uncontrolled membrane deacylation, activation of other second messenger systems, uncontrolled Ca^{2+} influx and ultimate lethal cellular injury. While these concepts have been well studied in non-neural systems, the role and significance of PLA$_2$ activation in neural systems is poorly documented. In this review we will examine the principal mechanisms initiating and modulating intracellular PLA$_2$ activation and examine the contribuion of these mechanisms to initiating lethal neuronal injury.

MODULATION AND ACTIVATION OF PLA$_2$

PLA$_2$ is a paradigm for Ca^{2+}-mediated hydrolytic reactions at lipid-aqueous interfaces. Scott *et al.*[1] have described the molecular mechanism of PLA$_2$ action and reveal that PLA$_2$ is more active at the lipid-aqueous interface than in solution. Moreover, they suggest that the phospholipid molecule undergoing hydrolysis leaves the aggregate and reaches the catalytic surface by facilitated diffusion through a hydrophobic channel. This is not surprising when it is remembered that the polymorphic state of membrane lipids serves to determine its biological properties and functions. Temperautre-dependent or Ca^{2+}-induced transitions from bilayer to nonbilayer structures exhibit increased phospholipid motion leading to selective PLA$_2$ attack.[2,3]

As indicated in TABLE 1, enzymic activity may be influenced by a variety of factors. The polymorphic state of the membrane lipid will modulate PLA$_2$ activity. Numerous structural interconversions may arise from the aggregation of mixed lipids, lipid hydration, presence of Ca^{2+}, temperature and peroxidation (see below). Dawson[4] observed a change in the structural organization of the phospholipid mixture on the introduction of phosphatidylethanolamine (PE) to vesicle preparations of phosphatidylcholine (PC). Sevanian and Kim[5] demonstrated differential activity of PLA$_2$ as a consequence of change in the ratio of PC and PE. The selectivity of PLA$_2$ for phospholipid organization was appreciated by Butler and

[a] Address for correspondence: M. Anthony Verity, M.D., Department of Pathology (Neuropathology), UCLA School of Medicine, Los Angeles, CA 90024-1732; FAX (310)206-5178.

Abood[6] who used the enzyme to examine phospholipid organization in synaptic membranes, myelin and liposomes. It is clear, therefore, that the phospholipid composition of the membrane, the degree of unsaturation and the relative bilayer/non-bilayer configuration has a major influence on the apparent activity of PLA_2.

An association between enhanced PLA_2 activity and membrane lipid peroxidation has been demonstrated in various membranes including mitochondria,[7] lysosomes,[8] red cells,[9] and microsomes.[10] Hence, fatty acyl-hydroperoxides may be preferred substrates for endogenous or added phospholipase thereby explaining the enzyme activation in response to peroxidation.[5,11–13] These studies were extended using artificial liposomes prepared from PC and PE. Induced peroxidation by a variety of methods (measured by the thiobarbituric acid reaction) revealed that PLA_2 hydrolysis was highly correlated with the degree of peroxidation; that preparations containing the highest proportion of PE were most susceptible to peroxidation and, therefore, enhanced PLA_2 activity and the extent of hydrolysis was found to correlate with the degree of fatty acid unsaturation.[5]

An opportunity to examine the relationship between membrane peroxidation and PLA_2 activation was recently provided by our studies on the pathogenesis of methyl mercury–induced neurotoxicity. These studies had revealed significant lipoperoxidation in cerebellar granule cell suspensions and culture.[14,15] Moreover,

TABLE 1. Phospholipase A_2: Factors Controlling Activity

- Hydrolysis at sn-2 position fatty acyl group phosphate
- Enzyme activity influenced by:
  - a) Phospholipid state-structure
    - i) Bilayer polymorphism
    - ii) Composition
    - iii) State of peroxidation
  - b) Ca^{2+}
  - c) G-protein

we had demonstrated MeHg activation of PLA_2 in cerebellar granule cell culture.[16] Because of these associations, we hypothesized that MeHg-induced PLA_2 activation was a result of membrane lipoperoxidation (see Schema, FIG. 1). If the hypothesis was tenable, then inhibition of lipoperoxidation (by the antioxidant α-tocopherol) would be associated with diminished PLA_2 activity. Incubation of cerebellar granule cell cultures with 20 μM MeHg, 20 μM alpha-tocopherol succinate or in combination for 60 min, 37°C was performed (TABLE 2). α-Tocopherol succinate significantly reduced the MeHg induced lipoperoxidation as measured by thiobarbituric acid reacting substance but failed to protect against cytotoxicity or the activation of PLA_2 as determined by [³H]-arachidonate release. These data indicate that the PLA_2 activation induced by MeHg was not causally related to the associated membrane lipoperoxidation, but may be coupled to Ca^{2+} influx.

Cytoplasmic $[Ca^{2+}]$ has been established as a primary *in vivo* activator of PLA_2 activity.[17,18] *In vitro* studies with purified PLA_2 reveal a Ca^{2+} concentration-dependent activation[19,20] and Ca^{2+} ionophores promote PLA_2 activation in a variety of cells.[21–23] The relative roles of external Ca^{2+} and the mobilization of intracellular Ca^{2+} in the activation of PLA_2 with formation of arachidonic acid or eicosanoids is uncertain. On the one hand, Brooks *et al.*[24] demonstrated that receptor-stimulated PLA_2 in C62B glioma cells was coupled to the influx of external Ca^{2+} and not

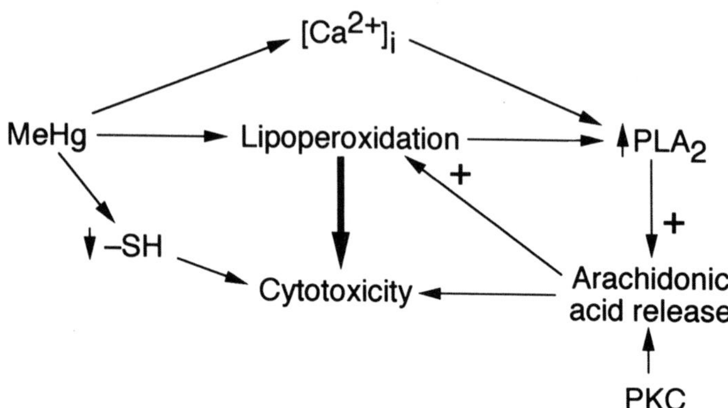

FIGURE 1. Schema for hypothesis coupling methyl mercury activation of phospholipase A_2 to mercurial-induced lipoperoxidation and/or increase of intracellular Ca^{2+}. See text for experimental details.

mobilization of intracellular Ca^{2+}. However, the participation of receptor-mediated *intracellular* Ca^{2+} mobilization in PLA_2 activation and arachidonate release was demonstrated in cultured astrocytes by Pearce *et al.*[25] Moreover, NMDA receptor activation induces a Ca^{2+} mediated arachidonic acid release in primary cultures of cerebellar granule cells.[26,27] 100 μM aspartate was able to induce a significant release of arachidonate in the absence of extracellular Ca^{2+}, such release being inhibited by TMB-8, a blocker of inositol 1,4,5-triphosphate–induced intracellular Ca^{2+} mobilization. Further evidence in support of receptor-mediated interaction on PLA_2 activation rather than as a consequence of a stimulated influx of extracellular Ca^{2+} was obtained in studies of epidermal growth factor (EGF) receptor stimulation of PLA_2 in cultured rat kidney cells.[28] Specifically, neither chelation of extracellular Ca^{2+} nor the addition of 1 mM Ca^{2+} affected basal arachidonate release nor modified the approximatley 10-fold stimulation induced by EGF. The release of [³H]-arachidonate from prelabeled amnion cell culture is markedly stimulated by superoxide anion (O^2) generated by the addition of xanthine oxidase to hypoxanthine.[29] Such arachidonate release was dependent on the increase of internal Ca^{2+}

TABLE 2. Effect of Methyl Mercury on Phospholipase A_2 Activity, Membrane Lipoperoxidation and Cytotoxicity in Cerebellar Granule Cell Culture

	[3H]-Arachidonate Release %	TBAR %	Cytotoxicity %
Control	2.8 ± 0.5	(100)	7
Methyl mercury, 20 μM	6.3 ± 0.8	157	33
α-tocopherol succinate, 20 μM	2.5 ± 0.4	84	2
MeHg + α-tocopherol succinate	6.5 ± 0.9	91	52

For experimental details see text. Values are mean ± SEM (culture wells, 3–7).

at least partially due to increase of internal pH and extracellular Ca^{2+}. Recently, provocative observations have been made by Piomelli and Greengard[30] which have revealed a Ca^{2+}-dependent *inhibition* of PLA₂ activity in synaptosomes. The inhibitory effect resulted from phosphorylation of a synaptosomal protein substrate suggesting that the Ca^{2+}-dependent inhibition in intact nerve endings was produced by activation of the multi-functional Ca^{2+}/calmodulin-dependent protein kinase 2, invoking the possibility of bidirectional control.

We have documented that PLA₂ may be activated *in vivo* and *in vitro* by elevated cytoplasmic Ca^{2+}, likely acting as the major regulator of this enzyme. However, numerous reports have now suggested that PLA₂ may be regulated directly through a G-protein. While it is established that the breakdown of inositol phospholipids is regulated via G-proteins, the question of separate or interrelated G-protein mediated activities of phospholipase C and phospholipase A₂ appear relevant. PLA₂ may be activated by the introduction of GTP analogs into permeabilized cells.[31,32] Moreover, arachidonate production was dissociated from phospholipase C activity. For instance, arachidonate production was inhibited by prior incubation with pertussis toxin which had no effect on inositol phosphate production whereas neomycin (an inhibitor of phospholipase C) prevented IP production but not arachidonate. Jelsema[33] has also shown that light activated PLA₂ through

TABLE 3. Fluoroaluminate Stimulation of PLA₂ is Neurotoxic in Cerebellar Granule Cell Culture

	[³H]-Arachidonate Release %	Cytotoxicity %
Control	0.83 ± 0.11	6 ± 3
AIF₄⁻, 10 mM	4.3 ± 0.3	9 ± 4
AIF₄⁻, 20 mM	6.3 ± 0.6	34 ± 7

AIF₄⁻ stimulation induced by 10 μM Al Cl₃ plus 10 or 20 mM NaF, 20 min, 37°C in control saline medium (CSS). Values are mean ± SEM (n = 4).

the action of the G-protein, transducin in rod outer segments of bovine retina. Narasimhan *et al.*[34] demonstrated GTPᵧS activation of endogenous PLA₂ in a permeabilized leukemia cell system. Such 5-to-6–fold activation occurred when free $[Ca^{2+}]$ was buffered at 10^{-7}–10^{-5} M. While the G-protein involved in PLA₂ activation is unknown, it may be a *ras* proto-oncogene. Micro-injection of the H-*ras* oncogene into fibroblasts had no effect on phosphoinositide metabolism but activated phospholipase A₂.[35]

Gilman[36] included stimulation by the non-hydrolizable analogs of GTP or aluminum fluoride among the criteria proposed for the involvement of a G-protein in a signaling process. For instance, fluoroaluminate stimulated basal and EGF-stimulated arachidonate production in kidney tubule cells.[28] Similarly, we have observed significant stimulation of PLA₂ measured as [³H]-arachidonate release from prelabeled cerebellar granule cell cultures by fluoroaluminate in a dose- and time-dependent manner (TABLE 3). Teitelbaum[28] observed that pre-treatment of renal tubule cells with pertussis toxin blocked EGF stimulation of arachidonate release. This observation couples PLA₂ activity to a specific set of pertussis-toxin inhibitable guanine nucleotide-binding regulatory proteins. There is an interesting paradox in these relationships. Numerous studies have revealed that cyclic AMP inhibits PLA₂ activity.[37] Moreover, in intact cells fluoroaluminate inhibits the stimulation of adenylate cyclase (and thereby production of cyclic AMP) by agonists whose receptors are coupled to G-protein.[38,39] Hence, fluoroaluminate stimulation of arachidonate release in cerebellar granule cells must occur either in the absence of cyclic AMP generation and/or through the selective activation of a G-protein, likely to be G_i capable of down regulating cAMP. A partial reconciliation of these observations was provided by Inoue *et al.*[40] who demonstrated differential activation of the stimulatory (G_s) and inhibitory (G_i) guanine nucleotide-binding proteins by fluoroaluminate. These authors concluded that fluoroaluminate activated G_i but not G_s in cells but activates both G-proteins in membrane preparations. These observations demonstrate the unique, dual modulation of two sets of G-proteins in the state of activity of PLA_2.

Activation of the α_1-adrenergic or hormone receptors for bradykinin commonly releases arachidonic acid and activates phospholipase C thereby releasing the second messengers inositol triphosphate and diacyl glycerol (DG). The former releases Ca^{2+} from intracellular stores whereas diacyl glycerol activates protein kinase C. Weiss *et al.*[41] demonstrated that α_1-adrenergic stimulated arachidonic acid release is almost completely dependent on the activation of PKC in a clonal isolate of a kidney cell line. The regulation of arachidonic acid release by PKC is also suggested from studies showing that phorbol esters release arachidonic acid in pinealocytes,[21] platelets,[42] and neutrophils.[43] It has been suggested that an elevation of intracellular Ca^{2+} and activation of PKC cooperatively regulate PLA_2 activity.[44] It has been shown recently that PKC acts to increase the sensitivity of PLA_2 to Ca^{2+}.[45,46] Channon and Leslie[47] have revealed a Ca^{2+}-mediated association of soluble PLA_2 with cell membranes leading to select membrane arachidonate release. Conceptually, therefore, the bulk of data suggests that the ability of an agonist to mobilize Ca^{2+} along with its ability to activatge PKC via G-protein interaction will determine its efficacy as a stimulator of PLA_2.

ROLE OF PLA_2 IN CELL AND NEURAL INJURY

Stimulated hydrolysis has been associated with ischemia,[48,49] chemical anoxic,[50,51] and cytolytic toxins.[52] The results are consistent with stimulated hydrolysis of arachidonate containing phospholipids mediated by elevated intracellular Ca^{2+}. Shier and DuBourdieu[23] examined the role of phospholipid hydrolysis in the mechanism of cell death by the Ca^{2+} ionophor A23187. Analysis of the rates of the two processes indicates that phospholipid hydrolysis triggers cell killing which may be inhibited by reduction of extracellular Ca^{2+} or addition of manganese ions (TABLE 4). Ca^{2+} plays a prominent role in excitatory amino acid neurotoxicity[53] and PLA_2 activation has been shown to occur during NMDA receptor activation.[26,27]

TABLE 4. Effect of Ionophore A23187 on Phospholipid Hydrolysis and Cytotoxicity in Cultures of 3T3 Fibroblasts

	20 Minutes		60 Minutes	
Concentration	Phospholipid Hydrolysis, %	Cytotoxicity %	Phospholipid Hydrolysis, %	Cytotoxicity %
Control	6 ± 0.5	1	4.5 ± 0.5	1
A23187, 5 μM	31 ± 1.6	3	29 ± 1.3	96

Mean values of phospholipid hydrolysis and cytoxicity assessed by trypan blue exclusion at 20 and 60 min in culture. Modified from Shier and DuBourdieu (1982).[23]

TABLE 5. Potentiation of PLA$_2$ Activation by A23187 in Low External $[Na^+]_e$

	[^{3}H]-Arachidonate Release % [Na]$_e$	
	120	12
Control	3.9 ± 0.2 (12)	4.3 ± 0.4 (9)
A23187, 5 μM	6.3 ± 0.3 (16)	27.4 ± 0.8 (72)

Values are mean ± SEM (n = 3–6) of percent [^{3}H]-arachidonate released into medium after 2 hours, 37°C. Values in parenthesis are percent cytotoxicity assessed by trypan blue exclusion.

Mattson *et al.*[54] demonstrated that hippocampal neurons and NCB-20 cells responded differently to A23187 in showing a prolonged or transient rise in Ca^{2+}, respectively. Moreover, the ability of NCB-20 cells to reduce the Ca^{2+} load was dependent on extracellular $[Na^+]$ suggesting that an active Na^+/Ca^{2+} exchange mechanism was important in protecting against neuron death. We have performed an analogous experiment using cerebellar granule cells in culture in which the activity of PLA$_2$ and cytotoxicity was correlated as a function of external $[Na^+]$ in the presence of the Ca^{2+} ionophor, A23187. In cultures supplemented with 120 mM Na^+, and 1.8 mM Ca^{2+}, addition of 5 μM A23187 induced a modest, 2-fold release of [^{3}H]-arachidonate after 2 hours incubation, 37°C (TABLE 5). No significant increase in cytotoxicity was observed. In this respect, the mature cerebellar granule cell appears relatively "resistant" to ionophoric mediated Ca^{2+} flux and suggests the presence of a highly efficient Na^+/Ca^{2+} exchanger in the cell membrane controlling the intracytoplasmic elevation of Ca^{2+}. In this respect the cells behaved analogously to the NCB-20 cells[54] in contrast to the more sensitive hippocampal neurons, confirmed following replacement of external Na^+ with choline which then demonstrated marked activation of PLA$_2$ and accompanying cytotoxicity (TABLE 5).

Pharmacologic inhibition of phospholipid degradation associated with ATP depletion has resulted in cytoprotection.[55–57] For instance, iodoacetate treatment of myocytes in culture resulted in marked reduction of ATP and many fold increase in [^{3}H]-arachidonate release. Inhibition of PLA$_2$ by mepacrine or U26384 produced substantial inhibition of [^{3}H]-arachidonate release and markedly attenuated abnormal cytoplasmic Ca^{2+} and K^+ levels. Such data supports the hypothesis that reduction of free fatty acid accumulation by inhibition of accelerated phospholipid degradation is associated with myocyte protection from Ca^{2+} loading.

Our attention to date has been focused on the cytotoxic role of phospholipase activation in the mediation of cell injury and data has been presented to show that abusive, high levels of PLA$_2$ activation causally reinforce lethal cell injury. Moreover, abnormal lipoperoxidation *per se* is known to activate PLA$_2$ (see above). Paradoxically, but of great interest is the observation that phospholipase A$_2$ activation may protect membranes from ongoing lipid peroxidation damage.[12] Membrane free radical or oxidant attack will produce lipid peroxides with subsequent disorganization of the bilayer. Under these circumstances PLA$_2$ selectively removes the oxidized fatty acids thereby decreasing membrane disruption and allowing "repair" of the oxidized fatty acid by glutathione peroxidase. Repair is further completed by reacylation with fatty acyl co-enzyme A. These observations identify an essential role for PLA_2 in the detoxification of phospholipid hydroperoxides. While this mechanism may act under perturbed, physiological states of membrane transduction states, moderate abusive stimulation will undoubtedly lead to focal rapid membrane cytolysis incapable of repair by the glutathione peroxidase/reacylation mechanism.

ROLE AND EFFECT OF ARACHIDONATE

As previously discussed PLA_2 is believed to be the main enzyme responsible for arachidonic acid release, suggested to be the rate-limiting step in the biosynthesis of the eicosanoids.[58] The metabolism of arachidonic acid by the cyclo-oxygenase or lipoxygenase pathways gives rise to many biologically active metabolites including the prostaglandins known to act on cell surface receptors. While it may be considered that the primary role of arachidonic acid is the rate limiting step in the production of lipid second messengers including the prostaglandins, thromboxanes, and leukotrines, the primary product of PLA_2 activation is known also to exert numerous effects *per se*. In addition to activating phospholipase C, arachidonic acid has been shown to stimulate or modulate numerous intracellular processes (TABLE 6). The activation of phospholipase C[59,60] may also represent an

TABLE 6. Cellular Effects of Arachidonic Acid

• Rate limiting for prostaglandin synthesis
• Activation of phospholipase C (PLC)
• Stimulate: —adenylate cyclase
—guanylate cyclase
—protein kinase C
• Stimulated release of intracellular Ca^{2+}
• Inhibit glutamate and GABA uptake

autocatalytic cycle as PLC activation followed by DG lipase and monoacylglycerol lipase activity leads to arachidonate production. Evidence has also been produced to show that arachidonic acid itself may stimulate adenylate cyclase,[61] guanylate cyclase,[62] and protein kinase C.[63,64] It is likely that these actions of arachidonate singly or in concert are responsible for the stimulation of secretion from anterior pituitary[65] or mast cells.[66] Wolf *et al.*[67] have demonstrated arachidonate induced release of Ca^{2+} from intracellular stores thereby directly contributing synergistically with the known mobilization and actions of Ca^{2+} in modulating PLA_2 activity. Finally, the polyunsaturated fatty acids, especially arachidonic acid, preferentially inhibit glutamate uptake in neurons.[68] These observations assume greater significance with recognition that phospholipids and arachidonic acid are membrane components changed early during cerebral edema.

CONCLUSION

There is no doubt that physiological modulation of endogenous phospholipase A_2 activity is responsible for the controlled hydrolysis of membrane linked phosphatides at the SN-2 position. Such activity will produce the rate limiting primary molecule, arachidonic acid from which an appropriate cascade of second messengers may be produced. Abusive activation of phospholipase A_2 via uncontrolled Ca^{2+} influx and/or release or prolonged G-protein activation will be instrumental in production of irreversible cell injury via focal membrane distortion. In this respect, the state of membrane lipoperoxidation confers both a mechanism for controlled repair and reacylation or abusive uncontrolled PLA_2 activation and subsequent membrane disintegration. Future studies will concentrate on factors modifying neuronal PLA_2 activation, coupling of specific neuronal excitotoxic receptors to PLA_2 activation, the interactive roles of adenylate/guanylate cyclase or protein kinase C activation and most importantly reduction of causal mechanisms relating to neuronal irreversible injury to the inception and magnitude of PLA_2 activation. Although likely not to be a single causal event in cell injury, the possibilities of appropriate therapeutic intervention afford an exciting avenue in the treatment of acute and delayed neuronal injury.

REFERENCES

1. SCOTT, D. L., S. P. WHITE, Z. OTWINOWSKI, W. YUAN, M. H. GELB & P. B. SIGLER. 1990. Interfacial catalysis: The mechanism of phospholipase A_2. Science **250:** 1541–1546.
2. NOORDHAM, P. C., C. J. A. VAN ECHFELD, B. DEKRUIJFF & J. DEGIER. 1981. Rapid transbilayer moment of phosphatidyl choline in unsaturated phosphatidyl ethanolamine containing model membrane. Biochim. Biophys. Acta **646:** 483–490.
3. SEVANIAN, A. 1988. Lipid peroxidation, membrane damage, and phospholipase A_2 action. *In* Cellular Antioxidant Defense Mechanisms, C. K. Chow, Ed. Vol. 2. CRC Press, Inc. Boca Raton, FL.
4. DAWSON, R. M. C. 1982. Phospholipid structure as a modulator of intracellular turnover. J. Am. Oil Chem. Soc. **59:** 401–418.
5. SEVANIAN, A. & E. KIM. 1985. Phospholipase A_2-dependent release of fatty acids from peroxidized membranes. J. Free Radical Biol. Med. **1:** 263–271.
6. BUTLER, M. & L. G. ABOOD. 1982. Use of phospholipase A to compare phospholipid organization in synaptic membrane myelin and liposomes. J. Membr. Biol. **66:** 1–12.
7. YASUDA, M. & T. FUJITA. 1977. Effect of lipid peroxidation on phospholipase A_2 activity of rat liver mitochondria. Japan J. Pharmacol. **27:** 429–435.
8. WEGLICKI, W. B., B. F. DICKENS & T. MAK. 1984. Enhanced liposomal phospholipid degradation and lysophospholipid production due to free radicals. Biochem. Biophys. Res. Commun. **124:** 229–235.
9. BARKER, M. O. & M. BRIN. 1975. Mechanism of lipid peroxidation of erythrocytes of vitamin E deficient rats and in phosphatidyl model system. Arch. Biochem. Biophys. **166:** 32–40.
10. SEVANIAN, A., S. F. MUAKKASSAH-KELLY & S. MONTESTRUQUE. 1983. The influence of phospholipase A_2 and glutathione peroxidase on the elimination of membrane lipid peroxides. Arch. Biochem. Biophys. **223:** 441–450.
11. SEVANIAN, A., R. A. STEIN & J. F. MEAD. 1981. Metabolism of epoxidized phosphatidylcholine by phospholipase A_2 and epoxide hydrolase. Lipids **16:** 781–792.
12. VAN KUIJK, F. G. M., A. SEVANIAN, G. J. HANDELMAN & E. A. DRATZ. 1987. A new role for PLA_2: Protection of membranes from lipid peroxidation damage. TIBS. **12:** 31–34.
13. BECKMAN, J. A., S. M. BOROWITZ & I. M. BURR. 1987. The role of phospholipase A activity in rat liver microsomal lipid peroxidation. J. Biol. Chem. **262:** 1479–1481.
14. SARAFIAN, T. & M. A. VERITY. 1991. Oxidative mechanisms underlying methyl mercury neurotoxicity. Int. J. Devel. Neurosci. **9:** 147–153.
15. VERITY, M. A. & T. SARAFIAN. 1991. Role of oxidative injury in the pathogenesis of methyl mercury neurotoxicity. Advances in Mercury Toxicology. T. Suzuki & T. Clarkson, Eds.: 209–222. Plenum Press. New York.

16. VERITY, M. A., A. SEVANIAN, T. SARAFIAN & P. HOCHSTEIN. 1991. Methyl mercury activates neuronal PLA$_2$ in a Ca^{2+} independent manner. J. Neurochem. **57:** S64.

17. BILLAH, M. M., E. G. LAPETINA & P. CUATRECASAS. 1980. PLA$_2$ and phospholipase C activities of platelets. J. Biol. Chem. **255:** 10227–10231.

18. VAN DEN BOSCH, H. 1980. Intracellular phospholipases A. Biochem. Biophys. Acta **604:** 191–246.

19. JESSE, R. L. & R. C. FRANSON. 1979. Modulation of purified phospholipase A$_2$ activity from human platelets by Ca^{2+} and indomethacin. Biochem. Biophys. Acta **575:** 467–470.

20. ONO, T., H. TOJO, S. KURAMITSU, H. KAGAMIYAMA & M. OKAMOTO. 1988. Purification and characterization of a membrane associated phospholipase A$_2$ from rat spleen. J. Biol. Chem. **263:** 5732–5738.

21. HO, A. K. & D. C. KLEIN. 1987. Activation of alpha-1-adrenoceptors, protein kinase C, or treatment with intracellular free Ca^{2+} elevating agents increases pineal phospholipase A$_2$ activity. J. Biol. Chem. **262:** 11764–11770.

22. DEGEORGE, J. J., B. MORELL, K. D. MCCARTHY & E. G. LAPENTINA. 1986. Cholinergic stimulation of arachidonic acid and phosphatidic acid metabolism in C62B glioma cells. J. Biol. Chem. **261:** 3428–3433.

23. SHIER, W. T. & D. J. DUBOURDIEU. 1982. Role of phospholipid hydrolysis in the mechanism of toxic cell death by Ca^{2+} and ionophor A23187. Biochem. Biophys. Res. Commun. **109:** 106–112.

24. BROOKS, R. C., K. D. MCCARTHY, E. G. LAPATINA & P. MORELL. 1989. Receptor-stimulated PLA$_2$ activation is coupled to influx of external Ca^{2+} and not to mobilization of intracellular Ca^{2+} in C62B glioma cells. J. Biol. Chem. **264:** 20147–20153.

25. PEARCE, B., S. MURPHY, J. JEROME, C. MORROW & P. DANDONA. 1989. ATP-evoked Ca^{2+} mobilization and prostanoid release from astrocytes: P$_2$-purinergic receptors linked to phosphoinositide hydrolysis. J. Neurochem. **52:** 971–977.

26. LAZAREWICZ, J. W., J. T. WROBLEWSKI & V. COSTA. 1990. N-methyl-D-aspartate sensitive glutamate receptors induced Ca^{2+}-mediated arachidonic acid release in primary cultures of cerebellar granule cells. J. Neurochem. **55:** 1875–1881.

27. SANFELIU, C., A. HUNT & A. J. PATELL. 1990. Exposure to N-methyl-D-aspartate increases release of arachidonic acid in primary cultures of rat hippocampal neurons and not in astrocytes. Brain. Res. **526:** 241–248.

28. TEITELBAUM, I. 1990. The epidermal growth factor receptor is coupled to a phospholipase A$_2$-specific pertussis toxin-inhibitable guanine nucleotide-binding regulatory protein in cultured rat inner medullary collecting tubule cells. J. Biol. Chem. **265:** 4218–4222.

29. IKEBUCHI, Y., N. MASUMOTO, K. TASAKA, K. KOIKE, K. KASAHARA, A. MIYAKE & O. TANIZAWA. 1991. Superoxide anion increases intracellular pH, intracellular-free Ca^{2+} and arachidonate release in human amnion cells. J. Biol. Chem. **266:** 13233–13237.

30. PIOMELLI, D. & P. GREENGARD. 1991: Bidirectional control of phospholipase A$_2$ activity by Ca^{2+}/calmodulin-dependent protein kinase II, cAMP-dependent protein kinase, and casein kinase II. Proc. Natl. Acad. Sci. USA **88:** 6770–6774.

31. BURCH, R. M., A. LUINI & J. AXELROD. 1986. Phospholipase A$_2$ and phospholipase C are activated by distinct GTP-binding proteins in response to α_1-adrenergic stimulation in FRTL thyroid cells. Proc. Natl. Acad. Sci. USA **83:** 7201–7205.

32. NAKASHIMA, S., A. SUGANUMA, A. MATSUI, H. HATTORI, M. SATO, A. TAKENAKA & Y. NOZAWA. 1989. Primary role of calcium ions in arachidonic acid release from rat platelet membranes. Comparison with human platelet membranes. Biochem. J. **259:** 139–144.

33. JELSEMA, C. L. 1987. Light activation of phospholipase A$_2$ in rod outer segments of bovine retina and its modulation by GTP-binding proteins. J. Biol. Chem. **262:** 163–168.

34. NARASIMHAN, V., D. HOLOWKA & B. BAIRD. 1990. A guanine nucleotide-binding protein participates in IgE receptor-mediated activation of endogenous and reconstituted phospholipase A$_2$ in a permeabilized cell system. J. Biol. Chem. **264:** 1459–1464.

35. BAR-SAGI, D. & J. R. FERAMISCO. 1986. Induction of membrane ruffling and fluid-phase pinocytosis in quiescent fibroblasts by ras proteins. Science **233:** 1061–1068.

36. GILMAN, A. G. 1987. G proteins; Transducers of receptor-generated signals. Ann. Rev. Biochem. **56:** 615–649.

37. TEITELBAUM, I. & T. BERL. 1986. Effects of Ca^{2+} on vasopressin-medicated cyclic adenosine monophosphate formation cultured rat inner medullary collecting tubule cells. J. Clin. Invest. **77:** 1574–1583.

38. KATADA, T., G. M. BOKOCH, J. K. NORTHUP, M. UI & A. G. GILMAN. 1984. The inhibiting guanine nucleotide-binding regulatory component of adenylate cyclase. J. Biol. Chem. **259:** 3568–3577.

39. BLACKMORE, P. F. & J. H. EXTON. 1986. Studies on the hepatic calcium-mobilizing activity of aluminum fluoride and glucagon. Modulation by cAMP and phorbol myristate acetate. J. Biol. Chem. **261:** 11056–11063.

40. INOUE, Y. P. H. FISHMAN & R. V. REBOIS. 1990. Differential activation of the stimulatory and inhibitory guanine nucleotide-binding proteins by fluoroaluminate in cells and in membranes. J. Biol. Chem. **265:** 10645–10651.

41. WEISS, B. A., S. R. SLIVKA & P. A. INSEL. 1989. Defining the role of protein kinase C in epinephrine- and bradykinin-stimulated arachidonic acid metabolism in Madin-Darby canine kidney cells. Mol. Pharmacol. **36:** 317–326.

42. HALENDA, S. P., G. B. ZAVOICO & M. B. FEINSTEIN. 1985. Phorbol esters and oleoyl acetyl glycerol enhance release of arachidonic acid in platelets stimulated by Ca^{2+} ionophore A23187. J. Biol. Chem. **260:** 12484–12491.

43. McINTYRE, T. M., S. L. REINHOLD, S. M. PRESCOTT & G. A. ZIMMERMAN. 1987. Protein kinase C activity appears to be required for the synthesis of platelet activating factor and leukotriene B_4 by human neutrophils. J. Biol. Chem. **262:** 15370–15376.

44. WHATLEY, R. E., P. NELSON, G. A. ZIMMERMAN, D. L. STEVENS, C. J. PARKER, T. M. McINTYRE & S. M. PRESCOTT. 1989. The regulation of platelet-activating factor production in endothelial cells. The role of Ca^{2+} and protein kinase C. J. Biol. Chem. **264:** 6325–6333.

45. CARTER, T. D., T. J. HALLAM & J. D. PEARSON. 1989. Protein kinase C activation alters the sensitivity of agonist-stimulated endothelial-cell prostacyclin production to intracellular Ca^{2+}. Biochem. J. **262:** 431–437.

46. BAULDRY, S. A., R. L. WYKLE & D. A. BASS. 1988. Phospholipase A_2 activation in human neutrophils. Differential actions of diacylglycerols and alkyl acylglycerols in primary cells for stimulation by *N*-formyl-Met-Leu-Phe. J. Biol. Chem. **263:** 16787–16795.

47. CHANNON, J. Y. & C. C. LESLIE. 1990. A Ca^{2+}-dependent mechanism for associating a soluble arachidonoyl-hydrolyzing PLA_2 with membrane in the macrophage cell line RAW264.7. J. Biol. Chem. **265:** 5409–5413.

48. CHIEN, K. R., J. ABRAMS, A. SERRONI, J. T. MARTIN & J. L. FARBER. 1978. Accelerated phospholipid degradation and associated membrane dysfunction in irreversible ischemic liver cell injury. J. Biol. Chem. **253:** 4809–4817.

49. SIESJO, B. K. 1981. Cell damage in the brain: A speculative synthesis. J. Cereb. Blood Flo. Metab. **1:** 155–166.

50. JONES, R. L., J. C. MILLER, H. K. HAGLER, K. R. CHIEN, J. T. WILLERSON & L. M. BUJA. 1989. Association between inhibition in arachidonic acid release and prevention of Ca^{2+} loading during ATP depletion in cultured rat cardiac myocytes. Am. J. Pathol. **135:** 541–556.

51. ARMSTRONG, S. C. & C. E. GANOTE. 1991. Effecs of the phospholipase inhibitor mepacrine on injury in ischemic and metabolically inhibited adult isolated myocytes. Am. J. Pathol. **138:** 545–555.

52. SHIER, W. T. 1979. Activation of high levels of endogenous PLA_2 in cultured cells. Proc. Natl. Acad. Sci. USA **75:** 195–199.

53. CHOI, D. W. 1988. Ca^{2+}-mediated neurotoxicity: Relationship to specific channel types and role in ischemic damage. T.I.N.S. **11:** 465–469.

54. MATTSON, M. P., P. B. GUTHRIE & S. B. KATER. 1989. A role for Na^{+}-dependent Ca^{2+} extrusion in protection against neuronal cytotoxicity. FASEB J. **3:** 2519–2526.

55. BEST, L., A. SENER, P. C. F. MATHIAS & W. J. MALAISSE. 1984. Inhibition by mepa-

crine and p-bromophenacylbromide of phosphoinositide hydrolysis, glucose oxidation, Ca^{2+} uptake and insulin release in rat pancreatic islets. Biochem. Pharmacol. **33:** 2657–2662.

56. SEN, A., J. C. MILLER, R. REYNOLDS, J. T. WILLERSON, L. M. BUJA & K. R. CHIEN. 1988. Inhibition of the release of arachidonate acid prevents the development of sarcolemmal membrane defects in cultured rat myocardial cells during adenosine triphosphate depletion. J. Clin. Invest. **82:** 1333–1338.

57. JONES, R. L., J. C. MILLER, H. K. HAGLER, K. R. CHIEN, J. T. WILLERSON & L. M. BUJA. 1989. Association between inhibition of arachidonic acid release and prevention of calcium loading during ATP depletion in cultured rat cardiac myocytes. Am. J. Pathol. **135:** 541–556.

58. DENNIS, E. A. 1987. The regulation of eicosanoid production: Role of phospholipases and inhibitors. Bio/Technology **5:** 1294–1300.

59. IRVINE, R. F., A. J. LETCHER & R. M. C. DAWSON. 1979. Fatty acid stimulation of membrane phosphatidylinositol hydrolysis by brain phosphatidylinositol phosphodiesterase. Biochem. J. **178:** 497–500.

60. ZEITLER, B. & S. HANDWERGER. 1985. Arachidonic acid stimulates phosphoinositide hydrolysis and human placental lactogen release in an enriched fraction of placental cells. Mol. Pharmacol. **28:** 549–554.

61. POON, R., J. M. RICHARDS, W. R. CLARK. 1981. The relationship between plasma membrane lipid composition and physical-chemical properties. II. Effect of phospholipid fatty acid modulation on plasma membrane physical properties and enzymatic activities. Biochem. Biophys. Acta **649:** 58–66.

62. GERZER, R., A. R. BRASH & J. G. HARDMAN. 1986. Activation of soluble guanylate cyclase by arachidonic acid and 15-lipoxygenase products. Biochem. Biophys. Acta **886:** 383–389.

63. McPHAIL, L. C., C. C. CLAYTON, & R. SNYDERMAN. 1984. A potential second messenger role for unsaturated fatty acids: Activation of Ca^{2+}-dependent protein kinase. Science **224:** 622–625.

64. MURAKAMI, K. & A. ROUTTENBERG. 1985. Direct activation of purified protein kinase C by unsaturated fatty acids (oleate and arachidonate) in the absence of phospholipids and Ca^{2+}. FEBS **192:** 189–193.

65. CHANG, J. P., J. GRAETER & K. J. CATT. 1986. Coordinate actions of arachidonic acid and protein kinase C in gonadotrophin releasing hormone-stimulated secretion of luteinizing hormone. Biochem. Biophys. Res. Commun. **134:** 134–139.

66. NAKAO, A., A. BUCHANAN & P. POTOBAR. 1980. Possible involvement of phospholipase A_2 in A23187-induced histamine release from purified rat mast cells. Int. Arch. Allergy Appl. Immunol. **63:** 30–43.

67. WOLF, B. A., J. TURK, W. R. SHERMAN & M. L. McDANIEL. 1986. Intracellular Ca^{2+} mobilization by arachidonic acid. Comparison with myo-inositol 1.4.5-trisphosphate in isolated pancreatic islets. J. Biol. Chem. **261:** 622–625.

68. YU, A. C. H., P. H. CHAN & R. A. FISHMAN. 1986. Effects of arachidonic acid on glutamate and gamma-amino butyric acid uptake in primary cultures of rat cerebral cortical astrocytes and neurons. J. Neurochem. **47:** 1181–1189.

Neurotrophic Factor Deprivation–induced Death

THOMAS L. DECKWERTH AND
EUGENE M. JOHNSON, JR.
Washington University School of Medicine
Department of Molecular Biology and Pharmacology
660 South Euclid Avenue, Box 8103
St. Louis, Missouri 63110

After the terminal division of the neuroblast, the now postmitotic neuron differentiates and establishes functional connections to the target. During this critical developmental period of neuronal death, the neuron becomes dependent for survival upon neurotrophic factors that are secreted by the innervated target and are only available to the neuron in limiting amounts. Insufficient access to the trophic factor causes degeneration and subsequent death of the dependent neuron. On average, the number of neurons in a population is reduced to about one half during this critical period. In molecular terms, intraneuronal processes, which maintain long-term stability and viability, are transiently under the control of the neurotrophic factor during this critical developmental period such that insufficient access to the trophic factor triggers the onset of regressive events that result in death of the neuron. The degeneration of a neuron proceeds in an autonomous, controlled manner and has apparently no negative impact on neighboring neurons or other cells. The understanding of the molecular processes underlying degeneration and death will add a new dimension to our knowledge of cellular physiology and may aid in elucidating the pathological mechanisms underlying acute neuronal injury, neurodegenerative diseases, and aging. Furthermore, the selective induction of these degenerative events in transformed cells may allow controlled tumor regression.[1]

The molecular mechanisms of degeneration and death caused by nerve growth factor (NGF) deprivation have been studied in neurons from spinal and sympathetic ganglia using morphological and biochemical approaches. Electron-microscopic images of sympathetic neurons dying after injection of anti-NGF antiserum into newborn rodents reveal degenerative changes[2–4] consistent with what has come to be termed apoptotic death.[5] NGF deprivation *in vitro* leads to nuclear alterations reminiscent of apoptosis in some of the neurons examined.[6] Early biochemical investigations of NGF actions on responsive neurons, conducted with intact ganglia or cell suspensions of freshly dissociated ganglia, focused on metabolic parameters and homeostasis of ionic gradients across the plasma membrane.[7,8] The results of these studies are difficult to interpret because the neuronal preparations were suffering from mechanical injury and axotomy and not many neurons were capable of long-term survival even in the presence of NGF.[7,9] However, it is not necessary to use freshly prepared neuronal preparations to study the effects of NGF withdrawal. Established cultures of embryonic sympathetic neurons can be maintained for months and are dependent upon NGF for survival in a qualitatively similar way as *in vivo*.[10,11] In such cultures, degeneration and death after NGF deprivation are prevented by inhibitors of RNA and protein synthesis.[6] The dependence of death on macromolecular synthesis has been reproduced in this and other neuronal systems *in vitro*[12,13] and *in vivo*.[14] One possible explanation for the ability of inhibitors of protein and RNA synthesis to prevent death is the suppression of the synthesis of gene products that mediate the coordinated death of the cell. Other possible interpretations of this observation have been discussed previously in detail.[15] Two other classes of compounds capable of preventing death, whose most effective members include potassium ion and cyclic 8-(4-chlorophenyl-thio)adenosine-3':5'-monophosphate (CPTcAMP), moderately increase the concentration of free intracellular calcium[16] or raise or mimic elevated cytoplasmic cAMP levels,[13,17,18] respectively. Interferon γ is able to retard the onset of NGF deprivation-induced death, but does not prevent death.[19] Recently, data have been reported that suggest that NGF, potassium ion, and CPTcAMP halt degeneration initiated by NGF deprivation by a posttranslational mechanism.[13] Thus a translation-independent mechanism may exist capable of stopping the progression of degeneration and thereby preventing neuronal death.

TEMPORAL ANALYSIS OF THE SEQUENCE OF MOLECULAR CHANGES UNDERLYING NGF DEPRIVATION-INDUCED DEGENERATION AND DEATH

Previous studies from our laboratory used the release of the cytosolic enzyme adenylate kinase into the medium as a measure of neuronal death.[6] Release of adenylate kinase starts relatively late after NGF removal consistent with the visual impression of a delay prior to onset of cell loss. The existence of such a lag phase is confirmed by counting viable neurons using both refractility (data not shown) and crystal violet staining (FIG. 1) as criteria for viability. Cell loss begins 18 h after NGF deprivation and is essentially complete by 48 h; half the cells have died by 27 h. This time-course of loss of viability is considerably different from the time-course reported for serum deprivation-induced death of PC12 cells.[20] PC12 cells, a rat pheochromocytoma cell line that can acquire a sympathetic neuron-like phenotype upon exposure to NGF, does not require NGF for survival in the presence of serum. Under serum-free conditions, PC12 cells die rapidly but their death can be prevented by NGF[20] and other growth factors.[21] The lack of a substantial delay and the first-order exponential loss of viability of PC12 cells suggests that serum deprivation triggers a single rate-limiting stochastic process that leads to death. In contrast, the delay seen in neuronal death is indicative of at least one, possibly several, processes that are required to trigger loss of viability. The existence of such a sequence of degenerative events is substantiated further by the dependence of death upon protein and RNA synthesis,[6] which may indicate the active participation of gene products in the degenerative process. No such requirement for macromolecular synthesis is observed for death of serum-deprived PC12 cells.[21] The ability of interferon γ to retard the rate of death[19] was interpreted to indicate that the inhibition of a putative cascade of degenerative events is analogous to the cascade of events initiated by viral replication or mitogenic stimulation.

Evidence for a sequence of degenerative processes can be obtained by measuring when and how different morphological and biochemical parameters change after onset of NGF deprivation. FIGURE 2 illustrates such a series of time-courses of hypothetical parameters which increase or decrease prior loss of viability. The order in which parameters change is determined by the time of onset of change and the time or half-maximal change for each parameter. A temporal sequence of changes of different parameters would define in which order and with what rate different functional compartments within the cell become affected by removal of growth factor. In further experiments, the characterization of a sequence of degenerative events will allow one to determine whether the changes of different parameters are connected causally to death. Such an analysis is currently in progress.

The presence of a temporally resolvable sequence of degenerative events predicts that neuroprotective agents, which halt particular steps of this degenerative cascade, will only be active during certain periods, *i.e.*, before the execution of the process they inhibit specifically is completed. The width of the therapeutic

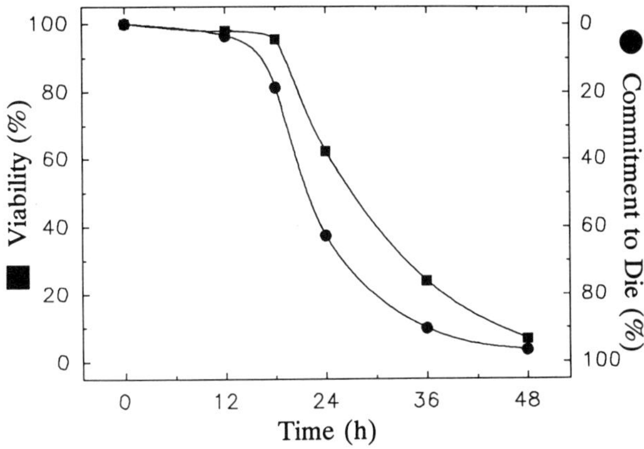

FIGURE 1. Time-courses of viability (■) and commitment to die (●) of sympathetic neurons deprived of NGF. Cultures of embryonic rat superior cervical ganglion (SCG) neurons maintained for 8 d were deprived of NGF for various times between 0 and 48 h as indicated on the abscissa. To measure the time-course of viability, cultures were fixed with 4% buffered paraformaldehyde, stained with crystal violet, dehydrated, and mounted permanently. Neuronal cell bodies were counted as viable if they stained with crystal violet more strongly than did the debris. To measure the time-course of commitment to die, after various times of NGF deprivation NGF was added back and the neurons maintained for one more week. After this period, only neurons able to respond to NGF with long-term survival at the time of readdition of NGF remained. The number of neurons was determined as described for the time-course of viability. The details of the procedure will be published elsewhere.[46] Half the neurons are committed to die and have died after 22 h and 27 h, respectively.

window for a neuroprotective agent is measured by determining the fraction of NGF-deprived neurons capable of responding to the agent with long-term survival after various times of NGF-deprivation. The decreasing curves in FIGURE 2 illustrate how such time-courses of rescue may look like. The presence of a cascade of events would predict that the time-courses of rescue with neuroprotective agents should neither be identical (but perhaps not be experimentally resolvable) nor be superimposable onto the time-course of loss of viability for agents acting by different mechanisms. Experimental evidence for this notion is emerging. In sympathetic neurons, the time-course of rescue with cycloheximide, an inhibitor of protein synthesis, has been reported to precede the time-course of rescue with

NGF;[13] thus, there appears to be a period during which inhibition of protein synthesis can no longer halt the progression of degeneration, while NGF is still capable of conferring protection. This suggests that NGF can act to prevent death at a time subsequent to the synthesis of all proteins necessary to kill the cell. Importantly, the time-course of rescue with NGF precedes the time-course of loss of viability by only 5 h (FIG. 1). This means, that upon loss of the ability to respond to NGF with survival, the neuron has become committed to die and will loose viability a few hours later (defined by crystal violet staining). Since this delay between loss of rescuability with NGF and loss of viability is very short, NGF acts as a neuroprotective agent for more than 80% of the time after NGF deprivation (for 22 h out of 27 h, FIG. 1). No agent has yet been found that protects against

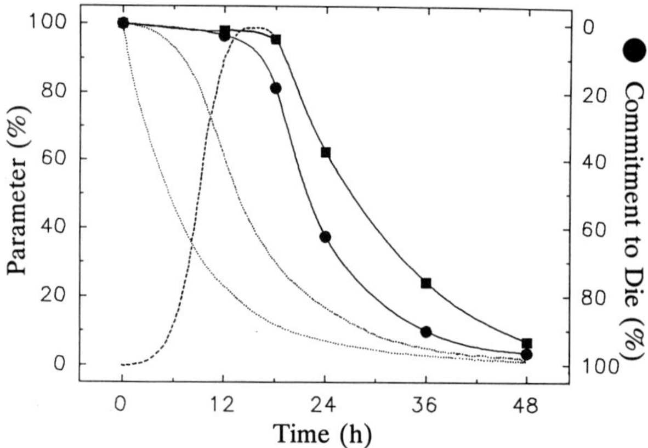

FIGURE 2. Construction of a map of the temporal sequence of changes initiated by NGF deprivation. Loss of viability (■) and commitment to die (●) are preceded by changes in other functional neuronal parameters. These parameters may either be acute changes, such as the amount or rate of turnover of specific cellular components, or more complex responses, such as the ability to respond to different neuroprotective agents with survival. NGF deprivation may cause parameters to decrease (·····) or increase (-----) with different time-courses prior to commitment to die and loss of viability. Time-courses of rescue with neuroprotective agents will only decrease monotonously (·····). The time-points of onset and half-maximal change of different parameters can be used to construct a map of the temporal sequence underlying neuronal degeneration.

death at later times than does NGF. Therefore, measured by the length of the period starting with onset of NGF deprivation and ending with loss of the ability of a neuroprotective agent to maintain survival, NGF is the most effective neuroprotective compound for sympathetic neurons known.

In conclusion, determination of the time-courses of morphological and biochemical parameters should enable the construction of a temporal map of the acute degenerative changes that are initiated by NGF deprivation and lead to death. The order of the time-courses of rescue will define the temporal sequence of critical events whose inhibition halts progression of degeneration and will yield information about the therapeutic windows for neuroprotective agents in this paradigm of neurodegeneration.

TROPHIC FACTORS, THEIR MIMETICS, AND THEIR INDUCERS ARE POTENTIAL AGENTS FOR THE TREATMENT OF NEURODEGENERATIVE DISEASES AND NEURONAL INJURY

Depending upon their mode of action, neuroprotective agents not only differ in respect to their therapeutic windows but also in respect to the quality of protection they provide. Besides having a wide therapeutic window that lasts as long as possible toward loss of viability, an ideal neuroprotective agent would act to prevent death by halting the progression of degenerative changes and, in addition, initiate trophic events that repair and reverse the inflicted damage. Because degeneration progresses and worsens the condition of the neuron with increasing time after NGF deprivation, the trophic activity conferred by a neuroprotective agent will be the more important, the later after onset of degeneration rescue with a neuroprotective agent is attempted. For NGF-deprived sympathetic neurons, NGF, potassium ion, and CPTcAMP come close to this ideal *in vitro*. In contrast, cycloheximide halts NGF deprivation-induced degeneration and death but does not provide trophic support. In fact, its presence is incompatible with true long-term survival because it inhibits total cellular protein synthesis, a process obviously required for long-term survival of cells in general. Likewise, protection from death by aurintricarboxylic acid, an inhibitor of nucleases and numerous other enzymes, prevents death but shows toxic side effects and does not appear to provide trophic support.[22] Interferon γ is different from all these agents in that it does not halt degeneration and death but rather retards their initiation or slows the progression of the degenerative process.[19]

The presence of a period of degeneration that precedes the onset of death is not limited to neurotrophic factor deprivation-induced death but is also shared by neurodegenerative conditions and sequelae of neuronal injury. Cholinergic neurons of the basal forebrain, one of several neuronal populations affected by Alzheimer's disease, show pronounced atrophy as measured by a reduction of soma size and loss of cholinergic markers prior to loss of viability.[23] This atrophy and loss of cholinergic markers, such as choline acetyl-transferase (ChAT) staining, can be induced experimentally by a lesion to fimbria and fornix. The delayed onset of an intraventricular infusion of NGF weeks after placing the lesion, at which time ChAT staining is greatly diminished in the injured neurons, reverses the degenerative morphological changes and restores ChAT activity in a large fraction of the affected neurons.[24] This NGF-rescue paradigm clearly demonstrates that death of cholinergic neurons of the basal forebrain is preceded by an extensive period of degeneration. Evidence is increasing that the cause for these degenerative changes, either directly or indirectly, is the deposition of the β-amyloid protein, which in turn is caused by environmental and familial factors.[25,26] Thus, loss of viability of neurons affected by neurodegenerative diseases such as Alzheimer's is preceded by a series of slowly accumulating degenerative changes similar to those seen after neurotrophic factor deprivation prior to the death of the neuron. In the case of transient excitotoxic damage to hippocampal, cerebellar, or cortical neurons, for example, as a result of stroke, the onset of neuronal death starts after a considerable delay after termination of the excitotoxic insult. The degenerative changes underlying this delayed neuronal death have been tentatively divided into three phases: induction, amplification, and expression.[27] Each phase is characterized by the action of specific molecular mechanisms. Inherent in this model is a sequence of degenerative events that ultimately causes death. Furthermore, the specific pharmacological interventions proposed and proven to halt progression of excitotoxic damage should be effective during restricted temporal windows after the initial toxic insult is over. This has, in fact, been demonstrated both *in vivo* and *in vitro* for *N*-methyl-D-aspartate receptor antagonists that prevent delayed neuronal death when given subsequent to the excitotoxic or ischemic insult.[28-30]

These similarities with respect to the time-courses of degeneration and death in neurotrophic factor deprivation–induced death, neurodegenerative diseases, and delayed neuronal death suggest that the idea of a cascade of degenerative events leading to death may be a common underlying principle in neurodegeneration. This is not to say that the molecular details underlying neurotrophic factor deprivation–induced death, neurodegenerative diseases, and delayed neuronal death are identical. However, evidence is accumulating that suggests that neurotrophic factors act as neuroprotecive agents in all these paradigms of neuronal death. NGF protects forebrain cholinergic neurons from degeneration and death caused by neuronal injury and aging and reverses the decrease of cognitive abilities that parallels these processes.[31] NGF has been reported to reduce delayed neuronal death of hippocampal neurons caused by transient ischemia *in vivo*[32] and to block hypoglycemia-induced death of hippocampal neurons *in vitro*.[33] Brain-derived neurotrophic factor (BDNF) is a neurotrophic factor for retinal ganglion cells,[34] septal cholinergic neurons,[35] and ventral mesencephalic dopaminergic neurons *in vitro*[36] and protects the latter neurons from MPP$^+$-induced damage.[36] Ciliary neurotrophic factor (CNTF) enhances the survival of selected populations of hippocampal neurons[37] and protects central motorneurons[38] and medial septal neurons[39] from death after axotomy. Thus, neurotrophic factors can reverse degenerative processes in neurons compromised by various different insults, suggesting that the molecular mechanisms triggered by neurotrophic factors can reverse a wide spectrum of degenerative conditions. Taken together, the high quality of protection conferred by neurotrophic factors, their wide temporal window for neuroprotective action, and the responsivity of populations of central neurons affected by neurodegenerative disease and acute injury to neurotrophic factors suggest, that trophic factors, compounds that mimic their action closely, or agents that induce their synthesis in appropriate locations[40] should display rather optimal properties as neuroprotective compounds.

DNA FRAGMENTATION MAY BE A MARKER FOR AND PART OF THE MECHANISM UNDERLYING THE COMMITMENT OF NEURONS TO DIE

In vivo, a neuron is committed to die during the critical developmental period if, after a period of insufficient supply with trophic factor, it can no longer be rescued from death by the physiological trophic factor. By analogy, the time-course of commitment to die for sympathetic neurons *in vitro* is defined as the time-course of rescue with NGF (FIG. 1). This definition can be extended to include other neuroprotective agents in which case the commitment to die becomes a function of the particular neuroprotective agent chosen.[18] The molecular mechanisms underlying the commitment to die are not known but are accessible to investigation.

The molecular hallmark of apoptotic death, a commonly seen mode of physiologically appropriate cell death, is the degradation of the nuclear DNA by a Ca^{++}/Mg^{++}-activated endonuclease to oligonucleosomal fragments.[5] DNA fragmentation precedes lysis and is not seen in physiological settings after lysis has occurred. While it is not understood, if or how DNA fragmentation leads to subsequent death, it has not been possible to dissociate DNA fragmentation from death. In sympathetic neurons, NGF deprivation induces DNA fragmentation after a delay of 19 h (FIG. 3) in close temporal association with the onset of commitment to die (FIG. 1). The detection of fragmented DNA in sympathetic neurons deprived of NGF has been reported, while this work was in progress,[13]

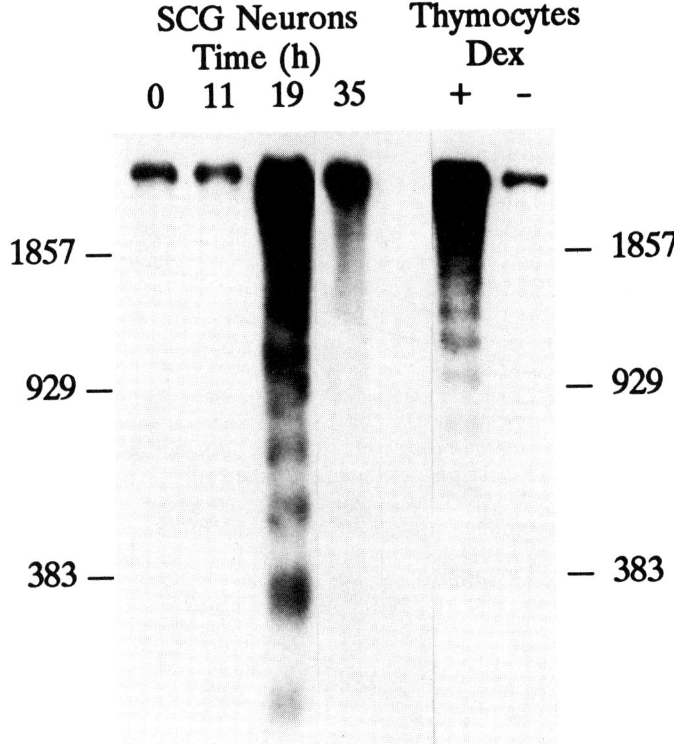

FIGURE 3. The time-course of DNA fragmentation in sympathetic neurons induced by NGF deprivation. Total neuronal DNA was prepared from cultures containing equal numbers (about 5000 neurons) of SCG neurons deprived of NGF for various times between 0 and 35 h, separated on a 3% agarose gel, transferred to a nylon membrane and hybridized with a [^{32}P]-labeled probe prepared from total rat genomic DNA by random priming. As comparison, the two right lanes show genomic DNA prepared from equal numbers of rat thymocytes, which can be induced to fragment their genome upon exposure to the glucocorticoid dexamethasone. The details of the procedure will be published elsewhere.[46]

although a time-course of DNA fragmentation and correlation with commitment was not presented. The possible presence of DNA fragmentation was also suggested by the finding, that aurintricarboxylic acid, an inhibitor of nucleases among many other enzymes, prevents NGF deprivation–induced death.[22]

The temporal correlation between the onset of DNA fragmentation and commitment to die suggests a functional role for DNA fragmentation in the process of commitment to die. Such a role is supported by the time-course of DNA fragmentation seen upon serum deprivation of PC12 cells,[22] DNA fragmentation starts as early as 3 h after onset of serum deprivation, consistent with the lack of a substantial delay prior to onset of loss of viability. The time-course of rescue with serum has not yet been reported for PC12 cells; however, one would expect this time-course to be very similar to and possibly indistinguishable from the time-course of loss of viability because there is no substantial delay between serum deprivation and onset of cell loss.[20] Furthermore, addition of NGF after various times of serum deprivation immediately halts further cell death suggesting that the time-courses of NGF rescue and viability may not be experimentally resolvable.[20] Since long-term survival of most cells requires coordinated RNA and protein synthesis, fragmentation of the genome appears inconsistent with long-term survival. However, inhibition of RNA and protein synthesis *per se* is not likely to be the cause of the rapid demise of the cells since synthesis of RNA and protein itself decreases precipitously immediately after onset of NGF deprivation (T. L. Deckwerth, unpublished) and since sympathetic neurons survive extended periods of complete inhibition of RNA and protein synthesis.[18,41] Thus, DNA fragmentation may possibly trigger other, so far, uncharacterized processes inside the neuron, which lead to death. A potential candidate may be the activation of poly(ADP-ribose) synthetase.[42] Alternatively, DNA fragmentation may be an epiphenomenon not directly linked to cell death.

The occurrence of DNA fragmentation may be of diagnostic value in other systems of neuronal degeneration as well, since it may serve as a marker for the critical phase in which trophic factors lose the ability to halt and reverse progression of degeneration. DNA fragmentation has also been observed in nervous tissue during both developmental cell death[43] and upon intoxication.[44,45] Thus, it appears possible that in some neurodegenerative diseases and conditions of neuronal injury, DNA fragmentation in neurons may indicate the state of degeneration and predict the response to treatment with trophic factors.

SUMMARY

Deprivation of sympathetic neurons of their physiological neurotrophic factor, nerve growth factor (NGF), leads to degeneration of soma and neurites, followed by loss of viability. The progression of degeneration and death are dependent upon macromolecular synthesis indicating an active participation of neuronal metabolism. Loss of viability begins only after a considerable delay after onset of NGF deprivation suggesting the presence of a sequence of degenerative events that triggers death. Such a sequence of degenerative events predicts that the activity of neuroprotective agents functioning by different mechanisms will be restricted to particular windows in time. The time-course of commitment to die as measured by the ability of NGF-deprived neurons to respond to NGF with long-term survival precedes the time-course of loss of viability by only a few hours, demonstrating that NGF displays neuroprotective properties for most of the time between onset of deprivation and death. Furthermore, NGF repairs and reverses the degenerative changes caused by prolonged periods of NGF deprivation. Because of these two aspects of NGF action, NGF demonstrates superior properties as a neuroprotective agent. NGF deprivation initiates DNA fragmentation of the neuronal genome into oligonucleosomal fragments in close temporal association with the onset of commitment to die. This is consistent with the idea that DNA fragmentation may be instrumental in causing the commitment to die. Thus, DNA fragmentation may serve as a marker of the physiologically most relevant critical step occurring during degeneration and may indicate the end of the period during which trophic factors are useful as neuroprotective agents. These results may be transferable to neurodegenerative diseases or sequelae of neuronal injury because of similarities in the phenomenology of degeneration and death.

REFERENCES

1. TRAUTH, B. C., C. KLAS, A. M. J. PETERS, S. MATZKU, P. MÖLLER, W. FALK, K.-M. DEBATIN, & P. H. KRAMMER. 1989. Monoclonal antibody-mediated tumor regression by induction of apoptosis. Science **245:** 301–304.
2. ANGELETTI, P. U., R. LEVI-MONTALCINI & F. CARAMIA. 1971. Analysis of the effects of the antiserum to the nerve growth factor in adult mice. Brain Res. **27:** 343–355.
3. LEVI-MONTALCINI, R., F. CARAMIA & P. U. ANGELETTI. 1969. Alterations in the fine strucure of nucleoli in sympathetic neurons following NGF-antiserum treatment. Brain Res. **12:** 54–73.
4. WRIGHT, L. L., T. J. CUNNINGHAM & A. J. SMOLEN. 1983. Developmental neuron death in the rat superior cervical sympathetic ganglion: Cell counts and ultrastructure. J. Neurocytol. **12:** 727–738.
5. ARENDS, M. J. & A. H. WYLLIE. 1991. Apoptosis: Mechanisms and roles in pathology. Int. Rev. Exp. Pathol. **32:** 223–254.
6. MARTIN, D. P., R. E. SCHMIDT, P. S. DiSTEFANO, O. H. LOWRY, J. G. CARTER & E. M. JOHNSON, JR. 1988. Inhibitors of protein synthesis and RNA synthesis prevent neuronal death caused by nerve growth factor deprivation. J. Cell Biol. **106:** 829–844.
7. THOENEN, H. & Y. A. BARDE. 1980. Physiology of nerve growth factor. Physiol. Rev. **60:** 1284–1335.
8. VARON, S. & S. D. SKAPER. 1983. The Na^+, K^+ pump may mediate the control of nerve cells by nerve growth factor. TIBS **8:** 22–25.
9. SENDTNER, M., H. GNAHN, A. WAKADE & H. THOENEN. 1985. Is activation of the Na^+K^+ pump necessary for NGF-mediated neuronal survival? J. Neurosci. **8:** 458–462.
10. LAZARUS, K. J., R. A. BRADSHAW, N. R. WEST & R. P. BUNGE. 1976. Adaptive survival of rat sympathetic neurons cultured without supporting cells or exogenous nerve growth factor. Brain Res. **113:** 159–164.
11. KOIKE, T. & S. TANAKA. 1991. Evidence that nerve growth factor dependence of sympathetic neurons for survival *in vitro* may be determined by levels of cytoplasmic free Ca^{2+}. Proc. Natl. Acad. Sci. USA **88:** 3892–3896.
12. SCOTT, S. A. & A. M. DAVIES. 1990. Inhibition of protein synthesis prevents cell death in sensory and parasympathetic neurons deprived of neurotrophic factor *in vitro*. J. Neurobiol. **21:** 630–638.
13. EDWARDS, S. N., A. E. BUCKMASTER & A. M. TOLKOVSKY. 1991. The death programme in cultured sympathetic neurones can be suppressed at the posttranslational level by nerve growth factor, cyclic AMP, and depolarization. J. Neurochem. **57:** 2140–2143.
14. OPPENHEIM, R. W. 1991. Cell death during development of the nervous system. Ann. Rev. Neurosci. **14:** 453–501.
15. JOHNSON, E. M., JR. & T. L. DECKWERTH. 1993. Molecular mechanisms of developmental neuronal death. Ann. Rev. Neurosci. **16:** 31–46.
16. KOIKE, T., D. P. MARTIN & E. M. JOHNSON, JR. 1989. Role of Ca^{2+} channels in the ability of membrane depolarization to prevent neuronal death induced by trophic-factor deprivation: Evidence that levels of internal Ca^{2+} determine nerve growth factor dependence of sympathetic ganglion cells. Proc. Natl. Acad. Sci. USA **86:** 6421–6425.
17. RYDEL, R. & L. A. GREENE. 1988. cAMP analogs promote survival and neurite out-

growth in cultures of rat sympathetic and sensory neurons independently of nerve growth factor. Proc. Natl. Acad. Sci. USA **85:** 1257–1261.

18. MARTIN, D. P., A. ITO, K. HORIGOME, P. A. LAMPE & E. M. JOHNSON, JR. 1992. Biochemical characterization of programmed cell death in NGF-deprived sympathetic neurons. J. Neurobiol. **23:** 1205–1220.

19. CHANG, J. Y., D. P. MARTIN & E. M. JOHNSON, JR. 1990. Interferon suppresses sympathetic neuronal cell death caused by nerve growth factor deprivation. J. Neurochem. **55:** 436–445.

20. L. A. GREENE. 1978. Nerve growth factor prevents the death and stimulates the neuronal differentiation of clonal PC12 pheochromocytoma cells in serum-free medium. J. Cell Biol. **78:** 747–755.

21. RUKENSTEIN, A., R. E. RYDEL & L. A. GREENE. 1991. Multiple agents rescue PC12 cells from serum-free cell death by translation- and transcription-independent mechanisms. J. Neurosci. **11:** 2552–2563.

22. BATISTATOU, A. & L. A. GREENE. 1991. Aurintricarboxylic acid rescues PC12 cells and sympathetic neurons from cell death caused by nerve growth factor deprivation: Correlation with suppression of endonuclease activity. J. Cell Biol. **115:** 461–471.

23. KOLIATSOS, V. E., R. E. CLATTERBUCK, G. K. GOURAS & D. L. PRICE. 1991. Biologic effects of nerve growth factor on lesioned basal forebrain neurons. Ann. N.Y. Acad. Sci. **640:** 102–109.

24. HAGG, T., M. MANTHROPE, H. L. VAHLSING & S. VARON. 1988. Delayed treatment with nerve growth factor reverses the apparent loss of cholinergic neurons after acute brain damage. Exp. Neurol. **101:** 303–312.

25. SELKOE, D. J. 1991. The molecular pathology of Alzheimer's disease. Neuron **6:** 487–498.

26. HARDY, J. A. & HIGGINS, G. A. 1992. Alzheimer's Disease: The amyloid cascade hypothesis. Science **256:** 184–185.

27. CHOI, D. W. 1990. Methods for antagonizing glutamate toxicity. Cerebrovasc. Brain. Metab. Rev. **2:** 105–147.

28. HARTLEY, D. M. & D. W. CHOI. 1989. Delayed rescue of N-methyl-D-aspartate receptor-mediated neuronal injury in cortical culture. J. Pharm. Exp. Therap. **250:** 752–758.

29. FOSTER, A. C., R. GILL & G. N. WOODRUFF. 1988. Neuroprotective effects of MK-801 in vivo: Selectivity and evidence for delayed degeneration mediated by NMDA receptor activation. J. Neurosci. **8:** 4745–4754.

30. GILL, R., A. C. FOSTER & G. N. WOODRUFF. 1988. MK-801 is neuroprotective in gerbils when administered during the post-ischaemic period. Neuroscience **25:** 847–855.

31. GAGE, F. H., M. H. TUSZYNSKI, K. S. CHEN, A. M. FAGAN & G. A. HIGGINS. 1991. Nerve growth factor function in the central nervous system. Curr. Top. Microbiol. Immunol. **165:** 71–93.

32. SHIGENO, T., T. MIMA, K. TAKAKURA, D. I. GRAHAM, G. KATO, Y. HASHIMOTO & S. FURUKAWA. 1991. Amelioration of delayed neuronal death in the hippocampus by nerve growth factor. J. Neurosci. **11:** 2914–2919.

33. CHENG, B. & M. P. MATTSON. 1991. NGF and bFGF protect rat hippocampal and human cortical neurons against hypoglycemic damage by stabilizing calcium homeostasis. Neuron **7:** 1031–1041.

34. JOHNSON, J. E., Y.-A. BARDE, M. SCHWAB & H. THOENEN. 1986. Brain-derived neurotrophic factor supports the survival of cultured rat retinal ganglion cells. J. Neurosci. **6:** 3031–3038.

35. ALDERSON, R. F., A. L. ALTERMAN, Y.-A. BARDE & R. M. LINDSAY. 1990. Brain-derived neurotrophic factor increases survival and differentiated functions of rat septal cholinergic neurons in culture. Neuron **5:** 297–306.

36. C. HYMAN, M. HOFER, Y.-A. BARDE, M. JUHASZ, G. D. YANCOPOULOS, S. P. SQUINTO & R. M. LINDSAY. 1991. BDNF is a neurotrophic factor for dopaminergic neurons of the substantia nigra. Nature **350:** 230–232.

37. IP, N. Y., Y. LI, I. VAN DE STADT, N. PANAYOTATOS, R. F. ALDERSON & R. M. LINDSAY. 1991. Ciliary neurotrophic factor enhances neuronal survival in embryonic rat hippocampal neurons. J. Neurosci. **11:** 3124–3134.

38. M. SENDTNER, G. W. KREUZBERG & H. THOENEN. 1990. Ciliary neurotrophic factor prevents the degeneration of motor neurons after axotomy. Nature **345:** 440–441.

39. T. HAGG, D. QUON, J. HIGAKI & S. VARON. 1992. Ciliary neurotrophic factor prevents neuronal degeneration and promotes low affinity NGF receptor expression in the adult rat CNS. Neuron **8:** 145–158.

40. H. THOENEN, F. ZAFRA, B. HENGERER & D. LINDHOLM. 1991. The synthesis of nerve growth factor and brain-derived growth factor in hippocampal and cortical neurons is regulated by specific transmitter systems. Ann. N. Y. Acad. Sci. **640:** 86–90.

41. CLARKE, P. G. H. 1990. Developmental cell death: Morphological diversity and multiple mechanisms. Anat. Embryol. **181:** 195–213.

42. CARSON, D. A., S. SETO, B. WASSON & C. J. CARRERA. 1986. DNA strand breaks, NAD metabolism, and programmed cell death. Exp. Cell Res. **164:** 273–281.

43. ILSCHNER, S. U. & P. WARING. 1992. Fragmentation of DNA in the retina of chicken embryos coincides with retinal ganglion cell death. Biochem. Biophys. Res. Commun. **183:** 1056–1061.

44. KURE, S., T. TOMINAGA, T. YOSHIMOTO, K. TADA & K. NARISAWA. 1991. Glutamate triggers internucleosomal DNA cleavage in neuronal cells. Biochem. Biophys. Res. Commun. **179:** 39–45.

45. DIPASQUALE, B., A. M. MARINI & R. J. YOULE. 1991. Apoptosis and DNA degradation induced by 1-methyl-4-phenylpyridinium in neurons. Biochem. Biophys. Res. Commun. **181:** 1442–1448.

46. DECKWERTH, T. L. & E. M. JOHNSON, JR. In preparation.

Glutamate, Immediate-Early Genes, and Cell Death in the Nervous System

MONTSERRAT VENDRELL, TOM CURRAN, AND
JAMES I. MORGAN[a]

Roche Institute of Molecular Biology
Roche Research Center
Nutley, New Jersey 07110

Neurons possess several morphological and physiological characteristics that set them apart from other cell types and permits them to receive, process and relay information. However, this level of specialization seems to have been developed at the expense of making neurons vulnerable to the very signaling mechanisms that support these unique physiological properties. For example, excessive exposure of neurons to excitatory amino acid (EAA) neurotransmitters, (one of the primary classes of intercellular signalling molecules of the brain) or the ingress of abnormally large amounts of calcium (a major intracellular second messenger in neurons) can result in neuronal damage. Indeed, several pathological conditions that have neuronal death as a component, such as cerebral ischemia and epilepsy, seem to involve activation of the NMDA (*N*-methyl-D-aspartate) subtype of the glutamate receptor which directly gate calcium. In addition, a number of environmental neurotoxins, such as kainic and domoic acids, act through other classes of glutamate receptors to cause neuronal damage and loss. This class of glutamate receptor can lead to elevated intracellular ionized calcium levels via indirect gating through voltage-sensitive calcium channels opened as a consequence of depolarization.

These observations have led to an aggressive search for agents that can prevent or attenuate neuronal loss. While most studies have investigated agents that act to block glutamate receptors or inhibit calcium uptake, several studies have shown that protein synthesis inhibitors can be neuroprotective.[1] This suggests that the insults that lead to neuronal death activate, or require, gene expression. Indeed, we and others, have shown that several neurotoxins, including kainic acid and lindane (gamma-hexachlorocyclohexane), as well as cerebral ischemia and surgical lesions, activate the transcription of cellular immediate-early (cIE) genes in the brain. Since many cIE genes encode transcription factors that control the expression of target genes, they could provide a key mechanistic link between neuronal activation and transcriptional programs that may be involved in cell death. While there is evidence of an association between activation of a cIE response and cell death, the precise significance of this correlation is unknown. However, these data are sufficiently compelling to review them here and to propose a scheme that might provide the basis for future experiments aimed at elucidating the molecular mechanisms contributing to the process of cell death in the nervous system.

---

[a] Address correspondence to James I. Morgan, Ph.D.; Tel.: (201)235-5999.

WHAT IS THE CELLULAR IMMEDIATE-EARLY RESPONSE?

In response to transynaptic excitation, neurons can exhibit both short-term and long-term responses. Rapid, (often short-lived), transcription-independent changes are elicited by the modification of pre-existing substrates, such as phosphorylation of ion channels, enzymes, receptors or cytoskeletal proteins by protein kinases. By contrast, relatively short periods of excitation can also bring about responses that persist over a longer time-frame and often require *de novo* protein synthesis. In the nervous system, such transcription-dependent responses appear to contribute to synaptic plasticity, neuronal sprouting and long-term modifications of the output of a neuronal system, as might occur, for instance, in learning and memory.[2,3] This has been taken to imply that gene expression may play a role in these processes. While an understanding of the molecular mechanisms that couple short-lived, second messenger-mediated, events to long-term adaptive alterations in neurons is obviously of extreme relevance, it is only recently that the details of stimulus-transcription coupling have begun to be unraveled.

Extracellular stimuli elicit the rapid, transient, transcriptional activation of a class of genes known as cellular immediate-early (cIE) genes.[4] Many of these genes encode nuclear proteins, that are known, or putative, transcription factors such as Fos and Jun.[5] Fos, the protein encoded by the proto-oncogene c-*fos,* forms a dimeric complex with Jun, the product of another proto-oncogene, c-*jun.* This association occurs through an α-helical domain called a leucine zipper, that contains a heptad repeat of leucine residues.[6] Fos-Jun heterodimers bind to a specific DNA sequence TGACTCA which is known to be the consensus binding site for the transcription factor, activator protein 1 (AP-1). In fact, Fos and Jun, as well as the products of other members of the *fos* and *jun* gene families, are known to be constituents of AP-1.[7] Furthermore, any individual member of the *fos* family can form heterodimers with any individual member of the *jun* family. In addition, members of the *jun* family can dimerize amongst themselves, although members of the *fos* family cannot. However, it is now recognized that the *fos* and *jun* families are members of a larger superfamily of genes that encode proteins that possess a leucine zipper and a basic DNA binding domain. This class of genes is referred to as the basic-zipper superfamily and contains members of the activating transcription factor (ATFs) and cAMP response element binding protein (CREB) families. This greatly increases the range of potential dimers and means that both inducible and constitutive transcription factors can be involved in the cIE response. Thus, Fos and Jun can display AP-1 or CREB binding activities depending upon the other protein with which they are complexed. Since AP-1 and CRE sites are known to be important for both basal and stimulated transcription from a number of genes it is supposed that cIE gene products can interact with other inducible and constitutive transcription factors to bring about alterations in expression of these target genes. In this sense the cIE gene products behave as if they were nuclear third messengers, coupling short term extracellular stimuli to longer term alterations in cellular phenotype by changing target gene expression.[3]

REGULATION OF INTRACELLULAR CALCIUM LEVELS IN NEURONS

Calcium ions are an important intracellular second messenger in neurons, and are used ubiquitously in signal transduction at the synapse. In principle, calcium ions come from two sources during signaling events; by gating from the extracellular milieu and by controlled release from intracellular stores and pools. Once in the cytosol, the calcium ions activate calmodulin, thereby regulating the many calmodulin-dependent processes; additionally the ions interact directly with many enzymes and other proteins to modify their properties. As noted above, excessively high levels of intracellular calcium are deleterious and thus, free calcium concentrations within most cells are maintained within very strict limits.

Several intracellular mechanisms cooperate to maintain the intracellular free calcium concentration in the nanomolar range, representing a chemical gradient of some 1:10,000 to the millimolar levels present in the extracellular milieu. For example, calcium can be pumped out of the cell through energy-dependent mechanisms involving sodium-calcium exchange proteins or calcium ATPases. Alternatively calcium may be actively sequestered into intracellular compartments, such as the endoplasmic reticulum (ER) or mitochondria, by the action of distinct forms of calcium ATPases. In addition, calcium may be buffered by cytosolic calcium-binding proteins, such as calmodulin or calbindin 28 K,[8] which are frequently present at particularly high levels in neurons.

Calcium enters the cell through two types of channels: those that are voltage-dependent and those that are receptor-operated. Several classes of pharmacological agents act upon the voltage-sensitive calcium channel, amongst which are the dihydropyridines (DHP)[9,10] which interact with the so-called L-type channels. DHP agonists such as BAY K8644, can elicit convulsions,[11] while antagonists such as nimodipine and nifedipine are able to prevent the seizures induced by pentylenetetrazole (PTZ)[12,13] and lindane.[14] Both PTZ and lindane are believed to act on the chloride channel associated with the gamma-aminobutyric acid receptor (GABA$_A$) receptor. Suppression of the GABA system results in hyperactivity of neurons with a subsequent depolarization leading to the opening of L-type, voltage-dependent, calcium channels. For example, lindane has been reported to produce both time- and dose-dependent increases in intracellular free calcium levels[15] that can be blocked by antagonists of the L-type calcium channel.[16] Calcium can also enter the cell through receptor-operated channels. While a number of neurotransmitter receptors are calcium gating channels, the most relevant for this discussion are those that involve the excitatory amino acid receptors and will be discussed below.

Transient elevation of intracellular calcium levels also results from the liberation of sequestered calcium from organelles.[17] The main intracellular calcium storage compartment, the ER, contains at least two distinct pools of releasable calcium. One of the pools is released by the action of inositol 1,4,5-triphosphate (InsP3) while the other is released by calcium itself.[18] InsP3 is generated following agonist binding at metabotropic receptors in the plasma membrane via the hydrolysis of phosphatidylinositol 4,5-bisphosphate (PIP2) to yield InsP3 and diacyglycerol. The latter activates protein kinase C, while InsP3 induces calcium release by binding to an intracellular ligand-operated calcium channel in the ER membrane, the InsP3 receptor. Cytosolic calcium can also trigger further calcium release from a second pool in the ER. This occurs by calcium activation of the ryanodine receptor (RyanR).[19]

Since calcium is an important second messenger in the neuron, multiple mechanisms have evolved to permit its levels to be modulated rapidly in response to synaptic activity. However, considerable evidence points to the fact that calcium is a deleterious ion when present at elevated concentrations for extended periods of time. Thus many mechanisms are also present to expel, sequester and bind free calcium and maintain calcium levels within a strict range within the neuron.

A critical issue pertaining to the thesis being developed here is whether calcium plays any role in the activation of cIE genes.

ROLE OF CALCIUM IN THE ACTIVATION OF cIE GENES

The majority of our knowledge concerning the role of Ca^{2+} in the regulation of cIE gene expression comes from studies in PC12, pheochromocytoma cells. In PC12 cells, both nerve growth factor (NGF) and membrane depolarization induce the rapid and transient expression of c-*fos*.[20–23] Pharmacological and Fura-2 imaging analyses have established that, in PC12 cells, depolarization causes the influx of calcium through L-type voltage-sensitive calcium channels. This calcium transient is essential for the induction of c-*fos* since the cIE response is blocked by removal of extracellular calcium or the addition of DHP antagonists, while it is mimicked by DHP agonists such as BAY K8644. Subsequently the elevated calcium concentration is thought to activate calmodulin, since the cIE response is blocked by all calmodulin antagonists (*e.g.* W7, trifluoroperazine). Studies from Greenberg and his colleagues have shown that calmodulin subsequently activates a calmodulin-dependent protein kinase which phosphorylates a transcription factor complex associated with the c-*fos* promoter.[24] This regulatory element, called the Ca^{2+}-cAMP response element (CARE sequence : TGACGTCA), is situated at -60 bp relative to the start of transcription of c-*fos* and mediates induction by both calcium and cAMP and binds a protein belonging to the CREB family. Both the cAMP-dependent protein kinase and calmodulin kinase II can phosphorylate and activate this CREB[25,26] protein thereby stimulating transcription of c-*fos*. Thus two second messenger pathways converge upon a common transcription factor to induce c-*fos*.

THE EXCITATORY AMINO ACIDS

The excitatory amino acids, glutamate and aspartate, are important neurotransmitters in the vertebrate nervous system and they have been implicated in many neurophysiological and neuropathological processes. Not unexpectedly, therefore, their receptors are found throughout the CNS.[27] While, the ligands for the EAA receptors are two simple amino acids, the receptors themselves make up a growing gene family whose products appear to be able to associate in multimeric complexes and interact with various signal transduction systems.[28] Indeed, there appear to be three general classes of EAA receptors that are characterized by their selectivity for the glutamate agonists, NMDA, kainic acid, and quisqualate.[29] The class of genes encoding the NMDA receptor comprises at least four members (and several splice variants) and their products give rise to a glutamate receptor that can directly gate calcium ions. It is the NMDA receptor that has been particularly implicated in acute models of neuronal death.[30] Another class of glutamate receptors, the GluR family, contains several members (as well as splice variants and mRNA edited species) that are not ligand-gating calcium channels. Included in this family is the AMPA or kainate receptor, which is thought to mediate the excitotoxicity of kainic acid. While this class of receptor does not gate calcium *per se,* it can gate monovalent cations which depolarize the neuron and lead to the subsequent influx of calcium through voltage-sensitive channels. Finally, the quisqualate, or metabotropic, glutamate receptor is another distinct molecular entity.[31] Activation of this receptor frequently stimulates phosphoinositide turnover which leads to the production of InsP3 and the triggering of calcium release from intracellular stores, notably the endoplasmic reticulum. Thus a common feature of all glutamate receptor subclasses is that they can elicit an increase in intracellular calcium, albeit by distinct mechanistic routes.

The demonstration of calcium's role in cIE gene activation led us to consider whether neuronal depolarization *in vivo* resulted in a cIE response. The most common paradigm has been to alter calcium homeostasis by administration of different convulsants. In the case of c-*fos* induction, these treatments include electrical stimulation,[32–35] administration of GABA receptor antagonists, such as PTZ,[36] picrotoxin[37] or lindane,[14] or stimulation of NMDA[37,38] and non-NMDA excitatory amino acid receptors.[37,39,40]

EXPRESSION OF THE cIE GENES AFTER SEIZURE

One of the most useful models in the study of cIE gene expression *in vivo* has been the administration of PTZ to rodents. PTZ elicits seizures and convulsions within 2 minutes of injection and these can persist for half an hour. Within a few minutes of PTZ administration a dramatic increase in the expression of several cIE genes, including c-*fos*, c-*jun*, *jun*B, *erg*-1 and NGFI-B[36,37,41,42] can be detected in the CNS. As in PC12 cells, these transcriptional responses are transient and c-*fos* mRNA and Fos are eliminated within 4 hours of treatment. Despite this, total AP-1 binding activity remains elevated for at least 8 hours in the brain after PTZ seizures.[41] This protracted AP-1 like activity is explained by the appearance of other Fos-like antigens in brain that bind at the AP-1 consensus site, leading to two major conclusions. First, short periods of stimulation can result in much more persistent alterations in the level of a known transcription factor, AP-1. Second, the composition of AP-1 varies with time due to a sequential induction and disappearance of Fos and several Fos-related proteins. This dynamic alteration in AP-1 composition suggests a temporal ordering of the response that might provide for different target gene specificities or different consequences upon transcription of the same set of genes.

In vivo studies show that the NMDA-type of glutamate receptors mediate c-*fos* induction in the brain by PTZ.[37,43] Although the kainate type of receptors are not as widely distributed, treatment of rodents with kainic acid also elicits seizures and the induction of c-*fos* and other cIE genes in several brain regions.[37,39,40] Furthermore, both types of EAA receptors have been suggested to play a role in c-*fos* induction during ischemia,[44–46] and EAA receptor antagonists are effective in inhibiting cIE gene expression elicited by brain injury.[47,48] The gating of calcium through NMDA receptors, can also cause adaptive changes. In areas where the number of these receptors is high, such as the dentate gyrus of the hippocampus, repeated seizures (such as occurs in the kindling model of epilepsy), can lead to alterations in receptor numbers.[49] Therefore, it has been suggested that cIE gene products might couple the seizure stimulus to changes in receptor gene expression. To date there is no conclusive proof that any cIE gene directly regulates any target gene in the brain, although some indirect evidence has been presented for the preproenkephalin, preprodynorphin, and NGF genes being targets for AP-1 complexes.

One valuable application of cIE gene technology has been the development of mapping techniques to detect the temporal and spatial pattern of cIE gene activation. Furthermore, this has been used as a form of activity mapping analogous to 2'-deoxyglucose uptake.[50,51] These methods are based mainly on immunohistochemistry or *in situ* hybridization. Recently, our lab has developed a transgenic *fos*-lacZ mouse strain that provides an unambiguous model to identify the cell types that express c-*fos* either constitutively, or in response to extracellular stimulation.[52] This mouse has allowed a better characterization of the role of c-*fos* in developing and adult brain.[53,54]

CELL DEATH

Naturally occurring cell death is a physiological phenomenon that is essential for normal development, maintenance of tissue shape and size, formation of certain tissues, and cell selection in the immune system.[55] Pathologists have classified cell death into several categories based upon ultrastructural and morphological criteria. Necrotic cell death is characterized by a swelling of the cell, the disruption of internal and external membranes and lysis. It is known that acute EAA neurotoxicity can elicit an uncontrolled, sustained, elevation of cytosolic free calcium that may contribute to this process. In programmed cell death, or "apoptosis," cells undergo nuclear condensation and fragmentation and the nuclear fragments along with intracellular organelles are extruded. In some instances, nuclear DNA may be cleaved into fragments (nucleosomal ladder) as a consequence of the activation of an endogenous Ca^{2+}-Mg^{2+}-dependent endonuclease. Apoptosis is energy dependent and in some instances requires ongoing RNA and protein synthesis.[56] This has been taken to indicate that it is a suicide program that may require new gene expression.[57]

One of the strongest pieces of evidence for the activation of a "suicide program" comes from studies in *Caenorhabditis elegans (C. elegans)*. In this nematode, two genes have been identified, *ced*-3 and *ced*-4, that must be active in cells that are destined to die.[58] Both genes are thought to be involved in signal transduction, with *ced*-3 encoding a phosphoprotein and *ced*-4 a calcium-binding protein. The *unc*86 gene of *C. elegans,* which is responsible for signaling terminal differentiation of neurons, encodes a transcription factor.[59] Furthermore, another gene has been described, *ced*-9, that seems to act as a brake on the suicide program, thus resembling the mammalian gene *bcl*-2. The latter gene is the best candidate in a vertebrate for a component of a suicide program. The *bcl*-2 product is a mitochondrial protein that protects B and T lymphocytes against programmed cell death and when overexpressed in certain cells, can prevent programmed cell death and lead to tumor formation.[60] In the B cell, it has been established that *bcl*-2 transcription requires the presence of IL3. This is interesting since a number of neurotrophic factors (*e.g.* NGF and BDNF) are obligatory for the survival of neurons in the developing nervous system.

cIE GENES EXPRESSION AND CELL DEATH

cIE genes have been proposed to play a major role in the cascade of signalling events linking extracellular stimuli to long-term changes in gene expression. As we have seen, their induction is associated with processes such as neuronal activation and cell differentiation, however, there is also evidence that some members of the cIE gene class might be involved in the suicide program that leads to cell death. Overexpression of c-*myc* induces apoptosis in cells deprived of growth factors.[61] Conversely, blocking c-*myc* expression in T cell hybridomas with antisense oligonucleotides has been shown to prevent apoptosis.[62] The protein product of another proto-oncogene, bcl-2, seems to prevent apoptotic death induced by growth factor withdrawal and overexpression of c-*myc*.[63] c-*fos* has been suggested to be expressed in some situations involving cell death.[64–67] Using a transgenic *fos*-lacZ mouse strain as a model we have been able to detect c-*fos* induction in cellular populations undergoing programmed or induced cell death. For instance, Fos-lacZ is expressed in interdigital web cells and in the medial edge epithelium at the time of fusion of the palate during mouse development. Both cell populations are thought to undergo programmed cell death. We have also found Fos-lacZ continuously expressed in hypertrophic chondrocytes in the developing bone which also undergo hypertrophy and cell death in the bone core after blood vessel invasion.

In order to investigate the correlation between neuronal degeneration and c-*fos* expression, we crossed the *fos-lac*Z mice with a genetic mutant, *weaver,* in which cerebellar granule cells die.[68] We found cells expressing β-galactosidase activity precisely in the locations where granule cells degenerate in this strain of mouse. Using kainic acid, we have also examined the relationship between excitotoxic cell death and c-*fos* expression. Two to four hours after treatment with kainic acid, Fos-lacZ was expressed in several brain regions. Like authentic Fos, the β-galactosidase was also confined to neuronal nuclei. After 24 hours, no Fos-lacZ expression could be detected in the CNS. At 4 to 7 days post-treatment, Fos-lacZ expression reappeared in neurons located in specific regions of the limbic system: CA1 and CA3 of the hippocampus and the dorsomedial nucleus of the amygdala. This pattern of expression corresponds with the distribution of kainate receptors and the known neurotoxic profile of kainic acid. At this time, marked cytoarchitectural disorganization was observed and β-galactosidase activity ws distributed throughout the whole cell.[54] Thus *fos-lac*Z was reinduced by events associated with delayed neurotoxic cell death.

At present it is not possible to demonstrate whether c-*fos* expression is a cause or a consequence of the signaling cascade leading to cell death. However, we can state that the mechanisms that induce cIE gene expression are triggered prior to cell death in many situations. Clearly, c-*fos* expression could simply reflect the breakdown of intracellular signaling mechanisms, however, Fos could be a required component of the mechanisms that lead to programmed cell death. Mice that lack c-*fos* survive and, therefore, Fos cannot be essential for cell death in most circumstances. However, it is probably naive to think that any single gene is responsible for cell death in all cell types. Rather it is likely to be the interaction of complex networks of gene products that may vary on a cell-to-cell basis. In some cases Fos may play some direct role in the process, in other circumstances its activation may be peripheral to the program that leads to death. However, it does provide a tool with which the signaling pathways involved in cell death may be analyzed.

A MODEL OF NEUROTOXICITY

Under certain conditions, EAA receptors can become neurotoxic.[30] Indeed, they have been implicated in several pathological processes such as epilepsy and ischemia.[69] All these pathologies share as a common trait a massive entry of calcium into the cell beyond the buffering capacities of the mechanisms described above. After an initial influx of calcium through either voltage-dependent or NMDA-gated calcium channels, there is a membrane depolarization with opening of sodium channels. This produces a secondary, passive, influx of chloride and water, with subsequent neuronal swelling. A further entry of calcium leads to activation of second messenger systems, mobilization of internal calcium stores, activation of lipases and proteases, generation of free radicals, mitochondrial dysfunction and depletion of energy stores.[70] The rundown of ATP levels will result in impairment of re-uptake systems for EAAs, and other neurotransmitters.

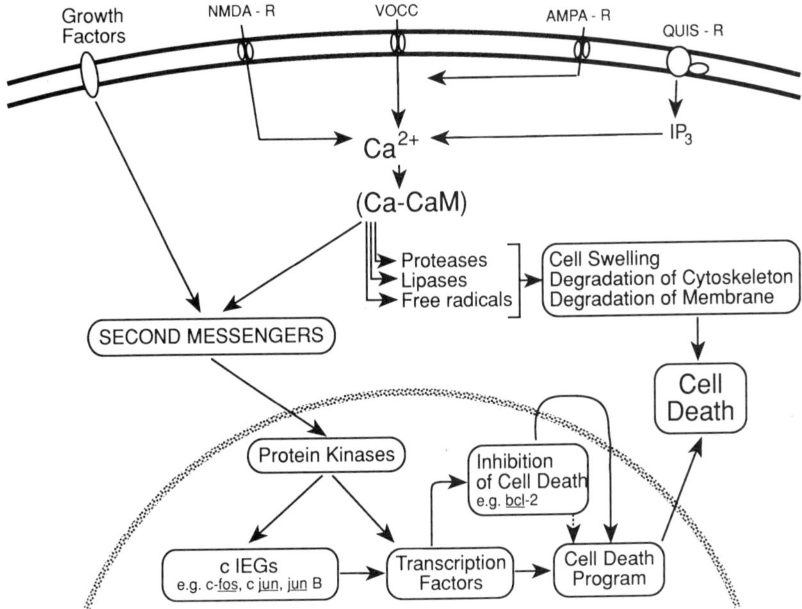

FIGURE 1. Model for the cIE response in cell death. See text for explanation. VOCC: voltage-operated calcium channels; NMDA-R: NMDA receptor; AMPA-R: AMPA receptor; QUIS-R: quisqualate receptor; IP$_3$: inositol 1,4,5-triphosphate; CaM: calmodulin; cIEGs: cellular immediate-early genes.

The EAAs will accumulate in the synaptic cleft causing continuous depolarization and constant calcium influx, a classical feed-forward mechanism that leads to destruction of the neuronal cytoskeleton and ultimately neuronal death. Such a process seems to underlie several pathological states including stroke.

In addition to the above mechanism, which represents the necrotic type of cell death, a disruption in intracellular calcium homeostasis can affect various protein kinase signaling pathways. This results in alterations in the levels and patterns of phosphorylated products with concomitant increases and decreases in the activity of numerous cellular enzymes. As elucidated above, these pathways can influence the expression of cIE genes, which are known to be expressed prior to neuronal death. Therefore, we suggest that the cIE response is involved in the process of programmed cell death. Their most likely role is to transactivate other genes that either contribute to the death program or are, perhaps, neuroprotective. The evaluation of these latter considerations may provide insights into the cellular mechanisms that contribute to cell death and yield novel substrates for pharmacological intervention in this process.

REFERENCES

1. WYLLIE, A. H., R. G. MORRIS, A. L. SMITH & D. DUNLOP. 1984. J. Pathol. **142:** 67–77.
2. GOELET, P., V. F. CASTELLUCCI, S. SCHACHER & E. R. KANDEL. 1986. Nature **322:** 419–422.
3. CURRAN, T. & J. I. MORGAN. 1987. Bioessays **7:** 255–258.
4. LAU, L. F. & D. NATHANS. 1987. Proc. Natl. Acad. Sci. USA **84:** 1182–1186.
5. MORGAN, J. I. & T. CURRAN. 1991. Ann. Rev. Neurosci. **14:** 421–451.
6. LANDSCHULZ, W. H., P. F. JOHNSON & S. L. MCKNIGHT. 1988. Science **240:** 1759–1764.
7. CURRAN, T. & B. R. FRANZA, JR. 1988. Cell **55:** 395–397.
8. MEANS, A. R., J. S. TASH & J. G. CHAFOULEAS. 1982. Physiol. Rev. **62:** 1–39.
9. BECHEM, M., S. HEBISCH & M. SCHRAMM. 1988. TIPS **9:** 257–261.
10. WIBO, M. & T. GODFRAIND. 1988. *In* Calcium and Calcium binding proteins. C. H. Gerday, L. Bolis & R. Giles, Eds.: 243–254. Springer-Verlag. Berlin.
11. SHELTON, R. C., J. A. GREBB & W. J. FREED. 1987. Brain Res. **492:** 399–402.
12. MEYER, F. B., R. E. ANDERSON, T. M. SUNDT, JR., T. L. YASH & F. W. SHARBROUGH. 1987. Epilepsia **28:** 409–414.
13. O'NEILL, S. K. & G. T. BOLGER. 1990. Brain Res. Bull. **25:** 211–214.
14. VENDRELL, M., J. M. TUSELL & J. SERRATOSA. 1991. J. Neurochem **58:** 862–869.
15. JOY, R. M. & V. W. BURNS. 1988. Neurotoxicology **9:** 637–644.
16. VENDRELL, M., M. J. PUJOL, J. M. TUSELL & J. SERRATOSA. 1992. Mol. Brain Res. **14:** 285–292.
17. WALZ, B. & O. BAUMANN. 1989. Prog. Histochem. Cytochem. **20:** 1–47.
18. HENZI, V. & B. MACDERMOTT. 1992. Neuroscience **46:** 251–273.
19. KASAI, H. & G. J. AUGUSTINE. 1990. Nature **348:** 735–738.
20. CURRAN, T. & J. I. MORGAN. 1985. Science **229:** 1265–1268.
21. GREENBERG, M., L. A. GREENE & E. B. ZIFF. 1985. J. Biol. Chem. **260:** 14101–14110.
22. KRUIJER, W., D. SCHUBERT & I. M. VERMA. 1985. Proc. Natl. Acad Sci. USA **82:** 7330–7334.
23. MORGAN, J. I. & T. CURRAN. 1986. Nature **322:** 552–555.
24. SHENG, M., G. MCFADDEN & M. E. GREENBERG. 1990. Neuron **4:** 453–460.
25. SHENG, M., M. A. THOMPSON & M. E. GREENBERG. 1991. Science **252:** 1427–1430.
26. DASH, P. K., K. A. KARL, M. A. COLICOS, R. PRYWES & E. R. KANDEL. 1991. Proc. Natl. Acad. Sci. USA **88:** 5061–5065.
27. COTMAN, C. W. & L. L. IVERSEN. 1987. TINS **10:** 263–265.
28. NAKANISHI, N., N. A. SHNEIDER & R. AXEL. 1990. Neuron **5:** 569–581.
29. FOSTER, A. C. & G. E. FAGG. 1984. Brain Res. Rev. **7:** 103–164.
30. ROTHMAN, S. M. & J. W. OLNEY. 1987. TINS **10:** 299–302.
31. MASU, M., Y. TANABE, K. TSUCHIDA, R. SHIGEMOTO & S. NAKANISHI. 1991. Nature **349:** 760–765.
32. DRAGUNOW, M. & H. A. ROBERTSON. 1987. Nature **329:** 441–442.
33. DAVAL, J. L., T. NAKAJIMA, C. H. GLEITER, R. M. POST & P. J. MARANGOS. 1989. J. Neurochem. **52:** 1954–57.
34. WHITE, J. D. & C. M. GALL. 1987. Mol. Brain Res. **3:** 21–29.
35. SHARP, F. R., M. F. GONZALEZ, J. W. SHARP & S. M. SAGAR. J. Comp. Neurol. **284:** 621–636.
36. MORGAN, J. I., D. R. COHEN, J. HEMPSTEAD & T. CURRAN. 1987. Science **237:** 192–197.

37. SONNENBERG, J. L., C. MITCHELMORE, P. F. MACGREGOR-LEON, J. HEMPSTEAD, J. I. MORGAN & T. CURRAN. 1989. J. Neurosci. Res. **24:** 72–80.
38. MCDONALD, J. W. & M. V. JOHNSTON. 1990. Brain Res. Rev. **15:** 41–70.
39. LE GAL LA SALLE, G. 1988. Neurosci. Lett. **88:** 127–130.
40. POPOVICI, T., G. BARBIN & Y. BEN ARI. 1988. J. Pharmacol. **150:** 405–406.
41. SONNENBERG, J. L., P. F. MACGREGOR-LEON, T. CURRAN & J. I. MORGAN. 1989. Neuron **3:** 359–365.
42. WATSON, M. A. & J. MILBRANDT. 1989. Mol. Cell. Biol. **9:** 4213–19.
43. COLE, A. J., D. W. SAFFEN, J. M. BARABAN & P. F. WORLEY. 1989. Nature **340:** 474–476.
44. POPOVICI, T., A. REPRESA, V. CREPEL, G. BARBIN, M. BEAUDOIN & Y. BEN-ARI. 1990. Brain Res. **536:** 183–194.
45. NOWAK, T. S., J. IKEDA & T. NAKAJIMA. 1990. Stroke **21:** 107–111.
46. JORGENSEN, M. B., J. DECKERT, D. C. WRIGHT & D. R. GEHLERT. 1989. Brain Res. **484:** 393–398.
47. HERRERA, D. G. & H. A. ROBERTSON. 1990. Neurosci. **35:** 273–281.
48. SHARP, J. W., S. M. SAGAR, K. HISANAGA, P. JASPER & F. R. SHARP. 1990. Exp. Neurol. **109:** 323–332.
49. SHIN, C., H. B. PEDERSEN & J. O. MCNAMARA. 1985. J. Neurosci. **5:** 2696–2701.
50. SAGAR, S. M., F. R. SHARP & T. CURRAN. 1988. Science **240:** 1328–1331.
51. DRAGUNOW, M. & R. FAULL. 1989. J. Neurosci. Methods **29:** 261–265.
52. SMEYNE, R. J., K. SCHILLING, L. ROBERTSON, D. LUK, J. OBERDICK, T. CURRAN & J. I. MORGAN. 1992. Neuron **8:** 13–23.
53. SMEYNE, R. J., T. CURRAN & J. I. MORGAN. 1992. Mol. Brain Res. **16:** 158–162.
54. SMEYNE, R. J., M. VENDRELL, M. HAYWARD, S. J. BAKER, G. G. MIAO, K. SCHILLING, L. M. ROBERTSON, T. CURRAN & J. I. MORGAN. 1993. Nature. In press.
55. SAUNDERS, J. W. 1966. Science. **154:** 604–612.
56. MARTIN, D. P. *et al.* 1988. J. Cell Biol. **106:** 829–844.
57. RAFF, M. C. 1992. Nature **356:** 397–400.
58. ELLIS, R. E. & H. R. HORVITZ. 1986. Cell **44:** 817–829.
59. HERR, W., R. A. STURM, R. G. CLERC, L. M. CORCORAN, D. BALTIMORE, P. A. SHARP, *et al.* 1988. Genes and Dev. **2:** 1513–1516.
60. STRASSER, A., A. W. HARRIS & S. CORY. 1991. Cell **67:** 889–899.
61. EVAN, G. I., A. H. WYLLIE, C. S. GILBERT, T. D. LITTLEWOOD, H. LAND, M. BROOKS, *et al.* 1992. Cell **69:** 119–128.
62. SHY, Y. *et al.* 1992. Science **257:** 212–214.
63. BISSONNETTE, R. P., F. ECHEVERRI, A. MAHBOUBI & D. R. GREEN. 1992. Nature **359:** 552–554.
64. BUTTYAN, R., Z. ZAKERY, R. LOCHSHIN & D. WOLGEMUTH. 1988. Molec. Endocrinol. **2:** 650–657.
65. GONZALES-MARTIN, C., I. DE DIEGO, D. CRESPO & A. FAIREN. 1992. Dev. Brain Res. **68:** 83–95.
66. COLOTTA, F., N. POLENTARUTTI, M. SIRONI & A. MANTOVANI. 1992. J. Biol. Chem. **267:** 18278–18283.
67. DONY, C. & P. GRUSS. Nature **328:** 711–714.
68. SMEYNE, R. J. & D. GOLDOWITZ. 1989. J. Neurosci. **9:** 1608–1620.
69. MELDRUM, B. & J. GARTHWAITE. 1990. TIPS **11:** 379–387.
70. CHOI, D. W. 1988. TINS **11:** 465–469.

Synthesis of Heat Shock/Stress Proteins during Cellular Injury

THADDEUS S. NOWAK, JR.

Department of Neurology
University of Tennessee College of Medicine
855 Monroe Avenue, Room 415
Memphis, Tennessee 38163

Expression of hsp72, a member of the 70 kDa heat shock/stress protein family, has now been evaluated in a number of brain injury models. Transient global ischemia results in an entirely neuronal distribution of both hsp72 mRNA and its encoded protein, while hyperthermic stress induces a predominantly glial and vascular expression with more limited neuronal involvement. Focal ischemic and traumatic insults can induce a stress response in numerous cell types within and around the site of the lesion. It is therefore apparent that hsp72 expression can provide a marker for ongoing injury in diverse cell populations within the brain. Recent studies also suggest that mild insults that induce a stress response may also confer protection against otherwise damaging ischemic insults, comparable to the expression of thermotolerance following moderate heat shock in other experimental models. This overview will therefore consider transcriptional and translational aspects of stress protein induction in brain, and the potential association between the stress response and tolerance to injury, with an emphasis on studies of experimental ischemia. Many conceptual and methodological issues that arise in a consideration of the postischemic stress response will be generally applicable to the evaluation of other changes in gene expression as markers of cellular injury.

THE STRESS RESPONSE

The stress response has been identified as a highly conserved mechanism of coordinated reprogramming of gene expression in response to environmental challenges,[1-4] and considerable evidence suggests that it is a component of the reaction to diverse injuries in brain.[5,6] It should be noted, however, that there are other well-documented response mechanisms, including for example the induction of proto-oncogene transcription factors,[7] and overlap of stress protein and proto-oncogene expression is evident in brain and other tissues after many stimuli, including ischemia.[8-12] In addition there are multiple regulatory mechanisms by which heat shock genes can be regulated, so expression of mRNAs and proteins encoded by these genes does not necessarily indicate a classical heat shock response.[13-15] Nevertheless, the notion of a stress response following potentially injurious stimuli remains a useful conceptual framework for evaluating much of the experimental work on gene expression after ischemia and other insults.

At the molecular level heat shock genes are identified by the presence of defined heat shock sequence elements in their upstream regulatory regions[16] that provide binding sites for known heat shock factors[17-21] and mediate transcriptional responses. While triggering events such as generation of oxygen radicals[22,23] or accumulation of damaged proteins[24-27] have been proposed to participate in the initiation of the stress response, the signal transduction mechanisms that can lead to activation of heat shock factors remain to be fully identified. There appear to be conformational changes associated with activation,[28,29] and phosphorylation of a yeast heat shock factor has been demonstrated.[18] While some work suggests that intracellular calcium elevation is not an obligate component of the stress response,[30] there is recent evidence of a requirement for calcium and protein kinase in the activation of heat shock factors in response to temperature elevation.[31] In addition to heat shock elements, a well-characterized human hsp70 promoter includes functional serum and calcium/cyclic AMP response elements comparable to those present upstream of the c-*fos* gene,[13-15] and these may contribute to the frequent coinduction of these genes noted above. Similar multiplicity of regulatory elements has been identified in additional genes of the human hsp70 family,[32,33] as well as in a mouse hsp70 promoter,[34] although the rodent gene most studied in models of brain injury has not been explicitly characterized (see below). Anoxic/ aglycemic insults sufficient to deplete ATP levels in cell culture result in the activation of heat shock factors,[35] but comparable studies have yet to be done after ischemia *in vivo*.

With regard to the proteins induced by heat shock, translation products of distinct size classes have been reproducibly detected in many studies, giving rise to a nomenclature based on apparent molecular weight (*e.g.*, hsp27, hsp90). The demonstration that ubiquitin expression can be regulated by heat shock identifies a protein of known function as a component of the stress response,[36-38] and emphasizes its close association with proteolytic mechanisms. Although numerous proteins may show increased expression in response to hyperthermia or other stresses,[39] the presence of heat shock elements in regulatory sequences has been demonstrated for only a limited number of genes. Most studies of the stress response in brain have focused on the 70 kDa proteins that are among those most prominently induced.[5,6]

The 70 kDa stress protein family consists of a group of closely related proteins that function as molecular chaperones during the intracellular processing of other proteins, with recognized involvement in the transport of proteins across membranes of mitochondria and endoplasmic reticulum.[40-43] Major members of this family are listed in TABLE 1, which also indicates some of the variations in terminology that have been used. Brain tissue provides a particularly rich source of the constitutively expressed proteins, including clathrin uncoating ATPase activity (hsc70) that has yielded much information regarding the function of this class of proteins,[44,45] and the same protein has been studied in other contexts as a microtubule-associated protein, β-internexin.[46,47] Information regarding the structure and function of this family of molecules is based primarily on studies of the constitutively expressed proteins. Notable features include the binding and hydrolysis of ATP,[48] as well as the presence of conserved calmodulin binding domains.[49,50] The tertiary structure of the ATPase domain of hsc70 shows many features similar to hexokinase and actin, although the primary sequences bear little resemblance to these proteins.[51,52]

METHODOLOGICAL CONSIDERATIONS

The need to distinguish among the various members of the hsp70 family is of particular importance in studies of the nervous system since heat shock cognate

TABLE 1. Proteins of the Mammalian hsp70 Family

Name	Synonyms	Properties	References
hsc70	p73, hsp73	Abundant constitutively expressed protein; clathrin uncoating ATPase, β-internexin.	44, 45, 47
hsp70	p72	Major inducible 70 kDa stress protein, but also constitutively expressed particularly in brain.	13, 48, 53, 54
hsp72		Strictly inducible protein in most models, with rare constitutive expression that is tissue- and species-dependent.	13, 54, 56
hsp75	p75	Mitochondrial heat shock protein, also constitutively expressed.	48
grp78	BiP	"Glucose-regulated" protein, constitutively expressed in endoplasmic reticulum.	124, 125

proteins are abundant in normal brain.[53,54] Such distinctions may be of fundamental interest should the several proteins eventually be understood to have unique functional roles and differential stimulus/response characteristics. As a practical issue there is an advantage to using a marker that is absent from normal cells and selectively indicates a response to injury, so that a robust signal is obtained.

There are a number of commercially available monoclonal antibodies with differing specificities for members of the 70 kDa stress protein family. Most widely used is an antibody originally characterized by Welch and Suhan[55] (Amersham RPN.1197; StressGen SPA-810) that selectively detects the hsp72 induced in rodent cells following diverse insults. It should be noted that some cell types in some species do show constitutive expression of a protein recognized by this antibody; prominent staining is noted in gerbil ependymal cells[54] and kidney medulla (M. Kozuka and T. S. Nowak, unpublished observations), and in blots of rat kidney medulla and numerous guinea pig tissues.[56] This is not a confounding issue under typical experimental conditions provided the necessary controls are in place, and in some cases may reflect responses to acute behavioral stresses,[57] the significance of which could otherwise be easily overlooked. Conversely, there appear to be situations in which a protein corresponding to hsp72 is induced but remains undetected with the hsp72-selective monoclonal.[12,58] Staining anomalies have occasionally been noted in cell cultures, with evidence for masking of epitopes by protein-protein interactions.[59] Pan-hsp70 antibodies recognizing most members of the family are available (Affinity BioReagents, Neshanic Station, NJ) that when applied with two-dimensional electrophoresis may be useful in detecting cryptic hsp72 expression.

Parallel issues arise with respect to the specificity of probes used for hybridization studies of the stress response at the transcriptional level. Oligonucleotides of defined sequence have been identified that are selective for inducible and constitutively expressed RNAs of the hsp70 family.[60] The oligonucleotide that recognizes stress inducible sequences is effective in detecting mRNAs in rat, mouse and gerbil tissues after hyperthermic and ischemic insults.[60–63] In addition there are cDNAs that show similar specificity obtained from rat,[64] and more recently from gerbil libraries.[65] In no case has it been unambiguously demonstrated that the induced mRNA detected with these selective probes encodes the hsp72 protein that is detected after inducing insults, but this appears to be a reasonable inference and 'hsp72' is used here in reference to this major inducible mRNA in rodent brain.

EXPRESSION OF HSP72 AFTER BRAIN INJURY

Global Ischemia, Excitotoxic Insults and Hyperthermia

Postischemic hsp72 expression was first identified in studies employing *in vitro* and *in vivo* amino acid incorporation methods to the analysis of proteins synthesized in brain after global and focal ischemia.[66–69] Its potential utility as a marker of neuronal injury was recognized in subsequent immunocytochemical analysis in the gerbil that showed expression restricted to neurons of hippocampus as well as other brain regions.[54] Generally comparable results have been obtained in studies using other global ischemia models.[70–72]

It is apparent that hsp72 immunoreactivity for the most part provides an index of neuron populations destined to survive an ischemic insult. This result is particularly clear in the gerbil,[54] since minimal expression is detected in the CA1 hippocampal neurons destined to be lost in this model (FIG. 1A). Comparable results have been obtained for ubiquitin immunoreactivity after ischemia, characterized by an initial depletion that progressively recovers in surviving cell populations.[73] Such observations are consistent with the long lasting deficits in protein synthesis activity known to occur in vulnerable neurons in both gerbil and rat transient ischemia models.[74–76] Attenuated hsp72 expression in injured neurons is also evident after kainic acid lesions in the rat, in that CA3 neurons that will be killed by the excitotoxin fail to express hsp72, while the less affected population in CA1 shows more prominent staining.[77] Widespread hsp72 expression in surviving neurons is also found after global ischemia in the rat, but in addition there is prominent immunoreactivity detected in CA1 neurons, most of which will also be lost.[70,72] When the effect of insult duration is examined in detail it is evident that very brief ischemia results in selective accumulation of hsp72 immunoreactivity in the most vulnerable neurons of dentate hilus and CA1, with gradual involvement of other populations as the length of the ischemic interval is increased, showing finally a decrease in staining intensity in vulnerable populations only after the longest insults.[72] From the above studies it can be concluded that hsp72 induction provides an index of cells that have experienced potentially damaging stress, that translational recovery can be a factor limiting hsp72 accumulation in vulnerable neurons, but that successful hsp72 expression provides no absolute indicator of the potential for neuron survival. Similar conclusions have been reached in recent studies of hsp72 expression in an electrical stimulation model of hippocampal injury.[78]

In situ hybridization studies of hsp72 mRNA expression provide complementary information regarding the transcriptional component of the stress response. In contrast to the limited protein synthesis recovery that may be possible in vulnerable neurons, there is rapid normalization of RNA synthesis upon postischemic recirculation. This allows significant accumulation of hsp72,[62] c-*fos* and c-*jun*,[11,79,80] superoxide dismutase,[81] and presumably other induced mRNAs in both vulnerable and resistant neurons after ischemia. Expression of hsp72 mRNA therefore provides a sensitive means of localizing the stress response, uncomplicated by the issue of translational recovery, that is more generally useful for the mapping of responsive cells (FIG. 1B). With the use of non-radioactive probes, differences in hsp72 expression in subpopulations of dentate granule cells have

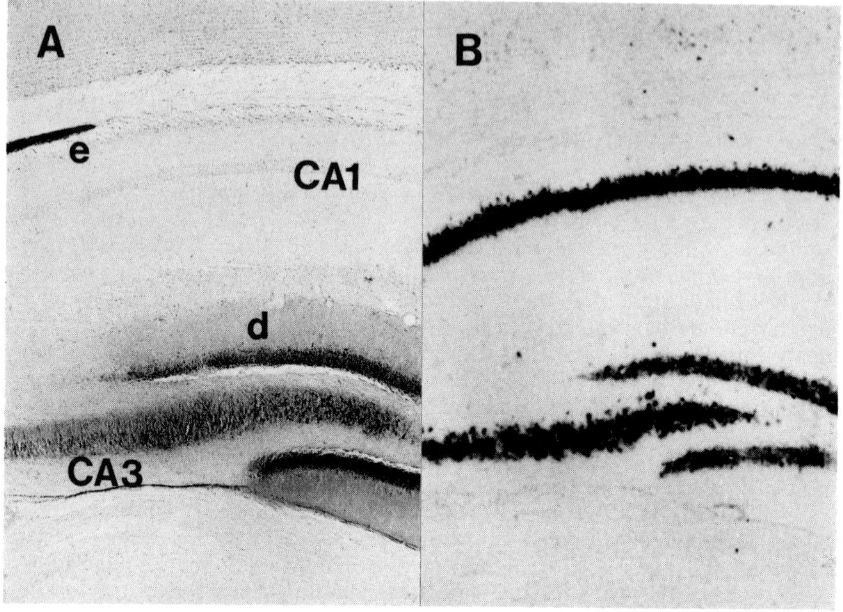

FIGURE 1. Comparison of hsp72 protein and mRNA expression after transient ischemia in the gerbil. **A:** Hsp72 immunoreactivity in hippocampus 24 h after 5 min global ischemia, demonstrating staining of neurons in dentate (d) and CA3, but not in the vulnerable CA1 region. Positive ependyma (e) seen here is also present in control gerbils. **B:** *In situ* hybridization of hsp72 mRNA at 24 h recirculation, illustrating strong induction in CA1 neurons. Considerable hybridization also persists in dentate and CA3 which is not typical at such a late time point, indicating that there was an unusually severe insult in this animal. Ependymal hybridization is absent from this animal but is variably detected in the gerbil, suggesting that its transient expression may be sufficient to account for the accumulation of immunoreactive protein routinely observed.

been detected after neonatal hypoxia-ischemia.[82] Recent studies have also identified increases in a heat shock cognate mRNA in postischemic gerbil brain.[65]

Several agents result in neuron-specific expression of hsp72 in brain. Kainic acid induces hsp72 in hippocampus and other brain regions,[77,83,84] and under conditions that result in selective loss of CA3 neurons there is prominent expression of hsp72 immunoreactivity in CA1.[77] This observation complements the above results after global ischemia, and provides further evidence associating accumulation of hsp72 with neuron survival. A recent literature has also developed documenting hsp72 expression in neurons of cingulate cortex, associated with transient neuropathological changes that occur following administration of N-methyl-D-aspartate (NMDA) receptor antagonists such as MK-801.[85,86] The robust expression of hsp72 immunoreactivity in these cells is again consistent with their ultimate survival. Of considerable interest is the finding that pharmacological interventions that attenuate the pathological changes in these cells also block induction of hsp72, further validating its utility as a marker of neuronal injury under these conditions.[86]

In contrast to the neuronal expression seen after global ischemia and neurotoxic insults, hyperthermic stress results in a preferential localization of hsp72 immunoreactivity in glial cells and in the endothelium of the vasculature,[63,87] although prominent neuronal expression in discrete brain regions is evident by both immunocytochemistry and *in situ* hybridization.[63,87,88] *In vitro* studies in cultured cells also indicate a more robust stress response in astrocytes than in neurons.[63,89] There are few detailed studies of the neuropathological correlates of hyperthermia *in vivo*, but it is of interest that more striking blood-brain barrier changes are noted in response to moderately hyperthermic ischemic insults,[90] and glial activation indicated by increased expression of glial fibrillary acidic protein is seen after acute systemic hyperthermia.[91]

Focal Ischemia and Traumatic Injury

While only brief periods of global ischemia are compatible with survival, long-lasting or permanent loss of blood flow to a discrete brain region is a key feature of clinical stroke and of the animal models of this condition. Under such conditions a central core of poorly perfused tissue suffers infarction, with eventual loss of most cellular elements, while a "penumbra" of intermediate perfusion experiences varied degrees of selective neuronal injury.[92] A complex pattern of hsp72 expression is observed in brain following such focal ischemic insults. After permanent occlusions neuronal hsp72 immunoreactivity is prominent in the zone adjacent to an infarct, but its expression is restricted to surviving vascular elements within the densely ischemic core.[84] Similar distributions characterize the pattern of hsp72 staining in necrotic foci that can sometimes occur after global insults.[71,93,94] A rim of positive astrocytes is frequently observed at the edge of an infarct.[94] If the focal insult is sufficiently brief, then neuronal hsp72 expression is evident throughout the ischemic territory, while 60–90 min ischemia reproduces the pattern seen after permanent occlusions.[95,96] These observations suggest that hsp72 expression defines a hierarchy of vulnerability (neurons > astrocytes > endothelium) after focal insults. Available studies at the transcriptional level lack the cellular resolution necessary to characterize the responses of these distinct cell types, but are generally consistent with the above findings.[96,97]

Induction of the stress response has been studied after other focal injuries with generally comparable results. Incisions in the cortical surface result in increased expression of an hsp70 mRNA in both glia and neurons at the site of injury.[98] Immunoreactive hsp72 accumulates in both neurons and glia in the zone of surviving tissue around the injury focus after spinal cord trauma.[99] Recent studies in a fluid percussion brain injury model also demonstrating staining of neurons and glia surrounding the region of focal injury and vascular hsp72 expression within the necrotic focus.[100] Rare positive cells were reported in distant brain regions, suggesting that hsp72 expression may provide a marker for localizing the distribution of diffuse injury after such insults.

INDUCED ISCHEMIC TOLERANCE

There is now evidence in a number of models that brief ischemic or even hyperthermic insults may reduce the impact of subsequent, otherwise damaging

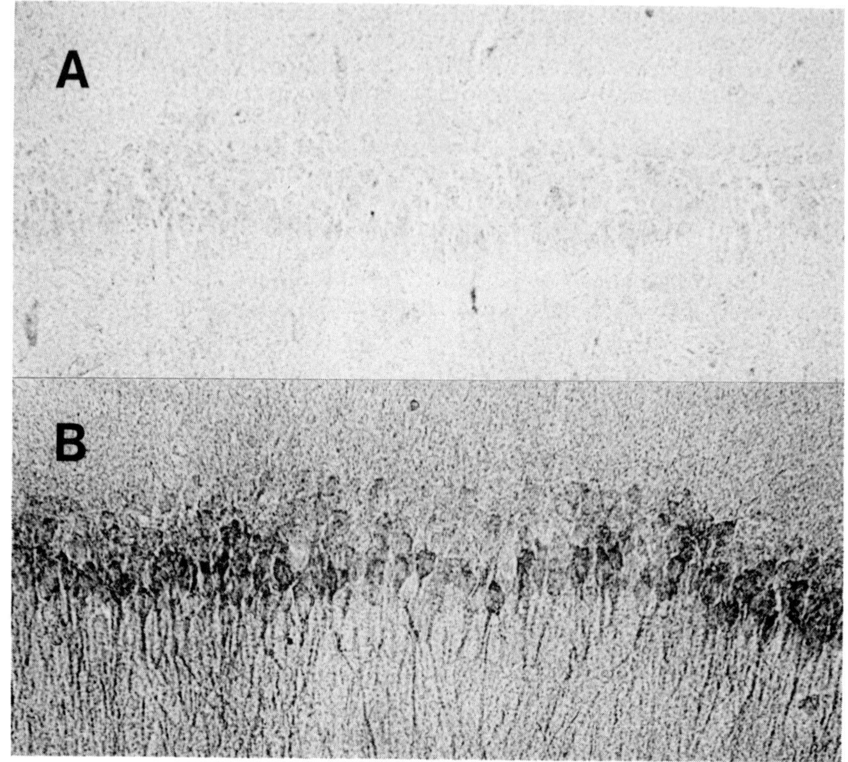

FIGURE 2. Comparison of hsp72 immunoreactivity in gerbil CA1 neurons after lethal and non-lethal insults. **A:** Ischemia of 5 min duration results in negligible staining of vulnerable CA1 pyramidal cells in the gerbil at 24 h recirculation. **B:** After a brief insult (2.5 min) significant hsp72 accumulates in CA1 neurons, and may be associated with induction of ischemic tolerance.

periods of ischemia.[101–105] There are related *in vitro* experiments indicating that glutamate neurotoxicity may also be reduced by prior hyperthermic stress.[106,107] The driving hypothesis in these studies is that the stress response may contribute to the expression of tolerance, by analogy with related phenomena of induced thermotolerance following heat shock, and it is clear that hsp72 immunoreactivity can accumulate in CA1 neurons after brief insults in the gerbil[101] (FIG. 2). Although the body of evidence from rat studies cited above indicates that hsp72 is expressed in CA1 neurons even after longer insults that result in loss of these cells, it may be argued that prior accumulation of stress proteins may be necessary so that they are available at the time of the ischemic challenge, and the delayed time course of tolerance expression is consistent with such a requirement. Other reports indicate that brief hyperthermic insults can induce tolerance to light-induced injury in retina[108] and may reduce ischemic injury in the brain,[103] although interpretation of the latter results are complicated by the differences in localization of hsp72 expression after hyperthermic and ischemic insults noted above.

Two main factors preclude any firm conclusions regarding the role of the stress response in ischemic tolerance. In the first place, changes in gene expression in neurons after ischemia continue to be documented in ever increasing numbers, including transcription factors,[109] growth factors,[79] as well as enzymes that may be of functional importance such as ornithine decarboxylase[110,111] and superoxide dismutase.[81] Although for most of these there have been no detailed comparisons of transcriptional and translational expression as it relates to the duration of ischemia, there is now good evidence that a Jun-immunoreactive protein accumulates in CA1 neurons after 2 min but not after 5 min ischemia in the gerbil.[12,112,113] It may be presumed that increased expression of this transcription factor may have consequences for the spectrum of mRNAs and proteins subsequently expressed in CA1 neurons after brief insults. Apart from inferring influences on subsequent transcriptional regulation, this finding further allows the generalization that translational recovery in CA1 neurons after short periods of ischemia must result in expression of a wide range of proteins encoded by the mRNAs induced after ischemia. Future studies may be expected to document more fully the range of gene expression that could contribute to the tolerant state.

A second factor that limits interpretation of *in vivo* ischemic tolerance studies is the complexity of the models themselves. Brain temperature, for example, is well documented as a potential source of variability in all ischemia models,[114,155] and is particularly a factor in pharmacological studies of neuroprotection.[116,117] A significant hyperthermic response has been identified during early recirculation in the gerbil and has been suggested to be a critical determinant of cellular injury,[118] although there are also negative reports.[119] In our own studies we have demonstrated that postischemic temperature is a critical variable determining the expression of hsp72 mRNA after 2 min ischemia in the gerbil model.[117] Hyperthermia above 39°C during 3 h recirculation, that itself does not induce a robust stress response, is an absolute requirement for hsp72 expression after such threshold insults. Future studies of induced ischemic tolerance must give particular attention to temperature as a variable, both during the inducing stress and after subsequent test challenges.

THE STRESS RESPONSE IN HUMAN DISEASE

An evolving literature has begun to address the potential relevance of the stress response to human neuropathology. It would be expected that ischemic insults in man would result in patterns of stress protein expression comparable to that seen in animal models, but no data is currently available. There are reports of increased 70 kDa stress protein expression (hsp72 and grp78) localized to the plaques and tangles of Alzheimer's disease brain,[120] with increased protein staining on immunoblots of the pathological tissue. In our own hands the hsp72-selective antibody detected comparable immunoreactivity in two-dimensional blots from a wide range of normal and pathological human postmortem brain samples (G. Stoner and T. S. Nowak, Jr., unpublished observations). Weak astrocytic hsp72 staining has been described in brains of both normal controls and multiple sclerosis patients and no association with demyelinating plaques was observed,[121] although antibodies directed against the hsp60 family detected reactive oligodendrocytes bordering such lesions.

In contrast to the somewhat equivocal results obtained for hsp72, numerous studies demonstrate ubiquitin immunoreactivity in association with pathological structures present in a range of degenerative diseases.[122] Hsp72 and ubiquitin immunoreactivities have been reported to be expressed with different distributions in amyotrophic lateral sclerosis.[123] It is possible that ubiquitin staining reflects an abnormal accumulation of this otherwise normally expressed protein, rather than manifestation of a disease-associated stress response. Further studies of these and other proteins are clearly necessary to establish the relevance of the stress response to diseases affecting the human nervous system.

SUMMARY AND CONCLUSIONS

Several conclusions can be drawn from available data on the expression of stress proteins in brain with respect to their utility as markers of cellular injury. First, it is evident that all cell types in brain are capable of expressing stress proteins, although there is striking specificity in the population responding to a given insult. The apparent hierarchy of responsiveness indicated by hsp72 expression correlates well with the relative vulnerability of specific cell populations in a given model. With increasing severity of injury there can be an attenuation of the translational component of the stress response, in that hsp72 immunoreactivity fails to accumulate even though its mRNA is abundantly expressed. For this reason, hsp72 immunoreactivity provides an index of cell populations that have responded to an insult with a functional stress response. Such a response is not sufficient to guarantee survival, since many CA1 neurons that show significant hsp72 staining are eventually lost after global ischemia in the rat. However, brief insults that result in expression of hsp72 and other proteins encoded by induced mRNAs do result in tolerance to subsequent insults. Future studies may be expected to reveal the contributions of specific gene products to the tolerant state. Meanwhile, complementary evaluations of hsp72 mRNA and protein expression provide practical means of identifying cell populations responding to diverse injuries.

REFERENCES

1. SCHLESINGER, M. J., M. ASHBURNER & A. TISSIERES, Eds. 1982. Heat Shock from Bacteria to Man. Cold Spring Harbor Laboratory. Cold Spring Harbor, NY.
2. LINDQUIST, S. 1986. The heat-shock response. Annu. Rev. Biochem. **55:** 1151–1191.
3. LINDQUIST, S. & E. A. CRAIG. 1988. The heat-shock proteins. Annu. Rev. Genet. **22:** 631–677.
4. MORIMOTO, R., A. TISSIERES & C. GEORGOPOULOS. 1990. Stress Proteins in Biology and Medicine. Cold Spring Harbor Laboratory. Cold Spring Harbor, NY.
5. BROWN, I. R. 1990. Induction of heat shock (stress) genes in the mammalian brain by hyperthermia and other traumatic events: A current perspective. J. Neurosci. Res. **27:** 247–255.
6. NOWAK, T. S., Jr. 1990. Protein synthesis and the heat shock/stress response after ischemia. Cerebrovasc. Brain Metab. Rev. **2:** 345–366.
7. MORGAN, J. I. & T. CURRAN. 1991. Stimulus-transcription coupling in the nervous system: Involvement of the inducible proto-oncogenes *fos* and *jun*. Annu. Rev. Neurosci. **14:** 421–451.
8. ANDREWS, G. K., M. A. HARDING, J. P. CALVET & E. D. ADAMSON. 1987. The heat

shock response in HeLa cells is accompanied by elevated expression of the c-*fos* protooncogene. Mol. Cell Biol. **7:** 3452–3458.

9. GUBITS, R. M. & J. L. FAIRHURST. 1988. c-*fos* mRNA levels are increased by the cellular stressors, heat shock and sodium arsenite. Oncogene **3:** 163–168.

10. SCHIAFFONATI, L., E. RAPPOCCIOLO, L. TACCHINI, G. CAIRO & A. BERNELLI-ZAZZERA. 1990. Reprogramming of gene expression in postischemic rat liver: Induction of protooncogenes and hsp70 gene family. J. Cell. Physiol. **143:** 79–87.

11. NOWAK, T. S., JR., J. IKEDA & T. NAKAJIMA. 1990. 70 Kilodalton heat shock protein and c-*fos* gene expression following transient ischemia. Stroke **21**(Suppl. III): 107–111.

12. NOWAK, T. S., JR., O. C. OSBORNE & S. SUGA. 1993. Stress protein and protooncogene expression as indicators of neuronal pathophysiology after ischemia. *In* Neurobiology of Ischemic Brain Damage—Progress in Brain Research. K. Kogure & B. K. Siejö, Eds Vol. **96:** 195–208. Elsevier Science Publishers. Amsterdam.

13. WATOWICH, S. S. & R. I. MORIMOTO. 1988. Complex regulation of heat shock- and glucose-responsive genes in human cells. Mol. Cell. Biol. **8:** 393–405.

14. WU, B. J., R. E. KINGSTON & R. I. MORIMOTO. 1986. Human hsp70 promoter contains at least two distinct regulatory domains. Proc. Natl. Acad. Sci. USA **83:** 629–633.

15. CHOI, H.-K., B. LI, Z. LIN, L. E. HUANG & A. Y.-C. LIU. 1991. cAMP and cAMP-dependent protein kinase regulate the human heat shock protein 70 gene promoter activity. J. Biol. Chem. **266:** 11858–11865.

16. PELHAM, H. R. B. 1982. A regulatory upstream promoter element in the *Drosophila* hsp70 heat-shock gene. Cell **30:** 517–528.

17. WU, C., S. WILSON, B. WALKER, I. DAWID, T. PAISLEY, V. ZIMARINO & H. UEDA. 1987. Purification and properties of Drosophila heat shock activator protein. Science **238:** 1247–1253.

18. SORGER, P. K. & H. R. B. PELHAM. 1988. Yeast heat shock factor is an essential DNA-binding protein that exhibits temperature-dependent phosphorylation. Cell **54:** 855–864.

19. SCHARF, K.-D., S. ROSE, W. ZOTT, F. SCHÖFF & L. NOVER. 1990. Three tomato genes code for heat stress transcription factors with a region of remarkable homology to the DNA-binding domain of the yeast HSF. EMBO J. **9:** 4495–4501.

20. RABINDRAN, S. K., G. GIORGI, J. CLOS & C. WU. 1991. Molecular cloning and expression of a human heat shock factor, HSF1. Proc. Natl. Acad. Sci. USA **88:** 6906–6910.

21. SCHUETZ, T. J., G. J. GALLO, L. SHELDON, P. TEMPST & R. E. KINGSTON. 1991. Isolation of a cDNA for HSF2: Evidence for two heat shock factor genes in humans. Proc. Natl. Acad. Sci. USA **88:** 6911–6915.

22. SCIANDRA, J. J., J. R. SUBJECK & C. S. HUGHES. 1984. Induction of glucose-regulated proteins during anaerobic exposure and of heat-shock proteins after reoxygenation. Proc. Natl. Acad. Sci. USA **81:** 4843–4847.

23. COURGEON, A.-M., E. ROLLET, J. BECKER, C. MAISONHAUTE & M. BEST-BELPOMME. 1988. Hydrogen peroxide (H_2O_2) induces actin and some heat-shock proteins in *Drosophila* cells. Eur. J. Biochem. **171:** 163–170.

24. HIGHTOWER, L. E. 1980. Cultured animal cells exposed to amino acid analogues or puromycin rapidly synthesize several polypeptides. J. Cell Physiol. **102:** 407–427.

25. GOFF, S. A. & A. L. GOLDBERG. 1985. Production of abnormal proteins in E. Coli stimulates transcription of *lon* and other heat shock genes. Cell **41:** 587–595.

26. ANANTHAN, J., A. L. GOLDBERG & R. VOELLMY. 1986. Abnormal proteins serve as eukaryotic stress signals and trigger the activation of heat shock genes. Science **232:** 522–524.

27. LEE, K.-J. & G. M. HAHN. 1988. Abnormal proteins as the trigger for the induction of stress responses: Heat, diamide, and sodium arsenite. J. Cell. Physiol. **136:** 411–420.

28. ZIMARINO, V., S. WILSON & C. WU. 1990. Antibody-mediated activation of *Drosophila* heat shock factor in vitro. Science **249:** 546–549.

29. RABINDRAN, S. K., R. I. HAROUN, J. CLOS, J. WISNIEWSKI & C. WU. 1993. Regulation

of heat shock factor trimer formation: role of a conserved leucine zipper. Science **259:** 230–234.

30. DRUMMOND, I. A. S., D. LIVINGSTONE & R. A. STEINHARDT. 1988. Heat shock protein synthesis and cytoskeletal rearrangements occur independently of intracellular free calcium increases in *Drosophila* cells and tissues. Radiat. Res. **113:** 402–413.

31. PRICE, B. D. & S. K. CALDERWOOD. 1991. Ca^{2+} is essential for multistep activation of the heat shock factor in permeabilized cells. Mol. Cell. Biol. **11:** 3365–3368.

32. VOELLMY, R., A. AHMED, P. SCHILLER, P. BROMLEY & D. RUNGGER. 1985. Isolation and functional analysis of a human 70,000-dalton heat shock protein gene segment. Proc. Natl. Acad. Sci. USA **82:** 4949–4953.

33. LEUNG, T. K. C., M. Y. RAJENDRAN, C. MONFRIES, C. HALL & L. LIM. 1990. The human heat-shock protein family. Expression of a novel heat-inducible HSP70 (HSP70B′) and isolation of its cDNA and genomic DNA. Biochem. J. **267:** 125–132.

34. HUNT, C. & S. CALDERWOOD. 1990. Characterization and sequence of a mouse *hsp70* gene and its expression in mouse cell lines. Gene **87:** 199–204.

35. BENJAMIN, I. J., B. KRÖGER & R. S. WILLIAMS. 1990. Activation of the heat shock transcription factor by hypoxia in mammalian cells. Proc. Natl. Acad. Sci. USA **87:** 6263–6267.

36. BOND, U. & M. J. SCHLESINGER. 1985. Ubiquitin is a heat shock protein in chicken embryo fibroblasts. Mol. Cell Biol. **5:** 949–956.

37. BOND, U. & M. J. SCHLESINGER. 1986. The chicken ubiquitin gene contains a heat shock promoter and expresses an unstable mRNA in heat shocked cells. Mol. Cell Biol. **6:** 4602–4610.

38. FORNACE, A. L., JR., I. ALAMO, JR., M. C. HOLLANDER & E. LAMOREAUX. 1989. Ubiquitin mRNA is a major stress-induced transcript in mammalian cells. Nucl. Acids Res. **17:** 1215–1230.

39. MAYTIN, E. V., R. A. COLBERT & D. A. YOUNG. 1985. Early heat shock proteins in primary thymocytes. Evidence for transcriptional and translational regulation. J. Biol. Chem. **260:** 2384–2392.

40. CHIRICO, W. J., M. G. WATERS & G. BLOBEL. 1988. 70K heat shock related proteins stimulate protein translocation into microsomes. Nature **332:** 805–810.

41. DESHAIES, R. J., B. D. KOCH, M. WERNER-WASHBURNE, E. A. CRAIG & R. SCHEKMAN. 1988. A subfamily of stress proteins facilitates translocation of secretory and mitochondrial precursor polypeptides. Nature **332:** 800–805.

42. FLYNN, G. C., T. G. CHAPPELL & J. R. ROTHMAN. 1989. Peptide binding and release by proteins implicated as catalysts of protein assembly. Science **245:** 385–390.

43. BECKMANN, R. P., L. A. MIZZEN & W. J. WELCH. 1990. Interaction of hsp70 with newly synthesized proteins: Implications for protein folding and assembly. Science **248:** 850–854.

44. UNGEWICKEL, E. 1985. The 70-kd mammalian heat shock proteins are structurally and functionally related to the uncoating protein that releases triskelion from coated vesicles. EMBO J. **4:** 3385–3391.

45. CHAPPELL, T. G., W. J. WELCH, D. M. SCHLOSSMAN, K. B. PALTER, M. J. SCHLESINGER & J. E. ROTHMAN. 1986. Uncoating ATPase is a member of the 70 kilodalton family of stress proteins. Cell **45:** 3–13.

46. WHATLEY, S. A., T. LEUNG, C. HALL & L. LIM. 1986. The brain 68-kilodalton microtubule-associated protein is the cognate form of the 70-kilodalton mammalian heat-shock protein and is present as a specific isoform in synaptosomal membranes. J. Neurochem. **47:** 1576–1583.

47. GREEN, L. A. D. & R. K. H. LIEM. 1989. β-Internexin is a microtubule-associated protein identical to the 70-kDa heat-shock cognate protein and the clathrin uncoating ATPase. J. Biol. Chem. **264:** 15210–15215.

48. WELCH, W. J. & J. R. FERAMISCO. 1985. Rapid purification of mammalian 70,000-dalton stress proteins: affinity of the proteins for nucleotides. Mol. Cell. Biol. **5:** 1229–1237.

49. CLARK, B. D. & I. R. BROWN. 1986. A retinal heat-shock protein is associated with

elements of the cytoskeleton and binds to calmodulin. Biochem. Biophys. Res. Commun. **139:** 974–981.

50. STEVENSON, M. A. & S. K. CALDERWOOD. 1990. Members of the 70-kilodalton heat shock protein family contain a highly conserved calmodulin-binding domain. Mol. Cell. Biol. **10:** 1234–1238.

51. FLAHERTY, K. M., D. B. McKAY, W. KABSCH & K. C. HOLMES. 1991. Similarity of the three-dimensional structures of actin and the ATPase fragment of a 70-kDa heat shock cognate protein. Proc. Natl. Acad. Sci. USA **88:** 5041–5045.

52. FLAHERTY, K. M., C. DeLUCA-FLAHERTY & D. B. McKAY. 1990. Three-dimensional structure of the ATPase fragment of a 70K heat-shock cognate protein. Nature **346:** 623–628.

53. O'MALLEY, K. A., J. D. MAURON, J. D. BARCHAS & L. KEDES. 1985. Constitutively expressed rat mRNA encoding a 70-kilodalton heat-shock-like protein. Mol. Cell. Biol. **5:** 3476–3483.

54. VASS, K., W. J. WELCH & T. S. NOWAK, JR. 1988. Localization of 70 kDa stress protein induction in gerbil brain after ischemia. Acta Neuropathol. **77:** 128–135.

55. WELCH, W. J. & J. P. SUHAN. 1986. Cellular and biochemical events in mammalian cells during and after recovery from physiological stress. J. Cell Biol. **103:** 2035–2052.

56. DECHESNE, C. J., H. N. KIM, T. S. NOWAK, JR. & R. J. WENTHOLD. 1992. Expression of heat shock protein, HSP72, in the guinea pig and rat cochlea after hyperthermia: Immunocytochemical and in situ hybridization analysis. Hearing Res. **59:** 195–204.

57. BLAKE, M. J., R. UDELSMAN, G. J. FEULNER, D. D. NORTON & N. J. HOLBROOK. 1991. Stress-induced heat shock protein 70 expression in adrenal cortex: An adrenocorticotropic hormone-sensitive, age-dependent response. Proc. Natl. Acad. Sci. USA **88:** 9873–9877.

58. DWYER, B. E., R. N. NISHIMURA & I. R. BROWN. 1989. Synthesis of the major inducible heat shock protein in rat hippocampus after neonatal hypoxia-ischemia. Exp. Neurol. **104:** 28–31.

59. MILARSKI, K. L., W. J. WELCH & R. I. MORIMOTO. 1989. Cell cycle-dependent association of HSP70 with specific cellular proteins. J. Cell Biol. **108:** 413–423.

60. MILLER, E. K., J. D. RAESE & M. MORRISON-BOGORAD. 1991. Expression of heat shock protein 70 and heat shock cognate 70 messenger RNAs in rat cortex and cerebellum after heat shock or amphetamine treatment. J. Neurochem. **56:** 2060–2071.

61. NOWAK, T. S., JR., U. BOND & M. J. SCHLESINGER. 1990. Heat shock RNA levels in brain and other tissues after hyperthermia and transient ischemia. J. Neurochem. **54:** 451–458.

62. NOWAK, T. S., JR. 1991. Localization of 70 kDa stress protein mRNA induction in gerbil brain after ischemia. J. Cereb. Blood Flow Metab. **11:** 432–439.

63. MARINI, A. M., M. KOZUKA, R. L. LIPSKY & T. S. NOWAK, JR. 1990. 70-Kilodalton heat shock protein induction in cerebellar astrocytes and cerebellar granule cells in vitro: Comparison with immunocytochemical localization after hyperthermia in vivo. J. Neurochem. **54:** 1509–1516.

64. BROWN, I. R. & S. J. RUSH. 1990. Expression of heat shock genes (hsp70) in the mammalian brain: Distinguishing constitutively expressed and hyperthermia-inducible mRNA species. J. Neurosci. Res. **25:** 14–19.

65. KAWAGOE, J., K. ABE, S. SATO, I. NAGANO, S. NAKAMURA & K. KOGURE. 1992. Distributions of heat shock protein-70 mRNAs and heat shock cognate protein-70 mRNAs after transient global ischemia in gerbil brain. J. Cereb. Blood Flow Metab. **12:** 794–801.

66. NOWAK, T. S., JR. 1985. Synthesis of a stress protein following transient ischemia in the gerbil. J. Neurochem. **45:** 1635–1641.

67. DIENEL, G. A., M. KIESSLING, M. JACEWICZ & W. A. PULSINELLI. 1986. Synthesis of heat shock proteins in rat brain cortex after transient ischemia. J. Cereb. Blood Flow Metab. **6:** 505–510.

68. JACEWICZ, M., M. KIESSLING & W. A. PULSINELLI. 1986. Selective gene expression in focal cerebral ischemia. J. Cereb. Blood Flow Metab. **6:** 263–272.

69. KIESSLING, M., G. A. DIENEL, M. JACEWICZ & W. A. PULSINELLI. 1986. Protein synthesis in postischemic rat brain: a two-dimensional electrophoretic analysis. J. Cereb. Blood Flow Metab. **6:** 642–649.

70. CHOPP, M., Y. LI, M. O. DERESKI, S. R. LEVINE, Y. YOSHIDA & J. H. GARCIA. 1991. Neuronal injury and expression of 72-kDa heat-shock protein after forebrain ischemia in the rat. Acta Neuropathol. **83:** 66–71.

71. GONZALEZ, M. F., D. LOWENSTEIN, S. FERNYAK, K. HISANAGA, R. SIMON & F. R. SHARP. 1991. Induction of heat shock protein 72-like immunoreactivity in the hippocampal formation following transient global ischemia. Brain Res. Bull. **26:** 241–250.

72. SIMON, R. P., H. CHO, R. GWINN & D. H. LOWENSTEIN. 1991. The temporal profile of 72-kDa heat-shock protein expression following global ischemia. J. Neurosci. **11:** 881–889.

73. MAGNUSSON, K. & T. WIELOCH. 1989. Impairment of protein ubiquitination may cause delayed neuronal death. Neurosci. Lett. **96:** 264–270.

74. DIENEL, G. A., W. A. PULSINELLI & T. E. DUFFY. 1980. Regional protein synthesis in rat brain following acute hemispheric ischemia. J. Neurochem. **35:** 1216–1226.

75. KIRINO, T. & K. SANO. 1984. Fine structural nature of delayed neuronal death following ischemia in the gerbil hippocampus. Acta Neuropathol. (Berl.) **62:** 209–218.

76. THILMANN, R., Y. XIE, P. KLEIHUES & M. KIESSLING. 1986. Persistent inhibition of protein synthesis precedes delayed neuronal death in postischemic gerbil hippocampus. Acta Neuropathol. **71:** 88–93.

77. VASS, K., M. L. BERGER, T. S. NOWAK, JR., W. J. WELCH & H. LASSMANN. 1989. Induction of stress protein HSP70 in nerve cells after status epilepticus in the rat. Neurosci. Lett. **100:** 259–264.

78. SLOVITER, R. S. & D. H. LOWENSTEIN. 1992. Heat shock protein expression in vulnerable cells of the rat hippocampus as an indicator of excitation induced neuronal stress. J. Neurosci. **12:** 3004–3009.

79. LINDVALL, O., P. ERNFORS, J. BENGZON, Z. KOKAIA, M.-L. SMITH, B. K. SIESJÖ & H. PERSSON. 1992. Differential regulation of mRNAs for nerve growth factor, brain-derived neurotrophic factor, and neurotrophin 3 in the adult rat brain following cerebral ischemia and hypoglycemia coma. Proc. Natl. Acad. Sci. USA **89:** 648–652.

80. WESSEL, T. C., T. H. JOH & B. T. VOLPE. 1991. In situ hybridization analysis of c-*fos* and c-*jun* expression in the rat brain following transient forebrain ischemia. Brain Res. **567:** 231–240.

81. MATSUYAMA, T., H. MICHISHITA, H. NAKAMURA, M. TSUCHIYAMA, S. SHIMIZU, K. WATANABE & M. SUGITA. 1993. Induction of copper-zinc superoxide dismutase in gerbil hippocampus after ischemia. J. Cereb. Blood Flow Metab. **13:** 135–144.

82. BLUMENFELD, K. S., F. A. WELSH, V. A. HARRIS & M. A. PESENSON. 1992. Regional expression of c-fos and heat shock protein-70 mRNA following hypoxia-ischemia in immature rat brain. J. Cereb. Blood Flow Metab. **12:** 987–995.

83. UNEY, J. B., P. N. LEIGH, C. D. MARSDEN, A. LEES & B. H. ANDERTON. 1988. Stereotaxic injection of kainic acid into the striatum of rats induces synthesis of mRNA for heat shock protein 70. FEBS Lett. **235:** 215–218.

84. GONZALEZ, M. F., K. SHIRAISHI, K. HISANAGA, S. M. SAGAR, M. MANDABACH & F. R. SHARP. 1989. Heat shock proteins as markers of neural injury. Mol. Brain Res. **6:** 93–100.

85. SHARP, F. R., P. JASPER, J. HALL, L. NOBLE & S. M. SAGAR. 1991. MK-801 and ketamine induce heat shock protein HSP70 in injured neurons in posterior cingulate and retrosplenial cortex. Ann. Neurol. **30:** 801–809.

86. OLNEY, J. W., J. LABRUYERE, G. WANG, D. F. WOZNIAK, M. T. PRICE & M. A. SESMA. 1991. NMDA antagonist neurotoxicity: Mechanism and prevention. Science **254:** 1515–1518.

87. SPRANG, G. K. & I. R. BROWN. 1987. Selective induction of a heat shock gene in fiber tracts and cerebellar neurons of the rabbit brain detected by in situ hybridization. Mol. Brain. Res. **3:** 89–93.

88. BLAKE, M. J., T. S. NOWAK, JR. & N. J. HOLBROOK. 1990. In vivo hyperthermia

induces expression of HSP70 mRNA in brain regions controlling the neuroendocrine response to stress. Mol. Brain Res. **8:** 89–92.

89. NISHIMURA, R. N., B. E. DWYER, K. CLEGG, R. COLE & J. DE VELLIS. 1991. Comparison of the heat shock response in cultured cortical neurons and astrocytes. Mol. Brain Res. **9:** 39–45.

90. DIETRICH, W. D., R. BUSTO, M. HALLEY & I. VALDES. 1990. The importance of brain temperature in alterations of the blood-brain barrier following cerebral ischemia. J. Neuropathol. Exp. Neurol. **49:** 486–497.

91. SHARMA, H. S., C. ZIMMER, J. WESTMAN & J. CERVOS-NAVARRO. 1992. Acute systemic heat stress increases glial fibrillary acidic protein immunoreactivity in brain: Experimental observations in conscious normotensive young rats. Neuroscience **48:** 889–901.

92. ASTRUP, J., B. K. SIESJÖ & L. SYMON. 1981. Thresholds in cerebral ischemia. The ischemic penumbra. Stroke **12:** 723–725.

93. FERRIERO, D. M., H. Q. SOBERANO, R. P. SIMON & F. R. SHARP. 1990. Hypoxia-ischemia induces heat shock protein-like (hsp72) immunoreactivity in neonatal rat brain. Dev. Brain Res. **53:** 145–150.

94. SHARP, F. R., D. LOWENSTEIN, R. SIMON & K. HISANAGA. 1991. Heat shock protein hsp72 induction in cortical and striatal astrocytes and neurons following infarction. J. Cereb. Blood Flow Metab. **11:** 621–627.

95. LI, Y., M. CHOPP, J. H. GARCIA, Y. YOSHIDA, Z. G. ZHANG & S. R. LEVINE. 1992. Distribution of the 72-kd heat-shock protein as a function of transient focal cerebral ischemia in rats. Stroke **23:** 1292–1298.

96. KINOUCHI, H., F. R. SHARP, M. P. HILL, J. KOISTINAHO, S. M. SAGAR & P. H. CHAN. 1993. Induction of 70-kDa heat shock protein and hsp70 mRNA following transient focal cerebral ischemia in the rat. J. Cereb. Blood Flow Metab. **13:** 105–115.

97. WELSH, F. A., D. J. MOYER & V. A. HARRIS. 1992. Regional expression of heat shock protein-70 mRNA and c-fos mRNA following focal ischemia in rat brain. J. Cereb. Blood Flow Metab. **12:** 204–212.

98. BROWN, I. R., S. RUSH & G. O. IVY. 1989. Induction of a heat shock gene at the site of tissue injury in the rat brain. Neuron **2:** 1559–1564.

99. GOWER, D. J., C. HOLLMAN, S. LEE & M. TYTELL. 1989. Spinal cord injury and the stress protein response. J. Neurosurg. **70:** 605–611.

100. TANNO, H., R. P. NOCKELS, L. H. PITTS & L. J. NOBLE. 1993. Immunolocalization of heat shock protein after fluid percussive brain injury and relationship to breakdown of the blood-brain barrier. J. Cereb. Blood Flow Metab. **13:** 116–124.

101. KIRINO, T., Y. TSUJITA & A. TAMURA. 1991. Induced tolerance to ischemia in gerbil hippocampal neurons. J. Cereb Blood Flow Metab **11:** 299–307.

102. KITAGAWA, K., M. MATSUMOTO, M. TAGAYA, R. HATA, H. UEDA, M. NIINOBE, N. HANDA, R. FUKUNAGA, K. KIMURA, K. MIKOSHIBA & T. KAMADA. 1990. "Ischemic tolerance" phenomenon found in brain. Brain Res. **528:** 21–24.

103. KITAGAWA, K., M. MATSUMOTO, M. TAGAYA, K. KUWABARA, R. HATA, N. HANDA, R. FUKUNAGA, K. KIMURA & T. KAMADA. 1991. Hyperthermia-induced neuronal protection against ischemic injury in gerbils. J. Cereb. Blood Flow Metab. **11:** 449–452.

104. LIU, Y., H. KATO, N. NAKATA & K. KOGURE. 1992. Protection of rat hippocampus against ischemic neuronal damage by pretreatment with sublethal ischemia. Brain Res. **586:** 121–124.

105. CHOPP, M., H. CHEN, K.-L. HO, M. O. DERESKI, E. BROWN, F. W. HETZEL & K. M. A. WELCH. 1989. Transient hyperthermia protects against subsequent forebrain ischemic cell damage in the rat. Neurology **39:** 1396–1398.

106. LOWENSTEIN, D. H., P. H. CHAN & M. F. MILES. 1991. The stress protein response in cultured neurons: Characterization and evidence for a protective role in excitotoxicity. Neuron **7:** 1053–1060.

107. RORDORF, G., W. J. KOROSHETZ & J. V. BONVENTRE. 1991. Heat shock protects cultured neurons from glutamate toxicity. Neuron **7:** 1043–1051.

108. BARBE, M. F., M. TYTELL, D. J. GOWER & W. J. WELCH. 1988. Hyperthermia protects against light damage in the rat retina. Science **241:** 1817–1820.

109. ABE, K., J. KAWAGOE, S. SATO, M. SAHARA & K. KOGURE. 1991. Induction of the 'zinc finger' gene after transient focal ischemia in rat cerebral cortex. Neurosci. Lett. **123:** 248–250.

110. MÜLLER, M., M. CLEEF, G. RÖHN, P. BONNEKOH, A. E. I. PAJUNEN, H.-G. BERNSTEIN & W. PASCHEN. 1991. Ornithine decarboxylase in reversible cerebral ischemia: an immunohistochemical study. Acta Neuropathol. **83:** 39–45.

111. DEMPSEY, R. J., J. M. CARNEY & M. S. KINDY. 1991. Modulation of ornithine decarboxylase mRNA following transient ischemia in the gerbil. J. Cereb. Blood Flow Metab. **11:** 979–985.

112. SUGA, S. & T. S. NOWAK, JR. 1991. Localization of immunoreactive Fos and Jun proteins in gerbil brain: Effect of transient ischemia (Abstract). J. Cereb. Blood Flow Metab. **11:** S352.

113. NOWAK, T. S., JR., O. C. OSBORNE & S. SUGA. 1992. Changes in gene expression after transient ischemia as potential markers for excitotoxic pathology. *In* The Role of Neurotransmitters in Brain Injury. M. Y.-T. Globus & W. D. Dietrich, Eds.: 227–232. Plenum Press. New York.

114. CHURN, S. B., W. C. TAFT, M. S. BILLINGSLEY, R. E. BLAIR & R. J. DELORENZO. 1990. Temperature modulation of ischemic neuronal death and inhibition of calcium/calmodulin-dependent protein kinase II in gerbils. Stroke **21:** 1715–1721.

115. GINSBERG, M. D., L. L. STERNAU, M. Y. GLOBUS, W. D. DIETRICH & R. BUSTO. 1992. Therapeutic modulation of brain temperature: Relevance to ischemic brain injury. Cerebrovasc. Brain Metab. Rev. **4:** 189–225.

116. BUCHAN, A. & W. A. PULSINELLI. 1990. Hypothermia but not the N-methyl-D-aspartate antagonist, MK-801, attenuates neuronal damage in gerbils subjected to transient global ischemia. J. Neurosci. **10:** 311–316.

117. SUGA, S. & T. S. NOWAK, JR. 1993. Pharmacology of the postischemic stress response: Effects of temperature on hsp70 expression after transient ischemia and hypothermic action of NBQX in the gerbil. *In* Pharmacology of Cerebral Ischemia 1992. J. Krieglstein & H. Oberpichler-Schwenk, Eds.: 279–286. Wissenschaftliche Verlag. Stuttgart.

118. KUROIWA, T., P. BONNEKOH & K.-A. HOSSMANN. 1990. Prevention of postischemic hyperthermia prevents ischemic injury of CA_1 neurons in gerbils. J. Cereb. Blood Flow Metab. **10:** 550–556.

119. WELSH, F. A. & V. A. HARRIS. 1991. Postischemic hypothermia fails to reduce ischemic injury in gerbil hippocampus. J. Cereb. Blood Flow Metab. **11:** 617–620.

120. HAMOS, J. E., B. OBLAS, D. PULASKI-SALO, W. J. WELCH, D. G. BOLE & D. A. DRACHMAN. 1991. Expression of heat shock proteins in Alzheimer's disease. Neurology **41:** 345–350.

121. SELMAJ, K., C. F. BROSNAN & C. S. RAINE. 1992. Expression of heat shock protein-65 by oligodendrocytes in vivo and in vitro: Implications for multiple sclerosis. Neurology **42:** 795–800.

122. LOWE, J., R. J. MAYER & M. LANDON. 1993. Ubiquitin in neurodegenerative diseases. Brain Pathol. **3:** 55–65.

123. GAROFALO, O., P. G. KENNEDY, M. SWASH, J. E. MARTIN, P. LUTHERT, B. H. ANDERTON & P. N. LEIGH. 1991. Ubiquitin and heat shock protein expression in amyotrophic lateral sclerosis. Neuropath. Appl. Neurobiol. **17:** 39–45.

124. MUNRO, S. & H. R. B. PELHAM. 1986. An hsp70-like protein in the ER: Identity with the 78 kd glucose-regulated protein and immunoglobulin heavy chain binding protein. Cell **46:** 291–300.

125. WELCH, W. J., J. I. GARRELS, G. P. THOMAS, J. J.-C. LIN & J. R. FERAMISCO. 1983. Biochemical characterization of the mammalian stress proteins and identification of two stress proteins as glucose- and Ca^{++}-ionophore-regulated proteins. J. Biol. Chem. **258:** 7102–7111.

Molecular Mechanisms of Selective Neurotoxicants: Studies on Organotin Compounds[a]

STEPHANIE M. TOGGAS,[b] J. KYLE KRADY,[c]
THERESA A. THOMPSON, AND
MELVIN L. BILLINGSLEY[d]

Department of Pharmacology
Pennsylvania State University College of Medicine
Milton S. Hershey Medical Center
Hershey, Pennsylvania 17033

INTRODUCTION

Determination of the mechanisms of action of selective neurotoxicants is a major issue in neurotoxicology. Because of the heterogeneity of cell types in the CNS, conclusions regarding the neurotoxic actions of a given series of compounds and the patterns of such damage are difficult to make. Several selective neurotoxicants have proven valuable as agents for producing animal models of neurodegenerative diseases; the cellular and molecular actions of MPTP (1-methyl-4-phenyl-1,2,5,6-tetrahydropyridine), provide one such example.[1] Selective toxicity to dopaminergic systems is a combination of metabolism to the reactive intermediate MPP^+ (1-methyl-4-phenylpyridinium) by the enzyme monoamine oxidase B and uptake via the dopamine reuptake pump. Consequently, for this neurotoxicant at least two gene products, the dopamine uptake pump and monoamine oxidase B, must be present for toxicity to occur. A third gene product, tyrosine hydroxylase, is also present in damaged cells, and serves as a marker for monoaminergic neurons. In this particular paradigm, a molecular genetic approach designed to isolate gene products related to MPTP toxicity would be predicted to isolate at least three genes; two directly related to toxicity and a third, tyrosine hydroxylase, a biomarker for dopaminergic neurons.

A number of heavy metals are neurotoxic, and some show rather selective patterns of damage. Organotin compounds are widely used industrial chemicals that are introduced into the environment in significant quantities.[2] Two organotin compounds, trimethyltin (TMT) and triethyltin (TET) produce neuropathologic

[a] This work was supported by PHS Grant RO1-ES05450 and EPA Grant R818002-01-0 to M.L.B.

[b] Current Address: Department Neuropharmacology, The Scripps Research Institute, La Jolla, CA 92037.

[c] Current Address: Department of Human Genetics, Yale University School of Medicine, New Haven, CT 06510.

[d] Address for correspondence: Dr. Melvin L. Billingsley, Department of Pharmacology, Hershey Medical Center, P.O. Box 850, Hershey, PA 17033; Tel.: (717)-531-6289; FAX: (717)-531-5013.

effects. A single exposure to TMT produces a specific pattern of neuronal damage and destruction in man and rodents, characterized by accumulation of dense bodies and autophagic vacuoles in the cytoplasm, vacuolization of the Golgi apparatus, and cell necrosis.[3-7] The selective nature of the lesion cannot be explained by a preferential distribution of TMT or tin to sensitive areas;[8,9] moreover, elemental tin and other metabolites of TMT do not display this pattern of neurotoxicity.[10,11] While increased glutamate release has been associated with TMT intoxication and suggested to contribute to TMT's neurotoxic effects, TMT itself does not appear to be an excitotoxin.[12-14] In spite of the numerous neurochemical changes that have been characterized in response to TMT intoxication, the mechanism of TMT-induced toxicity remains unknown.

In contrast, TET causes damage to myelin. The most dramatic human exposure occurred in France in 1954, when over 200 people ingested TET, as TET iodide, a contaminant of an oral preparaton of diethytin diiodide. This preparation, called Stalinon, was intended for treatment of acne and boils. Victims displayed interstitial brain edema, resulting in death in almost half of those exposed.[15] In rats, the effects of TET appear to be similar, with vacuolization and destruction of the myelin sheath resulting in a generalized edema and, often, death.[16] Thus, despite chemical similarity between organotins, specific and differential patterns of neuropathologies result following exposure.

MOLECULAR APPROACHES TO STUDY SELECTIVE NEUROTOXICANTS

Numerous approaches have proved beneficial for assessment of neurotoxicity; indeed, a multidisciplinary approach, ranging from behavioral through molecular approaches is needed in order to fully characterize selective neurotoxicants. In the case of organotins such as TMT, considerable information has accrued concerning the behavioral, histologic, and electrophysiologic consequences of exposure; however, mechanisms have remained elusive. We formulated a strategy, shown schematically in FIGURE 1, for addressing the selective mechanism of TMT neurotoxicity. At the regional level, initial studies mapped the extent of neurodegeneration by using silver stains for degenerating neurons.[17] The resulting maps focused attention on several areas of rat brain, most notably hippocampus and limbic cortex (FIG. 1B). The next level of analysis reduces the focus to the cellular level; this requires that specific cDNA or antibody probes are available for assays. The subsequent levels of analysis proceed from the subcellular level to the protein level and ultimately, to the level of gene expression (FIG. 1, D–F). Although this reductionist approach allows hypotheses to be tested at more specific levels, it requires that a battery of macromolecular probes are available for use in such experiments.

In the case of TMT, we hypothesized that sensitive neurons expressed a gene product(s) which predisposed them to the effects of TMT. This hypothesis led to development of the strategy shown in FIGURE 2, which was designed to isolate cDNAs that would identify gene products unique to TMT-sensitive cells. Subtractive hybridization, as previously described,[18] allowed removal of mRNAs common to sensitive and insensitive cells, and enriched for cDNAs preferentially expressed in TMT-sensitive neurons. Several criteria were used to screen presumptive TMT-specific cDNAs; such cDNAs should be present in control mRNA pools, but virtually absent following TMT lesions, and *in*

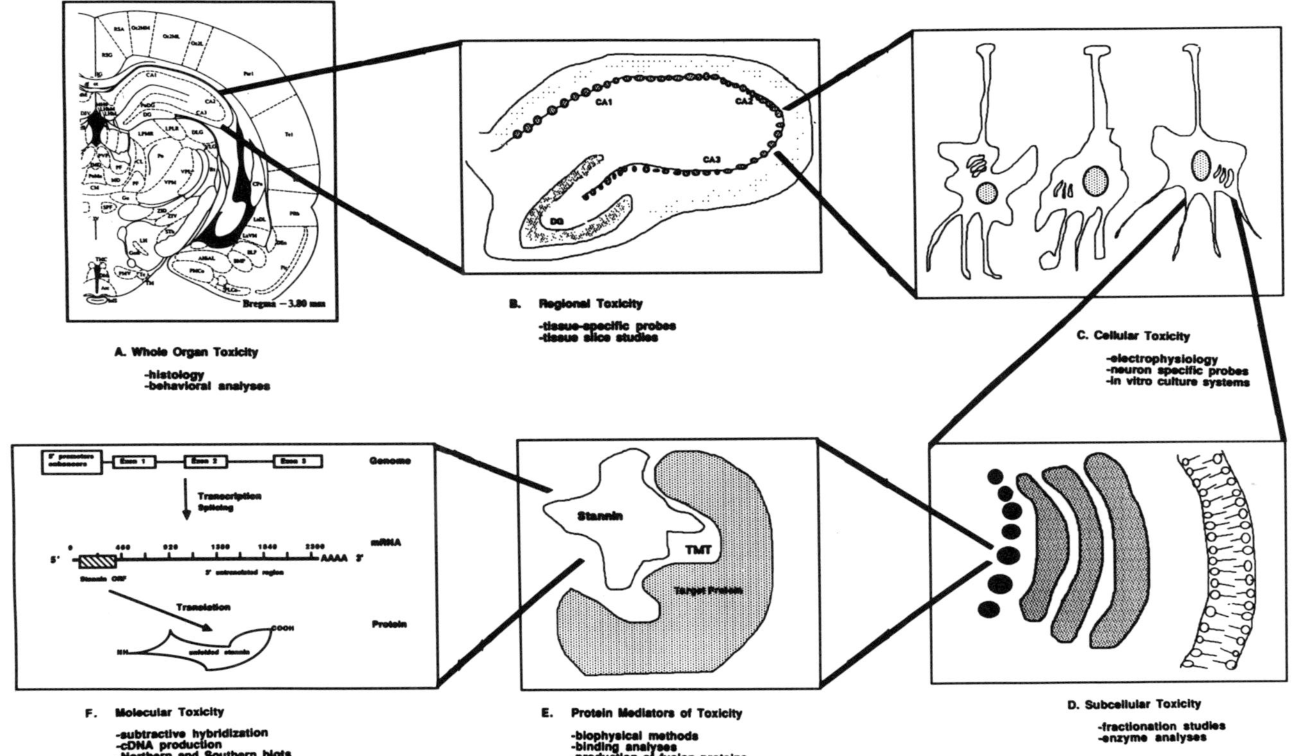

FIGURE 1. Schematic depicting the progression and interdependence of cellular and molecular strategies in neurotoxicology.

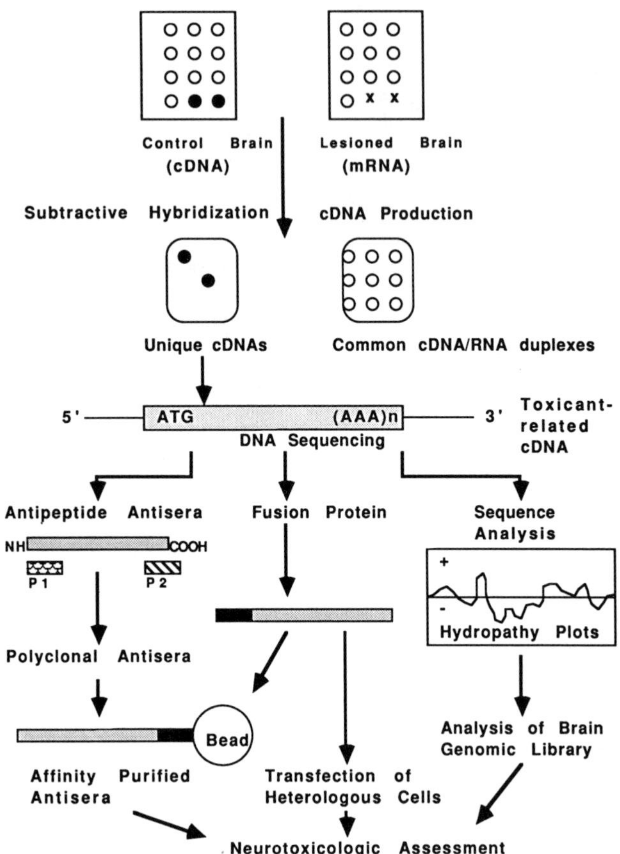

FIGURE 2. Strategy for developing molecular probes in neurotoxicology. This approach is designed to isolate gene products which are preferentially located in neurons sensitive to toxicants. The common cDNA/RNA duplexes isolated following subtractive hybridization are usually discarded.

situ hybridization analysis should localize the cDNAs to TMT-sensitive neurons. This approach has proved successful, resulting in the isolation and characterization of a unique cDNA, termed pr9T-19-37, which met the criteria listed above. The characterization of this cDNA and its protein product, termed "stannin" has been described in detail.[19]

Several types of experiments were performed with the full-length clone, using the molecular tools generated for further analysis. The following strategy was used after full-length clones were isolated from rat brain libraries and completely sequenced. In one set of studies, antipeptide antisera were raised against a synthetic peptide corresponding to the N-terminal of stannin; the amino acid sequence of stannin and the corresponding peptide is shown in FIGURE 3. The polyclonal antisera were purified using a novel approach described below, and used for identification of stannin in neurons. A second strategy involved production of a stannin fusion protein in bacteria. This construct has proved useful; 1) as an affinity ligand for purification of antisera; 2) as a source of considerable quantities of stannin protein and 3) as a rapid means for determining whether expression of stannin in heterologous cells induced TMT sensitivity. A third approach was to use sequence analysis to identify features of stannin common to other known cDNAs and proteins in databases; to date, no homologies have been determined. Our currently focus is to isolate genomic clones, in order to identify regions which may control the neuronal subtype expression of stannin.

Thus, by pursuing this strategy for isolation of genes specific to TMT-sensitive neurons, we have developed several valuable reagents to test the hypothesis that stannin mediates TMT toxicity. An outline of several studies using these tools is shown in FIGURE 4. The cDNA clone can be inserted into expression vectors, and used to transfect TMT-insensitive cells in culture. If stannin expression is necessary and sufficient for TMT toxicity, selected transformants are predicted to have greater sensitivity to the lethal effects of TMT, manifested as a lowered IC_{50} to the agent. Key variables include whether stannin expression is species-specific, whether stannin must be expressed in a neuronal phenotype and whether additional gene products need to be present in a given cell to manifest toxicity mediated by stannin. These variables can be addressed by using cell lines of rat and human origin, and by using neuroblastoma and glioma cell lines as well as somatic cells.

Affinity-purified antibodies can be used to map changes in stannin following TMT intoxication. Stannin-positive cells should decline subsequent to TMT intoxication. This can be assessed using Western blot analysis and immunocytochemistry. Finally, riboprobes derived from the cDNA can be used to study gene expression in various biologic and toxicologic studies using *in situ* hybridization and Northern blot analysis. Thus, once sequence-derived information is available and specific probes are generated, a wide range of experiments can be conducted to test hypotheses relating to the correlation between gene expression and susceptibility of toxicity.

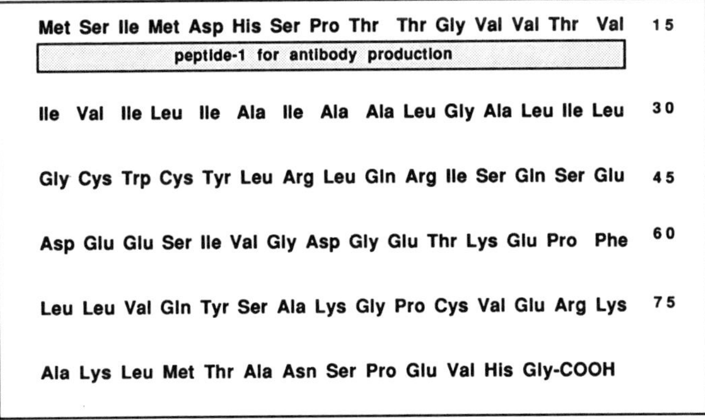

FIGURE 3. Amino acid sequence of stannin. The boxed region under residues 1–15 were used for production of polyclonal antipeptide antisera.

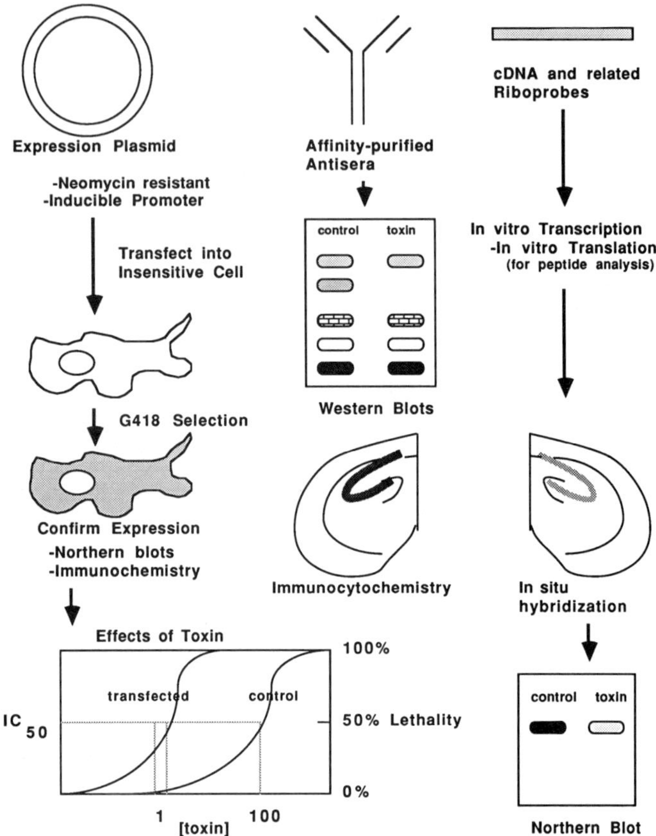

FIGURE 4. Specific uses of molecular probes in neurotoxicology. Three approaches are shown, focusing on expression of the putative gene product in heterologous cells, use of affinity-purified antisera to determine patterns of protein expression in brain, and use of riboprobes for *in situ* and Northern blot analysis.

SPECIFIC APPLICATION OF MOLECULAR APPROACHES USING STANNIN

We have applied several molecular biologic techniques to study the cellular and molecular basis of TMT toxicity. Several specific illustrations are outlined below, for purposes of demonstrating how some issues in selective neurotoxicity can be addressed via application of molecular biologic techniques and production of molecular probes.

Production of a Stannin Fusion Protein and Antisera Purification

Several plasmid vectors are available which allow expression of specific gene products as fusion proteins in bacteria. In general, such vectors allow rapid screening of recombinants based on color (interruption of gene fusions to the β-galactosidase gene), facilitate easy purification of the fusion protein, and allow recovery of the peptide of interest via selective proteolysis. We chose to express stannin in the pMAL-c vector; this plasmid produces a maltose binding protein (MBP) fused to β-galactosidase. In-frame insertion of stannin cDNA at a site which disrupts the MBP–β-galactosidase fusion yields a stannin peptide that is susceptible to proteolytic removal from MBP via Factor Xa, adds only two additional N-terminal amino acids to the putative protein, and allows rapid affinity purification of MBP/stannin fusions via MBP's strong affinity for amylose affinity resins. A schematic of this vector is shown in FIGURE 5. Expression of the MBP/ stannin fusion protein is induced by adding isopropyl-β-D-thiogalactoside (IPTG) to the cultures.

In one experiment, the MBP domain was cleaved from the affinity purified MBP/stannin fusion protein using the endopeptidase Factor Xa (New England Biolabs) at a fusion protein : enzyme ratio of 20 : 1. Following digestion, cleavage products were visualized by staining 15% SDS-PAGE gels with Coomassie brilliant blue, destaining and subsequently silver staining (Pierce). To determine optimum substrates for cleavage, one set of reactions was performed using the native MBP/ stannin fusion protein, and one set was performed using a denatured preparation of this protein. Denaturation was carried out by dialyzing the affinity-purified, native fusion protein against two changes of 20 mM Tris, pH 8.0, 6 M guanidine HCl at 4°C for 2 hours, followed by two 4-h dialyses against 20 mM Tris, pH 8.0, 100 mM NaCl. This dialysate was used in the Factor Xa cleavage reactions.

Digestion with Factor Xa of the native MBP/stannin fusion and the denatured form was performed to cleave the MBP domain from the stannin domain. As shown in FIGURE 6, distinct peptides migrating at approximately 17.5 kDa were visible in the 72-h and 84-h lanes for both the undenatured and denatured fusion reactions. Interestingly, the stannin peptide migrates anomalously in SDS-PAGE gels, and fails to stain with Coomassie blue, suggesting that the protein exists in an unusual conformation. Biophysical characterization of this protein is currently in progress.

The affinity-purified fusion protein was also used as a ligand for purification of antisera generated against synthetic peptides. A common strategy is to immobilize the peptide immunogen as an affinity matrix. We used a variant of this technique to purify antipeptide antisera; this scheme is shown in FIGURE 7. MBP/ stannin fusion proteins were induced in bacteria, purified via amylose columns, and immobilized on CnBr-activated Sepahrose 4B. Crude antisera raised against residues 1–15 of stannin (coupled via a C-terminal cysteine to keyhole limpet hemocyanin) was diluted 1 : 1 in Tris-buffered saline and incubated with the fusion protein affinity matrix. After extensive washing, elution via the chaotrope urea was used to obtain the affinity-purified antibody. This preparation was relatively devoid of background, and recognized a ~10 kDa peptide on Western blots of hippocampal homogenate. An advantage of this approach is that antipeptide antibodies are prepared which recognize the peptide antigen in a conformation linked to the remainder of the stannin protein. Also, such antibodies give additional evidence that the predicted open reading frame of stannin corresponds to the peptide used to generate the crude antiserum.

A third strategy is to use the fusion protein as an affinity ligand for exploring protein-protein interactions. In the case of stannin-MBP, an oriented affinity matrix can be made using amylose resin; the MBP domain attaches to the column, leaving the stannin domain free for interactions. One limitation of this approach is that the fusion protein may not interact with appropriate cellular protein targets because

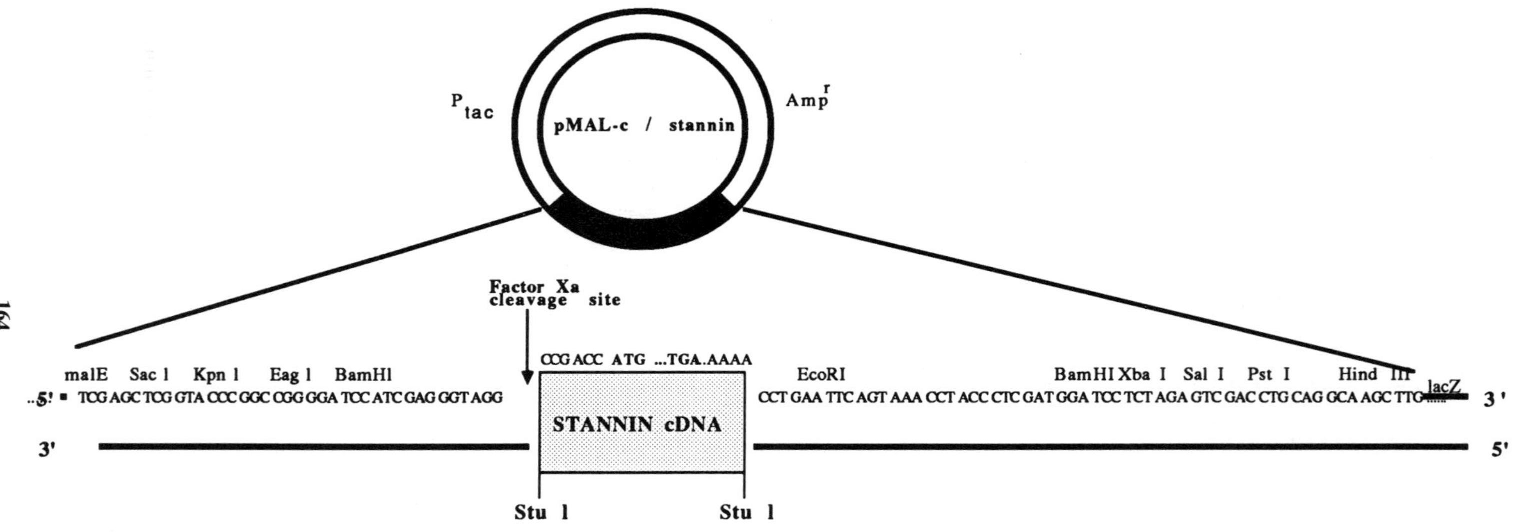

FIGURE 5. Stannin CDNA/pMAL-c bacterial expression vector. Map of stannin cDNA subcloned into the pMAL-c bacterial expression vector (New England Biolabs). Recombinants were selected by means of a blue/white color screen (interruption of malE-lacZα gene fusion) and restriction analysis. The Factor Xa site encoded by the vector allowed for cleavage of the MBP domain from the stannin domain.

of steric hindrance. A second consideration is that the conditions for eluting putative target proteins may be sufficiently harsh as to cause removal of the fusion protein from the support. This latter technical obstacle can be overcome by covalently attaching the fusion protein to a support bead. Thus, fusion proteins can be used to determine cellular targets which mediate toxicity (see FIG. 1E).

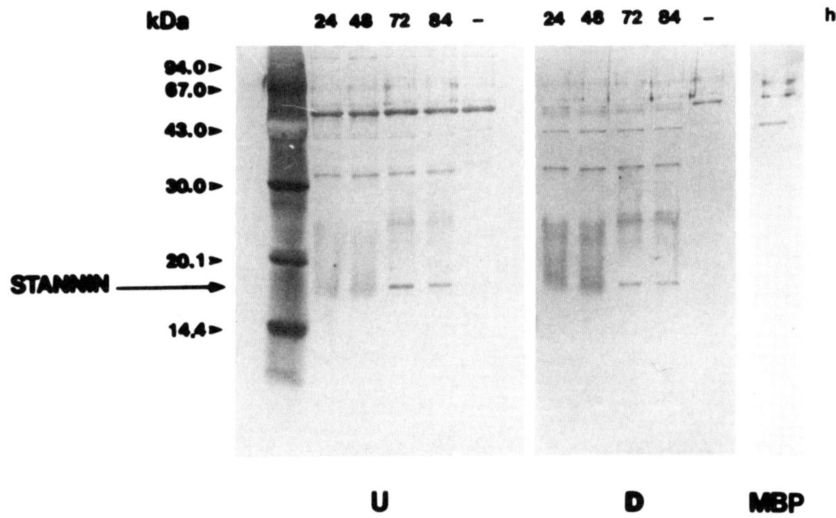

FIGURE 6. Factor Xa cleavage analysis of the MBP/stannin fusion protein. Undenatured and denatured forms of the affinity-purified MBP/stannin fusion protein were subjected to digestion with Factor Xa for 24–84 hours and products electrophoresed on 15% SDS gels. After silver staining, but not Coomassie staining, gels were found to contain a small molecular weight cleavage product (stannin) in the 72- and 84-h lanes, for both the undenatured and denatured substrates (*arrow*). The electrophoretic mobility of this product is estimated to be 17.5 kDa. The 32 kDa species visible in all reaction lanes is Factor Xa. (–): Negative control for protein stability to 84 h, no Factor Xa added; U: undenatured substrate reactions; D: denatured substrate reactions; MBP: purified maltose-binding protein.

Use of Affinity-purified Antibodies to Stannin

One prediction related to the hypothesis that stannin is related to TMT toxicity is that stannin immunoreactivity should be decreased in brain tissue of rats treated with TMT. To investigate this hypothesis, coronal brain sections (50 μm) from TMT-treated rats (8 mg/kg; i.p. 7 days prior to analysis) were incubated with either crude or affinity-purified stannin antipeptide antisera. Immunoreactivity was detected using a horseradish peroxidase-linked secondary antibody in conjunction with diaminobenzidine (DAB) and hydrogen peroxide. Marked decreases in immunoreactivity were seen in hippocampus, entorhinal cortex, and amygdala.

FIGURES 8 and 9 show results of this analysis for 3 TMT-treated animals.

FIGURE 8A demonstrates the pattern of immunoreactivity obtained in Ammon's horn (*magnification:* × 100) using affinity-purified stannin antipeptide antisera. This section, from a rat that did not display an overt TMT lesion as determined behaviorally and histologically, exhibited a pattern of immunoreactivity that ap-

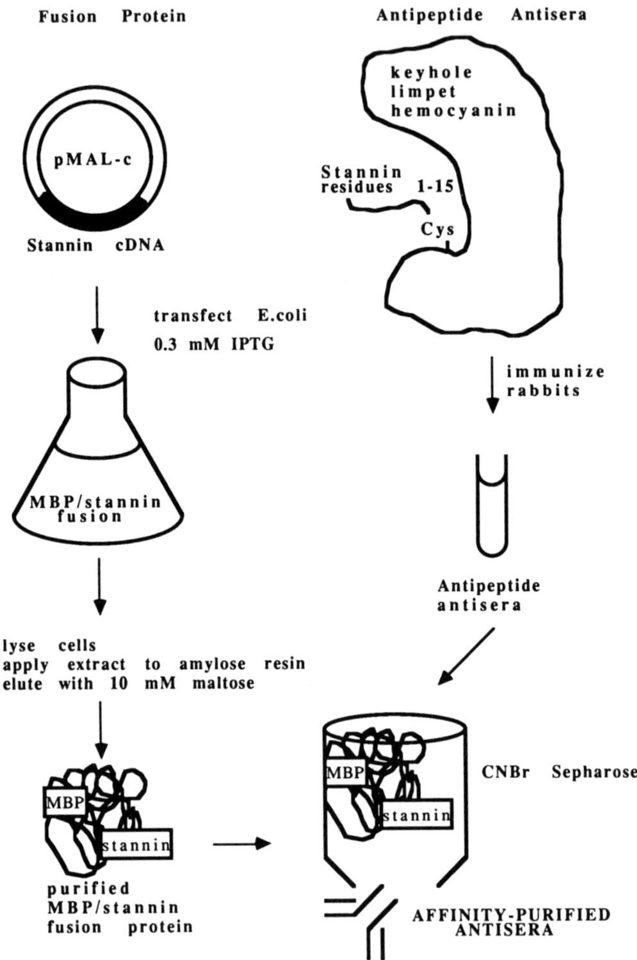

FIGURE 7. Antisera affinity purification scheme. Strategy used to purify antipeptide antisera against stannin peptides via immobilized stannin-MBP fusion proteins.

peared normal. In contrast, FIGURE 8B illustrates stannin immunostaining in representative TMT-treated brain section from a rat with a behaviorally and histologically detectable TMT lesion (*magnification:* × 100). Decreases in stannin immunoreactivity, as well as regions devoid of immunoreactivity, were observed.

FIGURE 9 shows the pattern of stannin immunostaining for a TMT-treated section from a different rat (*magnification:* × 40). In this animal, an almost total loss of staining was seen in the CA1 region, with a net decrease in staining observed throughout the hippocampal fields. For each animal analyzed, similar sections were stained with hematoxylin/eosin for histological detection of cellular damage. Areas of histologically verified damage corresponded well with areas of decreased stannin immunoreactivity. From this, one interpretation was that stannin was expressed in neurons affected by TMT, but that it was unclear whether stannin was a marker for or causal of damage.

Effects of Stannin Expression on TMT Sensitivity in Bacteria

One test for differentiating whether stannin is either a marker or a causal agent of TMT toxicity is to determine if expression of this protein in heterologous cells results in sensitization to TMT. We have exploited the expression of the MBP/stannin fusion protein in bacteria to test this possibility. Cultures of TB1 *E. coli* containing non-recombinant plasmids, plasmids with inserts in the reverse orientation, and plasmids with inserts in the correct orientation were induced to produce MBP/β-galactosidase-α, MBP, and MBP/stannin proteins, respectively. A schematic of these constructs is shown in FIGURE 10. SDS-PAGE analysis illustrated similar levels fusion protein induction among all cultures.

Culture growth was measured by determining the optical density at 600 nm of a 1 ml sample. For this bacterial strain, the conversion factor listed by the supplier (New England Biolabs) was 1 $OD_{600} = 4 \times 10^8$ cells/ml. An initial reading after IPTG induction but before TMT treatment was recorded as OD_{600} at time 0. Responses to TMT administration were monitored by measuring the OD_{600} at 30-min intervals for 4 hours, followed by measurements at 14 and 38 hours. These later time points were assayed to determine maximum growth levels reached for each culture. FIGURE 10 displays plots of OD_{600} versus time obtained for each of the three culture types at a concentration of 100 μM TMT, compared with plots obtained for equivalent cultures which received no TMT. Interestingly, the culture containing the plasmid induced to produce the MBP/stannin fusion protein clearly demonstrates enhanced sensitivity to TMT as shown by its decreased growth rate. When growth was examined at later times, stannin-expressing cultures failed to achieve the same level as other cultures. This same trend was observed when the experiment was repeated. These results suggest that, at least in bacteria, presence of the stannin domain can cause cellular sensitivity to TMT.

Although the stannin peptide exists as only a portion of the fusion protein construct produced in these cells, results form the other types of cultures suggest that this portion is responsible for conferring TMT sensitivity. If the MBP portion were responsible, then cultures producing either the reverse stannin construct (which produces MBP) and/or the control non-recombinant construct (which produces MBP/β-galactosidase-α) should have shown responses to 100 μM TMT similar to those producing the MBP/stannin construct. However, these two cultures had growth rates and saturation levels at 100 μM much like cultures that received no TMT. The presence of MBP alone or MBP fused to another 10 kDa-protein (β-galactosidase-α) does not appear to be sufficient to induce sensitivity. In addition, SDS-PAGE analysis of the amount of induced protein present in each culture indicated that cultures were induced to similar levels. Toxicity was not due to the presence of higher levels of induced MBP/stannin fusion in relation to the other fusions. In this system, TMT appears to require the stannin amino acid

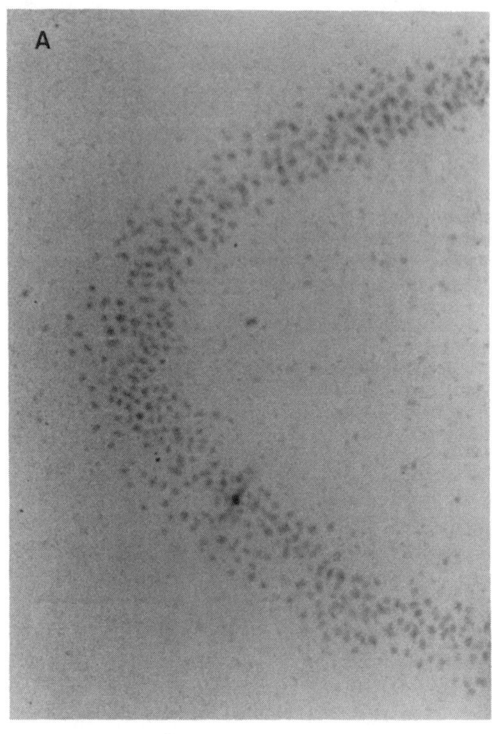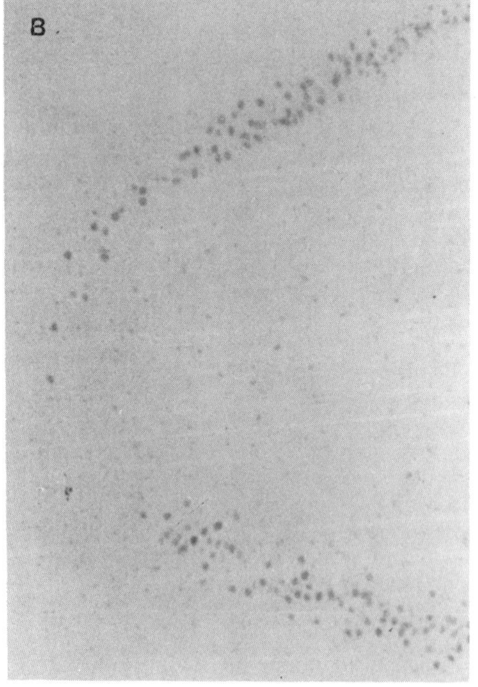

FIGURE 8. Stannin immunoreactivity in Ammon's horn 7 days following TMT administration (8 mg/kg; i.p.). **A** shows immunoreactivity in a rat which failed to show behavioral or histologic signs after TMT administration. **B** shows a loss of stannin immunoreactivity in a rat which showed both behavioral (aggression, self-mutilation, hyperactivity, tremors) and histologic evidence of TMT-induced toxicity. (*Magnification:* × 100)

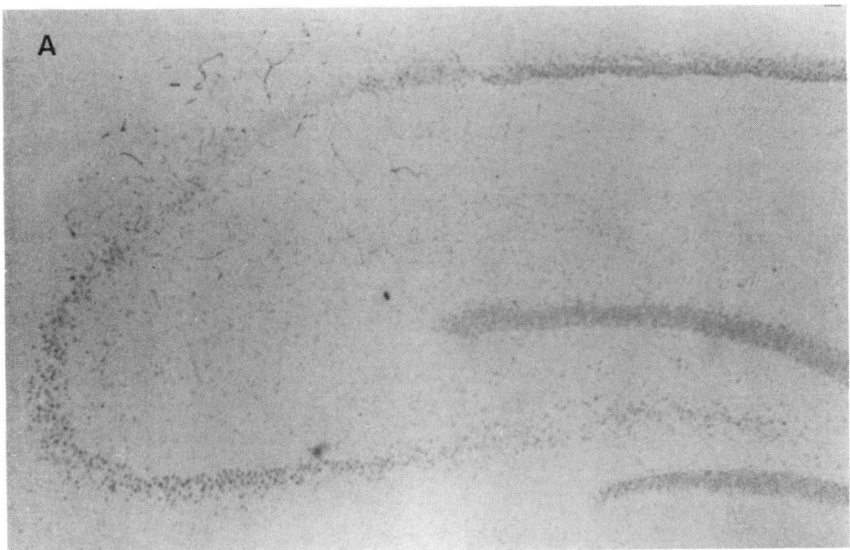

FIGURE 9. Stannin immunoreactivity in CA1 pyramidal cells 7 days following TMT administration. This rat showed both behavioral and histologic evidence of TMT-induced neurotoxicity; a marked loss of stannin immunoreactivity was noted in the CA1 hippocampal fields. (*Magnification:* **A** = × 40; **B** = × 100)

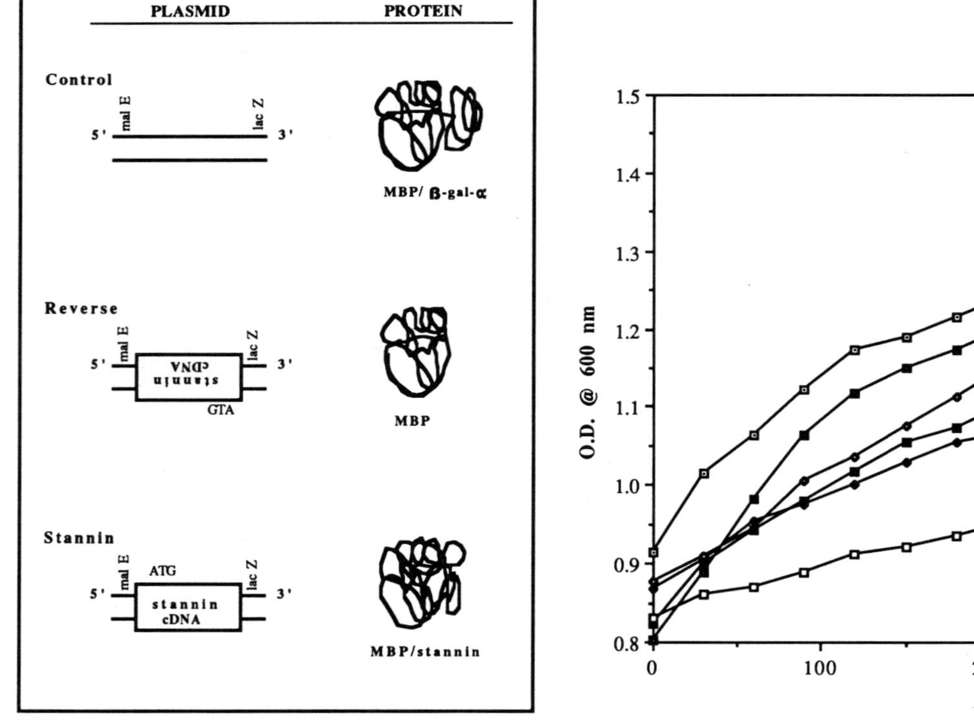

FIGURE 10. Expression of stannin-MBP fusion protein induces TMT sensitivity in bacteria. The schematic shown in the left panel outlines the orientation of the three plasmids used for bacterial transfection, and shows the fusion proteins produced by these cultures. The right panel shows growth curves of TB1 *E. coli.* bacteria containing control MBP plasmids (control), reversed MBP-stannin plasmids (reverse), and stannin-MBP fusion plasmids (stannin). Growth curves were determined for each culture in the presence and absence of TMT (100 μM).

sequence to produce its toxic efects. Although provocative, these findings need to be confirmed in eukaryotic cell systems.

Determination of TMT Toxicity in Cultured Eukaryotic Cells

In order to determine which eukaryotic cells would best serve as hosts for transfection studies, a series of *in vitro* toxicity assays were performed on a series of cell lines (TABLE 1). A fluorescence-based viability assay, in which live cells exclude ethidium homodimer (red fluorescence) but take up calcein-AM (green fluorescence) was used to determine sensitivity to TMT. After 48-h exposures to a range of concentrations of TMT, viability levels were determined. As shown in TABLE 1, human HTB-14 glioma cells were most resistant to the lethal effects of TMT, followed by the murine 3T3 fibroblasts. Human SMS-KCNR neuroblastomas and monkey TC7 kidney cells were considerably more sensitive to TMT. The latter cell line is often used for transient transfection assays. Based on these preliminary results, both HTB-14 and 3T3 cell lines will be used for heterologous transfections with stannin cDNA.

TABLE 1. Effects of TMT on Cell Viability in Several Cell Lines

		Percentage Non-viable Cells	
Cell Line	Species	10 μM TMT	100 μM TMT
HTB-14 Glioma	Human	17	31
NIH 3T3 Fibroblasts	Murine	28	50
SMS-KCNR Neuroblastoma	Human	67	78
TC7 Kidney	Monkey	61	90

Non-viable cells fluoresced red with ethidium homdimer; viable cells fluoresced green with calcien-AM. Each value represents the mean of 2 separate experiments, performed in duplicate.

DEVELOPMENTAL EXPRESSION OF STANNIN mRNA

The approach used in this study afforded a series of molecular probes, including stannin cDNA contained in a riboprobe vector system. The details and molecular cloning of stannin into this vector system are presented elsewhere.[18] Radio-labeled sense strand (control) and antisense strand riboprobes corresponding to stannin were generated using ^{35}S-UTP. The specific activities were approximately 10^9 dpm/μg RNA. *In situ* hybridization studies using adult and developing rat brain were carried out as previously described.[18,19]

FIGURE 11 shows the pattern of hybridization of antisense stannin riboprobes in the lateral septal nuclei; sense riboprobes failed to generate a signal. The septal nuclei are very sensitive to TMT; this region is among the earliest regions to show degeneration. Previous studies found both stannin peptide and mRNA in hippocampus and other limbic regions. Thus, stannin is present in neurons known to be sensitive to TMT.

Developing rats are more sensitive to TMT than adults, and show a more global range of damage following exposure.[21,22] If stannin expression relates to this developmental sensitivity, one prediction is that its expression would be more widespread in neonates. FIGURE 12 illustrates the pattern of stannin hybridization during hippocampal development. On postnatal day 1 (PND 1), expression is seen throughout the hippocampal region, and persists at high levels on PND 5. By PND 20, a marked reorganization is seen, and resembles the adult pattern. Examination of CA3 neurons is also shown in FIGURE 12; stannin hybridization is strong in this region, and progresses from a diffuse staining on PND 1 to a more focal pattern by PND 20. Previous studies indicated that stannin mRNA is expressed

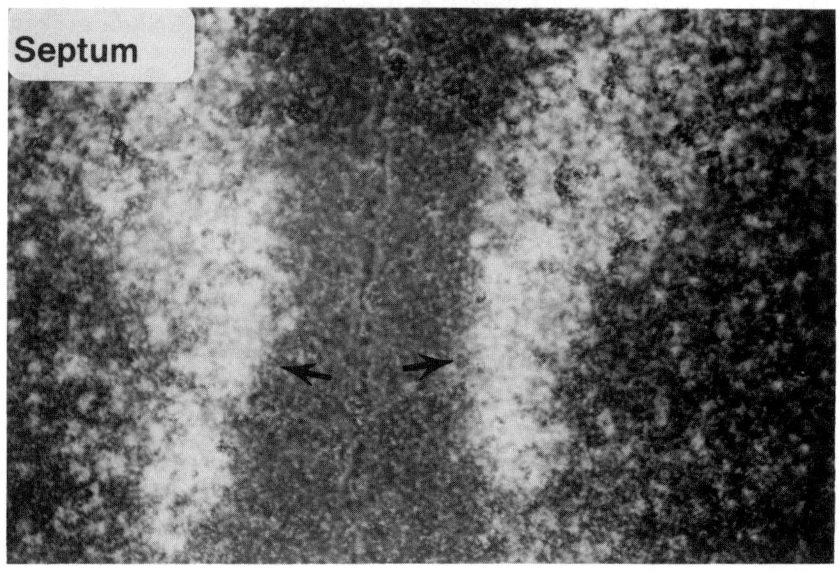

FIGURE 11. Pattern of stannin *in situ* hybridization in lateral septal nuclei. Coronal sections (interaural distance, 0.7 mm) of control adult rat brain were hybridized with ^{35}S-labeled antisense riboprobes to stannin. Slides were emulsion coated and exposed for 1 week. Silver grains can be seen over the septal neurons. (Dark-field microscopy, × 100).

in the telencephalon of E15 embryos. Thus, stannin expression occurs early in development, and undergoes a marked pattern of reorganization during postnatal brain development.

CRITICAL ISSUES FOR MOLECULAR ASSESSMENT OF NEUROTOXICANTS

The approaches discussed in this paper have wider applications in the field of neurotoxicology, providing that several global issues are addressed prior to undertaking an extensive molecular genetic approach. Specific critical issues need to be resolved in order to determine whether stannin is necessary and sufficient for TMT toxicity. The data presented suggest that stannin is present in TMT-sensitive neurons. Additional experiments have demonstrated that a stannin-like mRNA is present in kidney and lymphocytes; both organs show sensitivity to TMT.[19] Southern blot analysis of genomic DNA under stringent conditions has indicated that a conserved homolog is present in rats, rabbits, Drosophila, and humans.[19] These data suggest that stannin is conserved, and likely to subserve an important role in eukaryotic organisms.

Several speculations are possible regarding the role of stannin in TMT toxicity. First, stannin may directly interact with TMT, but not other organotins; the predicted structure has 3 cysteines and 2 histidines as possible metal-binding residues. Using the stannin fusion protein, we can directly determine if this protein binds TMT, and subsequently, whether a TMT-stannin complex can interact with other cellular macromolecules.

A second issue relates to whether stannin is a protein marker for damage or a causal gene product. Results in bacteria suggest that the stannin peptide domain can confer sensitivity to TMT, which supports the hypothesis that stannin can become a toxic protein in the presence of TMT. One possibility is that the stannin-TMT complex interfered with a critical cellular macromolecule that is common between bacteria and rat. However, there are important caveats which limit interpretation. First, there is considerable evolutionary distance between bacteria and brain; targets identified in bacteria may be unrelated to mammalian targets. Issues related to this issue are best addressed using transfection studies of mammalian cells.

Another aspect related to causality is that although evidence to date suggests that stannin is expressed in sensitive cells, more than one gene product may need to be present in a sensitive cell. Again, the parallel between MPTP and dopaminergic gene products bears notice. Issues related to a multigenic cause might be addressed by transfecting cDNAs into stannin insensitive cells which express a partial neuronal phenotype, such as rat PC-12 cells. However, if mammalian transfectants fail to be sensitized by stannin, one interpretation would be that stannin is a marker for sensitive cells.

Several global issues relate to use of molecular biologic techniques for neurotoxicology. First, not all selective neurotoxicants will be explained in molecular genetic terms; agents which acutely disrupt neurotransmission will resist characterization in this manner. However, some agents, such as excitotoxins, may yield to this approach.[22] Second, the approaches outlined allow development of specific molecular probes which can be used in studies of normal neuronal function. In this case, neurotoxicants can be used as effective molecular dissection tools for removing selective populations of cells.

A third issue relates to using the outlined strategies for identification of gene products which are induced following neuronal injury. By reversing the subtraction paradigm, one would select for those genes expressed most prominently in damaged brain. Screens would look for expression, via Northern blots, of the target in treated, but not control tissues. *In situ* hybridization may identify glial cells which express injury-related cDNAs.[23] Finally, the use of heterologous cell systems to test whether a specific molecule enhances toxicity is a key step in use of the outlined protocols.

In the future, molecular biologic techniques in neurotoxicology are likely to expand to include the use of specific transgenic mouse models and gene deletion models for testing neurotoxicants. Such murine models may prove useful for

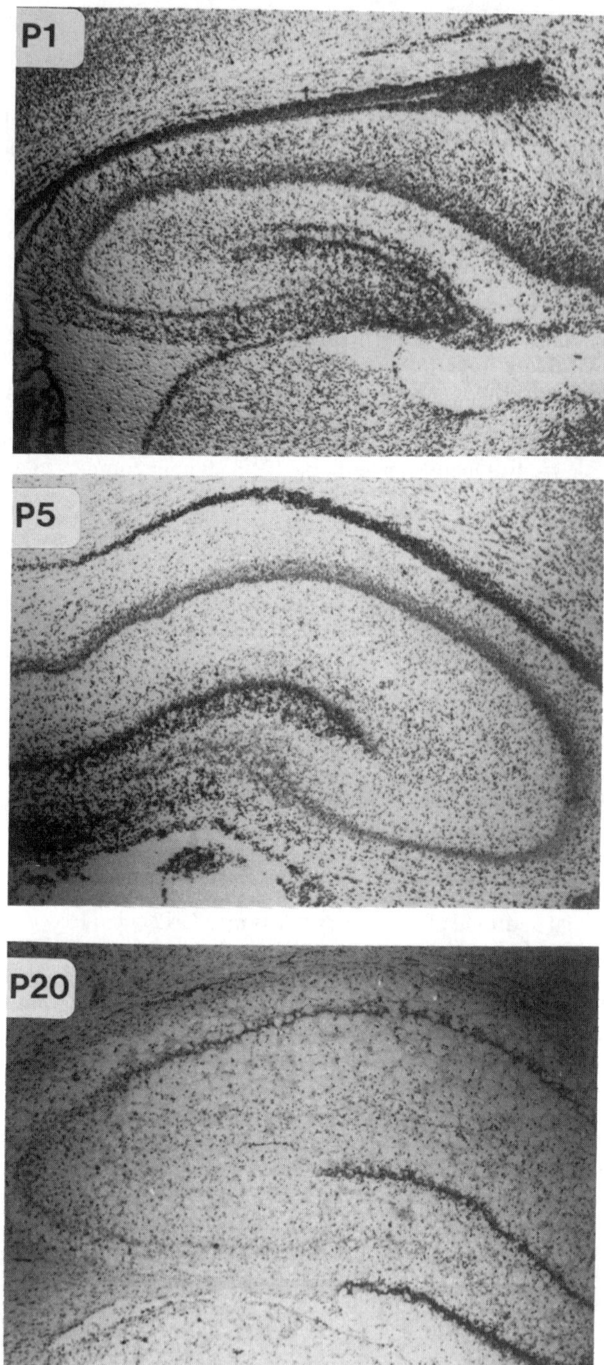

FIGURE 12. *In situ* hybridization pattern of stannin in developing rat hippocampus. Coronal sections of rat hippocampus were prepared from postnatal day 1 (PND 1), PND 5 and PND 20 rats, and hybridized with ^{35}S-labeled antisense riboprobes to stannin. Sections in the left panel show a bright-field image of whole hippocampus at various developmental epochs;

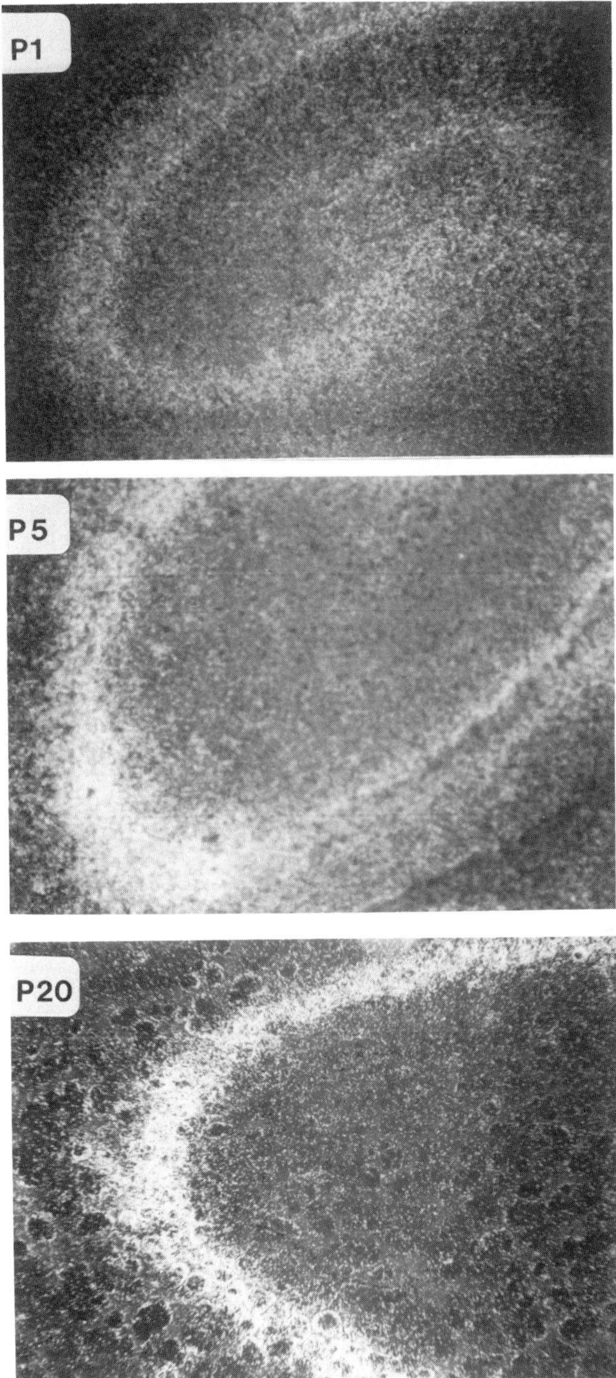

sections were emulsion-dipped and counterstained with cresyl violet. Sections in the right panel are dark-field images of stannin hybridization in Ammon's horn. (*Magnification:* × 100)

testing novel toxicants as well as determining the function of specific neuronal genes. In addition, it may be possible to construct specific cell lines which express characteristics related to a range of toxicities. Cell lines expressing sensitivity to a variety of toxicants may be useful *in vitro* systems for determining actions of unknown agents. Finally, heterologous cell lines can be used to determine whether effective treatments can be devised which reverse or block the actions of selected neurotoxicants. By developing molecular models using a defined selective toxicant such as TMT, we hope to shed light on both the mechanism of action and treatment strategies which blunt organometal toxicities.

ACKNOWLEDGMENT

The authors wish to thank Ms. Christine Patanow for expert technical assistance.

REFERENCES

1. ZIGMOND, M. J. & E. M. STRICKER. 1989. Animal models of parkinsonism using selecive neurotoxins: Clinical and basic implications. Int. Rev. Neurobiol. **31:** 1–79.
2. SNOEIJ, N. J., A. H. PENNINKS & W. SEINEN. 1987. Biological activity of organotin compounds—an overview. Environ. Res. **44:** 335–353.
3. NOLAN, C. C., A. W. BROWN & J. B. CAVANAGH. 1990. Regional variations in nerve cell responses to trimethyltin intoxication in mongolian gerbils and rats; further evidence for involvement of the Golgi apparatus. Acta Neuropathol. **81:** 204–212.
4. BROWN, A. W., W. N. ALDRIDGE, B. W. STREET & R. D. VERSCHOYLE. 1979. The behavioral and neuropathologic sequelae of intoxication by trimethyltin compounds in the rat. Am. J. Pathol. **97:** 59–82.
5. BROWN, A. W., J. B. CAVANAGH, R. D. VERSCHOYLE, M. F. GYSBERS, H. B. JONES & W. N. ALDRIDGE. 1984. Evolution of the intracellular changes in neurons caused by trimethyltin. Neuropathol. Appl. Neurobiol. **10:** 267–283.
6. BESSER, R., G. KRAMER, R. THUMLER, J. BOHL, L. GUTMANN & H. C. HOPF. 1987. Acute trimethyltin limbic-cerebellar syndrome. Neurology **37:** 945–950.
7. BOULDIN, T. W., N. D. GOINES, C. R. BAGNELL & M. R. KRIGMAN. 1981. Pathogenesis of trimethyltin neuronal toxicity. Ultrastructural and cytochemical observations. Am. J. Pathol. **104:** 237–249.
8. COOK, L. L., S. M. HEATH & J. P. O'CALLAGHAN. 1984. Distribution of tin in brain subcellular fractions following administration of trimethyl tin and triethyl tin to the rat. Toxicol. Appl. Pharmacol. **73:** 564–568.
9. MUSHAK, P., M. R. KRIGMAN & R. B. MAILMAN. 1982. Comparative organotin toxicity in the developing rat: Somatic and morphological changes and relationship to accumulation of total tin. Neurobehav. Toxicol. Teratol. **4:** 209–215.
10. BOYER, I. J. 1989. Toxicity of dibutyltin, tributyltin, and other organotin compounds to humans and to experimental animals. Toxicology **55:** 253–298.
11. COOK, L. L., K. E. STINE & L. W. REITER. 1984. Tin distribution in adult rat tissues after exposure to trimethyltin and triethyltin. Toxicol. Appl. Pharmacol. **76:** 344–348.
12. NAALSUND, L. U. & F. FONNUM. 1986. The effect of trimethyltin on three glutamergic and gabaergic transmitter parameters *in vitro:* High affinity uptake, release and recpetor binding. NeuroToxicology **7:** 53–62.
13. PATEL, M., B. K. ARDELT, G. K. W. YIM & G. E. ISOM. 1990. Interaction of trimethyltin with hippocampal glutamate. NeuroToxicology **11:** 601–608.
14. ALLEN, C. N. & F. FONNUM. 1984. Trimethyltin inhibits the activity of hippocampal neurons recorded *in vitro*. NeuroToxicology **5:** 23–30.
15. BARNES, J. M. & H. B. STONER. 1958. Toxic properties of some dialkyl and trialkyl tin salts. Brit. J. Industr. Med. **15:** 15–22.

16. O'CALLAGHAN, J. P. 1988. Neurotypic and gliotypic proteins as biochemical markers of neurotoxicity. Neurotoxicol. Teratol. **10:** 445–452.

17. BALABAN, C. D., J. P. O'CALLAGHAN & M. L. BILLINGSLEY. 1988. Trimethyltin-induced neuronal damage in the rat brain: Comparative studies using silver degeneration stains, immunocytochemistry and immunoassay for neuronotypic and gliotypic proteins. Neuroscience **26:** 337–361.

18. KRADY, J. K., G. A. OYLER, C. D. BALABAN & M. L. BILLINGSLEY. 1990. Use of avidin-biotin subtractive hybridization to characterize mRNA common to neurons destroyed by the selective neurotoxicant trimethyltin. Mol. Brain Res. **7:** 287–297.

19. TOGGAS, S. M., J. K, KRADY & M. L. BILLINGSLEY. 1993. Molecular neurotoxicology of trimethyltin: identification of stannin, a novel protein expressed in trimethyltin-sensitive cells. Mol. Pharmacol. **42:** 44–56.

20. MILLER, D. B. & J. P. O'CALLAGHAN. 1984. Biochemical, functional and morphological indicators of neurotoxicity: Effects of acute administration of trimethyltin to the developing rat. J. Pharm. Exp. Ther. **231:** 744–751.

21. RUPPERT, P. H., K. F. DEAN & L. W. REITER. 1983. Developmental and behavioral toxicity following acute postnatal exposure of rat pups to trimethyltin. Neurobehav. Toxicol. Teratol. **5:** 421–429.

22. CHOI, D. W. & S. M. ROTHMAN. 1990. The role of glutamate neurotoxicity in hypoxic-ischemic neuronal death. Ann. Rev. Neurosci. **13:** 171–182.

23. BROCK, T. O. & J. P. O'CALLAGHAN. 1987. Quantitative changes in the synaptic vesicle proteins synapsin I and p38 and the astrocyte-specific protein glial fibrillary acidic protein are associated with chemical-induced injury to the rat central nervous system. J. Neurosci. **7:** 931–942.

Heterogeneity of Brain Gene Expression in Alzheimer's Disease[a]

JOHN R. DUGUID,[b-d] CHRISTOPHER TRZEPACZ,[d]
THOMAS KEMPER,[e] WALLACE W. TOURTELLOTE,[f] AND
LADISLAV VOLICER[g]

[c]Departments of Medicine, Neurology, and Medical Genetics
Indiana University School of Medicine
Indianapolis, Indiana 46202

[d]Research Service, VA Medical Center
1481 West 10th Street
Indianapolis, Indiana 46202

[e]Department of Neurology, Boston City Hospital
Boston, Massachusetts 02118

[f]Neurology and Research Services
VAMC W. Los Angeles, Wadsworth Division
Los Angeles, California 90073

[g]Geriatric Research, Education, and Clinical Center
VA Medical Center
Bedford, Massachusetts 01730

We have recently examined the transcript levels of differentially expressed genes in scrapie, a slow virus infection, and in Alzheimer's diseases (AD), and have found that these conditions share certain patterns of altered brain gene expression.[1] In this work we have studied the expression of glial fibrillary acidic protein (GFAP), metallothionein II, α_1-antichymotrypsin (ACT) and sulfated glycoprotein-2 (SGP-2) in a larger series of AD cases and have found differences among these cases. We have related the different patterns of gene expression to clinical and histopathological findings in each of the cases. Our results are consistent with previous studies which have found heterogeneity among AD cases on the basis of clinical,[2-9] histopathological,[10-15] neurochemical,[10-14,16,17] and genetic parameters.[18-22]

METHODS

Patients and Tissue

The sources of tissue, harvesting, and storage have been described.[1,23] Patients studied here had post-mortem intervals of less than 6 hours. Although this limited the number of patients available for study, all the RNAs used had intact rRNA

[a] This work was supported by a grant from the U.S. Department of Veterans Affairs.
[b] Please address correspondence to John Duguid, M.D. at the VA Medical Center; (317)635-7401, x2601.

after denaturing agarose gel electrophoresis, a measure of RNA integrity important in the analysis of RNA blot signals. Since no low autolysis time cases without neurological disease were available to us we studied gene expression in the hippocampus of AD patients and compared it to that in Parkinson's disease (PD) and Huntington's disease (HD). While the hippocampal formation is a region of the brain uniformly involved in AD,[24] there is no primary pathology in the hippocampus in either PD or HD,[25] which served as controls.

Neuropathological diagnoses were made using hematoxylin-eosin and Bodian stains.[26] Clinical data were collected from review of medical records. Dementia severity was assessed using the CDR scale,[27] which we have modified by adding a more advanced stage, CDR4: these patients had end-stage dementia, were mute and bedridden, and had no interaction with the environment except for primitive functions.

RNA Blots

RNA was prepared[28] from 2 g sections of the hippocampal formation, including subiculum, dentate gyrus and the CA zones. After electrophoresis,[29] 1.5% agarose gels were incubated for 30 min in 15 mN NaOH and blotted[30] from this solvent onto Immobilon-N membranes (Millipore, Bedford, MA) overnight at 20°C. The filters were washed twice in 0.3 M NaCl, 0.03 M sodium citrate, pH 7.0, and then baked, blocked and hybridized as described.[28] The cDNA probes were generated from previously described recombinant inserts using random primers and the Klenow fragment of *E. coli* polymerase I,[1] while probe from human rRNA was synthesized using random primers and MMLV reverse transcriptase.[28] Autoradiograms were quantitated using a Hoeffer (San Francisco, CA) scanning densitometer and analyzed using a SpectraPhysics (San Jose, CA) integrator.

Histology

Ten μ sections of formaldehyde-fixed paraffin embedded tissue were stained with hematoxylin and eosin[26] for evaluation of neuronal loss. This evaluation was performed independently by two experienced neuroanatomists who had no knowledge of the cases. Sections were stained with thioflavin S and viewed with fluorescence microscopy to determine the density of senile plaques and neurofibrillary tangles.[31] The number of plaques and tangles in a 0.64 mm^2 area of subiculum were counted in quadruplicate using an ocular grid (Don Santo, Natick, MA).

Immunohistochemistry

Peroxidase-conjugated sheep antibody against human ACT was obtained from Biodesign International (Kennebunkport, ME). Ten μ sections were mounted on slides, deparaffinized in xylene, hydrated through an ethanol series, and incubated in 5% bovine serum albumin in 0.15 M NaCl, 0.02 M sodium phosphate, pH 7.5 (PBS), for 30 min. The sections were then incubated with the antibody, diluted 1/20 in PBS for 1 hour. The sections were then washed with 5 changes of PBS over 20 min, and reacted with diaminobenzidine in the presence of imidazole and hydrogen peroxide.[32] Sections were then counterstained with Mayer's hematoxylin[26] to demonstrate nuclear morphology.

Statistical Analysis

Statistical analysis was performed using Statview II software (Abacus Concepts, Berkley, CA) running on a Macintosh II computer (Apple Computer, Cupertino, CA). Nonparametric statistics (Spearman's rank correlation) were used in all analyses because they are distribution independent; normality could not be adequately tested in the small sample sizes studied here.[33]

RESULTS

Hippocampal RNA from seven AD cases and five controls was subjected to RNA blot analysis and probed with cDNAs coding for GFAP, metallothionein, ACT and SGP-2. The blots were also hybridized with rRNA probe to control for RNA integrity, loading, and transfer. The signals from each blot were quantitated by scanning densitometry and normalized with the 18S rRNA signal from each lane and the results are presented in FIGURE 1. While GFAP expression was increased to different degrees in all of the AD patients, metallothionein and ACT had an increased expression in selected AD patients. SGP-2 expression was increased in two patients. No significant correlation was found among the signals for the different genes in the different patients.

The topographical distribution of the increased expression of these genes was studied. RNA was prepared from frontal, parietal, occipital and cerebellar cortex (patients 10 and 11) and compared to the hippocampal RNA using RNA blot analysis (FIG. 2). In each instance where there was significantly increased expression in the hippocampus in FIGURE 1 (GFAP and ACT, patient 11; metallothionein, patient 10), the hippocampus was the site of greatest expression. This finding is consistent with the greater involvement of the hippocampus in AD compared to the other regions of the brain sampled.[24] While we did not examine the topographical distribution of SGP-2, it has been shown to have an increased expression in regions prominently involved in AD.[34]

We examined both clinical and histopathological parameters of the patients studied, and compared these to the levels of gene expression determined above. The clinical features of the patients are summarized in TABLE 1. Because of the small sample sizes considered, a correlation would have to be quite strong to be statistically significant. Nevertheless, a significant Spearman rank correlation coefficient was found between age at onset and ACT expression ($r_s = 0.899$, $p = 0.045$). No significant correlation was found between age and level of ACT expression in the controls ($r_s = 0.462$, $p = 0.356$).

The pathological features of the different cases are summarized in TABLE 2, showing the heterogeneity in density of senile plaques, neurofibrillary tangles and neuronal loss in the different patients, a well-recognized phenomenon.[24] No statistically significant correlation was found between the levels of expression of these genes and the histopathological parameters.

Hippocampal ACT was localized immunohistochemically in sections from Patient 11, who had a high level of ACT expression. As can be seen in FIGURE 3A, the increased ACT mRNA expression in patient 11 was accompanied by cytoplasmic staining of this protein in neurons, identified by both nuclear and cellular morphology. This neuronal ACT staining was less intense in the AD patients with lower ACT mRNA levels, however the previously reported staining of senile plaques and astrocytes[35] was similar in all AD cases (not shown).

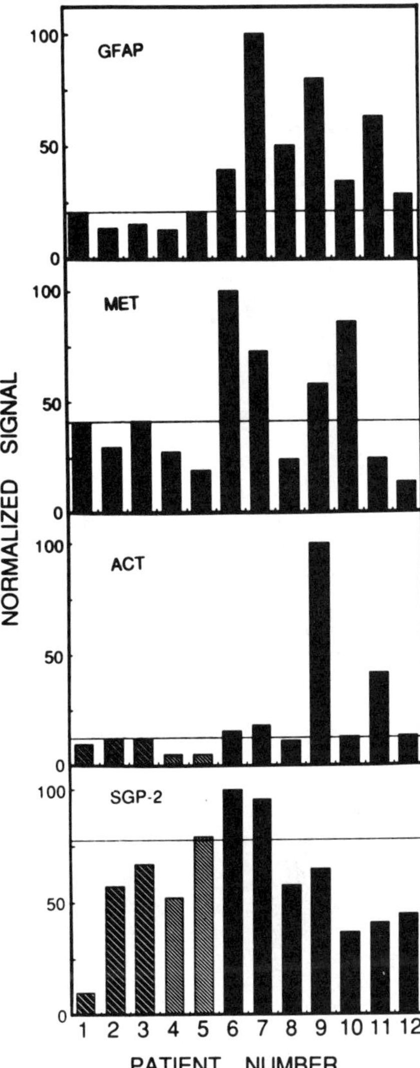

FIGURE 1. Hippocampal gene expression in Alzheimer's disease. The signals from 48-h autoradiograms of RNA blots (10 μg/lane) for the genes under study were quantitated by scanning densitometry and integration. These values were normalized by dividing the integrated signal intensities for each case by he 18S rRNA signal intensity (0.5-h exposure) for that case. Patients 1–3 had Parkinson's disease, patients 4–5 had Huntington's disease, and patients 6–12 had AD. The line in each panel indicates the value of the mean of the controls plus two times the standard error of the mean.

The relationship between the presence of neurofibrillary tangles and neuronal ACT levels was examined by the previous staining of the section photographed in FIGURE 3A with thioflavin S, the results of which is presented in FIGURE 3B. First, it was found that many apparently intact neurons with high levels of ACT did not have detectable neurofibrillary tangles, and *vice versa* (white arrows indicate the same landmarks in the two panels). Second, of the neurons that gave signals to both stains, some demonstrated a high level of ACT and a weak neurofibrillary tangle signal (lower black arrow), while others demonstrated a low level of ACT and a strong neurofibrillary tangle signal (upper black arrow).

DISCUSSION

We have found marked differences in the pattern of altered brain gene expression in different cases of AD. We did not find a correlation between the levels of expression of the different genes with each other in the different AD patients. The level of GFAP expression has been previously shown to correlate with the intensity of gliosis that occurs in this condition.[36] The increased expression of the

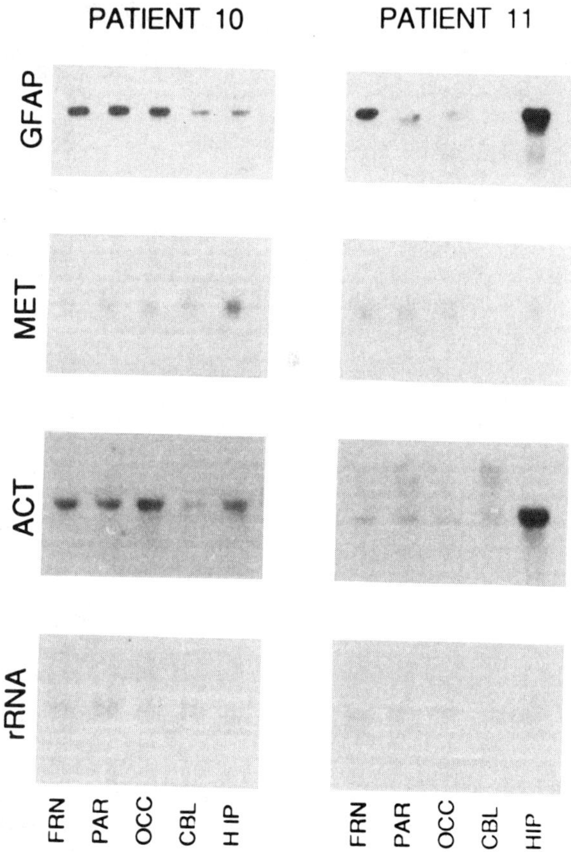

FIGURE 2. Topographical distribution of altered brain gene expression in Alzheimer's disease. 10 μg of RNA from frontal pole (FRN), parietal lobe (PAR), occipital pole (OCC), cerebellum (CBL) and hippocampus (HIP) were electrophoresed, blotted, and hybridized to the indicated probes. Exposure times were 48 hours.

GFAP gene in AD relative to controls we found is similar to that reported by May and co-workers.[34]

The variable expression of the metallothionein gene in the different AD patients had no significant correlation with either clinical or pathological severity, which argues against stage dependence of metallothionein expression, though the small sample size in this study limits the detection of weak correlations as significant.

TABLE 1. Clinical Parameters of Alzheimer's Disease Patients

Patient Number	Onset (yrs)	Course (yrs)	Dementia Severity (CDR)	Cause of Death
6	—/M[a]	—[a]	3	CHF[b]
7	63/M	10	4	pneumonia
8	52/M	11	4	pneumonia
9	86/F	7	3	pneumonia
10	63/M	8	3	asphyxia
11	68/M	4	3	pneumonia
12	61/M	6	3	CHF

There was no family history of dementia recorded for any of the AD cases. All AD cases and case 5 had received neuroleptic medication chronically. The age and sex of the control patients were: 1, 83M; 2, 75M; 3, 69F; 4, 30M; 5, 69F.

[a] Age at onset was not recorded in available medical records, therefore this patient was not included in statistical analyses related to age at onset of course.

[b] CHF represents congestive heart failure.

Metallothionein is a stress protein,[37] and its variably increased brain expression in Alzheimer's disease may result from variable stress suffered by degenerating neurons in different patients.

May and co-workers found that while SGP-2 was in general increased in AD, one of their controls had greater SGP-2 expression than did two of their AD cases on the basis of RNA blot analysis.[34] This is consistent with the variable SGP-2 expression reported here. Our previous finding of a uniformly increased SGP-2 expression in AD[1] was based on comparison to a control with very low levels of SGP-2 expression, similar to patient 1 in this study. SGP-2 has been shown to be a structural protein of the Sertoli cell, as well as its major secretory product.[38] It has recently been shown that the human homologue of SGP-2 is also a complement-associated protein.[39,40] This has led May and co-workers to suggest that complement may be involved in AD neurodegeneration.[34]

We found ACT mRNA to have a markedly increased level in two of the seven AD patients studied, compared to controls. The variable expression of ACT in the AD cases was not significantly correlated with either clinical or histopathological severity, which argued against stage dependency of ACT expression. However, we found that high levels of ACT mRNA expression were associated with later age at onset of AD, though our series was statistically small and definitive statements regarding this association should be deferred pending further studies. This caution is supported by our recent finding that there was no significant correlation between age at onset and neuronal ACT immunochemical signal in a series of 20 AD cases.

ACT is a component of senile plaques and has been shown to have an increased expression in AD,[41] but was also found to have an increased expression in neurolog-

TABLE 2. Histopathologic Parameters of Patients with Alzheimer's Disease

Patient Number	Neurofibrillary Tangles/mm^2	Senile Plaques/mm^2	Neuron Loss
6	46.1	5.9	+
7	145.0	9.4	+ + +
8	144.5	12.5	+ +
9	126.1	3.9	+
10	69.2	5.9	+
11	35.2	15.6	+
12	124.7	12.5	+

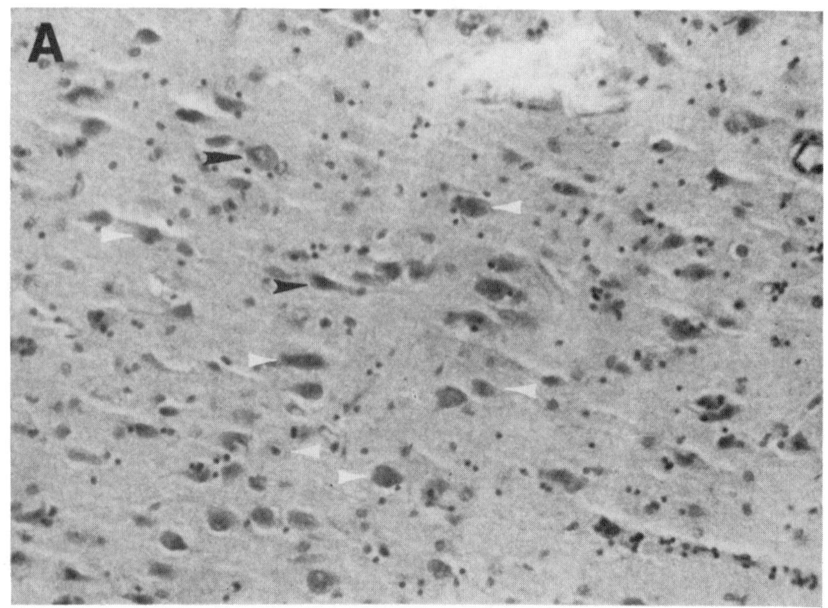

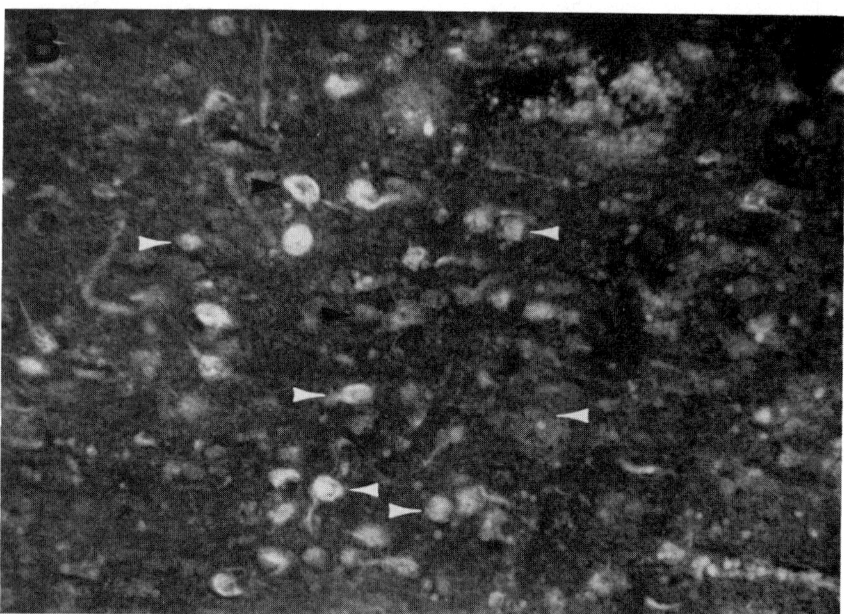

FIGURE 3. Immunohistochemical detection of ACT in hippocampus. **A:** ACT was localized in hippocampal sections from patient 11 by horseradish peroxidase signal followed by staining with hematoxylin. **B:** The relationship of neuronal ACT staining to the presence of neurofibrillary tangles was explored in the same section by first staining with thioflavin S and photographing the fluorescent image, followed by the immunohistochemical staining for ACT shown in **A**. White arrows identify identical landmarks in both panels while the black arrows identify neurons of interest, discussed in the text. *Magnification:* × 100.

ical conditions in which senile plaques are not found.[42] The increased expression of ACT in these other conditions was attributed to the fact that ACT is an acute phase reactant.[42] Our finding that ACT mRNA levels were not strongly correlated with plaque density suggests that increased ACT expression in certain cases of AD may result from additional factors in the disease, perhaps the equivalent of an acute phase response. This possibility is supported by the recent report that IL-1, a potent inducer of the systemic acute phase response, has an increased brain gene expression in AD.[43]

We found that a case with high levels of ACT mRNA expression demonstrated accumulation of ACT in neuronal cytoplasm, with lesser signals derived from senile plaques and astrocytes, previously reported as the major sites of ACT accumulation.[35] We expect that this discrepancy resulted from the heterogeneity of ACT expression in AD that we have reported here.

We explored the relationship of neuronal ACT staining to the presence of neurofibrillary tangles, a classic sign of neuronal involvement in AD. Our finding that there was discordance between ACT staining and neurofibrillary tangle staining suggests that the two parameters identify different stages or facets of the pathological process. ACT immunohistochemistry might therefore provide useful new information in the pathological study of AD. Further study of a larger series of cases may identify other clinical and histopathological characteristics associated with elevated ACT expression.

SUMMARY

We have examined the expression of several genes whose transcripts have increased levels in Alzheimer's disease and have found heterogeneity in these levels in different patients with this condition. The level of expression of these genes was compared to different clinical and pathological aspects of the disease. A case with markedly elevated α_1-antichymotrypsin mRNA levels demonstrated prominent neuronal accumulation of this protein. Many of the neurons which demonstrated α_1-antichymotrypsin staining did not have neurofibrillary tangles, and *vice versa*. This suggests that α_1-antichymotrypsin staining might identify a different facet of the pathology of Alzheimer's disease than does neurofibrillary tangle staining and may provide new information in the study of this condition.

ACKNOWLEDGMENTS

We would like to thank Drs. Cliff Barnes and Deepak Pandya for neuroanatomical consultation and suggestions, Dr. Devayani Lathi for providing tissue and Mr. Del Cain for assistance with reference materials; all are at the ENRM VA Hospital. We would like to thank Dr. Ray Gleason of the Massachusetts Institute of Technology for his help with the statistical analysis. Additional tissue was provided by the National Neurologic Research Specimen Bank located at VAMC W. Los Angeles, Los Angeles CA 90073, which is sponsored by NINDS/NIMH, National Multiple Sclerosis Society, Hereditary Disease Foundation, Comprehensive Epilepsy Program, Dystonia Medical Research Foundation, and Veterans Health Services and Research Administration, Department of Veterans Affairs.

REFERENCES

1. DUGUID, J. R., C. BOHMONT, N. LIU & W. W. TOURTELLOTTE. 1989. Proc. Natl. Acad. Sci. USA **86:** 7260–7264.
2. FILLEY, C. M., J. KELLY & R. K. HEATON. 1986. Arch. Neurol. **43:** 574–576.
3. CHUI, H. C., E. L. TENG, V. W. HENDERSON & A. C. MOY. 1985. Neurology **35:** 1544–1550.
4. FREED, D. M., S. CORKIN, J. H. GROWDON & M. J. NISSEN. 1989. Neuropsychologia **27:** 325–339.
5. NEARV, D., J. S. SNOWDEN, D. M. BOWEN, N. R. SIMS, *et al.* 1986. J. Neurol. Neurosurg. Psychiatry **49:** 163–174.
6. SELTZER, B. & I. SHERWIN. 1983. Arch. Neurol. **40:** 143–146.
7. SELTZER, B., M. J. K. BURRES & I. SHERWIN. 1984. Neurology **34:** 367–369.
8. SELTZER, B. & I. SHERWIN. 1986. Arch. Neurol. **43:** 665–668.
9. MAYEUX, R., Y. STERN & S. SPANTON. 1985. Neurology **35:** 453–461.
10. BIRD, T. D., S. M. SUMI, E. J. NEMENS, D. NOCHLIN *et al.* 1989. Ann. Neurol. **25:** 12–25.
11. BONDAREFF, W., C. Q. MOUNTJOY, M. ROTM, M. N. ROSSOR, *et al.* 1987. Arch. Gen. Psych. **44:** 412–417.
12. KATZMAN, R., R. TERRY, R. DETERESA, T. BROWN, *et al.* 1988. Ann. Neurol. **23:** 138–144.
13. MANN, D. M., P. O. YATES & B. MARCYNIUK. 1988. Arch. Gen. Psychiatry **45:** 962–963.
14. TERRY, R. D., A. PECK, R. DETERESA, R. SCHECHTER, *et al.* 1981. Ann. Neurol. **10:** 184–192.
15. VOGT, B. A., G. W. VAN HOESEN & L. J. VOGT. 1990. Acta Neuropathol. **80:** 581–589.
16. ZUBENKO, G. S., F. J. HUFF, J. BEYER, J. AUERBACH, *et al.* 1988. Arch. Gen. Psychiatry **45:** 889–893.
17. VOLICER, L., L. K. DIRENFELD, P. J. LANGLAIS, M. FREEDMAN, *et al.* 1985. J. Gerontol. **40:** 708–713.
18. FARRER, L. A., R. H. MYERS, L. A. CUPPLES, P. H. ST. GEORGE-HYSLOP, *et al.* 1990. Neurology **40:** 395–403.
19. PERICAK-VANCE, M. A., L. H. YAMAOKA, C. S. HAYNES, *et al.* 1988. Exp. Neurol. **102:** 271–279.
20. SCHELLENBERG, G. D., T. D. BIRD, E. M. WIJSMAN, *et al.* 1988. Science **241:** 1507–1510.
21. ST. GEORGE-HYSLOP, P. H., J. L. HAINES, L. A. FARRER, R. POLINSKY, *et al.* 1990. Nature **347:** 194–197.
22. GOATE, A., M. C. CHARTIER-HARLIN, M. MULLAN, J. BROWN, *et al.* 1991. Nature **349:** 704–706.
23. TOURTELLOTTE, W., H. H. ITABASHI, I. ROSARIO & K. BERMAN. 1984. Ann. N.Y. Acad. Sci. **436:** 513–516.
24. JAMADA, M. & P. MEHRAEIN. 1968. Arch. Psychi. **211:** 308–324.
25. ADAMS, J. H., Ed. 1984. Greenfield's Neuropathology, 4th edit. John Wiley and Sons. New York.
26. LUNA, L. G., Ed. 1968. Manual of Histologic Staining Methods of the Armed Forces Institute of Pathology, 3 edit. McGraw-Hill. New York.
27. HUGHES, C. P., L. BERG, W. L. DANZIGER, L. A. COBEN, *et al.* 1982. Br. J. Psychiatry **140:** 566–572.
28. DUGUID, J. R., R. G. ROHWER & B. SEED. 1988. Proc. Natl. Acad. Sci. USA **85:** 5738–5742.
29. MANIATIS, T., E. F. FRITSCH & J. SAMBROOK. 1982. Molecular Cloning: A Laboratory Manual. Cold Spring Harbor, NY. Cold Spring Harbor Laboratory.
30. THOMAS, P. S. 1980. Proc. Natl. Acad. Sci. USA **77:** 5201–5205.
31. HYMAN, B., G. W. VAN HOESEN & A. R. DAMASIO. 1990. Neurology **40:** 1721–1730.
32. TROJANOWSKI, J. Q., M. A. OBROCKA & V. M. LEE. 1983. J. Histochem. Cytochem. **31:** 1217–1223.

33. ZAR, J. E. 1984. Biostatistical Analysis. Englewood Cliffs, NJ. Prentice-Hall.
34. MAY, P. C., M. LAMPERT-ETCHELLS, S. JOHNSON, J. POIRIE, *et al.* 1990. Neuron **6:** 831–839.
35. PASTERNACK, J. M., C. R. ABRAHAM, B. J. VAN DYKE, H. POTTER, *et al.* 1989. Am. J. Pathol. **135:** 827–834.
36. CLARK, A. W., C. A. KREKOSKI, I. M. PARHAD, D. LISTON, *et al.* 1989. Ann. Neurol. **25:** 331–339.
37. KARIN, M. 1985. Cell **41:** 9–10.
38. COLLARD, M. W. & M. D. GRISWOLD. 1987. Biochemistry **26:** 3297–3303.
39. JENNE, P. E. & J. TSCHOPP. 1989. Proc. Natl. Acad. Sci. USA **86:** 7123–7127.
40. KRISZBAUM, L., J. A. SHARPE, B. MURPHY, A. J. F. D'APICE, *et al.* 1989. EMBO J. **8:** 711–718.
41. ABRAHAM, C. R., D. J. SELKOE & H. POTTER. 1988. Cell **52:** 487–501.
42. ABRAHAM, C. R. & H. POTTER. 1989. Biotechnology **7:** 147–153.
43. GRIFFIN, W. S. T., L. C. STANLEY, C. LING, L. WHITE, *et al.* 1989. Proc. Natl. Acad. Sci. USA **86:** 7611–7615.

Polyubiquitin Gene Expression following Cerebral Ischemia[a]

CORNELIO G. CADAY,[b] ROBERT M. SKLAR,[c]
DAVID J. BERLOVE,[b] AHMED KEMMOU,[b]
ROBERT H. BROWN, JR.,[c] AND SETH P. FINKLESTEIN[b]

[b]CNS Growth Factor Research Laboratory
[c]Day Neuromuscular Research Center
Department of Neurology
Massachusetts General Hospital and
Harvard Medical School
Boston, Massachusetts 02114

Cerebral ischemia is a major cause of disability and death in the United States with over 500,000 cases annually. Two general kinds of cerebral ischemia are identified—focal and global ischemia.[1-5] Focal ischemia, observed following thromboembolic stroke, causes damage to a discrete region of brain tissue (infarct). On the other hand, global ischemia, which occurs in conditions such as cardiac arrest, induces a phenomenon called "delayed neuronal death" among a defined population of vulnerable neurons in the brain.[5,6] Delayed neuronal death may also occur at the borders ("penumbra") of infarcts following focal ischemia.[1,3,4] This phenomenon raises the question: Is it possible to salvage neurons undergoing delayed neuronal death following ischemia?

A well-known animal model to study the phenomenon of delayed neuronal death is the gerbil model of transient global ischemia.[5-7] Temporary (5–10 minute) bilateral carotid artery occlusion in the gerbil induces global forebrain ischemia, causing selectively vulnerable neurons to undergo delayed neuronal death, especially neurons in the CA-1 sector of the hippocampus. Remarkably, these neurons appear histologically intact for about a day or two after ischemia. During this period, CA-1 neurons retain their ability to synthesize proteins and exhibit electrical excitability (although not to a normal degree). Subsequently, however, these vulnerable neurons go on to die within 2–4 days.[5-7] Protein synthesis inhibitors alleviate delayed death of CA-1 neurons following transient global ischemia, suggesting that this process requires protein synthesis.[8] Other cell death processes, including programmed cell death observed during development and apoptosis, also require protein synthesis.[9-14] It is possible, therefore, that delayed neuronal death following ischemia may share common mechanisms with programmed cell death observed in these other cell death processes.

A number of laboratories, including our own, have shown that brain ischemia modulates gene expression.[15-32] We have hypothesized that processes initiated by ischemia culminate in at least two general pathways. One pathway may be a "suicide pathway" leading to death of vulnerable neurons. Another pathway, a "survival pathway," may result in the synthesis of neuroprotective proteins,

[a] This work was supported by grants from the National Institutes of Health (NINDS NS-10828 and NIA AG-08207) and the American Heart Association.

sparing neurons from damage. Either enhancement of the "survival pathway" or antagonism of the "suicide pathway" may lead to increased neuronal survival.

Our laboratory has been engaged in identifying gene products that participate in programs of cell survival or cell death after ischemia. Several approaches used include: identification of known candidate proteins and analysis of their expression following ischemia, and application of differential screening methods to identify gene families coordinately modulated during ischemia.

One of the proteins we have studied following cerebral ischemia is ubiquitin. This choice was inspired by studies showing up-regulation of ubiquitin in programmed cell death during development.[16] Moreover, abnormal ubiquitin staining occurs in several neurodegenerative, chronic degenerative and viral diseases.[32] The precise role of ubiquitin in these diseases remains to be unraveled. A large body of studies, however, reveals that ubiquitin conjugation with proteins is a key step in diverse fundamental processes. These include protein degradation, cell cycle control, ribosome biogenesis, induced mutagenesis, DNA repair, and cell response to stress and injury.[32–36]

Ubiquitin is a highly conserved 76-residue protein found in all eukaryotic cells.[32–36] (Ubiquitin-like proteins have also been identified in viruses.[37,38]) The free ubiquitin monomer is a compact protein with a short protruding carboxy terminal tail. In contrast, the amino terminus (Met) of the free ubiquitin monomer is part of the compact ubiquitin structure that renders the amino terminal virtually inaccessible.[58]

The polymorphic ubiquitin genes are classified in two basic forms. Class I ubiquitin genes include monoubiquitin fusion genes that encode a single ubiquitin sequence fused to a "tail" peptide sequence.[39–45] These monoubiquitin fusion mRNAs are abundant during early stages of development and in actively dividing cells.[40,42,43] Class II ubiquitin genes include polyubiquitin genes that encode repeats of up to 100 of the monoubiquitin peptide.[32,40,47,48,55,56] Polyubiquitin mRNAs predominate in mature and later stages of development and in response to stress or trauma (*e.g.*, heat shock, starvation and injury).[40,49,52–54] Many organisms have several forms of monoubiquitin and polyubiquitin genes expressed at various stages of development.[32,40,42] In spite of ubiquitin gene polymorphism, however, the mature form of ubiquitin that conjugates with other proteins is always a monomeric 76-residue peptide.[32–36]

The physiological rationale for ubiquitin gene polymorphism is not fully understood. It is not clear, for example, why ubiquitin is fused with "tail" peptides in the Class I genes. One model proposed is that ubiquitin serves as a "chaperone" for the tail protein. Significantly, some of the monoubiquitin fusion genes are the sole sources of certain ribosomal proteins.[43–45] Deletion of the ubiquitin-coding sequence in these genes affects ribosome biogenesis.[44] Ubiquitin may facilitate incorporation of ribosomal proteins into nascent ribosomes, or may act to protect the tail ribosomal proteins from premature degradation.[44,45] Another model proposed is that the highly basic "tail" peptide of the fusion gene directs ubiquitin subcellular localization, or facilitates ubiquitin interaction with nucleic acids or other proteins.[39,41] The presence of a nuclear localization signal, as well as putative "Zn^{2+}-binding" domains in the tail peptides of the monoubiquitin fusion genes[40–42] are consistent with the latter model.

Under normal conditions, the polyubiquitin gene identified in yeast is not critical for cell viability. However, this gene is essential for cell survival during stress or trauma.[49] Up-regulation of polyubiquitin genes is an efficient mechanism to rapidly provide vast quantities of monomeric ubiquitin peptides under stress conditions. A "minigene" coding for the flanking sequences of the polyubiquitin gene and only a single ubiquitin coding sequence can substitute for the polyubiqui-tin gene.[49] Thus, aside from encoding multiple copies of ubiquitin monomers, the flanking regions of the polyubiquitin genes appear to code for regulatory informa-tion important for cell survival under stress conditions.[40,49,51–53,57] Interestingly, the 5'-flanking region of some polyubiquitin genes codes for a putative heat shock box element, suggesting that heat shock factors regulate the expression of polyubi-quitin following stress or trauma.[40,51,53,57] (There are polyubiquitin genes, however, which do not respond to heat shock factors or are not coordinately expressed with heat shock proteins.[55,56] These genes play more specific roles, *e.g.*, in sperma-togenesis.[56])

Ubiquitin confers its activity by conjugating with other proteins. Thus, other regulatory molecules involved in modulating ubiquitin-protein conjugations have pivotal roles in modulating the activity of ubiquitin (for recent reviews and mono-graphs see refs. 33–36). The ubiquitination process involves a sequence of ligation steps. First, an ATP-dependent ubiquitin-activating enzyme (E_1) catalyzes the formation of a thiolester between the carboxy terminus (Gly-76) of ubiquitin to a thiol site in the E_1 enzyme. This activated ubiquitin is then transferred to a thiol site of specific ubiquitin carrier proteins (E_2s). A final step involves the transfer of the activated ubiquitin from a specific carrier protein (E_2) to the ε-amino group (Lys) on the surface of the recipient protein. Certain ubiquitination processes require still another set of ubiquitin-protein ligases (E_3s) to complete the final step in the ubiquitination process.[33–36]

Protein ubiquitination plays an important role in rapid degradation of short-lived, denatured or damaged proteins. This degradation process requires an ATP-dependent protease (26S) complex.[59,60] This degradation process accounts for pivotal roles that ubiquitin plays in cell cycle control (*e.g.*, cyclin degradation), biochemical regulation of the activity of regulatory proteins, and elimination of damaged or denatured proteins.[33–36]

During degradation of ubiquitinated proteins, specific isopeptidases cleave the covalently bound ubiquitins through the carboxy terminus (Gly-76) amide bond. The compact structure of the ubiquitin prevents its destruction during the ATP-dependent degradation of ubiquitinated proteins, thus allowing liberated ubiquitins to be recycled.[33–36]

Induction of ubiquitin expression without concomitant induction or modulation of the aforementioned regulatory factors, in the ubiquitination and degradation processes, could alter the delicate balance between free and conjugated ubiqui-tins—thus also between free and ubiquitinated protein conjugates. It is possible, therefore, that abnormal ubiquitin staining in certain neurodegenerative tissues may be caused by a breakdown of the delicate equilibrium among the aforemen-tioned regulatory factors. Significantly, some of these regulatory factors have been implicated in neurodegenerative diseases.[32]

While protein ubiquitination plays an important role in protein degradation, many ubiquitinated proteins are fairly stable. These include specific histone pro-teins in the nucleus, ribosomal proteins, cytoskeletal proteins (*e.g.*, actin), mem-brane proteins, *etc.*[32,35] Current models propose that ubiquitination of proteins may be involved also in either chaperoning of proteins to specific subcellular compartments or modulation of protein activity or interaction.[32,35]

A summary of regulation and functions of the ubiquitin gene family is repre-sented schematically in FIGURE 1.

In recent studies, we have used the gerbil model to investigate the role of ubiquitin following transient global cerebal ischemia.[19] Using Northern blot tech-niques and a human cDNA probe for polyubiquitin[50] we observed three polyubiqui-

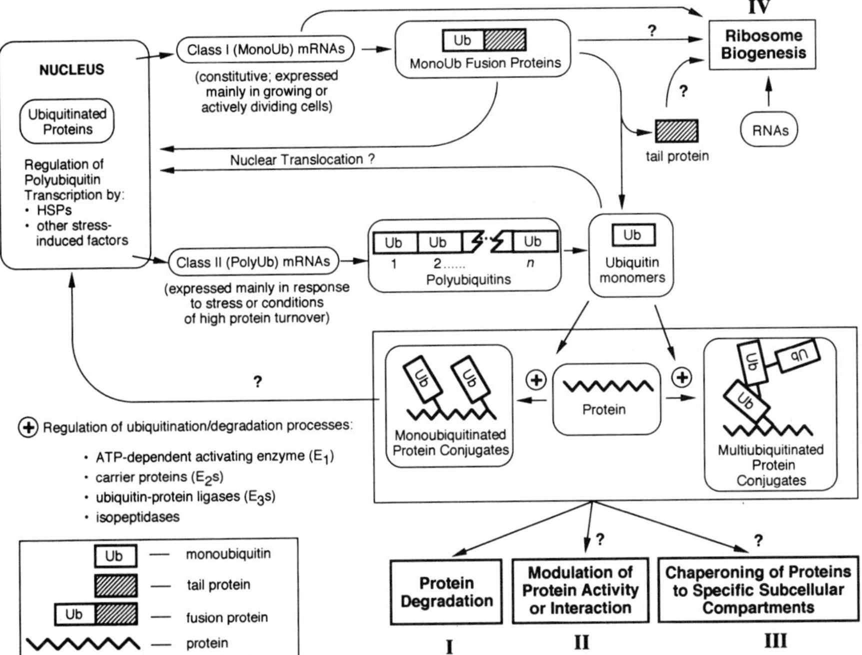

FIGURE 1. Regulation and functions of the ubiquitin gene family.

Monoubiquitin fusion proteins are formed through an amide bond between the carboxy terminus (Gly-76) of the ubiquitin monomer fused to the α-amino terminus of the tail peptide. Similarly, the primary translation products of polyubiquitin genes are fused through a carboxy terminus (Gly-76) to the α-amino terminus of the adjacent ubiquitin monomer.

The free ubiquitin monomer is a compact protein with a short protruding carboxy terminal tail. In contrast, the amino terminus (Met) of the free ubiquitin monomer is part of the compact ubiquitin structure that renders the amino terminal virtually inaccessible.

Ubiquitination of proteins involves an amide bond between the accessible carboxy terminus (Gly-76) of ubiquitin and a protruding ε-amino group (Lys) on the surface of the recipient protein. Formation of branched multiubiquitin chains in multiubiquitinated protein conjugates involves an amide linkage of the carboxy terminus (Gly-76) of ubiquitin covalently attached to the ε-amino group (Lys-48) of a ubiquitin previously linked to a ubiquitinated protein conjugate.

The ubiquitination process involves a sequence of ligation steps. First, an ATP-dependent ubiquitin-activating enzyme (E_1) catalyzes the formation of a thiolester between the carboxy terminus (Gly-76) of ubiquitin to a thiol site in the E_1 enzyme. This activated ubiquitin is then transferred to a thiol site of specific ubiquitin carrier proteins (E_2s). A final step involves the transfer of the activated ubiquitin from a specific carrier protein (E_2) to the ε-amino group (Lys) on the surface of the recipient protein. Certain ubiquitination processes require still another set of ubiquitin-protein ligases (E_3s) to complete the final step in the ubiquitination process.

Protein ubiquitination plays an important role in rapid degradation of short-lived, denatured or damaged proteins. This degradation process requires an ATP-dependent protease (26S) complex. This degradation process accounts for the pivotal role that ubiquitin plays in cell cycle control (*e.g.*, cyclin degradation), biochemical regulation of the activity of regulatory proteins, and elimination of damaged or denatured proteins.

During degradation of ubiquitinated proteins, specific isopeptidases cleave the covalently bound ubiquitins through the carboxy terminus (Gly-76) amide bond. The compact structure of the ubiquitin prevents its destruction during the ATP-dependent degradation of ubiquitinated proteins, thus allowing liberated ubiquitins to be recycled. [Legend continues overleaf.]

tin transcripts (at 3.6 kb, 2.2 kb, and 2.0 kb), and a single monoubiquitin transcript (at 0.6 kb) in the normal gerbil brain.[19] The 3.6 kb and 2.2 kb transcripts were major, while the 0.6 kb transcript was a minor component of the total ubiquitin transcripts in the intact hippocampus. We found that transient global ischemia up-regulated total polyubiquitin mRNA levels. Levels of the 3.6 kb and 2.2 kb mRNAs were especially increased at one day after ischemia. (Our data on the 2.0 kb mRNA were more variable and require confirmatory studies.) In contrast to levels of polyubiquitin mRNAs, levels of the monoubiquitin mRNA did not significantly increase following transient ischemia.[19]

Our study confirms and extends the findings of an earlier study that showed increase in total ubiquitin mRNA following transient global ischemia in the gerbil.[25] Our data further showed that this increase was due mainly to up-regulation of polyubiquitin mRNAs—especially the 3.6 kb and possibly the 2.2 kb transcripts.[19]

We then examined the detailed temporal expression of ubiquitin mRNAs following transient global ischemia.[19] Up-regulation of the 3.6 kb polyubiquitin transcript was evident by 4 hours and persisted for up to a day after ischemia; thereafter the levels began to decline. The temporal expression of the 2.2 kb transcript was similar to, although more variable than, that of the 3.6 kb transcript.

Our results showed that polyubiquitin gene expression was maximal in hippocampus *before* the onset of delayed neuronal death. However, it is not clear from our studies whether these genes play a role in cell *survival* or cell *death* after ischemia. Immunostaining studies in other laboratories have shown that ubiquitin immunoreactivity in gerbil hippocampus decreases initially following transient global ischemia, and then returns preferentially in neuronal populations (*e.g.*, CA-3) destined to survive.[20] This pattern is similar to the pattern of expression of heat shock proteins after ischemia,[24] and is consistent with other data showing regulation of ubiquitin expression by heat shock factors (see above). More complex patterns of ubiquitin and heat shock proteins immunoreactivity or expression were observed in other studies—especially at sublethal duration of forebrain ischemia.[21,27,28]

In contrast to the preceding observations, studies in the developing tobacco hawkmoth (*Manduca sexta*) show that polyubiquitin gene expression is increased in intersegmental muscles (and spinal neurons supplying these muscles) before programmed cell death.[16] Studies of cultured mammalian hippocampal neurons also show increased ubiquitin immunoreactivity preceding cell death.[61,62]

It thus remains unclear whether polyubiquitin mRNAs are expressed in neurons destined to survive or die after global ischemia. *In situ* hybridization studies are planned to address this question. Further studies are also planned to address the

---

Induction of ubiquitin expression without concomitant induction or modulation of the aforementioned regulatory factors, in the ubiquitination and degradation processes, could alter the delicate balance between free and conjugated ubiquitins—and thus also between free and ubiquitinated protein conjugates. It is possible, therefore, that abnormal ubiquitin staining in certain neurodegenerative tissues may be caused by a breakdown of the delicate equilibrium among the aforementioned regulatory factors.

While protein ubiquitination plays an important role in protein degradation, many ubiquitinated proteins are fairly stable. These include specific histone proteins in the nucleus, ribosomal proteins, cytoskeletal proteins (*e.g.*, actin), membrane proteins, *etc.* Current models propose that ubiquitination of proteins may be involved also in either chaperoning of proteins to specific subcellular compartments or modulation of protein activity or interaction.

role of specific ubiquitin-protein conjugates in molecular cascades contributing to cell survival versus cell death after ischemia.

ACKNOWLEDGMENTS

We thank Dr. Jens Vuust for providing the ubiquitin plasmid DNA; Dr. Jan Johannessen for reviewing the manuscript and preparing the figure illustration; Dr. Dan Rosen for technical assistance; and Dr. Mark Mattson for kindly sharing preprints of their work.

REFERENCES

(References adequately cited in reviews or monographs are not included in the citation, unless specifically discussed.)

1. ZIVIN, J. A. & D. W. CHOI. 1991. Sci. Am. **265:** 56–63.
2. COLLINS, R. C., Moderator. 1989. Ann. Intern. Med. **110:** 92–100.
3. CAPLAN, L. R. & R. W. STEIN. 1986. Stroke—A Clinical Approach. Butterworth Publishers. Stoneham, MA.
4. BARNETT, H. J. M., B. M. STEIN, J. P. MOHR & F. M. YATSU, Eds. 1986. Stroke—Pathophysiology, Diagnosis and Management. Churchill Livingston, Inc. New York.
5. SCHMIDT-KASTNER, R. & T. F. FREUND. 1991. Neuroscience **40:** 599–636.
6. KIRINO, T. 1982. Brain Res. **239:** 57–69.
7. SUZUKI, R., T. YAMAGUCHI, C.-L. LI & I. KLATZO. 1983. Acta Neuropathol. **60:** 217–222.
8. SHIGENO, T., Y. YAMASAKI, G. KATO, K. KUSAKA, T. MINA, K. TAKAKURA, D. I. GRAHAM & S. FURUKAWA. 1990. Neurosci. Lett. **120:** 117–119.
9. TOMEI, L. D. & F. O. COPE, Eds. 1991. Apoptosis: The Molecular Basis of Cell Death. Cold Spring Harbor Laboratory Press. Plainview, NY.
10. WARING, P., F. J. KOS & A. MULLBACHER. 1991. Med. Res. Rev. **11:** 219–236.
11. WILLIAMS, G. T. 1991. Cell **65:** 1097–1098.
12. OPPENHEIM, R. W. 1991. Annu. Rev. Neurosci. **14:** 453–501.
13. ELLIS, R. E., J. YUAN & H. R. HORVITZ. 1991. Annu. Rev. Cell Biol. **7:** 663–698.
14. DRISCOLL, M. & M. CHALFIE. 1992. Trends Neurosci. **15:** 15–19.
15. SCHWARTZ, L. M., L. KOSZ & B. K. KAY. 1990. Proc. Natl. Acad. Sci. USA **87:** 6594–6598.
16. SCHWARTZ, L. M., A. MYER, L. KOSZ, M. ENGLESTEIN & C. MAIER. 1990. Neuron **5:** 411–419.
17. FINKLESTEIN, S. P., C. G. CADAY, M. KANO, D. J. BERLOVE, C. Y. HSU, M. MOSKOWITZ & M. KLAGSBRUN. 1990. Stroke **21:** III-122–III-124.
18. CADAY, C. G., M. KANO, N. KOKETSU, D. J. BERLOVE, C. Y. HSU, M. A. MOSKOWITZ & S. P. FINKLESTEIN. Fibroblast growth factor levels after focal cerebral infarction in rats. Submitted, 1993.
19. CADAY, C. G., R. SKLAR, D. J. BERLOVE, A. KEMMOU, R. BROWN & S. P. FINKLESTEIN. Temporal expression of ubiquitin genes following transient global ischemia in the gerbil. Submitted, 1993.
20. MAGNUSSON, K. & T. WIELOCH. 1989. Neurosci. Lett. **96:** 264–270.
21. HAYASHI, T., K. TAKADA & M. MATSUDA. 1991. Mol. Chem. Neuropathol. **15:** 75–82.
22. KIESSLING, M., G. A. DIENIEL, M. JACEWICZ & W. A. PULSINELLI. 1986. J. Cereb. Blood Flow Metab. **6:** 642–649.
23. BROWN, I. R. 1990. J. Neurosci. **27:** 247–255.
24. VASS, K., W. J. WELCH & T. S. NOWAK, JR. 1988. Acta Neuropathol. **77:** 128–135.
25. NOWAK, JR., T. S., U. BOND & M. J. SCHLESINGER. 1990. J. Neurochem. **54:** 451–458.
26. ABE, K., R. E. TANZI & K. KOGURE. 1991. Neurosci. Lett. **125:** 166–168.

27. GONZALEZ, M. F., D. LOWENSTEIN, S. FERNYAK, K. HISANAGA, R. SIMON & F. R. SHARP. 1991. Brain Res. Bull. **26:** 241–250.
28. SIMON, R., H. CHO, R. GWYNN & D. LOWENSTEIN. 1991. J. Neurosci. **11:** 881–889.
29. UEMURA, Y., N. W. KOWALL & M. F. BEAL. 1991. Brain Res. **542:** 343–347.
30. UEMURA, Y., N. W. KOWALL & M. A. MOSKOWIZ. 1991. Brain Res. **552:** 99–105.
31. JORGENSEN, M. B., J. DECKERT, D. C. WRIGHT & D. R. GEHLERT. 1989. Brain Res. **484:** 393–398.
32. MAYER, R. J., J. ARNOLD, L. LASZLO, M. LANDON & J. LOWE. 1991. Biochim. Biophys. Acta **1089:** 141–157.
33. SCHLESINGER, M. & A. HERSHKO, Eds. 1988. The Ubiquitin System. Cold Spring Harbor Laboratory. Spring Harbor Press. Plainview, NY.
34. CIECHANOVER, A. & A. L. SCHWARTZ. 1989. Trends Biochem. Sci. **14:** 483–488.
35. JENTSCH, S., W. SEUFERT, T. SOMMER & H. A. REINS. 1990. Trends Biochem. Sci. 1990. **15:** 195–198.
36. HERSHKO, A. 1991. Trends Biochem. Sci. **16:** 265–268.
37. GUARINO, L. A. 1990. Proc. Natl. Acad. Sci. USA, **87:** 409–413.
38. MEYERS, G., N. TAUTZ, E. J. DUBOVI & H. J. THIEL. 1991. Virology **180:** 602–616.
39. LUND, P. K., P. B. M. MOATS-STAATS, J. G. SIMMONS, E. HOYT, A. J. D'ERCOLE, F. MARTIN & J. J. VAN WYK. 1985. J. Biol. Chem. **260:** 7609–7613.
40. OZKAYNAK, E., D. FINLEY, M. J. SOLOMON & A. VARSHAVSKY. 1987. EMBO J. **6:** 1429–1439.
41. REDMAN, K. L. & M. RECHSTEINER. 1988. J. Biol. Chem. **263:** 4926–4931.
42. MULLER-TAUBENBERGER, A., M. WESTPHAL, E. JAEGER, A. NOEGEL & G. GERISCH. 1988. FEBS Lett. **229:** 273–278.
43. MULLER-TAUBENBERGER, A., H. R. GRAACK, L. GROHMANN, M. SCHLEICHER & G. GERISCH. 1989. J. Biol. Chem. **264:** 5319–5322.
44. FINLEY, D., B. BARTEL & A. VARSHAVSKY. 1989. Nature **338:** 394–401.
45. REDMAN, K. L. & M. RECHSTEINER. 1989. Nature **338:** 438–440.
46. OHMACHI, T., R. GIORDA, D. R. SHAW & H. L. ENNIS. 1989. Biochem. **28:** 5226–5231.
47. OZKAYNAK, E., D. FINLEY & A. VARSHAVSKY. 1984. Nature **312:** 663–666.
48. DWORKIN-RASTI, E., A. SHRUTKOWSKI, & M. B. DWORKIN. 1984. Cell **39:** 321–325.
49. FINLEY, D., OZKAYNAK, E. & A. VARSHAVSKY. 1987. Cell **48:** 1035–1046.
50. WIBORG, O., M. S. PEDERSEN, A. WIND, L. E. BERGLUND, K. A. MARCKER & J. VUUST. 1985. EMBO J. **4:** 755–759.
51. NEVES, A. M., I. BARAHONA, L. GALEGO & C. RODRIGUES-POUSADA. 1988. Gene **73:** 87–96.
52. LEE, H. S., J. A. SIMON & J. T. LIS. 1988. Mol. Cell Biol. **8:** 4727–4735.
53. BOND, U., & M. J. SCHLEISINGER. 1986. Mol. Cell Biol. **6:** 4602–4620.
54. FORNACE, JR., A. J., I. ALAMO, JR., M. C. HOLLANDER & E. LAMOREAUX. 1989. Nucleic Acids Res. **17:** 1215–1230.
55. GRAHAM, A. W., D. JONES & E. P. CANDIDO. 1989. Mol. Cell Biol. **9:** 268–277.
56. MEZQUITA, J. & C. MEZQUITA. 1991. FEBS Lett. **279:** 69–72.
57. SWINDLE, J., J. AJIOKA, H. EISEN, B. SANWAL, C. JACQUEMOT, Z. BROWDER & G. BUCK. 1988. EMBO J. **7:** 1121–1127.
58. VIJAY-KUMAR, S., C. E. BUGG & W. J. COOK. 1987. J. Mol. Biol. **194:** 531–544.
59. HOUGH, R., G. PRATT, & M. RECHSTEINER. 1987. J. Biol. Chem. **262:** 8303–8313.
60. GANOTH, D., E. LESHINSKY, E. EYTAN, & A. HERSHKO. 1988. **263:** 12412–12419.
61. MATTSON, M. P. 1990. Neuron **4:** 105–117.
62. CHENG, B. & M. P. MATTSON. 1992. Exp. Neurol. **117:** 114–123.

Quantitative Features of Reactive Gliosis following Toxicant-induced Damage of the CNS[a]

JAMES P. O'CALLAGHAN[b]

Neurotoxicology Division (MD-74B)
Health Effects Research Laboratory
United States Environmental Protection Agency
Research Triangle Park, North Carolina 27711

INTRODUCTION

A characteristic feature of chemical-induced damage of the nervous system is selectivity; exposure to different nervous system toxicants results in damage to different brain regions and cell types.[1-3] The differential susceptibility of nervous system cell types to injury often is referred to as "selective vulnerability."[4,5] An implicit assumption underlying this concept is that intrinsic properties of individual neural cell types render them susceptible to damage by specific chemical exposures.[5] Unfortunately, our knowledge of the mechanisms that confer such vulnerability to specific toxic insults is limited. Thus, often there is no *a priori* basis for predicting the cell types affected by toxic exposures of the CNS. Given the extreme cellular and molecular heterogeneity of the nervous system,[6,7] the fact that targets of chemical-induced neurotoxicity are diverse and unpredictable should not be surprising. This biologically based situation does, however, make assessment of neurotoxicity difficult because one must face the problem of deciding where to look for damage. Overcoming this obstacle requires a "marker" of neural injury that can be used to localize (*i.e.*, "mark") loci of damage anywhere in the nervous system. The focus of the present paper is the proposal that the astrocyte-localized protein, glial fibrillary acidic protein (GFAP), can be used as one such marker of neural injury and degeneration. Recently, an excellent review has appeared that covers the quantitative aspects of gliosis resulting from all types of CNS injuries.[8] Thus, coverage here is limited to the quantitative features of gliosis resulting from toxicant exposures of the CNS. Portions of this article have appeared in expanded reviews of the same topic.[9-11]

WHY FOCUS ON GFAP?

One of the most widely documented cellular reactions to nervous system damage is proliferation and hypertrophy of astrocytes.[8,9,12-15] This response, often termed "reactive" gliosis or astrogliosis,[12,15] can be induced by a diversity of insults, including those resulting from physical damage, disease or chemicals.[8,15]

[a] This work was supported in part by NIDA IAG RA-ND-89-4.
[b] Address correspondence to James P. O'Callaghan, Ph.D.; Tel.: (919) 541-7779 or 541-4042; FAX: (919) 541-5175.

Reactive gliosis is an indirect response (*i.e.*, a reaction) to damage of a variety of neural cell types; it is not a response that occurs only as a consequence of neuronal damage. Indeed, damage to the myelin sheath of oligodendroglia is a well-known stimulus of astrogliosis.[16] Moreover, even damage to astrocytes themselves elicits reactive gliosis in surviving astrocytes.[17] Hence, reactive gliosis appears to be a generic response, that is, one triggered by damage to all types of neurons and glia.

The hallmark of reactive gliosis is accumulation of the intermediate filaments of astrocytes.[8,15] Glial fibrillary acidic protein (GFAP) is the major intermediate filament protein of astrocytes.[18] By definition, therefore, reactive gliosis is accompanied by an increase in GFAP.[15] Indeed, studies using antibodies to GFAP have firmly established the existence of reactive gliosis as a dominant response to CNS injury.[12,15] Thus, based on the accumulated morphological data, enhanced expression of GFAP appears to be a "marker" of all types of brain injuries.

THE NEED FOR QUANTITATIVE ASSESSMENT OF GLIOSIS

The existing data that describe the utilization of GFAP as a marker of neural injury have been obtained predominantly from studies of trauma (*e.g.*, stab wounds) or disease-induced astrogliosis;[14] little attention has been devoted to an examination of gliosis following chemical exposures. Moreover, as indicated above, most evaluations of reactive gliosis have placed an emphasis on qualitative (immunocytochemical) rather than quantitative analysis of GFAP. Reliance on immunocytochemical detection of GFAP has hampered our understanding of the features of reactive gliosis and the factors governing the expression of GFAP during neural injury. It is not difficult to see why this is the case, given the limitations of an immunocytochemistry-based approach. For example, while immunocytochemistry can reveal the pattern of enhanced immunostaining for GFAP, this technique does not easily lend itself to quantification, making analysis of large numbers of samples time-consuming and expensive. Undoubtedly, this has contributed to the prevalence of single time-point and, in the few studies involving toxicant exposures, single-dose investigations. Another significant drawback to immunocytochemical evaluations of GFAP is that fixatives and methods of fixation can dramatically influence the detectability of this protein in astrocytes of both grey and white matter.[19] In addition, specificity and source of antisera[19] and the effect of disease states on antibody-binding affinity[8] may contribute to the variations in GFAP immunoreactivity observed from one laboratory to another. The influence of drug pretreatments also may represent a significant variable that contributes to immunocytochemical artifacts.[20]

To overcome some of the inherent limitations of immunocytochemistry, we proposed that immunocytochemical evaluations of GFAP and other cell-type marker proteins be combined with immunoassays of the same proteins.[21] Implementation of this approach would permit a number of critical questions to be answered concerning the utility of GFAP as a marker of neurotoxicity. For example, is gliosis an all or none response as proposed by some,[22] or is it graded with respect to the degree of damage? Does the astrocyte response (as assessed by GFAP content) remain localized to the site of damage, or does it diffuse throughout the brain (*e.g.*, see ref. 23)? Is reactive gliosis due to chemical insult permanent, like the glial scar caused by trauma and disease,[13] or is it transient in nature? Can the efficacy of neuroprotective agents be assessed, indirectly, by quantification of reactive gliosis? The remainder of this article is devoted to a review of our efforts to resolve some of these issues by quantifying the amount of GFAP in tissue samples obtained from toxicant-exposed animals.

IMMUNOASSAYS OF GFAP

To examine the quantitative aspects of toxicant-induced gliosis requires an assay for GFAP. Given the emphasis on GFAP immunocytochemistry as the apparent endpoint of choice for demonstrating and evaluating astrogliosis, one would imagine that quantitative measures of GFAP have not been available. This is not the case. For nearly as long as antisera to GFAP have been available, assays have been described that demonstrate the feasibility of measuring the content of GFAP in a variety of tissues under both normal and pathological conditions.[24–26] With the advent of solid-phase immunoassays and microplate technology, a number of GFAP assays have been described that are suitable for processing large numbers of samples at low cost. We have developed two such assays, both of which are designed for analyzing the concentration of GFAP in detergent-based homogenates of brain tissue. The specifics of each procedure have been described.[28,29] The first relies on the propensity of GFAP to bind to nitrocellulose sheets. The amount of bound GFAP in a given sample is quantified by incubating with poly- or monoclonal antibodies followed by incubation with ^{125}I Protein A.[28,29] The second method relies on the ELISA technique in a sandwich format;[29] similar assays have been described by others.[26,30,31] The main advantage to the use of detergent-based assays is that homogenates of nervous tissue can be assayed directly without further fractionation or purification. Thus, the data obtained are indicative of effects that occurred in the intact tissue, not an extract of an operationally defined membrane or cytosol fraction. Because of the inherent sensitivity of immunoassays, only small amounts of tissue are needed. This permits analysis of discrete regions and cell layers, often at a level of sampling comparable to neuroanatomical evaluations.[28] Moreover, because sample amount is generally not limiting, aliquots of a given homogenate can be assayed for as many proteins as there are antibodies available. Another major advantage of solid-phase immunoassays is that the antigen does not need to be purified. Data can simply be presented as a percent of control. Finally, the need to develop antibodies to GFAP is obviated by the availability of monoclonal and polyclonal antibodies from commercial sources at relatively modest cost. When used in combination with microtiter plate readers, ELISA format assays are the method of choice because they are inexpensive, fast, do not require radioactive reagents and can be automated through the use of programmed liquid handling devices.

VALIDATION OF GFAP AS A MARKER OF NEURAL INJURY: FACTORS TO CONSIDER

Effects of Known CNS Toxicants

With assays in hand, the next step toward determining if increases in GFAP represent a common response to diverse neurotoxic insults was to assay its content in brain homogenates obtained from animals exposed to known CNS toxicants. Some of the toxic chemicals and injurious conditions used in this validation scheme

are shown in TABLE 1. These agents and conditions were chosen with two considerations in mind. First, we wanted to know if an increase in GFAP was a common
feature underlying damage to all brain regions and cell types. To that end, the
agents and conditions listed in TABLE 1 were chosen because they were known
to damage diverse regional, cellular and subcellular targets in the CNS. Second,
we wanted to know if subtle as well as severe toxicant-induced damage of the CNS
resulted in substantial increases in GFAP. Essentially, we were asking whether it
took outright cell death to increase the expression of GFAP or would damage not
apparent by routine histology, such as nerve terminal, myelin or axonal injury,
also increase tissue levels of GFAP? To address this issue, we chose toxicants
and toxicant dosages that ranged from those that caused obvious cell loss, to
those that caused damage to subcellular elements that would not be detected by
routine histopathology.

TABLE 1. Prototype Neurotoxicants or Injurious Conditions Used to Induce
Reactive Gliosis

Toxicants:	Toxicants continued:
MPTP	Amino-adipate
Trimethyltin	IDPN
Triethyltin	Methamphetamine
Tributyltin	MDA
Cadmium	MDMA
Methylmercury	
Bilirubin	Injuries:
Domoic acid	Stab wounds
Kainate	Nerve cut
6-OH Dopamine	Brain heating
5,7-Dihydroxytryptamine	Genetic mutations
Colchicine	Advanced age
3-Acetyl pyridine	Nocardia infection

Abbreviations: MPTP: 1-Methyl-4-Phenyl-1,2,3,6 tetrahydropyridine; IDPN: Iminodipropio-
nitrile; MDA: Methylenedioxyamphetamine; MDMA: Methylenedioxymethamphetamine;
Nocardia: Nocardia asteroides.

Having chosen the toxic or injurious conditions based on the above considerations, we began our attempt to validate GFAP as a marker of CNS toxicity by
examining prototype toxicants that would be classified in the most severe category:
those that cause neuronal loss revealed by light microscopy of Nissl-stained sections (for reviews see refs. 1 and 32). We also began by examining two brain
regions with layered cell structures, hippocampus and cerebellum, where neuronal
cell loss would be more obvious (*e.g.*, see refs. 28 and 33–36). In most of our
initial studies we divided brains from control and treated rats along the sagittal
plane. One side was then used for GFAP assays while the other side was used
for Nissl-based histology (*e.g.*, see refs. 28 and 35). In this way, qualitative
estimates of cell loss could be compared with quantitative estimates of astrogliosis.
In addition, assays of neuron-localized proteins were often included with assays
of GFAP to obtain quantitative estimates of neuronal damage (*e.g.* see refs. 28,
35, and 36). In some experiments, GFAP immunocytochemistry also was employed
to examine astrocyte morphology and number in brain regions with increased
levels of GFAP.[28,37]

Overt neuron loss manifested at the light microscopic level is not a subtle effect. That increases in GFAP reflect such effects, even quantitatively, would not be a major advance for neurotoxicology. The less obvious and, therefore, probably more common lesions are the ones for which sensitive markers are needed. Therefore, in our validation scheme, we assayed GFAP in homogenates of brain regions that did not exhibit lesions detectable by routine histology. We did this by examining brain regions known to have toxicant-induced damage to specific cell types that is not manifested by Nissl-based neuropathological changes.[38-40] Toxicants in this category, for example, would include those affecting only a small number of cells in a given region (*e.g.*, 3-acetyl pyridine), or those affecting subcellular elements not revealed by Nissl staining (*e.g.*, 5,7-DHT, MPTP, IDPN).

Effects of Pharmacological Agents

I indicated above that GFAP would not be a useful marker of neurotoxicity unless it revealed effects that were not obvious in routine neuropathological examinations. This addresses the need for a marker of neurodegeneration that is sensitive. A marker of neurodegeneration should also be specific, that is, it should only reveal the effects of agents that damage the nervous system. Thus, increases in GFAP should not be associated with exposure to chemicals not considered neurotoxic; for example, pharmacological agents at therapeutic dosages. Ideally, increases in GFAP also should not be observed in brain regions not affected by known neurotoxicants. A lack of specificity associated with either of these circumstances, especially the former, would limit the usefulness of GFAP as a marker of neurotoxicity. We have addressed both these issues with negative controls, as follows: First, in the course of evaluating prototype neurotoxicants, we included an assessment of GFAP levels in brain regions that were not thought to contain cellular elements damaged by the compound in question.[28,40,41] Second, although we have not conducted extensive studies of the effects of non-neurotoxic chemicals on levels of GFAP, we have examined the effects of a number of pharmacological agents at therapeutic dosages. Because these drugs were included as negative controls, they would not be expected to affect GFAP.

Effects of Physiological Variables

As would be the case for pharmacological effects, an influence of physiological factors on the concentration of GFAP also might confound the results of studies employing this protein as a marker of neural injury. Two physiological variables known to enhance the synthesis of GFAP are development[32] and aging.[42] In general, once adult levels are reached in mice and rats, GFAP concentration remains stable until it again increases with advanced age.[42] Thus, studies conducted in adult rats or mice would, in general, not be affected by age considerations. Moreover, the use of age-matched subjects would prevent age being a factor in any treatment effects on GFAP.

Recently, the concentration of GFAP has been shown to be under hormonal control by the adrenal gland. Adrenalectomy increases GFAP and its mRNA and this effect is reversed by glucocorticoid replacement therapy.[43-45] Corticosterone administered in high (non-physiological) daily dosages will down-regulate the expression of GFAP but environmental stressors (cold, noise, physical agitation) appear to be without effect.[44] Moreover, glucocorticoids do not affect injury- or toxicant-induced expression of GFAP.[44] These data indicate that, short of adrenalectomy, factors affecting endogenous glucocorticoid levels will not alter the concentration of GFAP. Castration has been reported to enhance the expression of GFAP[46] and reports of altered GFAP immunoreactivity due to estradiol treatment also have appeared.[47] What role testosterone or estradiol play in the regulation of injury-induced expression of GFAP, if any, has yet to be demonstrated.

FEATURES OF TOXICANT-INDUCED GLIOSIS

When we followed the strategy outlined above to validate the use of GFAP as a marker of neural injury and degeneration, a number of features associated with toxicant-induced gliosis emerged, as follows:

1. *Neurotoxic exposures cause large dose- and region-dependent increases in GFAP.* The initial agents used to induce gliosis were those known to kill cells as evidenced by Nissl staining. If these compounds did not induce large increases in GFAP, there would be no reason to proceed with the use of GFAP as prototype marker of neuronal damage. This strategy was implemented with the potent neuro-toxic organometal, trimethlytin (TMT). A single systemic administration of TMT results in a striking loss of pyramidal neurons in the hippocampal formation of the rat. We found this effect to be accompanied by a large dose-dependent increase in the concentration of GFAP.[28] In homogenates of whole hippocampus the effect of TMT on GFAP reached levels as great as 600% of control. Moreover, when the most affected region of hippocampus was microdissected and analyzed, GFAP levels reached values as great as 6000% of control. Not only were dosages of TMT that caused obvious cell death (8-9 mg/kg) capable of causing large increases in GFAP, but dosages below this threshold (5-6 mg/kg) did as well. Thus, at dosages of TMT below those necessary to cause evidence for neuronal loss based on Nissl stains, assays of GFAP were sensitive enough to reveal underlying damage.

Given that TMT was thought to selectively damage the hippocampus,[48] TMT-induced gliosis was expected to largely be limited to this region of the CNS. Instead, large increments in GFAP were seen in widespread areas of the brain.[28,41] These results were of some concern because they suggested that sites of enhanced expression of GFAP might not be limited to those that ''mark'' sites of underlying damage. To critically address this question, regions of TMT-induced neuronal damage were mapped using a cupric silver degeneration stain.[41] This technique is sensitive enough to reveal sites of damage that may have escaped detection with standard histological stains.[2] Areas showing silver impregnation (argyrophilia) were compared to GFAP levels obtained for the same region. A remarkably tight correspondence was found between the spatial distribution of argyrophilia and the regional pattern of increased expression of GFAP.[41] These data suggested that increments in GFAP indeed were linked to sites of damage.

The positive findings obtained with compounds that were overtly cytotoxic to the CNS provided the basis for examining compounds that damage subcellular elements of neural cells without causing cell death. Here, because the cell body would often remain intact, it was possible that the astrocyte response might not be as robust as it was following complete cellular destruction. 1-Methyl-4-phenyl-1,2,3,6-tetrahydropyridine (MPTP) appeared to be an ideal denervation tool to examine this issue. A single systemic administration of MPTP results in damage to dopaminergic nerve terminals in mouse striatum as evidenced by dopamine depletion,[49] loss of tyrosine hydroxylase (a marker of striatal dopaminergic neurons)[39] and a positive reaction with the de Olmos silver degeneration stain.[37] These effects are not associated with evidence of cytopathology based on Nissl staining (*e.g.*, see ref. 9). We found that dopaminergic terminal degeneration caused by MPTP, like the outright cytotoxicity induced by TMT, results in a large (350% of control) increase in GFAP.[39,40] Consistent with the known specificity of MPTP for nigrostriatal dopaminergic neurons, increases in GFAP were confined to the target regions, nigra and striatum.[9] These data again indicated that assays of GFAP were sensitive enough to reveal neurotoxicity in the absence of detectable cytopathology and specific enough to be limited to the regions containing the damaged cell type.

2. *Toxicant-induced increases in GFAP are not necessarily permanent.* The astrocyte response to traumatic injury or disease often is manifested by a persistent glial scar that is GFAP positive.[13] Based on this evidence we expected chemically

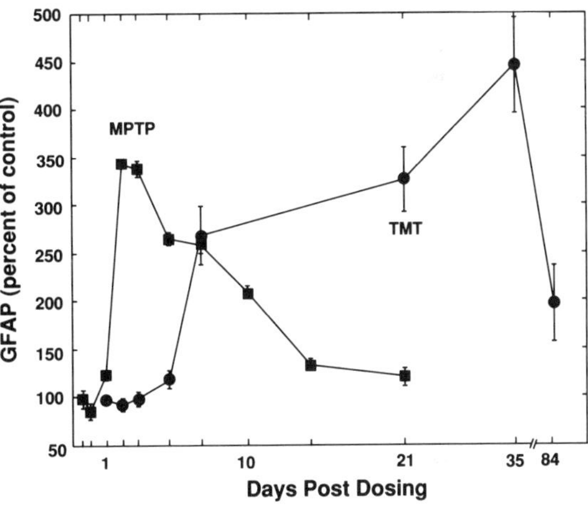

FIGURE 1. Time course of the effects of TMT (8.0 mg/kg, i.v.) and MPTP (12.5 mg/kg, s.c) on the concentration of GFAP in rat (Long-Evans) hippocampus (TMT) or mouse (C57B16/J) striatum (MPTP). (Adapted from Brock and O'Callaghan[28] and O'Callaghan *et al.*[39]

induced gliosis to result in similar scarring and, therefore, a long-lasting or permanent increase in GFAP. Based on our experience with several of the compounds listed in TABLE 1, we found just the opposite to be the case. The increase in GFAP was often transient in nature with the time-course of the both the onset and decline in this protein varying markedly from toxicant to toxicant. The data obtained with TMT and MPTP serve to illustrate this point (FIG. 1). The large increases in GFAP caused by both TMT and MPTP have different rates of onset and decline. The increase in GFAP due to TMT did not return to baseline until 12 weeks post-treatment whereas the increase due to MPTP returned to near control levels within two weeks of dosing. The most likely explanation for these disparate time-effect curves is that the continued presence of the toxic insult is required to maintain the astrocyte (GFAP) reaction. Thus, in the case of MPTP, its neurotoxic metabolite, MPP^+ is produced in a matter of minutes and subsequently eliminated from striatum over the course of a few hours.[50] TMT, on the other hand, has at least a half-life of 10 days in the brain[51] and the cell loss it causes occurs over several months.[52] It seems possible, therefore, that sustained cellular damage may be required to maintain the stimulus responsible for the continued increase in GFAP. Such a hypothesis would be consistent with the protracted cellular damage and glial scarring that occurs in chronic disease states, such as multiple sclerosis and Alzheimer's disease. Regardless of the mechanisms responsible for induction and maintenance of the GFAP response to brain injury, our findings with TMT, MPTP and other prototype neurotoxicants indicate that assessments of neurotoxicity using assays of GFAP should employ multiple time points in order to prevent false-negative results.

3. *Hypertrophy, not hyperplasia, appears to be the dominant response of astrocytes to neurotoxic injuries.* The initial studies by Cavanagh[53] indicated that astrocytes divide in response to penetrating wounds of the brain. Using ³H-thymidine autoradiography combined with GFAP immunocytochemistry, Latov and coworkers[27] confirmed that stab injuries caused astrocytes surrounding the wound site to divide. Using the same methodology we found that only a very small percentage of astrocytes (<1%) in hippocampus divided in response to TMT-induced neurotoxicity.[28] Likewise, the enhanced expression of GFAP in response to MPTP-induced damage to neostriatum does not appear to involve significant astrocyte division (J. P. O'Callaghan, K. F. Jensen and D. B. Miller, unpublished observation). Thus, at least for the neurotoxicants we have examined, the increase in GFAP reflects hypertrophy of astrocytes rather than hyperplasia. One possible reason for the disparity between the results using stab injuries and those using toxicants relates to disruption of the blood brain barrier. Stab injuries allow blood to enter the wound site. Blood contains known astrocyte mitogens,[54] which could result in their proliferation around the wound area. In toxicant injuries such as those caused by MPTP, the blood-brain barrier is not compromised,[39] blood-borne astrocyte mitogens do not enter the wound site,[39] and astrocyte proliferation does not appear to occur. Thus, if our data for TMT and MPTP can be applied to the general case, we expect that astrocytic hyperplasia will not be a major factor in the observed increases in GFAP. Given this possibility, it is doubtful that GFAP immunocytochemistry-based cell counts will be of much value in assessment of general neurotoxic responses because more GFAP per astrocyte, not more astrocytes, will be the predominant neurotoxic response.

4. *Increases in GFAP result from neurotoxic exposures during pre- and postnatal development.* Astrocytes of the developing CNS generally are thought to be less responsive to injury compared to their adult counterparts.[55] We have not found this to be the case based on the results of studies where toxicants were used to damage the rat CNS during either prenatal or postnatal development. Using a variety of developmental neurotoxicants, we found that exposure to these agents early in postnatal development results in large dose- time- and region-dependent increases in GFAP (reviewed in ref. 32). For example, exposure to TMT on postnatal day 5, which causes damage to the hippocampus qualitatively similar to that seen in the adult,[33] causes dose-dependent increases in GFAP that reach levels as great as 500% of control,[32] values comparable to those observed in the TMT-damaged adult hippocampus.[28] Also consistent with adult exposure to TMT, GFAP levels abate to near control levels with time.[32] Prenatal damage of the rat CNS also results in enhanced expression of GFAP. For example, damage to cortical neurons on gestational day 15 induced by the alkylating agent, methylazoxymethanol, results in an increase in GFAP as early as postnatal day 4.[56] Traumatic injury of the fetal rat brain also results in a positive GFAP response prior to parturition.[57] In aggregate, these findings allow for the tentative conclusion that GFAP may serve as a biochemical marker of developmental as well as adult

neurotoxicity. If the response of developing astrocytes to injury is similar to that observed in the adult, as is suggested by similar quantitative increments in GFAP, it is possible that cultured brain cells (typically prepared from rodents during the late gestational or early neonatal periods) may be useful for modeling astrogliosis *in vitro*. For example, the organotypic slice culture of the hippocampus retains the cytoarchitecture of the adult structure including differentiated GFAP-positive astrocytes arranged in a scaffold formation.[58] Such preparations may prove indispensable for determining the physiological and pharmacological factors regulating astrocyte responses *in situ*.

5. *Pharmacological agents do not increase GFAP*. The assumption underlying the use of GFAP as a marker of neural damage is that its enhanced expression is linked to neural damage. A corollary to this line of reasoning is that chemical exposures that do not damage the CNS should not induce the expression of GFAP. Given that astrocytes, *in vitro*, possess a multitude of receptors that might be responsive to physiological (see above) or pharmacological manipulation, *in vivo* (reviewed in ref. 59), it seemed prudent to consider the possibility that drugs administered at therapeutic dosages might increase GFAP without damaging the nervous system. To address this issue we used a variety of pharmacological agents

TABLE 2. Miscellaneous Agents Which Do Not Increase GFAP

Reserpine	Apomorphine
Tetrabenazine	Diethyldithiocarbamate
Phenobarbital	Muscimol
Pentobarbital	Scopolamine
Diethylether	Atropine
Ketamine	Corticosterone
Pargyline	2-Deoxyglucose
Nomifensine	Prazosin
Amfonelic acid	Indomethacin
Clorgyline	Difluoromethylornithine

as negative controls in our validation studies. None of these compounds, some of which are listed in TABLE 2, caused an increase GFAP. The number of drugs we have examined is not exhaustive. Moreover, comprehensive dose- and time-effect studies have not been attempted. Nevertheless, it is clear from these data that compounds from several pharmacological classes do not increase GFAP. These findings are consistent with the view that increases in GFAP occur as a consequence of cellular damage caused by chemical exposures, but do not result from drug exposures in the therapeutic range.

6. *The signal for toxicant-induced astrogliosis may emanate directly from the damaged cell*. Although toxicant-induced damage to neural cell types results in astrogliosis, it cannot be assumed that the damaged cell type is the only source of factors mediating the conversion of astrocytes into their reactive form. For example, for most of the agents listed in TABLE 1, we cannot rule out the possibility that these compounds may have affected astrocytes directly to induce the expression of GFAP. Moreover, it is also possible that toxicant-induced damage to neural cell types may result in astrogliosis through very indirect routes. For example, factors derived from serum or microglia are known to induce the growth of astrocytes, *in vitro* (discussed in ref. 39), findings which suggest that astrogliosis may

be mediated through a multi-step pathway involving cell types from within and outside the CNS, in addition to those damaged by the agent or injurious condition in question.

To begin to characterize the pathways and cell types involved in mediating toxicant-induced astrogliosis, we have focused on an examination of the origins of the astrocyte response to MPTP. A schematic of the MPTP model of astrogliosis is shown in FIGURE 2. According to this model, once MPTP is taken up by the brain, it is bioactivated into the active toxicant, MPP^+, predominantly through the catalytic action of monoamine oxidase B (MAO B).[60] Somewhat ironically, this reaction probably takes place in astrocytes because they are enriched in MAO B (see ref. 60). Because MPP^+ is a substrate for the dopamine transporter, it

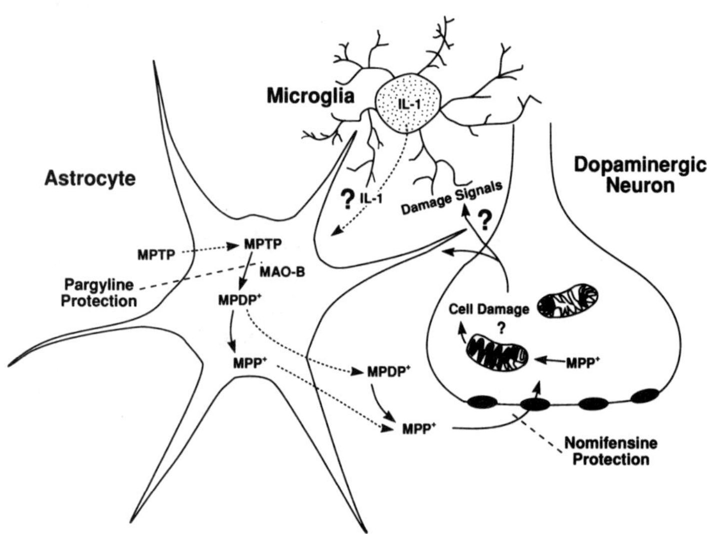

FIGURE 2. A schematic of the MPTP model for induction of reactive gliosis. See text for details. (Adapted from Sonsalla and Golbe.[65])

gains access to dopaminergic terminals where it inhibits Complex I respiration, with subsequent terminal damage presumably resulting from depletion of ATP.[61] The ensuing astroglial response, as reflected by an increase in GFAP (FIG. 1), theoretically results from release of ''damage'' factors from the MPP^+-damaged dopaminergic terminals. These factors, in turn, may activate resident astrocytes directly. Alternatively, they may recruit macrophages from the periphery or activate resident microglia. Together or separately, these additional cell types may trigger astrogliosis and the concomitant induction of GFAP. Because antagonists of MAO and the dopamine transporter were known to prevent MPTP-induced neurotoxicity through cell-type-specific neuroprotective mechanisms, we could use these agents to pharmacologically dissect the cellular origins of the MPTP-

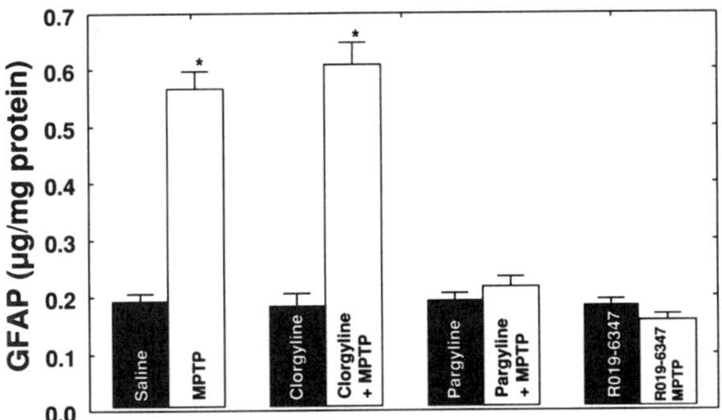

FIGURE 3. Inhibitors of MAO-B protect against MPTP-induced increase in GFAP. *Significantly different from corresponding control, $p < 0.05$. (Adapted from O'Callaghan *et al.*[39])

induced astrogliosis. Administration of the MAO B inhibitors, pargyline or RO19-6347, but not the MAO A inhibitor, clorgyline, completely blocked the MPTP-induced increase in GFAP (FIG. 3). Thus, preventing the formation of the active dopaminergic neurotoxicant, MPP+, prevented MPTP-induced gliosis. Likewise, protection of the dopaminergic terminal from MPP$^+$, by administration of the dopamine transporter inhibitors, nomifensine and amfonelic acid, also completely antagonized the MPTP-induced increase in GFAP (FIG. 4). Together these findings not only implicate the dopamine nerve terminal as the source of signals for initiating the observed gliosis, but they also indicate that induction of GFAP does not result from a direct effect of MPTP or MPP$^+$ on astrocytes. Circumstantial evidence obtained using the MPTP model of gliosis also indicated that astrocytes may be activated directly by factors emanating from the damaged dopaminergic nerve terminals without involvement of other cell types or mediators. The reasoning behind this contention is as follows: 1) the onset of the MPTP-induced increase

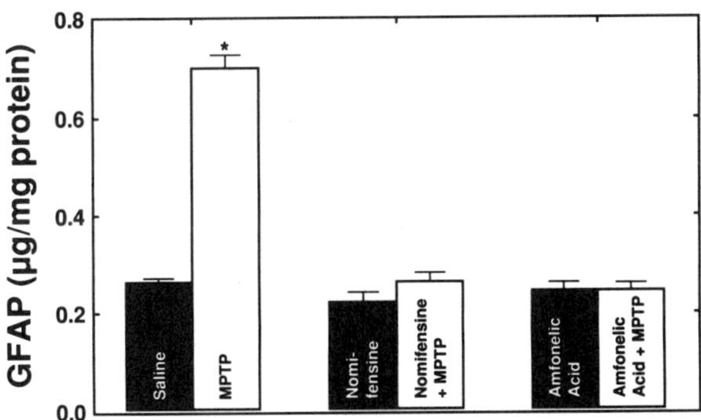

FIGURE 4. Inhibitors of the dopamine transporter protect against MPTP-induced increase in GFAP. *Significantly different from corresponding control, $p < 0.05$. (Adapted from O'Callaghan *et al.*[39])

in GFAP[39,40] and its mRNA (J. P. O'Callaghan and M. J. Mass, unpublished) occurred within 12-24 hours, a time frame that may be too short to involve a recruitment and activation of additional cell types; 2) as mentioned above, MPTP does not compromise the blood brain barrier, therefore, blood-borne mediators of injury or inflammation probably are not involved; and 3) elevated levels of brain IL-1, an astrocyte mitogen produced by microglia,[62] were not seen after MPTP,[39] findings suggesting that microglia were not required for the induction of gliosis. These observations are suggestive of the possibility that damaged cell types activate astrocytes directly through chemical messengers yet to be identified.

What then are the potential "damage factors" mediating astrogliosis? Damage to cell membranes is known to release free fatty acids through the aracidonate cascade.[63] Recent evidence suggests that cerebral eicosanoids formed through the lipoxygenase arm of aracidonate metabolism may play a role in mediating toxicant-

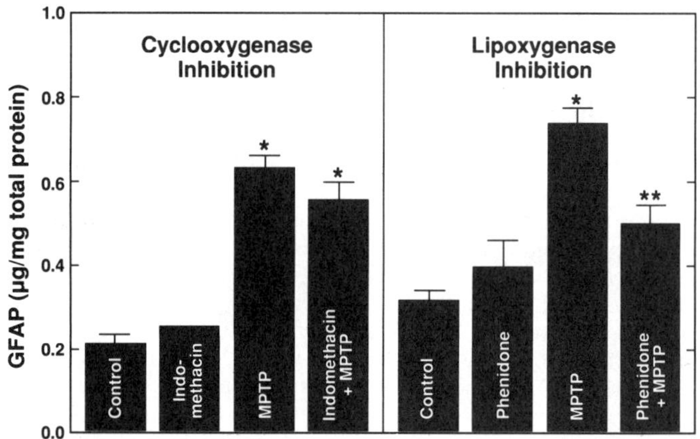

FIGURE 5. Lipoxygenase Inhibition attenuates the MPTP-induced increase in GFAP. See O'Callaghan *et al.*[66] for dosing regimens. *Significantly different from corresponding control, $p < 0.05$. **Significantly different from Control and MPTP groups, $p < 0.05$.

induced neuropathies.[64] To examine the role of aracidonate metabolites in the mediation of MPTP-induced astrogliosis, we co-administered MPTP with indomethacin or phenidone, inhibitors of the cyclooxygenase and lipoxygenase arms of arachidonate metabolism, respectively (FIG. 5). Co-administration of phenidone, but not indomethacin, with MPTP attenuated the MPTP-induced increase in GFAP (FIG. 5). These results raise the possibility that metabolites of the lipoxygenase arm of aracidonate metabolism may play a role in mediating MPTP-induced astrogliosis.

CONCLUSIONS

Our findings indicate that GFAP is a sensitive marker of toxicant-induced damage to the CNS. Assays of GFAP reveal dose- time- and region-dependent patterns of neural degeneration at toxicant dosages below those that cause light microscopic evidence of cell loss or damage. Areas exhibiting increased levels of GFAP are linked to sites of damage in the adult and developing CNS. Although an increase in GFAP appears to be a universal response to toxicant-induced damage of the CNS, it is by no means uniform. Its time of onset and its duration varies markedly from one toxicant to another. Moreover, baseline levels of GFAP vary from one brain region to another and across species. All of these differences may be a reflection of the diversity of astrocyte types,[8] which, in turn, provide the neurobiological basis for the diversity of astrocytic responses to injury. Whether common or diverse signaling mechanisms underlie conversion of astrocytes into their reactive state is an issue that needs to be resolved if we are to understand this dynamic cellular reaction to injury.

ACKNOWLEDGMENTS

The author thanks Drs. Stanley Barone, Jr. and D. B. Miller for valuable suggestions.

REFERENCES

1. O'CALLAGHAN, J. P. 1988. Neurotypic and gliotypic proteins as biochemical markers of neurotoxicity. Neurotoxicol. Teratol. **10:** 445–452.
2. SWITZER, R. C. 1991. Strategies for assessing neurotoxicity. Neurosci. Biobehav. Rev. **15:** 89–93.
3. BALABAN, C. D. 1992. The use of selective silver degeneration stains in neurotoxicology: Lessons from studies of selective neurotoxicants. *In* The Vulnerable Brain and Environmental Risks, Vol. 1, Malnutrition and Hazard Assessment. R. L. Issacson & K. F. Jensen. Eds.: 223–238, Plenum. New York.
4. SPENCER, P. S. & H. H. SCHAUMBURG. 1980. Experimental and Clinical Neurotoxicology, Williams and Wilkins. Baltimore, MD.
5. BAUMGARTEN, H. G. & B. ZIMMERMANN. 1992. Cellular and subcellular targets of neurotoxins: The concept of selective vulnerability. *In* Handbook of Experimental Pharmacology, Vol. 102 Selective Neurotoxicity. H. Herken & F. Hucho, Eds.: 1–28. Springer-Verlag. Heidelberg.
6. McKAY, R. D. G. & S. J. HOCKFIELD. 1982. Monoclonal antibodies distinguish antigenically discrete neuronal types in the vertebrate central nervous system. Proc. Natl. Acad. Sci. USA **79:** 6747–6751.
7. SUTCLIFFE, J. G. 1988. mRNA in the mammalian central nervous system. Ann. Rev. Neurosci. **11:** 157–198.
8. NORTON, W. T., D. A. AQUINO, I. HOZUMI, F.-C. CHIU & C. F. BROSNAN. 1992. Quantitative aspects of reactive gliosis: A review. Neurochem. Res. **17:** 877–885.
9. O'CALLAGHAN, J. P. 1991. Assessment of neurotoxicity: Use of glial fibrillary acidic protein as a biomarker. Biomed. Environ. Sci. **4:** 197–206.
10. O'CALLAGHAN, J. P. 1991. The use of glial fibrillary acidic protein in first-tier assessments of neurotoxicity. J. Am. Coll. Toxicol. **10:** 719–726.
11. O'CALLAGHAN, J. P. & D. B. MILLER. 1993. Quantification of reactive gliosis as an approach to neurotoxicity assessment. *In* Assessing Neurotoxicity of Drugs of Abuse, National Institute on Drug Abuse Monograph. L. Erinoff, Ed. U.S. Government Printing Office. Washington, D.C. In press.
12. LINDSAY, R. M. 1986. Reactive gliosis. *In* Astrocytes: Cell Biology and Pathology of Astrocytes, Vol. 3. S. Fedoroff & A. Vernadakis, Eds.: 231–262. Academic Press. Orlando, FL.
13. REIER, P. J. 1986. Gliosis following CNS injury: The anatomy of astrocytic scars and their influences on axonal elongation. *In* Astrocytes: Cell Biology and Pathology of

Astrocytes. S. Fedoroff & A. Vernadakis, Eds.: 263–324. Academic Press. Orlando, FL.

14. ENG, L. F. 1987. Experimental models for astrocyte activation and fibrous gliosis. *In* Glial-Neuronal Communication in Development and Regeneration. H. H. Althaus & W. Seifert, Eds.: 27–40. Springer-Verlag. Heidelberg.

15. ENG, L. F. 1988. Regulation of glial intermediate filaments in astrogliosis. *In* Biochemical Pathology of Astrocytes. M. D. Norenberg, L. Hertz & A. Schousboe, Eds.: 79–90. A. R. Liss. New York.

16. SMITH, M. E., F. P. SOMERA & L. F. ENG. 1983. Immunocytochemical staining for glial fibrillary acidic protein and the metabolism of cytoskeletal proteins in experimental allergic encephalomyelitis. Brain Res. **264:** 241–253.

17. TAKADA, M., Z. K. LI & T. HATTORI. 1990. Astroglial ablation prevents MPTP-induced nigrostriatal neuronal death. Brain Res. **509:** 55–61.

18. ENG, L. F. 1985. Glial fibrillary acidic protein (GFAP): The major protein of glial intermediate filaments in differentiated astrocytes. J. Neuroimmunol. **8:** 203–214.

19. SHEHAB, S. A. S., J. R. CRONLY-DILLON, S. N. NONA & C. A. STAFFORD. 1990. Preferential histochemical staining of protoplasmic and fibrous astrocytes in rat CNS with GFAP antibodies using different fixatives. Brain Res. **518:** 347–352.

20. HAYKAL-COATES, N., J. P. O'CALLAGHAN, J. F. REINHARD, JR. & K. F. JENSEN. 1991. Pargyline and gamma-butyrolactone enhance tyrosine hydroxylase immunostaining of nigrostriatal axons. Brain Res. **556:** 353–357.

21. O'CALLAGHAN, J. P. & D. B. MILLER. 1983. Nervous-system specific proteins as biochemical indicators of neurotoxicity. Trends Pharmacol. Sci. **4:** 388–390.

22. SCHIFFER, D., M. T. GIORDANA, A. MIGHELLI, G. GIACCONE, S. PEZZOTTA & A. MAURO. 1986. Glial fibrillary acidic protein and vimentin in the experimental glial reaction of the rat brain. Brain Res. **374:** 110–118.

23. MATHEWSON, A. J. & M. BERRY. 1985. Observations on the astrocyte response to a cerebral stab wound in adult rats. Brain Res. **327:** 61–69.

24. ENG, L. F., Y. L. LEE & L. E. M. MILES. 1976. Measurement of glial fibrillary acidic protein by a two-site immunoradiometric assay. Anal. Biochem. **71:** 243–259.

25. KRETZSCHMAR, H. A., S. J. DEARMOND & L. S. FORNO. 1985. Measurement of GFAP in hepatic encephalopathy by ELISA and transblots. J. Neuropathol. Exp. Neurol. **44:** 459–471.

26. ALBRECHTSEN, M. & E. BOCK. 1985. Quantification of glial fibrillary acidic protein (GFAP) in human body fluids by means of ELISA employing a monoclonal antibody. J. Neuroimmunol. **8:** 301–309.

27. LATOV, N., G. NILAVER, E. A. ZIMMERMAN, W. G. JOHNSON, A. SILVERMAN, R. DEFENDINDI & L. COTE. 1979. Fibrillary astrocytes proliferate in response to brain injury. Dev. Biol. **72:** 381–384.

28. BROCK, T. O. & J. P. O'CALLAGHAN. 1987. Quantitative Changes in the synaptic vesicle proteins synapsin I and p38 and the astrocyte-specific protein glial fibrillary acidic protein are associated with chemical-induced injury to the rat central nervous system. J. Neurosci. **7:** 931–942.

29. O'CALLAGHAN, J. P. 1991. Quantification of glial fibrillary acidic protein: Comparison of slot-immunobinding assays with a novel sandwich ELISA. Neurotoxicol. Teratol. **13:** 275–281.

30. STEWART, M. G., R. C. BOURNE & P. L. A. GABBOTT. 1986. Decreased levels of an astrocytic marker, glial fibrillary acidic protein, in the visual cortex of dark-reared rats: measurement by enzyme-linked immunosorbent assay. Neurosci. Lett. **63:** 147–152.

31. ENG, L. F., E. STOCKLIN, Y.-L. LEE, R. A. SHIURBA, R. CORIA, M. HALKS-MILLER, C. MOZSGAI, G. FUKAYAMA & M. GIBBS. 1986. Astrocyte culture on nitrocellulose membranes and plastic: detection of cytoskeletal proteins and mRNAs by immunocytochemistry and *in situ* hybridization. J. Neurosci. Res. **16:** 239–250.

32. O'CALLAGHAN, J. P. & D. B. MILLER. 1989. Assessment of chemically-induced alterations in brain development using assays of neuron- and glia-localized proteins. Neurotoxicology **10:** 393–406.

33. MILLER, D. B. & J. P. O'CALLAGHAN. 1984. Biochemical, functional and morphological

indicators of neurotoxicity: Effects of acute administration of trimethyltin to the developing rat. J. Pharmacol. Exp. Ther. **231:** 744–751.

34. O'CALLAGHAN, J. P. & D. B. MILLER. 1984. Neuron-specific phosphoproteins as biochemical indicators of neurotoxicity: Effects of acute administration of trimethyltin to the adult rat. J. Pharmacol. Exp. Ther. **231:** 736–743.

35. O'CALLAGHAN, J. P. & D. B. MILLER. 1985. Cerebeller hypoplasia in the Gunn rat is associated with quantitative changes in neurotypic and gliotypic proteins. J. Pharmacol. Exp. Ther. **234:** 522–533.

36. O'CALLAGHAN, J. P. & D. B. MILLER. 1988. Acute exposure of the neonatal rat to triethyltin results in persistent changes in neurotypic and gliotypic proteins. J. Pharmacol. Exp. Ther. **244:** 368–378.

37. O'CALLAGHAN, J. P. & K. F. JENSEN. 1991. Enhanced expression of glial fibrillary acidic protein and the cupric silver degeneration reaction can be used as sensitive and early indicators of neurotoxicity. Neurotoxicology **13:** 113–122.

38. REINHARD, J. F., JR., D. B. MILLER & J. P. O'CALLAGHAN. 1988. The neurotoxicant, MPTP (1-methyl-4-phenyl-1,2,3,6-tetrahydropyridine), increases glial fibrillary acidic protein and decreases dopamine levels of the mouse striatum: evidence for glial response to injury. Neurosci. Lett. **95:** 246–251.

39. O'CALLAGHAN, J. P., D. B. MILLER & J. F. REINHARD, JR. 1990. Characterization of the origins of astrocyte response to injury using the dopaminergic neurotoxicant, 1-methyl-4-phenyl-1,2,3,6-tetrahydropyridine. Brain Res. **521:** 73–80.

40. O'CALLAGHAN, J. P., D. B. MILLER & J. F. REINHARD, JR. 1990. 1-Methyl-4-phenyl-1,2,3,6-tetrahydropyridine (MPTP)-induced damage of striatal dopaminergic fibers attenuates subsequent astrocyte response to MPTP. Neurosci. Lett. **117:** 228–233.

41. BALABAN, C. D., J. P. O'CALLAGHAN & M. L. BILLINGSLEY. 1988. Trimethyltin-induced neuronal damage in the rat: Comparative studies using silver degeneration stains, immunocytochemistry and immunoassay for neuronotypic and gliotypic proteins. Neuroscience **26:** 337–361.

42. O'CALLAGHAN, J. P. & D. B. MILLER. 1991. The concentration of glial fibrillary acidic protein increases with age in the mouse and rat brain. Neurobiol. Aging **12:** 171–174.

43. O'CALLAGHAN, J. P., R. E. BRINTON & B. S. MCEWEN. 1989. Glucocorticoids regulate the concentration of glial fibrillary acidic protein throughout the brain. Brain Res. **494:** 159–161.

44. O'CALLAGHAN, J. P., R. E. BRINTON & B. S. MCEWEN. 1991. Glucocorticoids regulate the synthesis of glial fibrillary acidic protein in intact and adrenalectomized rats but do not affect its expression following brain injury. J. Neurochem. **57:** 860–869.

45. NICHOLS, N. R., H. H. OSTERBURG, J. N. MASTERS, S. L. MILLAR & C. E. FINCH. 1990. Messenger RNA for glial fibrillary acidic protein is decreased in rat brain following acute and chronic corticosterone treatment. Mol. Brain Res. **7:** 1–7.

46. DAY, J. R., N. J. LAPING, T. H. MCNEILL, S. S. SCHREIBER, G. PASINETTI & C. E. FINCH. 1990. Castration enhances expression of glial fibrillary acidic protein and sulfated glycoprotein-2 in the intact and lesioned-altered hippocampus of the adult male rat. Mol. Endocrinol. **4:** 1995–2002.

47. GARCIA-SEGURA, L. M., I. TORRES-ALEMAN & F. NAFTOLIN. 1989. Astrocytic shape and glial fibrillary acidic protein immunoreactivity are modified by estradiol in primary rat hypothalamic cultures. Dev. Brain Res. **47:** 298–302.

48. WALSH, T. J., D. B. MILLER & R. S. DYER. 1982. Trimethyltin, a selective limbic system neurotoxidant, impairs radial-arm maze performance. Neurobehav. Toxicol. Teratol. **4:** 177–183.

49. HEIKKILA, R. E., A. HESS & R. C. DUVOSIN. 1984. Dopaminergic neurotoxicity of 1-methyl-4-phenyl-1,2,3,6-tetrahydropyridine in mice. Science **224:** 1451–1453.

50. IRWIN, I., L. E. DELANNEY, D. DIMONTE & J. W. LANGSTON. 1989. The biodisposition of MPP+ in mouse brain. Neurosci. Lett. **101:** 83–88.

51. COOK, L. L., K. E. STINE & L. W. REITER. 1984. Tin distribution in adult rat tissues after exposure to trimethyltin and triethyltin. Toxicol. Appl. Pharmacol. **76:** 344–348.

52. CHANG, L. W. & R. S. DYER. 1983. A time course study of trimethyltin-induced neuropathology in rats. Neurobehav. Toxicol. Teratol. **5:** 443–459.

53. CAVANAGH, J. B. 1970. The proliferation of astrocytes around a needle wound in the rat brain. J. Anat. **106:** 471–487.

54. GIULIAN, D., J. WOODWARD, D. G. YOUNG, J. F. KREBS & L. B. LACHMAN. 1988. Interleukin-1 injected into mammalian brain stimulates astrogliosis and neovascularization. J. Neurosci. **8:** 2485–2490.

55. BARRETT, C. P., E. J. DONATI & L. GUTH. 1984. Differences between adult and neonatal rats in their astroglial response to spinal injury. Exp. Neurol. **84:** 374–385.

56. GOLDEY, E. S., M. E. STANTON, J. P. O'CALLAGHAN & K. M. CROFTON. 1992. Screening for developmental neurotoxicants: possible alternatives to existing guidelines. Toxicologist **12:** 348 (Abstract).

57. MOORE, I. E., J. M. BUONTEMPO & R. O. WELLER. 1987. Response of fetal and neonatal rat brain to injury. Neuropathol. Appl. Neurobiol. **13:** 219–228.

58. DEL RIO, J. A., B. HEIMRICH, E. SORIANO, H. SCHWEGLER & M. FROTSCHER. 1991. Proliferation and differentiation of glial fibrillary acidic protein-immunoreactive glial cells in organotypic slice cultures of rat hippocampus. Neuroscience **43:** 335–347.

59. KIMELBERG, H. K. 1988. Glial Cell Receptors. Raven Press. New York.

60. DIMONTE, D. A., E. Y. WU & J. W. LANGSTON. 1992. Role of astrocytes in MPTP metabolism and toxicity. Ann. N.Y. Acad. Sci. **648:** 219–228.

61. CHAN, P., L. E. DELANNEY, I. IRWIN, J. W. LANGSTON & D. DIMONTE. 1992. MPTP-induced ATP loss in mouse brain. Ann. N.Y. Acad. Sci. **648:** 306–308.

62. GIULIAN, D. & T. J. BAKER. 1985. Peptides released by ameboid microglia regulate astroglial proliferation. J. Cell Biol. **101:** 2411–2415.

63. ELLIS, E. F., K. F. WRIGHT, E. P. WEI & H. A. KONTOS. 1981. Cyclooxygenase products of arachidonic acid metabolism in cat cerebral cortex after experimental concussive brain injury. J. Neurochem. **37:** 892–896.

64. SIMMET, T. & B. TIPPLER. 1990. Cysteinyl-leukotriene production during limbic seizures triggered by kainic acid. Brain Res. **515:** 79–86.

65. SONSALLA, P. K. & L. I. GOLBE. 1988. Deprenyl as prophylaxis against Parkinson's disease? Clin. Neuropharmacol. **11:** 500–511.

66. O'CALLAGHAN, J. P., D. B. MILLER & K. F. JENSEN. 1991. Enhanced expression of glial fibrillary acidic protein (GFAP) induced by the neurotoxicant, 1-methyl-4-phenyl-1,2,3,6-tetrahydropyridine (MPTP), is attenuated by the lipoxygenase inhibitor, phenidone. J. Neurochem. **57**(Suppl.): S74.

Quinolinic Acid and Inflammation

MELVYN P. HEYES[a]

Section of Analytical Biochemistry
Laboratory of Clinical Science
Building 10, Room 3D40
Bethesda, Maryland 20892

INTRODUCTION

Quinolinic acid (QUIN) is an excitotoxic kynurenine pathway metabolite.[1,2] While the CNS concentrations of QUIN are low in normal subjects and patients with chronic non-inflammatory neurologic diseases,[3] substantial increases in the levels of QUIN occur in the CSF and CNS tissue of humans and non-human primates with inflammatory neurologic diseases.[3-11] The mechanisms responsible for the accumulation of QUIN are unclear, but induction of indoleamine-2,3-dioxygenase (IDO) and other kynurenine pathway enzymes has been implicated.[3,4,6,10,12-14] A stimulus for increased synthesis of QUIN may be cytokines, such as interferon-γ and tumor necrosis factor-α.[15,16] Therefore, increased synthesis of QUIN may be viewed both as a potential etiologic agent in the pathogenesis of neurologic deficits and brain injury in inflammatory neurologic diseases. QUIN and IDO measurements may also serve as a surrogate 'marker' of CNS inflammation.

HIV-1 Infection and AIDS

CSF QUIN levels were elevated 3.5-fold in the very early stages of HIV-1 infection[3,7,10] and correlated with the severity of motor deficits in a task sensitive to basal ganglia lesions.[7] In later stage patients with the AIDS dementia complex, opportunistic CNS conditions, or aseptic meningitis, the increases in CSF QUIN averaged over 20-fold.[10] Importantly, CSF QUIN levels correlated with quantitative measures of neuropsychologic deficits. Treatment with azidothymidine or anti-microbial therapy of opportunistic conditions appreciably reduced CSF QUIN levels and neurologic status improved. CSF QUIN levels correlated with both β_2-microglobulin and neopterin in CSF and serum,[3,4,17] which suggests that QUIN synthesis is activated in association with inflammation. There were no relationships between CSF QUIN with the ratio of serum: CSF albumin concentrations, which indicates that the increases in CSF QUIN was not dependent on a breakdown of the blood-brain barrier.[3,4] Further, although serum QUIN exceeded CSF levels by 20-fold in control subjects, we found that 14.4% of the later stage HIV-1-infected patients had higher CSF QUIN levels than serum, an observation which supports intracerebral QUIN synthesis.[10]

[a] Tel. (301)-496-3628; FAX: (301)-402-3049.

Other Inflammatory Neurologic Diseases

We have found markedly increased concentrations of QUIN in both lumbar CSF and *post mortem* brain tissue of patients with inflammatory diseases (bacterial, viral, fungal and parasitic infections, meningitis, autoimmune diseases and septicemia) independent of breakdown of the blood-brain barrier.[3,5,9] Correlations between CSF QUIN with markers of immune stimulation (neopterin, white blood cell counts and IgG levels) again indicates a relationship between accelerated kynurenine pathway metabolism and the degree of intracerebral immune stimulation. It is important to note that these increases in CSF QUIN cannot simply be attributed to brain atrophy, dementia, motor disturbances, disturbances in food intake, non-specific stress, gliosis or seizures as CSF QUIN and KYNA are not increased in patients with either Huntington's disease, Alzheimer's disease, seizures, depression, anorexia nervosa or bulimia nervosa.[3,18–23]

ANIMAL MODELS OF INFLAMMATORY NEUROLOGIC DISEASE

Generalized Immune Activation

In many of the inflammatory disease studied, immune stimulation was present not only within the CNS, but also in systemic tissues. Consequently it is difficult to differentiate CNS-restricted changes in kynurenine pathway metabolism from the contribution of systemic responses. We have proposed that changes in systemic kynurenine pathway metabolism influence changes in CNS QUIN level, particularly in circumstances where immune activation is predominantly or exclusively systemic.[3,12,24] A rodent model which replicates certain kynurenine pathway responses in both CNS and systemic tissues following systemic immune activation has been described and supports a contributory role for systemic kynurenine pathway responses in the CNS changes.[12,25–28] However, the following two studies in experimental models have clearly established that the CNS is indeed capable of synthesizing QUIN independent of systemic contributions.

CNS-restricted Immune Activation

Poliovirus Infection of Rhesus Macaques

Macaques received an intraspinal injection of poliovirus as a model of localized inflammatory neurologic disease.[6] Seventeen days later, spinal cord IDO activity and QUIN concentrations in both spinal cord and CSF were increased in proportion to the degree of inflammatory responses and neurologic damage in the spinal cord, as well as the severity of motor paralysis. There were also significant correlations between the severity of neuronal degeneration and inflammatory lesions in the spinal cord, brainstem, thalamus and motor cortex (average lesion score), with CSF concentrations of QUIN (FIG. 1). The absolute concentrations of QUIN in CSF and tissue (micromolar), exceeded levels reported to kill spinal cord neurons *in vitro* (nanomolar).[29] IDO activity was not affected in the frontal cortex, a region that is not a target for poliovirus. Spinal cord slices from poliovirus-infected macaques *in vitro* converted $[^{13}C_6]$-L-tryptophan to $[^{13}C_6]$-QUIN. Because spleen macrophages stimulated with interferon-γ were also able to convert $[^{13}C_6]$-L-tryptophan to $[^{13}C_6]$-QUIN, we postulated that QUIN may be produced in localized macrophage infiltrates into the CNS, and that such cells contain kynurenine-3-hydroxylase, kynureninease and 3-hydroxyanthranilate-3,4-dioxygenase. Subsequent studies established that the activities of kynurenine-3-hydroxylase and kynureninease were increased in the spinal cord of poliovirus-infected macaques; also, 3-hydroxyanthranilate-3,4-dioxygenase activity in spinal cord was unchanged (Saito and Heyes, in preparation).

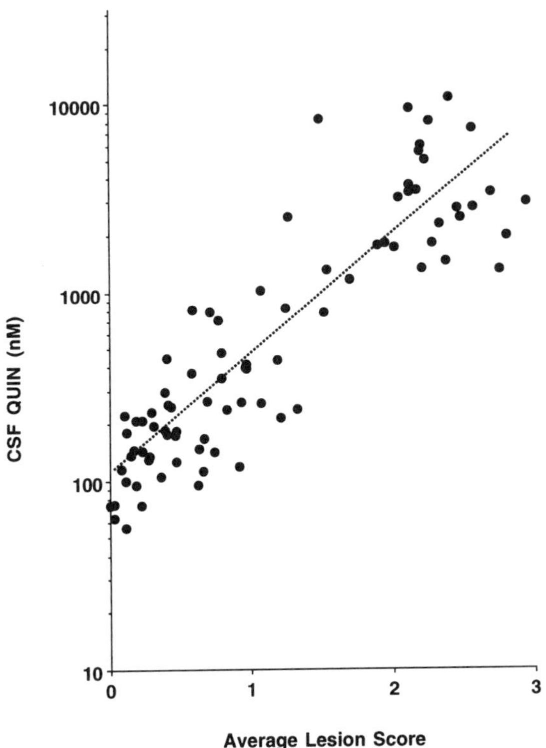

FIGURE 1. Significant correlations between the concentrations of the excitotoxin quinolinic acid (QUIN) and the severity of inflammatory responses and neurodegeneration in the spinal cord, brainstem, thalamus and cerebral cortex of macaques (average lesion score), 17 days following an intraspinal inoculation of live polivirus (from ref. 6).

Ischemic Brain Injury

Inflammatory lesions, including macrophage infiltrates and reactive gliosis, occur in damaged brain regions following transient cerebral ischemia. We have found proportional increases in IDO activity and QUIN concentrations in brain 4 days after 10 min of cerebral ischemia, with both responses in hippocampus >

striatum > cerebral cortex > thalamus. These increases paralleled the severity of local brain injury and inflammation. IDO activity and QUIN concentrations were unchanged in the cerebellum of post-ischemic gerbils, which is consistent with the preservation of blood flow and resultant absence of pathology in this region. Blood QUIN and L-kynurenine concentrations were unaffected by ischemia. Brain tissue QUIN levels at 4 days post-ischemia exceeded blood concentrations, minimizing a role for breakdown of the blood-brain barrier. Marked increases in the activity of kynureninase, kynurenine 3-hydroxylase and 3-hydroxyanthranilate-3,4-dioxygenase were also detected in hippocampus, but not in cerebellum. *In vivo* synthesis of $[^{13}C_6]$-QUIN from $[^{13}C_6]$-L-tryptophan but not $[^{13}C_6]$-anthranilic acid was demonstrated in hippocampus of 4 day post-ischemic animals.

Therapeutic Implications

Collectively, these observations support a role for QUIN in the pathogenesis of neurodegenerative changes in patients with a broad spectrum of inflammatory neurologic disease. The increases in QUIN are attributable to increased activities of IDO, kynureninase, kynurenine 3-hydroxylase and 3-hydroxyanthranilate-3,4-dioxygenase either within the CNS or systemic tissues. QUIN may contribute to neurologic dysfunction by interfering with NMDA receptor function. Strategies to attenuate the receptor mediated effects of QUIN, KYNA and other neuroactive kynurenines are potential avenues to therapy, although drugs which block NMDA receptors could conceivably accentuate neurologic deficits under some circumstances. Agents which attenuate QUIN formation may also be of benefit, including antibodies to interferon-γ and inhibitors of the kynurenine pathway, including 4-chloro-3-hydroxyanthranilate, 6-chlorotryptophan and norharmane.[12,15,30] Further, measures of CSF QUIN may serve as a useful 'marker' of CNS inflammation and brain injury.

REFERENCES

1. PERKINS, M. N. & T. W. STONE. 1983. Pharmacology and regional variations of quinolinic acid-evoked excitations in rat central nervous system. J. Pharmacol. Exp. Ther. **226:** 551–557.
2. SCHWARCZ, R., W. O. WHETSELL & R. E. M. MANGANO. 1983. Quinolinic acid: An endogenous metabolite can produce axon sparing lesions in rat brain. Science **219:** 316–318.
3. HEYES, M. P., K. SAITO, J. CROWLEY, L. E. DAVIS, M. A. DEMITRAK, M. DER, L. DILLING, M. J. P. KRUESI, A. LACKNER, S. A. LARSEN, K. LEE, H. LEONARD, S. P. MARKEY, A. MARTIN, S. MILSTIEN, M. M. MOURADIAN, M. R. PRANZATELLI, B. J. QUEARRY, A. SALAZAR, M. SMITH, S. E. STRAUS, T. SUNDERLAND, S. SWEDO & W. W. TOURTELLOTTE. 1992. Quinolinic acid and kynurenine pathway metabolism in inflammatory and non-inflammatory neurologic disease. Brain **115:** 1249–1273.
4. HEYES, M. P., B. J. BREW, K. SAITO, B. J. QUEARRY, R. W. PRICE, R. B. BHALLA, M. M. MOURADIAN, M. DER & S. P. MARKEY. 1992. Inter-relationships between neuroactive kynurenines, neopterin and β_2-microglobulin in cerebrospinal fluid and serum of HIV-1 infected patients. J. Neuroimmunol. **40:** 71–80.
5. SILVER, R. M., K. MCKINLEY, E. A. SMITH, B. J. QUEARRY, Y. HARATI, E. M. STERNBERG & M. P. HEYES. 1992. Tryptophan metabolism via the kynurenine pathway in patients with the eosinophilia-myalgia syndrome. Arthritis Rheumatol. **35:** 1097–1105.
6. HEYES, M. P., K. SAITO, D. JACOBOWITZ, O. TAKIKAWA, S. P. MARKEY & J. VICKERS.

1992. Poliovirus induces indoleamine-2,3-dioxygenase and quinolinic acid synthesis in macaque brain. FASEB J. **6:** 2977–2989.

7. MARTIN, A., M. P. HEYES, A. M. SALAZAR, D. L. KAMPEN, J. WILLIAMS, W. A. LAW, M. E. COATES & S. P. MARKEY. 1992. Progressive slowing of reaction time and increasing cerebrospinal fluid concentrations of quinolinic acid in HIV-infected individuals. J. Neuropsych. Clin. Neurosci. **4:** 270–279.

8. HEYES, M. P., E. K. JORDAN, K. LEE, K. SAITO, J. A. FRANK, P. J. SNOY, S. P. MARKEY & M. GRAVELL. 1992. Relationship of neurologic status in macaques infected with the simian immunodeficiency virus to cerebrospinal fluid and serum quinolinic acid and kynurenic acid. Brain Res. **570:** 237–250.

9. HALPERIN, J. J. & M. P. HEYES. 1992. Neuroactive kynurenines in Lyme borreliosis. Neurology **42:** 43–50.

10. HEYES, M. P., B. J. BREW, A. MARTIN, R. W. PRICE, A. M. SALAZAR, J. J. SIDTIS, J. A. YERGEY, M. M. MOURADIAN, A. E. SADLER, J. KEILP, D. RUBINOW & S. P. MARKEY. 1991. Quinolinic acid in cerebrospinal fluid and serum in HIV-1 infection: Relationship to clinical and neurologic status. Ann. Neurol. **29:** 202–209.

11. HEYES, M. P., M. GRAVELL, W. T. LONDON, M. EKHAUS, J. VICKERS, J. A. YERGEY, M. APRIL, D. BLACKMORE & S. P. MARKEY. 1990. Sustained increases in cerebrospinal fluid quinolinic acid concentrations in rhesus macaques *(Macaca Mulatta)* naturally infected with simian retrovirus type-D. Brain Res. **531:** 148–158.

12. SAITO, K., S. P. MARKEY & M. P. HEYES. 1992. Effects of immune activation on quinolinic acid and kynurenine pathway metabolism in the mouse. Neuroscience **51:** 25–39.

13. SAITO, K., A. LACKNER, S. P. MARKEY & M. P. HEYES. 1991. Cerebral cortex and lung indoleamine-2,3-dioxygenase activity is increased in type-D retrovirus infected macaques. Brain Res. **540:** 353–356.

14. HEYES, M. P. & B. J. QUEARRY. 1990. Quantification of kynurenic acid in cerebrospinal fluid: effects of systemic and central L-kynurenine administration. J. Chromatogr. **530:** 108–115.

15. SAITO, K., C. Y. CHEN, M. MASANA, J. CROWLEY, S. P. MARKEY & M. P. HEYES. 1993. 4-Chloro-3-hydroxyanthranilic acid, 6-chlorotryptophan and norharmane attenuate quinolinic acid formation by interferon-γ stimulated monocytes (THP-1) cells. Biochem. J. In press.

16. HEYES, M. P., K. SAITO & S. P. MARKEY. 1992. Human macrophages convert L-tryptophan to the neurotoxin quinolinic acid. Biochem. J. **283:** 633–635.

17. WILEY, C. A., C. L. ACHIM, R. D. SCHRIER, M. P. HEYES, J. A. McCUTCHEN & I. GRANT. 1992. Relationship of cerebrospinal fluid immune activation associated factors to HIV encephalitis. AIDS **6:** 1299–1307.

18. REYNOLDS, G. P., S. J. PEARSON, J. HALKET & M. SANDLER. 1988. Brain quinolinic acid in Huntington's disease. J. Neurochem. **50:** 1959–1960.

19. SCHWARCZ, R., C. A. TAMMINGA, R. KURLAN & I. SHOULSON. 1988. Cerebrospinal fluid levels of quinolinic acid in Huntington's disease and schizophrenia. Ann. Neurol. **24:** 580–582.

20. HEYES, M. P., K. J. SWARTZ, S. P. MARKEY & M. F. BEAL. 1991. Regional brain and cerebrospinal fluid quinolinic acid concentrations in Huntington's disease. Neurosci. Lett. **122:** 265–269.

21. MORONI, F., G. LOMBARDI, Y. ROBITAILLE & P. ETIENNE. 1986. Senile dementia and Alzheimer's disease: lack of changes of the cortical content of quinolinic acid. Neurobiol. Aging **7:** 249–253.

22. MOURADIAN, M. M., M. P. HEYES, J.-B. PAN, I. J. E. HEUSER, S. P. MARKEY & T. N. CHASE. 1989. No changes in central quinolinic acid levels in Alzheimer's disease. Neurosci. Lett. **105:** 233–238.

23. HEYES, M. P., A. R. WYLER, O. DEVINSKY, J. A. YERGEY, S. P. MARKEY & S. NADI. 1990. Quinolinic acid concentrations in brain and cerebrospinal fluid of patients with intractable complex partial seizures. Epilepsia **31:** 172–177.

24. HEYES, M. P. & A. LACKNER. 1990. Increased cerebrospinal fluid quinolinic acid, kynurenic acid and L-kynurenine in acute septicemia. J. Neurochem. **55:** 338–341.

25. HEYES, M. P., P. KIM & S. P. MARKEY. 1988. Systemic lipopolysaccharide and poke-weed mitogen increase quinolinic acid content of mouse cerebral cortex. J. Neurochem. **51:** 1946–1948.
26. HEYES, M. P., B. J. QUEARRY & S. P. MARKEY. 1989. Systemic endotoxin increases L-tryptophan, 5-hydroxyindoleacetic acid, 3-hydroxykynurenine and quinolinic acid content of mouse cerebral cortex. Brain Res. **491:** 173–179.
27. SAITO, K., T. S. NOWAK, JR., S. P. MARKEY & M. P. HEYES. 1993. Mechanism of delayed increases in kynurenine pathway metabolism in damaged brain regions following transient cerebral ischemia. J. Neurochem. **60:** 180–192.
28. SAITO, K., S. P. MARKEY & M. P. HEYES. 1991. Chronic effects of gamma-interferon on quinolinic acid and indoleamine-2,3-dioxygenase in brain of C57Bl6 mice. Brain Res. **546:** 151–154.
29. WHETSELL, W. O. & R. SCHWARCZ. 1989. Prolonged exposure to submicromolar concentrations of quinolinic acid causes excitotoxic damage in organotypic cultures of rat corticostriatal system. Neurosci. Lett. **97:** 271–275.
30. HEYES, M. P., B. HUTTO & S. P. MARKEY. 1988. 4-chloro-3-hydroxyanthranilic acid inhibits 3-hydroxyanthranilic acid oxidase in brain. Neurochem. Int. **13:** 405–409.

Release of Membrane-associated Growth Factors during Neural Injury[a]

GEORGE H. DE VRIES,[b,f] TIMOTHY J. NEUBERGER,[b]
ROOPA R. BAICHWAL,[c] JOHN W. BIGBEE,[d] LEE ZANE,[e]
AND JUN E. YOSHINO[e]

[b]Department of Biochemistry and Molecular Biophysics
[d]Department of Anatomy
Medical College of Virginia
Richmond, Virginia 23298-0614
[e]Department of Psychology
Colgate University
Hamilton, New York 13346

INTRODUCTION AND BACKGROUND

Growth factors serve tropic and trophic roles during the development of the nervous system.[1] When development is complete, basal levels of growth factors are maintained in the mature nervous system. However, after neural injury, growth factor activity is once again evident. For example, increased immunoreactivity of fibroblast growth factor (FGF) has been found after focal brain wounds,[2] after entorhinal-cortex lesion or fimbria-fornix lesion[3] or after forebrain ischemia.[4] We are investigating mechanisms by which membrane-associated growth factors can be made available after neural injury.

A major response to neural injury is the infiltration of phagocytic cells such as microglia and macrophages.[5] We have demonstrated that macrophages are able to release a growth factor(s) from ingested myelin membrane fragments in a subcellular fraction (myelin-enriched fraction, MEF) which is similar to debris produced as a consequence of the demyelination which often accompanies neural injury. We have shown that cultured macrophages ingest myelin debris[6] and release, into the supernatant, a mitogenic factor for Schwann cells.[7] In addition, we have shown that in Schwann cell cultures containing macrophages, the mitogenic potency of the supernatant is dependent on the number of macrophages in the culture.[8] Likewise, Schwann cells can also phagocytose the myelin to a limited extent,[6] and this phagocytosis may also generate a mitogen similar to the mitogen which is generated via macrophage phagocytosis. We have also observed that the greater mitogenic potency of CNS myelin compared to the mitogenic potency of PNS myelin correlates with the higher content of myelin basic protein (MBP) in

[a] The work in the authors' laboratories reviewed in this article has been supported by a grant from the National Multiple Sclerosis Society (RG2076-A-5) and Public Health Service grants NS10821 and NS15408.

[c] Present address: Department of Pathology, VA Medical Center, Palo Alto, CA 94304.

[f] Address correspondence to Dr. George H. De Vries, Department of Biochemistry and Molecular Biophysics, Medical College of Virginia, 1101 E. Marshall, Richmond, Virginia 23298-0614.

217

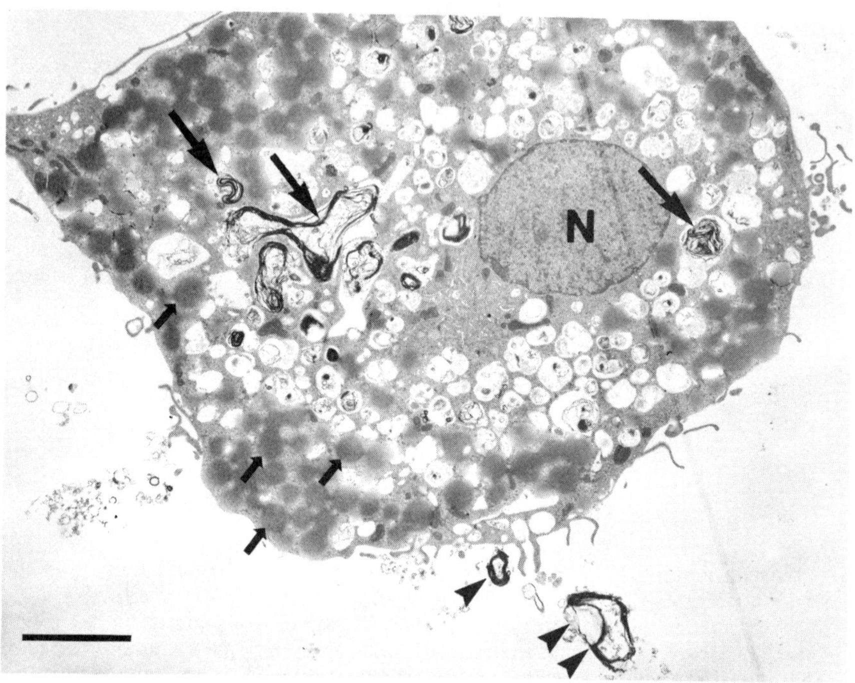

FIGURE 1. Electron micrograph of a microglial cell exposed for 48 h to a myelin-enriched fraction. Note the numerous phagocytosed myelin fragments (*large arrows*) as well as membrane-containing phagosomes at various stages of degradation. Abundant lipid vacuoles (*small arrows*) are also present. Note the nonphagocytosed myelin fragments on the culture substratum (*arrowheads*). N = nucleus. Bar equals 5 microns.

CNS myelin.[7] These data suggest that MBP itself may be related to the mitogen released when myelin is degraded. We subsequently demonstrated that myelin isolated from the Shiverer mutant, which lacks MBP, had limited mitogenicity.[9] Furthermore we showed that a polyvalent antisera to MBP could block the mitogenicity of the activated supernatant.[9] Finally, we have recently found that MBP peptides alone can serve as mitogens and we are attempting to exactly define the molecular nature of the MBP-related mitogen.[10] The parsimonious explanation for these observations is that during proteolytic degradation of myelin following trauma a peptide derived from MBP is released which then is mitogenic for the Schwann cells in the vicinity of the neural injury.

RELEASE OF MYELIN-ASSOCIATED GROWTH FACTORS IN THE CNS

Microglia are phagocytic cells which reside in the CNS, and are recruited to the site of injury after trauma. We were interested to determine if microglia recruited to the site of injury, are capable of generating membrane-related mitogens in a manner similar to the peripheral macrophages. Microglia were isolated from neonatal cerebral cortical cultures by differential adhesion.[11] In order to show that the microglia are able to ingest myelin, the cells were treated with a myelin-enriched fraction and examined by electron microscopy. As shown in FIGURE 1, microglia had a morphology consistent with active ingestion of myelin, including numerous phagocytosed myelin fragments as well as membrane-containing phagosomes. TABLE 1 summarizes the proliferation assays carried out with microglia conditioned supernatant. Treatment of the microglia with 200 μg/ml of a myelin fraction yielded a conditioned media that was mitogenic for neonatal astrocytes. If lysosomal processing by the microglia was impaired with ammonium chloride, the mitogenic activity of the conditioned medium was markedly decreased. Non-specific stimuli such as polystyrene beads and astrocytic membranes were not effective in producing a mitotically active supernatant.

Using an earlier study[12] which indicated that MBP by itself was mitogenic for astrocytes, we examined the possibility that a myelin membrane fraction could directly stimulate astrocyte proliferation. As shown in FIGURE 2, the myelin membranes induced a dose-dependent increase in ^{3}H-thymidine incorporation by astrocytes.

Our data indicate that myelin membranes can either directly stimulate proliferation of astrocytes or can be processed through the lysosomal compartment of microglia to produce a conditioned medium which is mitogenic for astrocytes. It is possible that a single mitogen for astrocytes is present in the myelin membranes. Alternatively, there may be two mitogens; one related to MBP that is released by microglia and a second mitogen which interacts directly with the astrocytes. Thus in both the CNS and PNS, phagocytic cells may release growth factors after neural injury by lysosomal processing of myelin membrane fragments. In both cases the growth factors produced by this processing serve as mitogens for glial cells located in the vicinity of the injured tissue.

TABLE 1. Conditioned Media from Microglia Treated with a Myelin-enriched Fraction are Mitogenic for Neonatal Astrocytes

Condition	[^{3}H]-Thymidine Incorporation, dpm	+6 mM Ammonium Chloride
Conditioned media, no myelin membranes	3950 ± 1200	4300 ± 1450
Conditioned media, myelin membranes, 200 μg/ml	15,500 ± 7100	5600 ± 1100
Conditioned media, fluorescent polystyrene beads, 50 ng/ml	2600 ± 650	
Conditioned media, astrocytic membrane at 50 μg/ml	3800 ± 1350	

Microglia were incubated with MEF (200 μg/ml), astrocyte membrane (50 μg/ml), polystyrene beads (50 ng/ml) or only media (0.25% fetal calf serum) for 48 h either in the presence or absence of ammonium chloride. Conditioned media was filtered (Gelman acrodisc, 0.2 μ pore size) and immediately added (100 μl) to neonatal astrocytes. The next day, 0.3 μC of [^{3}H]-thymidine in 25 μl of media was added to the cells. Twenty four h later, cells were harvested onto fiberglass filters and ^{3}H-thymidine incorporation was determined using a liquid scintillation counter.

POTENTIAL ROLE OF GROWTH FACTORS ASSOCIATED WITH THE NEURONAL SURFACE MEMBRANE

Another mechanism by which growth factors may be mobilized after neural injury involves release from the external surface of neuronal membranes. Some growth factors such as fibroblast growth factor (FGF) do not contain a classical signal sequence,[14] making it unlikely that this factor can be localized on the external surface of neuronal membranes. However, substantial quantities of FGF have been detected, both *in vivo* and *in vitro*, associated with extracellular matrix components.[15] In addition it has been demonstrated that FGF is not only present

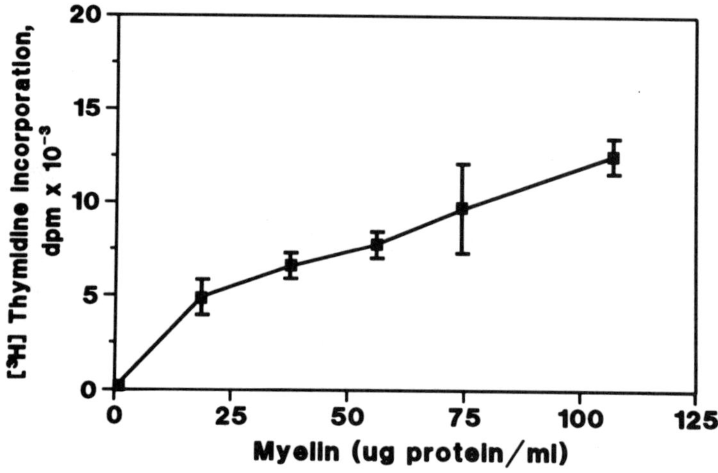

FIGURE 2. Dose response curve for myelin stimulation of neonatal rat astrocyte proliferation in serum-free N2 media. Purified neonatal rat astrocytes were prepared according to the methods of McCarthy and DeVellis[11] and plated on poly-D-lysine–coated 96-well cluster plates at a density of 5000 cells per well in 10% fetal calf serum (FCS)-containing media. The next day, wells were washed with serum free media and fed the serum-free media, N2.[13] Seventy-two hours later, MEF was added to wells at a final concentration of 9, 18, 36, 54, 72 or 108 μg/ml and the next day 0.3 μCi of ³H-thymidine was added to each well. After a 24-h pulse, cells were harvested onto fiberglass filters and ³H-thymidine incorporation was determined using a liquid scintillation counter.

within neurons[16] but also on the external surface of their plasma membranes.[17] We have recently carried out an immunocytochemical study of the distribution of FGF in cultured dorsal root ganglion (DRG) neurons.[17] When the embryonic neurons were cultured for less than 20 days, all of the FGF immunoreactivity was within the neuronal cell body and neuritic processes. However, after 30 days *in vitro* FGF was clearly found on the external surface of the neurons. An example of such localization is shown in FIGURE 3. Since these processes were stained in the living state prior to permeabilization, the FGF immunoreactivity must be localized on the external surface. In addition to finding FGF externally localized on peripheral neurons, we have determined that axolemma-enriched fractions

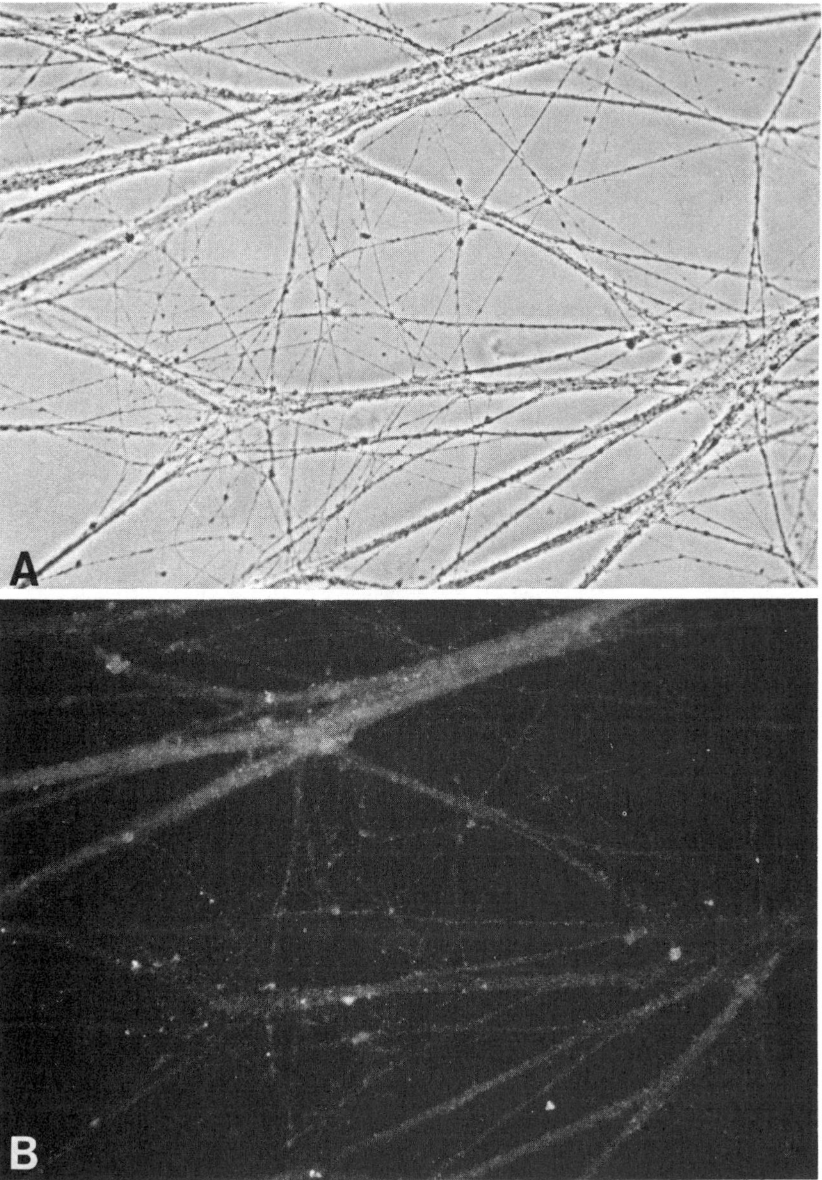

FIGURE 3. Phase **(A)** and fluorescence **(B)** photomicrograph of DRG neurites 30 days *in vitro* immunostained live with anti-basic FGF antibodies allowing detection of only extracellular basic FGF.

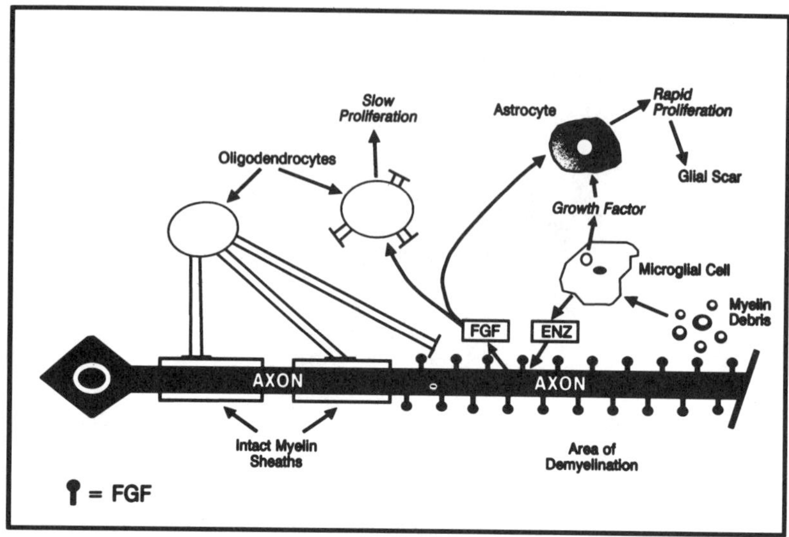

FIGURE 4. Schematic representation of the events which may occur after demyelination of CNS axons which results in the selective stimulation of astroglial proliferation.

(AEF) from both the CNS and PNS contain substantial quantities of external FGF.[18]

In neurons, FGF can be associated with the plasmalemma in two ways. Most often the FGF is associated with heparan sulfate proteoglycans (HSPG) which are integrally bound to the membrane either via a phosphatidyl inositol anchor which is sensitive to plasmin hydrolysis[19] or via a hydrophobic amino acid sequence which is sensitive to proteolytic cleavage by plasmin.[20] Alternatively FGF can be released from its HSPG association via heparitinase.[21] Invading phagocytic cells such as macrophages and microglia can secrete enzymes of this type which are capable of releasing the FGF from the membrane.[22,23] It is tempting to speculate that this externally disposed FGF may be released after neural injury by means of proteolytic enzymes secreted by invading phagocytic cells. In turn, this released growth factor could complement the myelin-related growth factor in serving as a potential mitogen for glial cells in the area of injury. Under the appropriate conditions, FGF has been shown to be a potent mitogen for both Schwann cells[24] and oligodendrocytes.[25]

UNIFYING THEMES IN THE RELEASE OF MEMBRANE-ASSOCIATED GROWTH FACTORS AFTER NEURAL INJURY

Under conditions in which there is demyelination with sparing of the neuronal process (as schematically depicted in FIG. 4), growth factors may be released via the myelin phagocytosis pathway and potentially by proteolytic release of factors such as FGF from the surface of the neuronal plasmalemma. However in cases where the axon is damaged and degenerates, (i.e., Wallerian degeneration) a "vesiculation" pathway for the release of membrane-associated growth factors may be operative. In this scenario, (depicted in FIG. 5) the plasma membrane of the damaged axon vesiculates in a manner so as to maintain its *in situ* orientation. As a result, the FGF which was bound to the outer surface of the intact axon is associated with the outside of the vesicles. The membrane vesicles then diffuse to nearby Schwann cells where they specifically bind and stimulate cell division. The interaction of these membrane vesicles (produced from damaged axons) with the glial cells is similar to the type of mitogenic stimulation resulting from the addition of axolemma-enriched fractions to cultured glial cells which has been extensively studied in our laboratory (for a recent review see ref. 26). We have also demonstrated the "membrane vesiculation" pathway in recent *in vitro* studies of co-cultures of DRG neurons and Schwann cells after crush injury to the neuritic field.[27] Thus, in this pathway growth factors are released after injury in the form of vesicles which then adhere to the appropriate glial cell in the vicinity and stimulate cell division. Although not depicted in FIGURE 4, the vesiculation pathway may also be operative in cases of trauma in the CNS. The specificity of the binding of these vesicles has been demonstrated by their failure to bind to nearby fibroblasts in the culture[27] and is illustrated in FIGURE 5. We have also noted that in the presence of astrocytes and oligodendrocytes, these vesicles preferentially bind to the oligodendrocytes.[28]

The data we present suggests at least three potential pathways for the release of membrane-associated growth factors after neural injury *in vivo:* 1) phagocytosis of the myelin membrane to release a growth factor; 2) vesiculation of the damaged neuronal membrane containing cell surface growth factors and subsequent binding of the vesicle to appropriate glial cells; and 3) proteolytic release of cell surface growth factors via enzymes released by invading phagocytes.

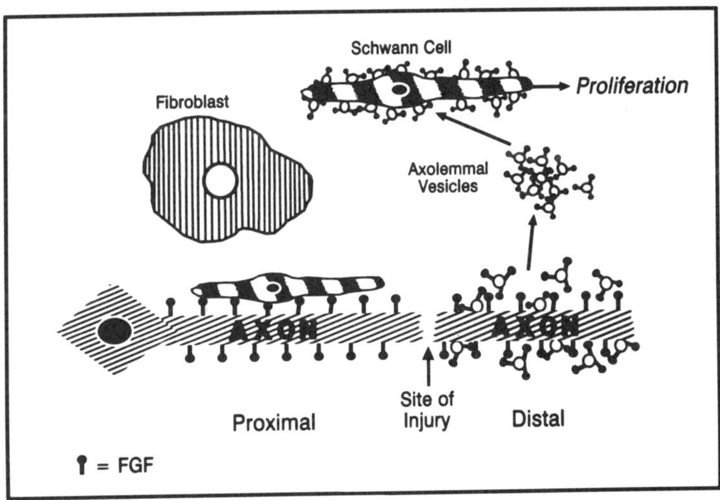

FIGURE 5. Schematic representation of events which may occur in an *in vitro* model of PNS injury which result in the accumulation of FGF on the outer plasma membrane of the Schwann cell.

SUMMARY AND CONCLUSIONS

The release of membrane-associated growth factors after neural injury may influence the outcome of the recovery. For example, for remyelination to occur after neural injury it is critical for the glial cell to proliferate prior to remyelination in both the PNS[29] and CNS.[30] In the CNS, the relative response of the oligodendrocytes and astroglia to growth factors mobilized during neural injury may play a role in the cellular dynamics of repair of neural injury or scarring and subsequent failure to repair neural injury. In support of this view, we have studied the mitotic potential[31] and cell cycle kinetics[32] of cultured adult oligodendrocytes and found that these adult cells respond only weakly to factors such as FGF which are known to be potent mitogens for neonatal cells. However, given the same dose of FGF, adult astrocytes are mitotically stimulated to a much greater degree than are the adult oligodendrocytes (Vick and De Vries, unpublished observations).

Given the pathways which may be operative in the release of growth factors after injury, it has not escaped our attention that, provided the released factors are in equilibrium with easily accessible and peripheral body fluids, these released factors may serve as new markers for neural injury. Further experiments are in progress to explore this possibility.

REFERENCES

1. GOLDFARB, M. 1990. The fibroblast growth factor family. Cell Growth Diff. **1:** 439–445.
2. FINKLESTEIN, S. P., P. J. APOSTOLIDES, C. G. CADAY, J. PROSSER, M. F. PHILIPS & M. KLAGSBRUN. 1988. Increased basic fibroblast growth factor (bFGF) immunoreactivity at the site of focal brain wounds. Brain Res. **460:** 253–259.
3. GÒMEZ-PINILLA, F., J. W-K. LEE & C. W. COTMAN. 1992. Basic FGF in adult rat brain: Cellular distribution and response to entorhinal lesion and fimbria-fornix transection. J. Neurosci. **12:** 345–355.
4. KIYOTA, Y., K. TAKAMI, M. IWANE, A. SHINO, M. MIYAMOTO, R. TSUKUDA & A. NAGAOKA. 1991. Increase in basic fibroblast growth factor-like immunoreactivity in rat brain after forebrain ischemia. Brain Res. **545:** 322–328.
5. BLIGHT, A. R. 1985. Delayed demyelination and macrophage invasion: A candidate for secondary cell damage in spinal cord injury. Cent. Nerv. Syst. Trauma. **2**(4): 299–315.
6. BIGBEE, J. W., J. E. YOSHINO & G. H. DEVRIES. 1987. Morphological and proliferative responses of cultured Schwann cells following rapid phagocytosis of a myelin-enriched fraction. J. Neurocytology. **16:** 487–496.
7. BAICHWAL, R., J. W. BIGBEE & G. H. DEVRIES. 1988. Macrophage-mediated myelin-related mitogenic factor for cultured Schwann cells. Proc. Natl. Acad. Sci. USA **85:** 1701–1705.
8. BAICHWAL, R. & G. DEVRIES. 1991. Peripheral nerve-induced mitogens and trophic factors and their potential role in peripheral nerve regeneration. Peripheral Nerve **2:** 25–31.
9. BAICHWAL, R. & G. H. DEVRIES. 1989. A mitogen for Schwann cells is derived from myelin basic protein. Biochem. Biophys. Res. Commun. **164:** 883–888.
10. TZENG, S.-F., G. E. DIEBLER & G. H. DEVRIES. 1993. Myelin basic protein related peptide involved in stimulation of Schwann cell proliferation. Trans. Am. Soc. Neurochem. In press.
11. McCARTHY, K. D. & J. DEVELLIS. 1980. Preparation of separate astroglial and oligodendroglial cell cultures from rat cerebral tissue. J. Cell Biol. **85:** 890–902.
12. BOLOGA, L. 1985. Myelin basic protein stimulates the proliferation of astrocytes: Possible explanation for multiple sclerosis plaque formation. Brain Res. **346:** 199–203.

13. BOTTENSTEIN, J. E. & G. H. SATO. 1979. Growth of a rat neuroblastoma cell line in serum-free supplemented medium. Proc. Natl. Acad. Sci. USA **76:** 514–517.

14. ABRAHAM, J. A., J. L. WHANG, A. TUMOLO, A. MERGIA, J. FRIEDMAN, D. GOSPODARO-WICZ & J. C. FIDDES. 1986. Human basic fibroblast growth factor: Nucleotide sequence and genomic organization. EMBO J. **5:** 2523–2528.

15. BAIRD, A. & N. LING. 1987. Fibroblast growth factors are present in the extracellular matrix produced by endothelial cells in vitro: Implications for a role of heparinase-like enzymes in the neovascular response. Biochem. Biophys. Res. Commun. **142:** 428–435.

16. ELDE, R., Y. CAO, A. CINTRA, T. C. BRELJE, M. PELTO-HUIKKO, T. JUNTTILA, K. FUXE, R. F. PETTERSSON & T. HÖKFELT. 1991. Prominent expression of acidic fibroblast growth factor in motor and sensory neurons. Neuron **7:** 349–364.

17. NEUBERGER, T. & G. H. DEVRIES. 1993. Developmental regulation of fibroblast growth factor expression in cultured dorsal root ganglion neurons. J. Neurocytol. In press.

18. NEUBERGER, T., T. RUSSELL, V. SERIO & G. H. DEVRIES. Fibroblast growth factor is associated with axolemma-enriched fractions. Biochem. Biophys. Res. Commun. Submitted.

19. BRUNNER, G., J. GABRILOVE, D. B. RIFKIN & E. L. WILSON. 1991. Phospholipase C release of basic fibroblast growth factor from human bond marrow cultures as a biologically active complex with a phosphatidylinositol-anchored heparan sulfate proteoglycan. J. Cell Biol. **114**(6): 1275–1283.

20. SAKSELA, O. & D. B. RIFKIN. 1990. Release of basic fibroblast growth factor-heparan sulfate complexes from endothelial cells by plasminogen activator-mediated proteolytic activity. J. Cell Biol. **110:** 767–775.

21. BASHKIN, P., S. DOCTROW, M. KLAGSBRUN, C. M. SVAHN, J. FOLKMAN & I. VLODAVSKY. 1989. Basic fibroblast growth factor binds to subendothelial extracellular matrix and is released by heparitinase and heparin-like molecules. Biochemisry **28:** 1737–1743.

22. PERRY, V. H., M. C. BROWN & S. GORDON. 1987. The macrophage response to central and peripheral nerve Injury: A posisble role for macrophages in regeneration. J. Exp. Med. **165:** 1218–1223.

23. NAKAJIMA, K., N. TSUZAKI, M. SHIMOJO, M. HAMANOUE & S. KOHSAKA. 1992. Microglial isolated from rat brain secrete a urokinase-type plasminogen activator. Brain Res. **577:** 285–292.

24. DAVIS, J. B. & P. STROOBANT. 1990. Platelet-derived growth factors and fibroblast growth factors are mitogens for rat Schwann cells. J. Cell Biol. **110:** 1353.

25. ECCLESTON, P. A. & D. H. SILBERBERG. 1985. Fibroblast growth factor is a mitogen of oligodendrocytes in vivo. Dev. Brain Res. **21:** 315–318.

26. DEVRIES, G. 1992. Schwann cell proliferation. *In* Peripheral Neuropathy. P. Dyck, P. K. Thomas, J. W. Griffin, P. A. Low & J. F. Poduslo, Eds. 3rd edit. Vol. 1: 290–298. W. B. Saunders Company. Philadelphia, PA.

27. NEUBERGER, T. & G. H. DEVRIES. 1993. Redistribution of fibroblast growth factor in cultured dorsal root neurons after injury. J. Neurocytol. In press.

28. VICK, R., T. NEUBERGER & G. H. DEVRIES. 1992. Role of adult oligodendrocytes in remyelination after neural injury. J. Neurotrauma. **9:** s93–s103.

29. HALL, S. M. & N. A. GREGSON. 1974. The effects of mitomycin c on remyelination in the peripheral nervous system. Nature **252:** 303–305.

30. WOOD, P. & R. P. BUNGE. 1991. The origin of remyelinating cells in the central nervous system: The role of the mature oligodendrocyte. Glia **4:** 225–232.

31. VICK, R. & G. H. DEVRIES. 1992. Mitotic potential of cultured adult oligodendrocytes. J. Neurosci. Res. **33:** 68–74.

32. VICK, R., J. M. COLLINS & G. H. DEVRIES. 1992. Cell cycle and proliferation dynamics of cultured adult rat oligodendrocytes. J. Neurosci. Res. **33:** 75–81.

Trophic Factor Production by Reactive Astrocytes in Injured Brain

JOAN P. SCHWARTZ,[a,c] JIN GEN SHENG,[b]
KUNIHIKO MITSUO, SUSUMU SHIRABE, AND
NOBUYOSHI NISHIYAMA

[a]Clinical Neuroscience Branch
[b]Surgical Neurology Branch
National Institute of Neurological Disorders and Stroke
National Institutes of Health
Bethesda, Maryland 20892

One important issue in terms of neural responses to injury is whether damage to the brain leads to re-expression of the same program and pattern of gene expression as occurred developmentally—that is, do some, or all, genes respond similarly during development and following injury. The one consistent response of the brain to injury is reactive gliosis, characterized as an increased expression of glial fibrillary acidic protein (GFAP) in astrocytes. A number of studies have demonstrated that physical damage,[1–4] or chemical toxins such as 1-methyl-4-phenyl-1,2,3,6-tetrahydropyridine (MPTP),[5–7] 6-hydroxydopamine (6-OHDA),[7–9] and kainic acid,[8] all of which induce neuronal degeneration, cause reactive gliosis.

Astrocytes can serve as a source of neurotrophic factors (NTFs) during development and recent studies have shown increased synthesis of two of these NTFs, basic fibroblast growth factor[10] and endothelins,[11] by astrocytes following brain injury. We were therefore interested in asking whether re-expression of NTFs could serve as another marker of neuronal injury, similar to the increased GFAP expression. We have examined the developmental time course of expression, as well as changes in the synthesis of specific NTFs in astrocytes derived from control or lesioned brain, with particular emphasis on nerve growth factor (NGF), brain-derived neurotrophic factor and neurotrophin-3, as well as the neuropeptides enkephalin and somatostatin (SS). All show distinct developmental patterns of expression, which vary depending on the brain region from which the astrocytes were prepared.[12] Following lesion of the substantia nigra (SN) dopaminergic pathway with MPTP, there are changes in the content of certain of these NTFs, which correlate with changes in GFAP content. We are currently examining the role which cytokines may play in the regulation of expression of these genes before and after brain injury.

MATERIALS AND METHODS

Drug Treatments

For 6-OHDA, male Sprague-Dawley rats weighing 300 ± 6 g were injected with 6-OHDA (2 μg/μl saline containing 0.2 mg/ml ascorbic acid) into the substan-

---

[c] Address correspondence to: Dr. Joan P. Schwartz, CNB, NINDS, NIH, Bldg. 9—Room 1W115, Bethesda, MD 20892; Tel.: (301)496-4049; FAX (301)402-0117.

tia nigra on the right side as described.[13] Sham-treated rats received the same volume of saline (0.9% NaCl).

For MPTP, young adult male C57/B16 mice (Charles River Laboratories) weighing 24–25 g were given either 24 mg/kg MPTP-HCl or saline i.p. twice/day for 4 days and sacrificed 10 days later.

Astrocyte Cultures

Astrocyte cultures were prepared from a litter of embryonic day 20 fetuses or postnatal day 3 or 8 rat pups, or from 3–4 adult (10–15 week old) Sprague-Dawley rats, and cultured in Dulbecco's Modified Eagle Medium, containing 10% fetal bovine serum, as described.[12]

Radioimmunoassays

Radioimmunoassays were carried out for met-enkephalin and SS as described.[12]

NGF 2-Site ELISA

NGF 2-site ELISA was carried out on cell extracts as described.[14]

RNA

RNA was analyzed by Northern and slot blot hybridization as has been described,[12-14] and is expressed in units of the specific mRNA relative to the non-changing mRNA for cyclophilin (1B15).

GFAP Immunohistochemistry

GFAP immunohistochemistry was carried out as(s) described[13] on formalin-fixed brain sections, using the primary antibody to GFAP (Dakopatts) at 1/250 followed by biotinylated goat anti-rabbit IgG (Vectastain Kit, Vector Labs, 1/200). Cell counts were determined in coronal sections, counting only GFAP(+) cell bodies, although the size of the cell bodies as well as the extent of processes were significantly increased.[13]

RESULTS

Comparison of the developmental time course of expression, in cerebellar astrocytes, of the genes for the two neuropeptides, enkephalin and SS, with that

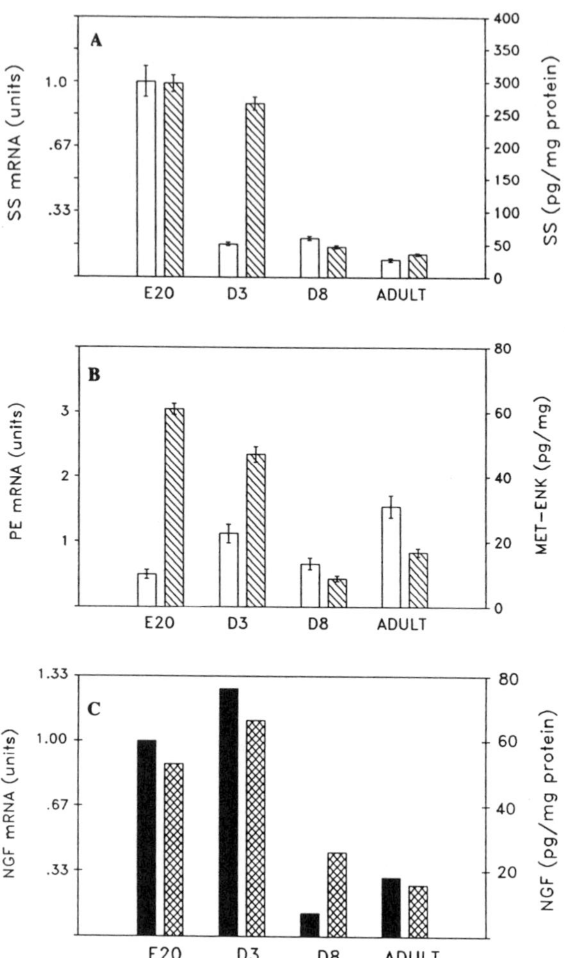

FIGURE 1. Somatostatin, proenkephalin, and nerve growth factor mRNA and peptide content in cerebellar astrocytes prepared from rats of different ages. Cerebellar astrocytes were prepared and cultured, and RNA and peptide analyses carried out, as described in MATERIALS AND METHODS. **A:** SS mRNA (*open bars*) and peptide (*striped bars*); **B:** PE mRNA (*open bars*) and met-enk (*striped bars*); **C:** NGF mRNA (*black bars*) and NGF (*hatched bars*).

of NGF, revealed striking similarities (FIG. 1). Peptide levels for all three decreased early developmentally: both SS (FIG. 1A) and met-enkephalin (FIG. 1B) were highest in astrocytes prepared from E20 animals, whereas NGF (FIG. 1C) peaked at postnatal day 3. By postnatal day 8, all three had decreased 8-to-10-fold, essentially to adult levels. However, regulation at the level of the mRNA differed. SS mRNA content had dropped to adult level by postnatal day 3 (FIG. 1A) and NGF mRNA by postnatal day 8 (FIG. 1C), thus preceding or mirroring the changes in the peptides themselves. However, PE mRNA actually increased 3-fold over this same developmental time period, in agreement with *in vivo* results obtained by Spruce *et al.*[15]

The results on the developmental expression of the peptides are in general agreement with results from other laboratories, which suggest that quiescent astrocytes produce significantly reduced amounts of neurotrophic factors. It was therefore of interest to see if expression increased in reactive astrocytes. One way to stimulate reactive gliosis is by lesion of the substantia nigra dopaminergic cells with 6-OHDA. When rats are injected unilaterally with 6-OHDA, reactive astrocytes (measured by increased GFAP immunohistochemistry) can be detected not only on the lesioned side but also on the contralateral side. The largest increase occurs in the lesioned SN itself (FIG. 2A), but increases are also seen in the striatum (FIG. 2B) and even in the cortex (FIG. 2C). Cell numbers increased most on the lesioned side, but significant changes were seen on the contralateral side as well. Saline injection induced changes on the injected side which were comparable or larger than those seen on the contralateral side of 6-OHDA-lesioned brain: in addition, small changes were detected on the contralateral side of saline-injected brains (FIG. 2).

Since some studies have reported the appearance of reactive astrocytes by immunohistochemistry without a corresponding increase in actual content of GFAP,[16–19] we also measured changes in GFAP, by immunoblot, and in GFAP mRNA. Both GFAP[13] and GFAP mRNA (FIG. 3A) increased following 6-OHDA, on both the ipsi- and contralateral sides of the striatum. GFAP content also increased after saline injection.[13] However, there was a specificity to the changes, since there was no change in the mRNA for S100β (FIG. 3B), another astrocyte-derived neurotrophic factor.[20]

Treatment with MPTP (1-methyl-4-phenyl-1,2,3,6-tetrahydropyridine) generates a second neurotoxic model, comparable to 6-OHDA, for inducing reactive gliosis in the striatum. Ten days after lesioning mice with a dose of MPTP sufficient to deplete striatal dopamine by 70%, the striata were removed and astrocytes prepared. Levels of NGF and PE mRNAs were compared in astrocytes from MPTP-lesioned striata with those from control striatal astrocytes. "Reactive" astrocytes (defined by their increased expression of GFAP), from MPTP-lesioned brain, contained increased amounts of NGF mRNA but decreased amounts of PE mRNA (TABLE 1).

DISCUSSION

It has become clear in recent years that neurons and glia communicate with and signal each other by release of a variety of transmitters, peptides, and other factors. Astrocytes express virtually all of the known neurotransmitter receptors,[21] but the recent discovery that they also express certain of the neuropeptide genes (reviewed in ref. 22) has greatly expanded the possibilities for neuronal-glial communication. The developmental patterns of both expression and precursor processing of the neuropeptide genes strongly suggest potential trophic roles for these peptides in early CNS development, particularly the enkephalins and somatostatins.[22] Thus, one of the primary circuits of information flow during CNS development may consist of neuronal regulation, via neurotransmitter release, of astrocyte production of NTFs such as NGF, enkephalin, and SS (FIG. 4).

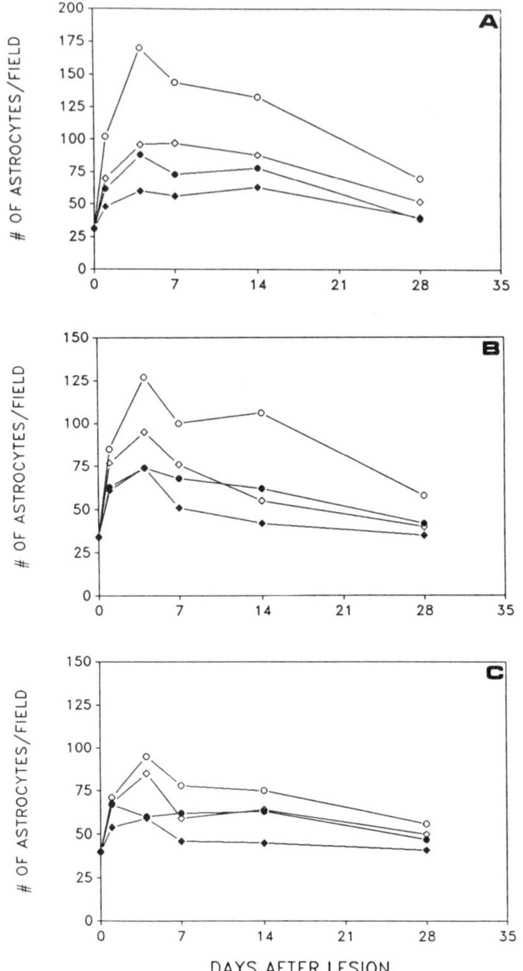

FIGURE 2. Time course of changes in ipsi- and contralateral GFAP expression following 6-OHDA lesion or saline injection. Animals were lesioned with 6-OHDA or injected with saline, and expression of GFAP analyzed by immunohistochemistry in substantia nigra **(A)**; in striatum **(B)**; and in cortex **(C)**; at the indicated days following lesion, as described in MATERIALS AND METHODS. The data at Day 0 are derived from uninjected control animals. 6-OHDA lesioned side (○); 6-OHDA contralateral side (●); saline-injected side (◇); saline-injected contralateral side (◆).

Developmentally, astrocytes produce and release the free peptides early. As was shown in FIGURE 1, in cerebellar astrocytes both enkephalin and SS peak at E20, while NGF is maximal at postnatal day 3. These data agree well with the developmental time courses seen *in vivo* for cerebellum.[12,22,23] Thus, as has been suggested, astrocyte synthesis of NTFs decreases in quiescent cells in the adult brain and it became of interest to ask whether synthesis turned back on in reactive astrocytes following injury.

One of the most consistent markers of neuronal injury is the induction of GFAP during reactive gliosis. Destruction of the dopamine neurons in the SN by direct unilateral injection of 6-OHDA results in the appearance of reactive astrocytes not only in the SN and striatum on the lesioned side, but also as far away as the cortex (FIG. 2C). In addition, reactive astrocytes increase in number on the contralateral side in all three of these brain regions (FIG. 2). How this regulation of GFAP expression occurs in reactive astrocytes during 6-OHDA-induced dopamine neuron degeneration is not yet understood. 6-OHDA injected into the SN is taken up into neurons by the catecholamine carrier system and produces its toxic effects following auto-oxidation, but does not act directly on glial cells. The alteration of GFAP expression must therefore be due to a product associated with neuronal degeneration, and can occur over long distances as seen in the striatum and cortex, both of which receive dopaminergic innervation. These results suggest that factors,

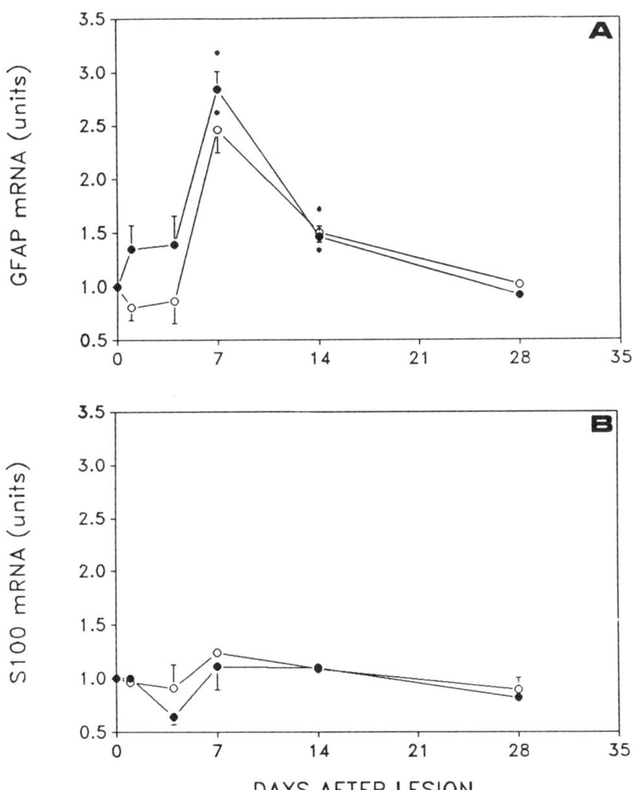

FIGURE 3. Time course of changes in ipsi- and contralateral striatal GFAP and S100β mRNA following 6-OHDA lesion. Animals were lesioned with 6-OHDA and sacrificed at the indicated days following lesion. GFAP mRNA **(A)** and S100β mRNA **(B)** were measured as described in MATERIALS AND METHODS for the lesioned side (●) and the contralateral side (○).

TABLE 1. Changes in Nerve Growth Factor and Proenkephalin mRNAs in "Reactive" Striatal Astrocytes from MPTP-lesioned Mouse Brain

Treatment	NGF mRNA (units)	PE mRNA (units)
Control	1.01 ± 0.11	2.77 ± 0.19
MPTP	1.81 ± 0.12^a	0.26 ± 0.01^a

Animals were injected with 20 mg/kg MPTP twice/day for 4 days. Astrocytes were prepared from striatum 10 days after the last injection.

[a] $p < .001$ vs. control.

as yet unidentified, may be released from damaged neurons into the extracellular space, where they could act directly on astrocytes, or indirectly via another cell, such as the microglia. This raises two important questions: 1) are the same factors involved as in development (*i.e.*, does Factor X_{DEV} = Factor X_{INJ}?—FIG. 4); and 2) could changes in astrocyte NTF production be used as another marker of neuronal injury?

Factors already known to activate GFAP expression and/or astrocyte division include hydrocortisone, putrescine, prostaglandin F2α, fibroblast growth factor,

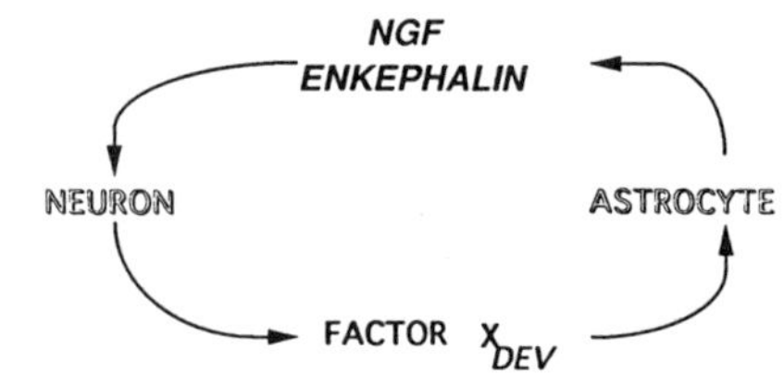

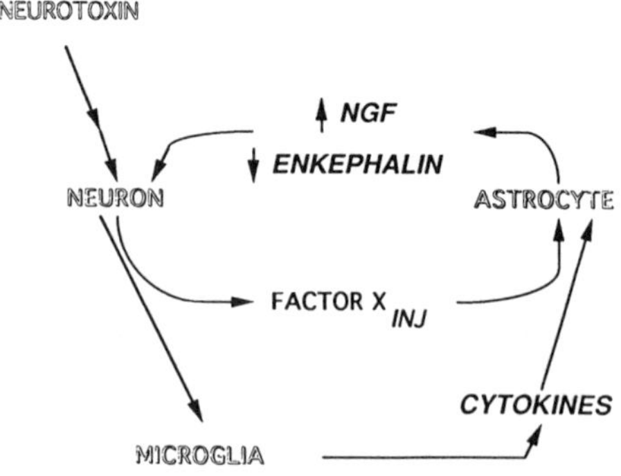

FIGURE 4. Hypothetical scheme for neuronal-glial interactions during development and following injury.

epidermal growth factor, and interleukin-1β.[24–26] These are potential candidates for inducing the glial reaction but most of them are not neuronally derived, suggesting the involvement of other cell types such as the microglia (FIG. 4). Developmentally, both NGF and PE decrease in striatal astrocytes.[27,28] Following MPTP treatment, NGF mRNA increased but PE mRNA decreased in "reactive" astrocytes derived from MPTP-lesioned striatum (TABLE 1), suggesting that not all NTFs are increased following injury. Furthermore, S100β mRNA was unchanged following 6-OHDA lesion (FIG. 3B). Since enkephalins appear to act as inhibitory modulators of CNS development (reviewed in ref. 22), one would not necessarily want an increased amount of astrocyte-derived enkephalins in the injured brain. In summary, astrocyte gene expression following injury does not perfectly mirror the developmental pattern (FIG. 4), suggesting that glia may be capable of selective and appropriate responses to injury. Understanding the factors involved in this regulation is essential if we wish to control the glial response in order to make it an appropriate one in terms of neuronal recovery.

REFERENCES

1. HOZUMI, I., F-C. CHIU & W. T. NORTON. 1990. Brain Res. **524:** 64–71.
2. HOZUMI, I., D. A. AQUINO & W. T. NORTON. 1990. Brain Res. **534:** 291–294.
3. MATHEWSON, A. J. & M. BERRY. 1985. Brain Res. **327:** 61–69.
4. TAKAMIYA, Y., S. KOHSAKA, S. TOYA, M. OTANI & Y. TSUKADA. 1988. Dev. Brain Res. **38:** 201–210.
5. REINHARD, J. F., D. B. MILLER & J. P. O'CALLAGHAN. 1988. Neurosci. Lett. **95:** 246–251.
6. SCHNEIDER, J. S. & F. J. DENARO. 1988. J. Neuropathol. Exp. Neurol. **47:** 452–458.
7. STROMBERG, I., H. BJÖRKLUND, D. DAHL, G. JONSSON, E. SUNDSTROM & L. OLSON. 1986. Brain Res. Bull. **17:** 225–236.
8. OGAWA, M., M. ARAKI, I. NAGATSU & M. YOSHIDA. 1989. Exp. Neurol. **106:** 187–196.
9. RATABOUL, P., N. FAUCON BIGUET, P. VERNIER, F. DE VITRY, S. BOULARAND, A. PRIVAT & J. MALLET. 1988. J. Neurosci. Res. **20:** 165–175.
10. GOMEZ-PINILLA, G., B. J. CUMMINGS & C. W. COTMAN. 1990. NeuroReport **1:** 211–214.
11. FUXE, K., E. ANGGARD, K. LUNDGREN, A. CINTRA, L. F. AGNATI, S. GALTON & J. VANE. 1989. Acta Physiol. Scand. **137:** 563–564.
12. SHINODA, H., A. M. MARINI & J. P. SCHWARTZ. 1992. Dev. Brain Res. **67:** 205–210.
13. SHENG, J. G., S. SHIRABE, N. NISHIYAMA & J. P. SCHWARTZ. 1993. Exp. Brain Res. In press.
14. SCHWARTZ, J. P. & K. MISHLER. 1990. Cell. Mol. Neurobiol. **10:** 447–457.
15. SPRUCE, B. A., R. CURTIS, G. P. WILKIN & D. M. GLOVER. 1990. EMBO J. **9:** 1787–1795.
16. AQUINO, D. A., F-C. CHIU, C. F. BROSNAN & W. T. NORTON. 1988. J. Neurochem. **51:** 1085–1096.
17. CHIU, F-C. & J. E. GOLDMAN. 1985. J. Neuroimmunol. **8:** 283–292.
18. KRAIG, R. P., L. DONG, R. THISTED & C. B. JAEGER. 1991. J. Neurosci. **11:** 2187–2198.
19. TRIMMER, P. A., P. J. REIER, T. H. OH & L. F. ENG. 1982. J. Neuroimmunol. **2:** 235–260.
20. SELINFREUND, R. H., S. W. BARGER, W. J. PLEDGER & L. J. VAN ELDIK. 1991. Proc. Natl. Acad. Sci. USA **88:** 3554–3558.
21. KIMELBERG, H. K. 1988. Glial Cell Receptors. Raven Press. New York.
22. SCHWARTZ, J. P. 1993. Neuropeptide expression in astrocytes. *In* Astrocytes: Pharmacology and Function. S. Murphy, Ed. Academic Press. San Diego, CA.
23. LARGE, T. H., S. C. BODARY, D. O. CLEGG, G. WESKAMP, U. OTTEN & L. F. REICHARDT. 1986. Science **234:** 352–355.
24. GIULIAN, D., K. VACA & B. JOHNSON. 1988. J. Neurosci. Res. **21:** 487–500.

25. MORRISON, R. S., J. DE VELLIS, Y. L. LEE, R. A. BRADSHAW & L. F. ENG. 1985. J. Neurosci. Res. **14:** 167–176.
26. ZINI, I., M. ZOLI, R. GRIMALDI, E. M. PICH, G. BIAGINI, K. FUXE & L. F. AGNATI. 1990. Neurosci. Lett. **27:** 13–16.
27. MITSUO, K. & J. P. SCHWARTZ. 1992. J. Mol. Neurosci. In press.
28. VILIJN, M-H., P. J-J. VAYSSE, R. S. ZUKIN & J. A. KESSLER. 1988. Proc. Natl. Acad. Sci. USA **85:** 6551–6555.

Sulfated Glycoprotein-2:
An Emerging Molecular Marker
for Neurodegeneration

PATRICK C. MAY[a]

CNS and Molecular Biology Research
Lilly Research Laboratories
Eli Lilly and Co.
Indianapolis, Indiana 46285

Efforts toward understanding mechanisms of neuronal cell death have intensified in the past several years in part driven by the increasing prevalence of Alzheimer's disease and other age-related neurodegenerative disorders. While frank neuron loss can be easily visualized by cell counting techniques, this approach provides little insight into the preceding neurodegenerative process. In contrast, characterization of biochemical and molecular changes accompanying neuronal degeneration may identify common pathways shared by various neuronal insults or point to novel mechanisms specific for a single disease process. In addition, biochemical markers identified by this approach may be more sensitive in assessing subtle manifestations of neuronal damage resulting in dysfunction but not overt cell loss.

Sulfated glycoprotein-2 (SGP-2) is a prominent marker of neurodegeneration emerging from this molecular approach.[1,2] SGP-2 RNA and related sequences have been repeatedly cloned from neural-derived cDNA libraries screened by differential or subtractive hybridization techniques (TABLE 1). For example, pADHC-9, a human cDNA related to SGP-2, was isolated from a hippocampal cDNA library by virtue of its overexpression in Alzheimer's disease hippocampus.[3–5] Hamster[6] and quail[7] cognates were isolated around the same time using related molecular techniques dependent upon overexpression in pathologic neural tissue. Most recently, SGP-2 was cloned from a human glioma[8] and degenerating retina from victims of retinitis pigmentosa.[9] The remarkable cloning of SGP-2 from these independent studies highlights its robust induction during neurodegenerative processes and also suggests a certain overlap in genes induced in response to neuronal injury.

SGP-2 EXPRESSION IN ALZHEIMER'S DISEASE

Altered expression of SGP-2 in Alzheimer's disease was confirmed by analysis of individual hippocampal RNA samples from AD and controls; these studies suggest an overall two-to-threefold increase in SGP-2 RNA albeit with some individual variability.[4–6] Limited analyses suggested that SGP-2 RNA levels were

[a] Address correspondence to: Patrick C. May, Ph.D., Lilly Research Laboratories, Lilly Corporate Center, Eli Lilly and Co., Indianapolis, IN 46285; FAX (317)276-9086.

not altered in cerebellum, a region less involved in Alzheimer's pathology (May *et al.*, unpublished data). *In situ* hybridization analyses identified a prominent laminar distribution of SGP-2 transcripts in the entorhinal cortex and hippocampal formation suggestive of localization to pyramidal neurons as well as dentate gyrus granule neurons (FIG. 1). High resolution emulsion autoradiography revealed prominent grain clusters over presumptive pyramidal and granule cell neurons, as well as over presumptive astrocytes in the hilus and molecular layer of the dentate gyrus.[5] Consistent with altered SGP-2 RNA expression, recent immunohistochemical studies detect SGP-2 protein that co-localizes to β-amyloid plaques within the parenchyma of Alzheimer's brain; little to no parenchymal expression was observed in aged-matched controls.[10,11] The function of SGP-2 in Alzheimer's disease brain is not known but likely relates to neurodegenerative and regenerative processes occurring in the hippocampus (see below).

TABLE 1. SGP-2-related Clones Isolated by Differential Screening of Neural-derived cDNA Libraries

cDNA Clone	Library Source	Differential Screen
pADHC-9[3,4,5]	Human hippocampus	Alzheimer's vs. CTL
T64[7]	Quail neuroretinal cell line	Transformed vs. CTL
SGP-2[6]	Hamster brain	Scrapie-infected vs. CTL
TB16[8]	Human glioma	Glioma vs. CTL
K661[9]	Human retina	Retinitis pigmentosa vs. CTL

SGP-2 REGULATION IN RODENT BRAIN

Rodent lesion models have been used extensively to assess dynamic changes in SGP-2 expression following brain injury (TABLE 2). Initially, these lesion studies attempted to model the intrinsic neuron loss or hippocampal deafferentation observed in Alzheimer's disease. Following direct injection of kainic acid, hippocampal pyramidal neurons degenerate within days.[12] The pyramidal neuronal degeneration is accompanied by a two-to-threefold increase in SGP-2 RNA and protein levels.[2,13] By *in situ* hybridization localization, much of the SGP-2 induction occurs in reactive astrocytes.[2,14] Immunocytochemical analyses localized SGP-2 protein to degenerating CA3 and CA4 pyramidal neurons in the hippocampus and hilus of the dentate gyrus; little SGP-2 immunoreactivity was observed in young intact controls.[5] Similar lack of neuronal SGP-2 immunoreactivity was observed in young (3–4 months) Sprague-Dawley rats but neuronal expression increases with age in several brain regions including hippocampus.[15]

Deafferentation of the hippocampus is also a prominent feature of Alzheimer's disease pathology.[16] This aspect of Alzheimer's neuropathology can be modeled in rodents by lesion of the entorhinal cortex which projects to the hippocampus.[17,18] Experimental deafferentation of the rat hippocampus results in increased expression of SGP-2 RNA[5,19,21] and protein[20] (TABLE 2). Induction of SGP-2 occurred early on in reactive astrocytes, but at later times, SGP-2 immunoreactive deposits appeared in the neuropil.[20] These changes in SGP-2 expression are coincident with

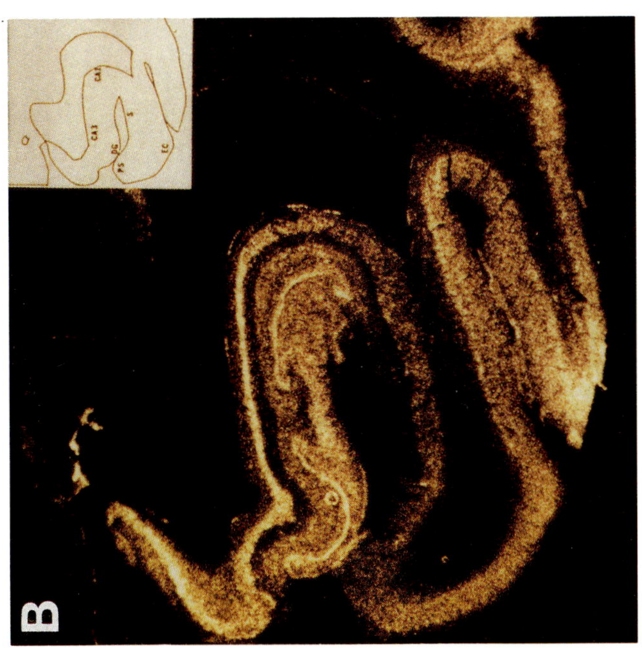

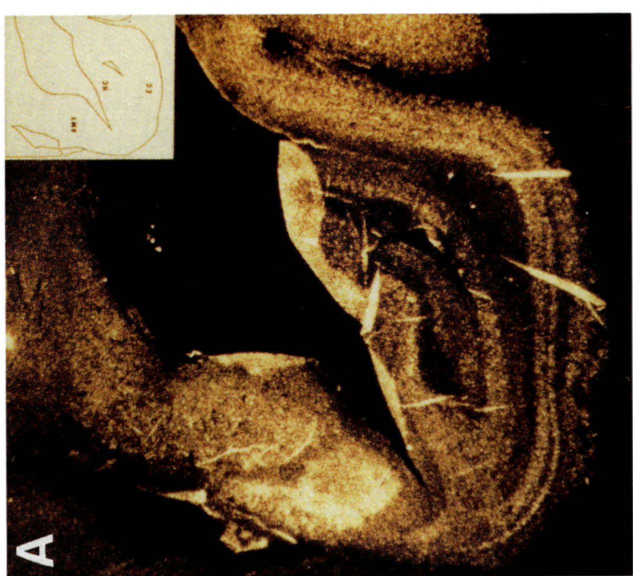

FIGURE 1. *In situ* mapping of pADHC-9/SGP-2 RNA transcripts in human temporal cortex. **(A)** Temporal lobe section from an 82-year-old male with Alzheimer's disease hybridized with an antisense 35S-cRNA probe for pADHC-9. Note the prominent laminar hybridization in layers of the entorhinal cortex (EC). **(B)** Temporal lobe section from a 78-year-old female with Alzheimer's disease hybridized with an antisense 35S-cRNA probe for pADHC-9. Note the prominent hybridization over the hippocampal pyramidal cell layer (CA) and granule cell layer of the dentate gyrus (DG). Hybridization with sense-strand cRNA probes for pAHDC-9/SGP-2 was not above background. (Reprinted with permission from May *et al.*,[5] 1990.)

TABLE 2. Experimental Lesions Affecting SGP-2 Expression in Brain

| | Lesion/Site | RNA Changes | | Protein Changes | |
		Northern	*In Situ* Localization	Blot	ICC Localization
KA	Hippocampal CA3 & CA4	2 fold[2,13]	Hilar cells, reactive astrocytes[2]	Elev.[13]	Atrophic CA3/CA4 pyramidal neurons[5]
IBO	Caudate nucleus interneurons	N.D.	Reactive astrocytes[14]	N.D.	N.D.
4VO	Hippocampal CA1 Caudate nucleus	2 fold[23]	N.D.	Elev.[23]	N.D.
ECL	Sprouting in molecular layer of DG	2–4 fold[5,19,21]	Reactive astrocytes in hilus and molecular layer of DG[19,21]	Elev.[20]	React. astro. in hilus & molec. layer of DG (early)[20] Punctate deposits in molec. layer of DG (late)[20]
CTX/ASP.	Sprouting in caudate nucleus	3–4 fold[26]	Reactive astrocytes[26]	Elev.[26]	N.D.
ADX	Granule cell loss in DG	N.D.	N.D.	N.D.	React. astro. adjacent to degenerating granule cells; Punctate deposits in molec. layer of DG[56]
ODX	Unknown	2 fold[19]	Reactive astrocytes[19]	N.D.	React. astro. in hilus and molec. layer of DG[19]

Abbreviations: KA–intraventricular kainate injection; IBO–intrastriatal ibotenate injection; 4VO–4 vessel occlusion; ECL–entorhinal cortex lesion; CTX/ASP–cortical aspiration; ADX–adrenalectomy; ODX–orchidectomy; N.D.–Not determined; DG–dentate gyrus; CA–hippocampal pyramidal cell layer.

the time course for lesion-induced sprouting and reactive synaptogenesis occurring in the molecular layer of the dentate gyrus.[22]

Studies examining SGP-2 expression in lesioned rodent brain have now extended beyond modeling of Alzheimer's disease hippocampal pathology (TABLE

A. SGP-2 RNA Blot: Caudate Nucleus

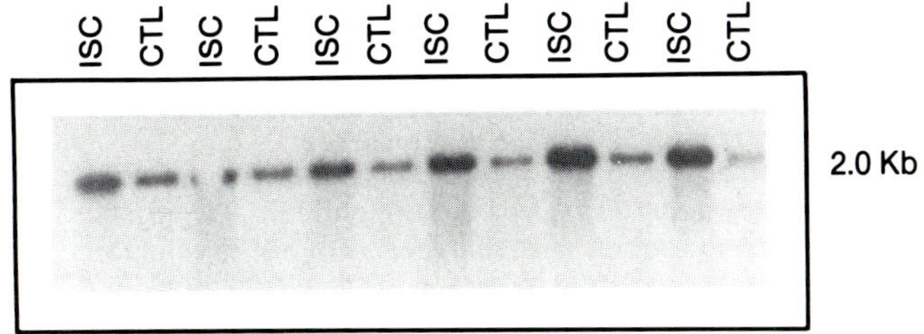

B. SGP-2 Immunoblot: Caudate Nucleus

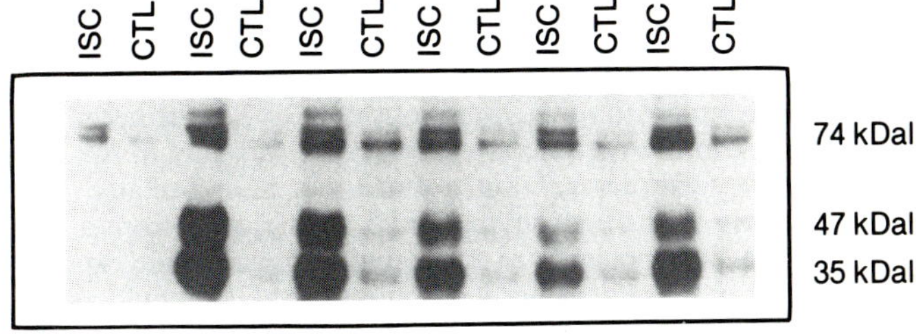

FIGURE 2. Induction of SGP-2 RNA and protein in rat caudate nucleus subjected to transient global ischemia. **(A).** Total RNA (3 μg) from individual caudate nucleus homogenates was size fractionated by denaturing agarose gel, blotted to nylon and hybridized with 32P-hexamer labeled SGP-2 DNA probes. SGP-2 mRNA transcripts were induced twofold by 30 min of ischemia. **(B)** Total protein (5 μg) from individual caudate homogenates was size fractionated by SDS-PAGE under reducing conditions, electroblotted to nitrocellulose and probed with anti-rat SGP-2. This antibody recognizes the intact precursor (74 kDal) and its two processed subunits (47 and 35 kDal) which normally associate via disulfide bonds. Global ischemia results in a marked increase in SGP-2 protein levels in the caudate. (SGP-2 cDNA and polyclonal antibody were kindly provided by Dr. Michael Griswold and Dr. Steven Sylvestor, Washington State University, Pullman WA. Reprinted with permission from May *et al.*,[23] 1992.)

2). For example, expression of SGP-2 increases in the caudate nucleus and hippocampus 3 days after 30 minutes of transient global ischemia (FIG. 2). In this model, the caudate nucleus degenerates within 24 hours, but hippocampal CA1 pyramidal neurons undergo a delayed neurodegeneration requiring 48–72 hours to be manifested.[23,24] Interestingly, SGP-2 RNA levels are already increased in the caudate

cytes.[5,19–21,42] Thus, reverse cholesterol transport by SGP-2 could serve a neurotrophic role for damaged neurons.

SGP-2 may have additional presumptive neurotrophic activities unrelated to lipid transport. SGP-2 could mediate cell : cell or cell : extracellular matrix interactions via predicted heparin-binding domains on SGP-2[37] which may facilitate adherence to heparan sulfate proteoglycans in the extracellular matrix. Following entorhinal cortex lesion, deposits of SGP-2 transiently appear in the terminal projection fields around the time of axonal sprouting and reactive synaptogenesis.[20] These neuropil deposits of SGP-2 are reminiscent of similarly transient deposits of J1/tenascin glycoprotein expressed during CNS development.[43] J1/tenascin expression defines boundaries in projection areas of CNS and may assist in pattern formation and synaptogenesis as J1/tenascin expression is altered in the cortex of genetically mutant mice.[43]

Neuroprotective Role

SGP-2 induced following neuronal injury may serve a neuroprotective function. Complement Lysis Inhibitor (CLI) and serum protein 40,40 (SP 40,40) are human serum-derived proteins related to rat SGP-2 that were isolated as components of the membrane attack complex of complement.[44,45] Hydrophobic domains predicted for SGP-2 protein may inhibit binding of nascent C5b-7 to membrane surfaces and thus attenuate complement-dependent cytolysis; such inhibition of complement lysis has been demonstrated *in vitro*.[44,46] Numerous proteins of the complement pathway have been localized to either β-amyloid plaques or surrounding dystrophic neurites in Alzheimer's disease brain.[47–52] In addition, β-amyloid plaques may initiate the complement cascade by binding and activating C1q protein.[53] Thus, increased expression of SGP-2 in Alzheimer's disease could be a compensatory response to limit ongoing complement-mediated damage.[5]

Somewhat unexpectedly, mRNAs encoding at least two of the early complement proteins (C1q and C4) are expressed endogenously in rat brain and markedly induced after lesions.[54,55] Whether lesion-induced expression of early complement factors is sufficient to trigger activation of the complete complement cascade will require demonstration of the active membrane attack complex in brain regions undergoing degeneration. Nonetheless, the potential for complement activation in rat brain after injury coupled with *in vitro* data showing complement inhibitory activity of human cognates of rat SGP-2 suggests a possible unique neuroprotective role for brain SGP-2.

CONCLUSION

This short review has explored the emerging neurobiology of SGP-2 as it relates to neurodegeneration. Induction of SGP-2 arises from a variety of neuronal insults and thus appears to be a reliable marker for neurodegeneration. Collectively, these studies also suggest some general involvement of SGP-2 in neurodegeneration and remodeling following neuronal injury. Understanding the function of SGP-2 in brain will require rigorous biochemical functional analysis using purified protein. Study of this neurodegeneration marker may ultimately identify common pathways for pharmacologic intervention which either retard neurodegenerative processes or accelerate neuronal recovery from injury.

REFERENCES

1. MAY, P. C. & C. E. FINCH. 1992. Trends in Neurosci. **15:** 391–396.
2. MICHEL, D., J-G. CHABOT, E. MOYSE, M. DANIK & R. QUIRION. 1992. Synapse **11:** 105–111.
3. MAY, P. C. & C. E. FINCH. 1988. *In* The Molecular Biology of Alzheimer's Disease. Current Communication Molecular Biology, C. E. Finch & P. Davies, Eds.: 43–46. Cold Spring Harbor Laboratory. Cold Spring Harbor, NY.
4. MAY, P. C., S. A. JOHNSON, J. POIRIER, M. A. LAMPERT-ETCHELLS & C. E. FINCH. 1989. Can. J. Neurol. Sci. **16:** 473–476.
5. MAY, P. C., M. A. LAMPERT-ETCHELLS, S. A. JOHNSON, J. POIRIER, J. N. MASTERS & C. E. FINCH. 1990. Neuron **5:** 831–839.
6. DUGUID, J. R., C. W. BOHMONT, N. LIU & W. W. TOURTELLOTTE. 1989. Proc. Natl. Acad. Sci. USA **86:** 7260–7264.
7. MICHEL, D., G. GILLET, M. VOLOVITCH, B. PESSAC, G. CALOTHY & G. BRUN. 1989. Oncogene Res. **4:** 127–136.
8. DANIK, M., J. G. CHABOT, C. MERCIER, A. L. DENABID, C. CHAUVIN, R. QUIRION & M. SUH. 1991. Proc. Natl. Acad. Sci. USA **88:** 8577–8581.
9. JONES, S. E., J. M. A. MEERABUX, D. A. YEATS & M. J. NEAL. 1992. FEBS **300:** 279–282.
10. MCGEER, P. L., T. KAWAMATA & D. WALKER. 1992. Brain Res. **579:** 337–341.
11. CHOI-MIURA, N-H., Y. IHARA, K. FUKUCHI, M. TAKEDA, N. NAKANO, T. TOBE & M. TOMITA. 1992. Acta Neuropathol. **83:** 260–264.
12. NADLER, J. N., B. W. PERRY & C. W. COTMAN. 1978. Nature **271:** 676–677.
13. MAY, P. C. & M. LAMPERT-ETCHELLS. 1990. Soc. Neurosci. Abs. **16:** 1267.
14. PASINETTI, G. M. & C. E. FINCH. 1991. Neuroscience Lett. **130:** 1–4.
15. SENUT, M. C., N. H. CHOI, F. OAZAT & Y. LAMOUR. 1992. Soc. Neurosci. Abs. **18:** 1489.
16. HYMAN, B. T., G. W. VAN HOESEN, A. R. DAMASIO & C. L. BARNES. 1984. Science **225:** 1168–1170.
17. COTMAN, C. W. & M. NIETRO-SAMPEDRO. 1985. Science **25:** 1287–1294.
18. GEDDES, J. W., D. T. MONAGHAN, C. W. COTMAN, I. T. LOTT, R. C. KIM & H. C. CHIU. 1985. Science **230:** 1179–1181.
19. DAY, J. R., N. J. LAPPING, T. H. MCNEIL, S. S. SCHREIBER, G. PASINETTI & C. E. FINCH. 1990. Mol. Endocrinol. **4:** 1995–2002.
20. LAMPERT-ETCHELLS, M., T. H. MCNEILL, N. LAPPING, C. ZAROW, C. E. FINCH & P. C. MAY. 1991. Brain Res. **563:** 101–106.
21. LAPING, N. J., N. R. NICHOLS, J. R. DAY & C. E. FINCH. 1991. Mol. Brain Res. **10:** 291–297.
22. STEWARD, O., S. L. VINSANT & L. DAVIS. 1988. J. Comp. Neurol. **267:** 203–210.
23. MAY, P. C., P. ROBISON, K. FUSON, B. SMALSTIG, D. STEPHENSON & J. A. CLEMENS. 1992. Mol. Brain. Res. **15:** 33–39.
24. PULSINELLI, W. A. 1985. Prog. Brain Res. **63:** 29–37.
25. FUSON, K. S., J. A. CLEMENS, J. A. PANETTA, E. B. SMALSTIG & P. C. MAY. 1992. Soc. Neurosci. Abs. **18:** 1261.
26. PASINETTI, G. M., H. W. CHENG, D. G. MORGAN, M. LAMPERT-ETCHELLS, T. H. MCNEILL & C. E. FINCH. 1993. Neuroscience. In press.
27. KISSINGER, C., M. K. SKINNER & M. D. GRISWOLD. 1982. Biol. Reprod. **27:** 233–240.
28. COLLARD, M. W. & M. D. GRISWOLD. 1987. Biochemistry **26:** 3297–3303.
29. LEGER, J. G., M. L. MONPETIT & M. P. TENNISWOOD. 1987. Biochem. Biophys. Res. Commun. **147:** 196–203.
30. BETTUZZI, S., R. A. HIIPAKKA, P. GILNA & S. LIAO. 1989. Biochem. J. **257:** 293–296.
31. BUTTYAN, R., C. A. OLSSON, J. PINTAR, C. CHANG, M. BANDYK. P-Y. NG & I. S. SAWCZUK. 1989. Mol. Cell. Biol. **9:** 3473–3481.
32. KYPRIANOU, N., R. B. ALEXANDER & J. T. ISAACS. 1991. J. Natl. Cancer Inst. **83:** 346–350.
33. GARDEN, G. A., M. BOTHWELL & E. W. RUBEL. 1991. J. Neurobiol. **22:** 590–604.

34. COPANI, A., D. T. LOO, C. J. PIKE, A. J. WALENCEWICZ & C. W. COTMAN. 1992. Soc. Neurosci. Abs. **18:** 1439.
35. FORLONI, G., R. CHIESA, N., ANGERETTI & S. SMIROLDO. 1992. Soc. Neurosci. Abs. **18:** 1439.
36. FRITZ, I. B., K. BURDZY, B. SETCHELL & O. BLASCHUK. 1983. Biol. Reprod. **28:** 1173–1188.
37. DE SILVA, H. V., J. L. HARMONY, W. D. STUART, C. M. GIL & J. ROBBINS. 1990. Biochemistry **29:** 5380–5389.
38. DE SILVA, H. V., W. D. STUART, C. R. DUVIC, J. R. WETTERAU, M. J. RAY, D. G. FERGUSON, H. W. ALBERS, W. R. SMITH & J. A. HARMONY. 1990. J. Biol. Chem. **265:** 13240–13247.
39. JENNE, D. E., B. LOWIN, M. C. PEITSCH, A. BOTTCHER, G. SCHMITZ & J. TSCHOPP. 1991. J. Biol. Chem. **266:** 11030–11036.
40. BOYLES, J. K., C. D. ZOELLNER, L. J. ANDERSON, L. M. KOSIK, R. E. PITAS, K. H. WEISGRABER, D. Y. HUI, R. W. MAHLEY, P. J. GEBICKE-HAERTER, M. L. IGNATIUS & E. M. SHOOTER. 1989. J. Clin. Invest. **83:** 1015–1031.
41. MAHLEY, R. W. 1988. Science **240:** 622–630.
42. POIRIER, J., M. HESS, P. C. MAY & C. E. FINCH. 1991. Mol. Brain Res. **11:** 97–106.
43. STEINDLER, D. A., T. F. O'BRIEN, E. LAYWELL, K., HARRINGTON, A. FAISSNER & M. SCHACHNER. 1990. Exp. Neurol. **109:** 35–56.
44. JENNE, D. E. & J. TSCHOPP. 1989. Proc. Natl. Acad. Sci. USA **86:** 7123–7127.
45. KIRSZBAUM, L., J. A. SHARPE, B. MURPHY, A. J. F. D'APICE, B. CLASSON, P. HUDSON & I. D. WALKER. 1989. EMBO J. **8:** 711–718.
46. CHOI, N.-H., T. MAZDA & M. TOMITA. 1989. Mol. Immunol. **26:** 835–840.
47. EIKELENBOOM P. & F. C. STAM. 1982. Acta Neuropathol. **57:** 239–242.
48. MCGEER, P. L., H. AKIYAMA, S. ITAGAKI & E. G. MCGEER. 1988. Can. J. Neurol. Sci. **16:** 516–527.
49. EIKELENBOOM, P., C. E. HACK, J. M. ROZEMULLER & F. C. STAM. 1989. Virchows Arch. (Cell Pathol.) **56:** 259–262.
50. MCGEER, P. L., H. AKIYAMA, S. ITAGAKI & E. G. MCGEER. 1989. Neuroscience Lett. **17:** 341–346.
51. MCGEER, P. L., D. G. WALKER, H. AKIYAMA, T. KAWAMATE, A. L. GUAN, C. J. PARKER, N. OKADA & E. G. MCGEER. 1991. Brain Res. **544:** 315–319.
52. ROGERS, J., J. LUBER-NAROD, S. D. STYREN & W. H. CIVIN. 1988. Neurobiol. Aging **9:** 330–349.
53. ROGERS, J., N. R. COOPER, S. WEBSTER, J. SCHULTZ, P. L. MCGEER, S. STYREN, W. H. CIVIN, L. BRACHOVA, B. BRADT, P. WARD & I. LIEBERBURG. 1992. Proc. Natl. Acad. Sci. USA **89:** 10016–10020.
54. JOHNSON, S. A., G. M. PASINETTI, M. LAMPERT-ETCHELLS & C. E. FINCH. 1992. Neurobiol. Aging. **13:** 641–648.
55. PASINETTI, G. M., S. A. JOHNSON, I. ROZOVSKY, M. LAMPERT-ETCHELLS, D. G. MORGAN, M. N. MORGAN, T. E. MORGAN, D. WILLOUGHBY & C. E. FINCH. 1992. Exp. Neurol. **118:** 117–125.
56. MCNEILL, T. H., J. N. MASTERS & C. E. FINCH. 1991. Exp. Neurol. **111:** 140–144.
57. PALMER, D. J. & D. L. CHRISTIE. 1990. J. Biol. Chem. **265:** 6617–6623.
58. HARTMANN, K., J. RAUCH, J. URBAN, K. PARCZYK, P. DIEL, C. PILARSKY, D. APPEL, W. HAASE, K. MANN, A. WELLER & C. KOCH-BRANDT. 1991. J. Biol. Chem. **266:** 9924–9931.
59. DIEMER, V. M. HOYLE, C. BAGLIONI & A. J. T. MILLS. 1992. J. Biol. Chem. **267:** 5257–5264.
60. JENNE, D. E. & J. TSCHOPP. 1992. Trends Biochem. Sci. **17:** 154–159.

Laminin-like and Laminin-binding Protein-like Immunoreactive Astrocytes in Rat Hippocampus after Transient Ischemia

Antibody to Laminin-binding Protein Is a Sensitive Marker of Neural Injury and Degeneration

MATHIAS JUCKER,[a,f,g] PAUL BIALOBOK,[b]
HYNDA K. KLEINMAN,[c] LARY C. WALKER,[d]
THEO HAGG,[e] AND DONALD K. INGRAM[a]

[a]Gerontology Research Center
National Institute on Aging
National Institutes of Health
Baltimore, Maryland 21224

[b]Fisons Corporation
755 Jefferson Road
Rochester, New York 14623

[c]Developmental Biology Laboratory
National Institute of Dental Research
National Institutes of Health
Bethesda, Maryland 20892

[d]Neuropathology Laboratory
Johns Hopkins University School of Medicine
Baltimore, Maryland 21205

[e]Department of Biology
University of California, San Diego
La Jolla, California 92093

[f]Department of Neurobiology
Swiss Federal Institute of Technology
CH-8093 Zürich, Switzerland

Laminin is a potent promoter of neurite outgrowth for neurons of the peripheral and central nervous systems.[1] The molecule was initially described as a distinct basement membrane glycoprotein composed of three disulfide-linked polypeptide chains[2,3] (B1-A-B2 chain; see FIG. 1). The discoveries of *S-laminin*, a homolog of the B1 chain,[4] and *merosin*, a variant of laminin with an M-chain instead of the homologous A chain,[5] imply a molecular heterogeneity within the laminin family. S-laminin is expressed in the synaptic basal lamina of the neuromuscular

[g] Address correspondence to Mathias Jucker, Ph.D. in Zürich; Tel.: 41-1-377 33 83; FAX: 41-1-371 02 35.

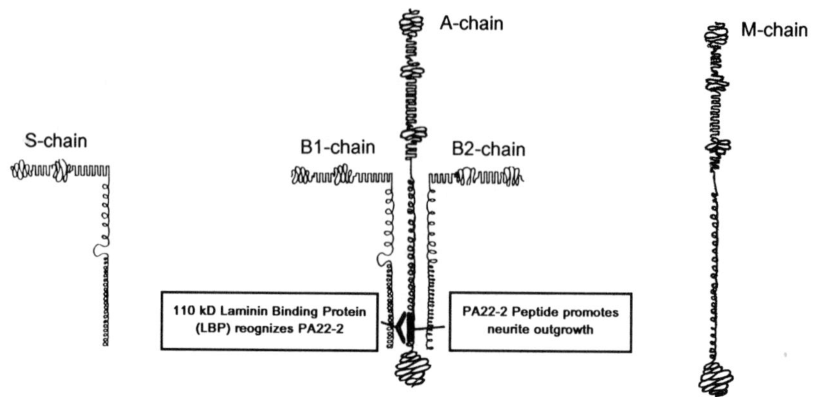

FIGURE 1. Schematic model of EHS laminin [B1-A-B2 chain] and the more recently discovered subunit homologs [S-chain; M-chain] (adapted from Sanes *et al.*[7]). In the present study, antibodies to laminin subunits and to the 110 kD laminin-binding protein (LBP), that interacts with a neurite-outgrowth promoting peptide from the laminin A chain, were used to study expression of laminin- and LBP-like molecules in response to transient ischemia.

junction, while merosin is expressed in the human placenta, in muscle and in peripheral nerve basal lamina and brain. Recently several new laminin isoforms assembled from the characterized subunits have been described that might serve spatially and temporally distinct functions.[6,7]

In normal brain, laminin can be immunohistochemically identified as a component of basement membrane—the thin, dense extracellular matrix structure that surrounds capillary elements.[8–10] Laminin-like molecules have also been demonstrated in neurons throughout the CNS[9–14] and associated with reactive glial cells in response to CNS injury.[9,15–17] In the developing mammalian CNS during periods of axonal growth, transient deposits of laminin-like molecules are observed.[13,18–20] Although the structure of CNS-derived laminin molecules has been only partially characterized, expression of laminin isoforms in the CNS is likely.[11,21,37]

A 19-amino acid synthetic peptide (PA22-2) derived from the C-terminal end of the laminin A chain (FIG. 1) has been identified as corresponding to a site on laminin with neurite–out growth activity for CNS neurons.[22,23] A putative receptor to this neurite outgrowth promoting site has been extracted from newborn mouse brain and identified as a non-integrin 110 kD laminin-binding protein[24] (LBP; FIG. 1). Antibody to LBP strongly immunostains fibers and distinct neuronal populations in normal adult brain while intense staining of reactive glial cells has been observed after CNS lesions.[25]

The role of reactive glial cells in damaged-induced reorganization and neurodegeneration has become increasingly important to analyze.[26–29] While the scar formed by reactive glial cells is believed to inhibit successful CNS regeneration, the expression of potential neurotrophic and neurite-promoting factors by reactive astrocytes might be beneficial for a lesion-induced restorative sprouting response.[26] The finding that reactive glial cells exhibit laminin-like and intense LBP-like immunoreactivities in response to CNS injury may suggest an interaction between laminin molecules and LBP in response to injury. This possibility prompted us to characterize reactive glial cell-derived laminin and LBP and to study their temporal expression in reactive glial cells in response to ischemia. Here we report the initial results of this ongoing study to suggest that antibody to LBP may be a suitable diagnostic marker in neuropathological evaluations of neural injury and degeneration.

Anesthetized 3-month old male Sprague-Dawley rats were subjected to 15 min of transient temperature-controlled ischemia by the method of 4-vessel occlusion.[30,31] After survival periods of 2 to 160 days, brains were perfusion-fixed and analyzed immunohistochemically as described elsewhere.[25] After transient and relatively moderate ischemia, the CA1 pyramidal neurons of the hippocampus have been shown to be selectively vulnerable, and delayed damage of these neurons has been observed to develop 24 to 72 hours after ischemia and beyond.[30,31] The loss of CA1 pyramidal cells 32 days after transient ischemia is demonstrated by thionin Nissl stain in FIGURE 2.

For the immunohistochemical evaluation of ischemic neuronal injury, the following antibodies were used: Polyclonal antibody to purified LBP;[24] polyclonal antibody to EHS laminin [B1-A-B2 chain];[32] monoclonal antibody (2E8) to the B2 laminin chain[33] (gift of E. Engvall); polyclonal and monoclonal (2G9) antibodies

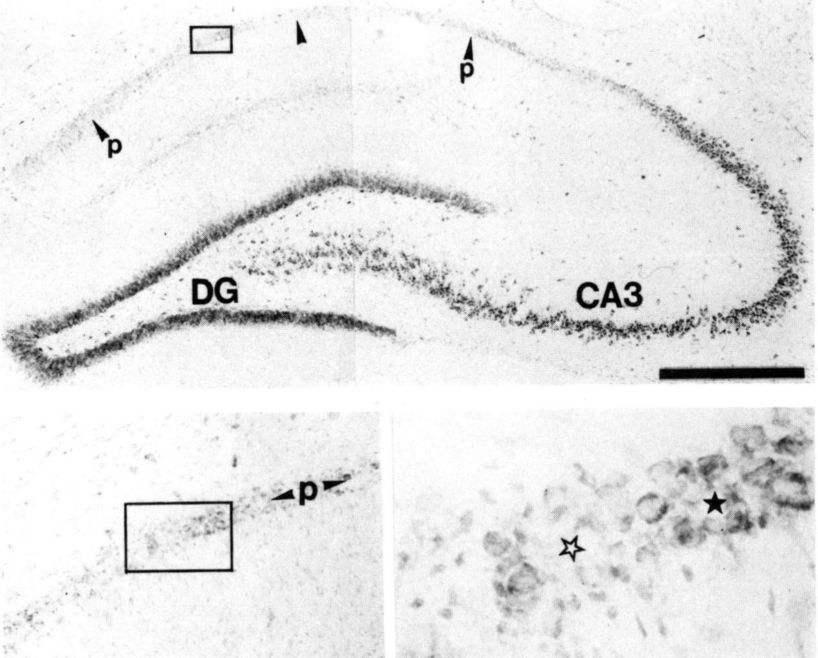

FIGURE 2. Thionin Nissl stain of a coronal section through the dorsal rat hippocampus 32 days after transient ischemia revealed degeneration of CA1 pyramidal cells (p) but sparing of CA3 pyramidal neurons and granules cells of the dentate gyrus (DG). Higher magnification of Nissl-stained CA1 pyramidal cells shows small clusters of surviving neurons (asterisk) among degenerated ones (open asterisk). The CA1 region is infiltrated by non-neuronal cells with small darkly stained nuclei. Scale is 500 μm.

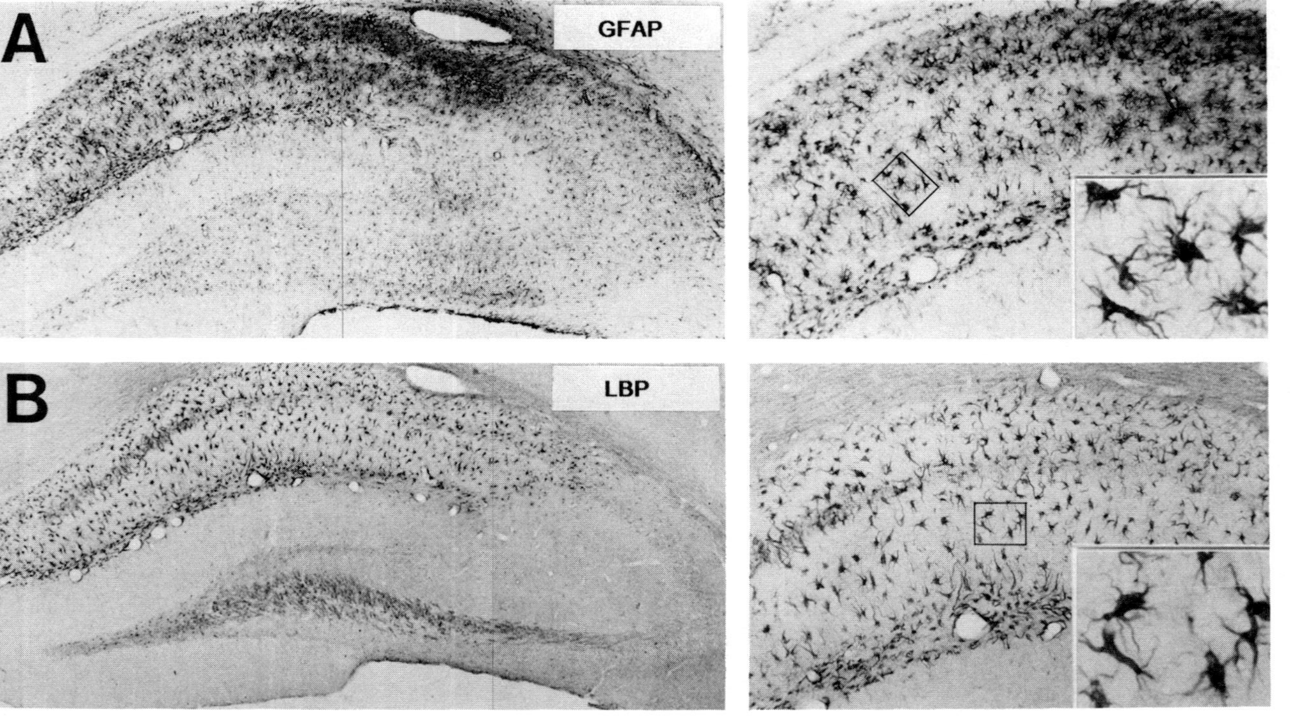

FIGURE 3. GFAP, LBP-like, and laminin-like immunoreactivities in rat dorsal hippocampus 32 days after transient ischemia. **A–D** are sections adjacent to the thionin Nissl stained section shown in FIGURE 2. The panels to the right are higher magnifications of the hippocampal CA1 subfields. **A:** Immunostaining with antibody to GFAP reveals hypertrophic reactive glial cells anatomically confined to the CA1 area where cell loss occurred (see FIG. 2). **B:** Polyclonal antibody to LBP distinctly labeled reactive astrocytes restricted to the damaged CA1 area. As in normal adult hippocampus, only a few and weakly stained glial cells were observed in undamaged regions of the hippocampus. Note the normal LBP-like immunostaining of mossy fibers in well formaldehyde-fixed tissue as reported previously.[25]

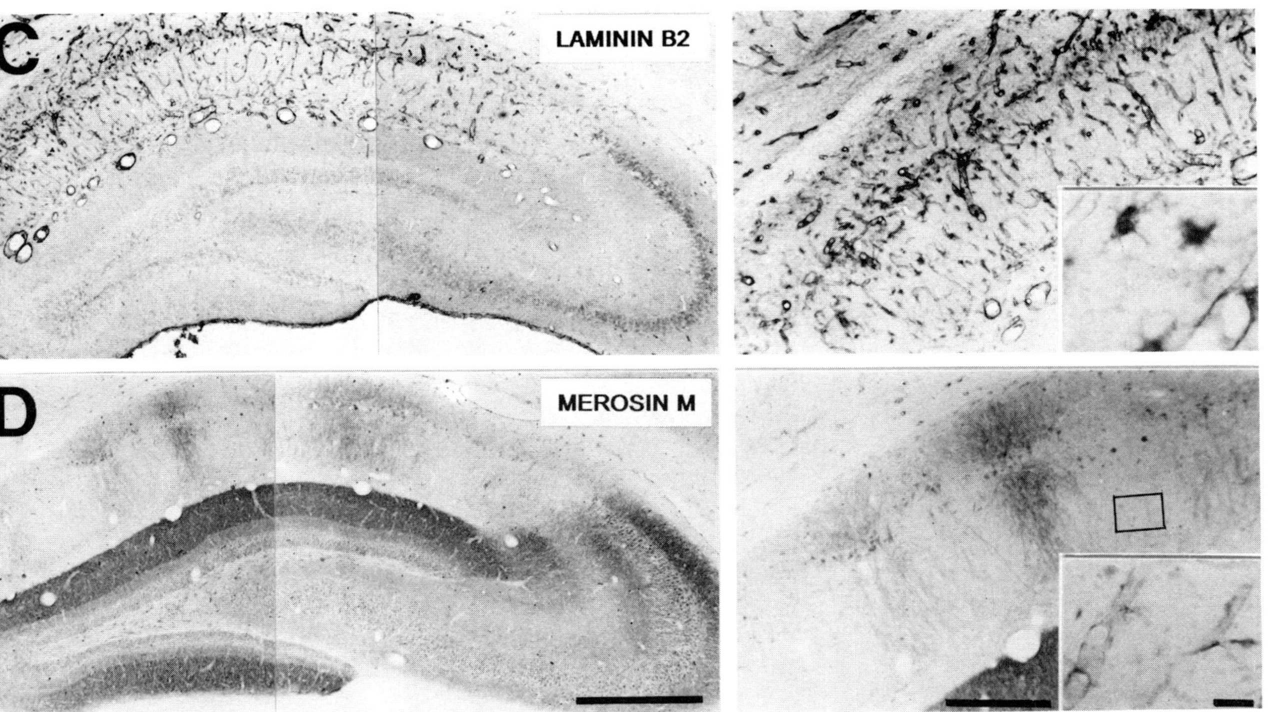

C: Monoclonal antibody to the B2 chain of laminin revealed immunopositive reactive astrocytes among laminin-positive vascular elements in the CA1 area. Immunostaining of reactive astrocytes is predominantly confined to the perykarya (insert). Note the normal (weak because of the high antibody dilution) intraneuronal laminin-like immunoreactivity of pyramidal neurons in CA2/CA3[9] and the loss of immunostaining in degenerating CA1 pyramidal neurons. **D:** Polyclonal antibody to the M-chain of human merosin did not reveal any staining of reactive astrocytes but revealed a loss of immunostaining in CA1. Note the immunoreactivity associated with fibers of surviving CA1 pyramidal cells (compare Nissl staining in FIG. 2). Distinct labeling of the outer two-thirds of the molecular layer of the dentate gyrus and the weak labeling of vascular basement membrane throughout the hippocampus are characteristic of merosin-like immunoreactivity in well-formaldehyde-fixed adult rat brain.[21] Scale bars in **D** are 500 μm, 200 μm and 20 μm for **A–D**.

to the M-chain of human merosin[6,7] (gift of E. Engvall); and polyclonal antibody to glial fibrillary acidic protein (DAKO). Controls included various normal rabbit sera and appropriate control mouse ascites.

Immunohistochemically stained sections through the rat hippocampus 32 days after transient ischemia are shown in FIGURE 3. Glial fibrillary acidic protein (GFAP) is a major protein of intermediate filaments specific to astroglia in the CNS, and the increase in GFAP-immunoreactivity in astrocytes has been used as a marker of CNS injury (e.g., ref. 26). In normal adult rats, GFAP-positive astrocytes are observed throughout the hippocampus with a comparable degree of immunoreactivity in CA1 and CA3, being slightly more intense in the hilus and slightly less intense in the molecular layers of the dentate gyrus.[34] In response to ischemia, intensely immunostained GFAP-positive astrocytes with enlarged cell bodies and thick, intensely labeled processes were observed anatomically restricted to CA1 where delayed neuronal cell loss occurred (FIG. 3A). GFAP-immunoreactivity in astrocytes increased in the first 2 days after ischemia throughout the hippocampus in a manner relatively nonspecific to the site of injury. At later times the intensity of astrocytic GFAP-staining progressed specifically in the CA1 subfield and somewhat in the hilus of the dentate gyrus, while the initial nonspecific increase of GFAP in hippocampal regions without evidence of postischemic damage (e.g., CA3) returned to baseline within 1–2 weeks. This observation agrees with findings from Petito et al.[35] and may indicate ischemia-induced transient initial changes throughout the hippocampus that are not detrimental to neurons but initiate a glial response. Reactive astrocytes with characteristically intense GFAP-immunostaining were still present at 160 days after ischemia, at a time when the CA1 field was shrunken to about 40% of its initial thickness.

Immunostaining for LBP in an adjacent section through the dorsal hippocampus is shown in FIGURE 3B. Thirty-two days after ischemia, LBP-positive astrocytes demarcate the CA1 subfield with the permanently damaged pyramidal neurons. In the remaining hippocampal subfields, at the most only faintly immunostained glial cells were seen, similar to that observed throughout the hippocampus in either sham-operated or normal adult rats.[25] Although at early time points (2–4 days after ischemia), LBP-positive reactive astrocytes could be detected in the CA3 region of the hippocampus, LBP-positive astrocytes appeared to be relatively early predictors for regions with permanent neuronal loss. Because of the clear difference in immunoreactivity of astrocytes observed in injured and uninjured brain regions as shown in FIG. 3B, anti-LBP would appear to be specific marker for neural injury and degeneration. Prominent LBP-like labeling of reactive astrocytes persisted up to 160 days after ischemia, the longest time point studied (data not shown).

Immunostaining with monoclonal antibody to the B2 chain of laminin revealed laminin-positive reactive glial cells among immunopositive capillary segments in CA1 of the hippocampus 32 days after ischemia (FIG. 3C). Similar results were observed with the polyclonal antibody to EHS laminin [B1-A-B2 chain]. The apparent upregulation of vascular basement membrane laminin in response to transient ischemia has been found to be related to differences in regional tissue fixation and might be largely a procedural artifact.[10] In contrast to LBP-like immunolabeled astrocytes (FIG. 3B insert), laminin-like immunostaining in reactive astrocytes was limited to somata and was not observed in distal glial processes (FIG. 3C, insert). Gial cells in normal adult hippocampus did not show laminin-like immunoreactivity with antibodies to EHS laminin and to the B2 laminin chain. Antibodies to the M-chain of merosin did not stain glial cells in either normal adult brain or in response to injury, but the polyclonal antibody revealed a significant loss of merosin-like immunostaining associated with fibers of CA1 pyramidal neurons 32 days after ischemia (FIG. 3D).

The present results suggest that the B2 laminin subunit and LBP-like molecules are expressed in reactive glial cells in response to CNS injury. Deposits of presumably glial-derived laminin are only transiently detectable in the developing mammalian CNS during a period of axonal growth but diminish thereafter.[18-20,36] Continued expression of laminin-like molecules has been found in glial cells of the optic nerve of the goldfish, a species that supports continuous retinal axonal growth and regeneration, and has been reported to correlate with regeneration *in vivo*.[36,37] Other studies have suggested that injury-induced CNS sprouting is promoted by astrocytes but is mediated by molecules other than laminin.[17] Glia-derived laminin has been reported to be a laminin isoform missing the A-chain.[38,39] A recent study, however, reports a laminin A chain-like immunoreactivity in glial cells in normal adult rat brain.[21] In culture, glial cells have been observed to express the laminin S-chain.[40] Thus, it might be that astrocytes express various laminin isoforms depending on their functional state or developmental age.[21] More molecular, biochemical and morphological characterization of glial-derived laminin molecules is necessary to move beyond speculation about their structure and function, their putative interaction with LBP, and their role after CNS injury.

In conclusion, antibody to LBP appears to be a highly specific marker for the onset and progression of astrogliosis following transient ischemia and other CNS injuries. LBP-immunoreactive astrocytes are restricted to the immediate lesion zone and appear more sensitive than GFAP-immunoreactive astrocytes in identifying areas of neuronal injury and degeneration. The antibody can be used as an early indicator of delayed neuronal degeneration and as a late indicator of past injuries. It has also been used successfully in identifying retrograde-induced secondary lesions following focal ischemia by photothrombosis (Spangler, Jucker, Ingram, unpublished results).

ACKNOWLEDGMENT

We would like to thank Eva Engvall for gifts of antibody to merosin and laminin.

REFERENCES

1. SANES, J. R. 1989. Ann. Rev. Neurosci. **12:** 491–516.
2. TIMPL, R., H. ROHDE, P. G. ROBEY, S. I. RENNARD, J.-M. FOIDART & G. R. MARTIN. 1979. J. Biol. Chem. **254:** 9933–9937.
3. MARTIN, G. R. & R. TIMPL. 1987. Ann. Rev. Cell Biol. **3:** 57–85.
4. HUNTER, D. D., V. SHAH, J. P. MERLIE & J. R. SANES. 1989. Nature **338:** 229–234.
5. EHRIG, K., I. LEIVO, W. S. ARGRAVES, E. RUOSLATHI & E. ENGVALL. 1990. Proc. Natl. Acad. Sci. USA **87:** 3264–3268.
6. ENGVALL, E., D. EARWICKER, T. HAAPARANTA, E. RUOSLATHI & J. R. SANES. 1990. Cell Reg. **1:** 731–740.
7. SANES, J. R., E. ENGVALL, R. BUTKOWSKI & D. D. HUNTER. 1990. J. Cell Biol. **111:** 1685–1699.
8. ERIKSDOTTER-NILSSON, M., H. BJÖRKLUND & L. OLSON. 1986. J. Neurosci. Meth. **17:** 275–286.
9. HAGG, T., D. MUIR, E. ENGVALL, S. VARON & M. MANTHORPE. 1989. Neuron **3:** 721–732.
10. JUCKER, M., P. BIALOBOK, T. HAGG & D. K. INGRAM. 1992. Brain Res. **586:** 166–170.

11. YAMAMOTO, T., Y. IWASAKI, H. YAMAMOTO, H. KONNO & M. ISEMURA. 1988. J. Neurol. Sci. **84:** 1–13.
12. SUZUKI, H., T. YAMAMOTO, H. YAMAMOTO, H. KONNO, Y. IWASAKI, Y. OHARA & H. TERUNUMA. 1990. Brain Res. **520:** 324–329.
13. ZHOU, F. C. 1990. Devel. Brain Res. **55:** 191–201.
14. SARTHY P. V. & M. FU. 1990. J. Cell Biol. **110:** 2099–2108.
15. LIESI, P., S. KAAKKOLA, D. DAHL & A. VAHERI. 1984. EMBO J. **3:** 683–686.
16. BERNSTEIN, J. J., R. GETZ, M. JEFFERSON & M. KELEMEN. 1985. Brain Res. **327:** 135–141.
17. GIFTOCHRISTOS, N. & S. DAVID. 1988. J. Neurocytol. **17:** 385–397.
18. MCLOON, S. C., L. K. MCLOON, S. L. PALM & L. T. FURCHT. 1988. J. Neurosci. **8:** 1981–1990.
19. LIESI, P. & J. SILVER. 1988. Devel. Biol. **130:** 774–785.
20. LETOURNEAU, P. C., A. M. MADSEN, S. L. PALM & L. T. FURCHT. 1988. Devel. Biol. **125:** 135–144.
21. HAGG, T., C. PORTERA-CAILLIAU, D. EARWICKER, S. VARON & E. ENGVALL. Submitted.
22. SEPHEL, G. C., K. TASHIRO, M. SASAKI, D. GREATOREX, G. R. MARTIN, Y. YAMADA & H. K. KLEINMAN. 1988. Biochem. Biophys. Res. Commun. **162:** 821–829.
23. JUCKER, M., H. K. KLEINMAN & D. K. INGRAM. 1991. J. Neurosci. Res. **28:** 507–517.
24. KLEINMAN, H. K., B. S. WEEKS, F. B. CANNON, T. M. SWEENEY, G. C. SEPHEL, B. CLEMENT, M. ZAIN, M. O. J. OLSON, M. JUCKER & B. A. BURROUS. 1991. Arch. Biochem. Biophys. **290:** 320–325.
25. JUCKER, M., H. K. KLEINMAN, C. F. HÖHMANN, J. M. ORDY & D. K. INGRAM. 1991. Brain Res. **555:** 305–312.
26. REIER, P. J., ENG, L. F. & L. JAKEMAN. 1989. Reactive astrocyte and axonal outgrowth in the injured CNS: Is gliosis really an impediment to regeneration? *In* Neural Regeneration and Transplantation. F. J. Seil, Ed.: 183–209. Alan R. Liss, Inc. New York.
27. GAGE, F. H., P. OLEJNICZAK & D. M. ARMSTRONG. 1988. Exp. Neurol. **102:** 2–13.
28. KIMELBERG, H. K. & M. D. NORENBERG. 1989. Sci. Am. **260**(4): 44–52.
29. FREDERICKSON, R. C. A. 1992. Neurobiol. Aging **13:** 239–253.
30. PULSINELLI, W. A., J. B. BIERLEY & F. PLUM. 1981. Ann. Neurol. **11:** 491–498.
31. ORDY, J. M., T. M. WENGENACK, P. BIALOBOK, P. D. COLEMAN, P. RODIER, R. B. BAGGS, W. P. DUNLAP & B. KATES. 1993. Exp. Neurol. **119:** 128–139.
32. MCGARVEY, M. L., A. BARON-VAN EVERCOOREN, H. K. KLEINAMN & M. DUBOIS-DALCQ. 1984. Devel. Biol. **105:** 18–28.
33. ENGVALL, E., G. E. DAVIS, K. DICKERSON, E. RUOSLATHI, S. VARON & M. MANTHORPE. 1986. J. Cell Biol. **103:** 2457–2465.
34. KALMAN, M. & F. HAJOS. 1989. Exp. Brain Res. **78:** 147–163.
35. PETITO, C. K., S. MORGELLO, J. C. FELIX & M. L. LESSER. 1990. J. Cereb. Blood Flow Metab. **10:** 850–859.
36. LIESI, P. 1985. EMBO J. **4:** 2505–2511.
37. HOPKINS, J. M., T. S. FORD-HOLEVINSKI, J. P. MCCOY & B. W. AGRANOFF. 1985. J. Neurosci. **5:** 3030–3038.
38. LIESI, P. & L. RISTELI. 1989. Exp. Neurol. **105:** 86–92.
39. WUJEK, J. R., H. HALEEM-SMITH, Y. YAMADA, R. LIPSKY, Y. T. LAN & E. FREESE. 1990. Devel. Brain Res. **55:** 237–247.
40. CHIU, A. Y., A. ESPINOSA DE LOS MONTEROS, R. A. COLE, S. LOERA & J. DE VELLIS. 1991. Glia **4:** 11–24.

Induction of a Neuroprotective State in Cerebellar Granule Cells following Activation of *N*-Methyl-D-Aspartate Receptors

ANN M. MARINI[a] AND STEVEN M. PAUL

Section on Molecular Pharmacology
Clinical Neuroscience Branch
National Institutes of Health
National Institute of Mental Health
Bethesda, Maryland 20892

Glutamate, the major excitatory neurotransmitter in brain, is also a potent excitotoxin to many neurons under a variety of experimental conditions.[1,2] At least three glutamate receptor subtypes have been described to date based upon their preferred affinity for agonists: *N*-methyl-D-aspartate (NMDA), quisqualate, and kainate.[3] Although all of the glutamate receptor subtypes have been implicated in glutamate-induced neurotoxicity, the NMDA receptor plays a pivotal role in mediating neuronal death in most primary culture neuronal excitotoxicity models following either brief or prolonged glutamate exposure. Excitotoxic injury has been suggested to be causally linked to ischemic brain injury (*e.g.*, stroke) and a variety of neurodegenerative disorders. In these disorders release of glutamate from damaged neuronal processes is thought to result in NMDA receptor-mediated toxicity. Because NMDA receptor-mediated neurotoxicity has been implicated in the pathogenesis of a variety of neurodegenerative disorders and ischemic brain injury, there has been considerable effort at delineating, and modulating the cellular and molecular events underlying NMDA receptor-mediated neurotoxicity. During the course of these studies, it has become apparent that certain populations of neurons are highly vulnerable to ischemic and/or neurotoxic insult (*e.g.*, CA_1 hippocampal neurons and dopaminergic neurons of the substantia nigra) whereas others are far less sensitive. At present, the biochemical factors responsible for differences in the vulnerability of various populations of neurons to neurotoxins are poorly understood.

Cultured cerebellar granule cells, the most abundant neuronal subtype in the mammalian brain,[4] are highly enriched in primary culture (~95% granule cells), and are susceptible to the excitotoxic actions of glutamate.[5] Cultured cerebellar granule cells are also susceptible to the neurotoxic effects of MPP^+,[6] the active neurotoxic metabolite of 1-methyl-1,2,3,6-tetrahydropyridine (MPTP) which produces a parkinsonian syndrome in man, and sub-human primates.[7]

In preliminary experiments we have shown that preincubation of cerebellar granule cells with NMDA reduced the toxicity observed following subsequent exposure to glutamate.[8,9] We assumed that the "neuroprotective" effect of NMDA against glutamate toxicity was due to an agonist-induced desensitization of NMDA

---

[a] Address correspondence and reprint requests to Dr. Marini.

receptors.[8] However, in further characterizing the mechanism(s) underlying the neuroprotective effects of NMDA against other neurotoxins, principally the chemical neurotoxin MPP$^+$, we have demonstrated the presence in these neurons of a novel NMDA receptor-mediated neuroprotective mechanism. We now report that in contrast to virtually all neurons studied to date, exposure of cerebellar granule cells to low (subtoxic) concentrations of NMDA or glutamate *in vitro* results in a robust neuroprotective effect against both MPP$^+$- and glutamate-induced neurotoxicity. The neuroprotective effects of NMDA and glutamate are blocked by the specific NMDA receptor antagonists 2-amino-5-phosphovalerate (APV) and (+)5-methyl-10,11-dihydro-5H-dibenzo[a,d] cyclohepten-5,10-imine maleate (MK-801), demonstrating a role for NMDA receptors in inducing the neuroprotective state.

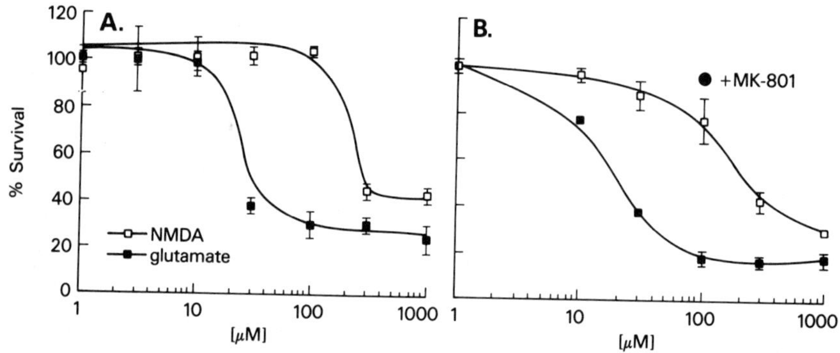

FIGURE 1. NMDA and glutamate toxicity of cerebellar granule cells in culture medium is concentration- and time-dependent. Cultured cerebellar granule cells were exposed to NMDA (1–1000 μM) or glutamate (1–1000 μM) for either **A** 60 min or **B** 24 h. In **A** cerebellar granule cells were exposed to NMDA or glutamate for 60 min followed by replacement of the medium with sister culture medium and assessment of neuronal viability with fluorescein diacetate measured 24 h later (see text for details). In **B** cells were exposed to NMDA or glutamate for 24 h prior to assessing neuronal viability. Concentrations of NMDA and glutamate of ≤ 100 μM and ≤ 10 μM, respectively, are subtoxic, whereas higher concentrations of either agonist resulted in a concentration and time-dependent toxicity. The NMDA receptor antagonist MK-801 completely blocks the neurotoxic effects of glutamate **(B)** and NMDA (data not shown). Data are from a representative experiment repeated twice with similar results.

Initial examination of the effects of glutamate and NMDA exposure on granule cell viability over a broad concentration range in culture medium containing magnesium and glucose showed a concentration-dependent neurotoxic response; toxicity was blocked by the selective NMDA receptor antagonist, MK-801 (FIG. 1). Exposure of granule cells for 60 min to NMDA or glutamate concentrations of ≤ 100 μM or ≤ 10 μM, respectively, was not neurotoxic under our culture conditions.

We then confirmed our previous observation that preincubation of cerebellar granule cells to subtoxic concentrations of NMDA antagonizes the neurotoxicity induce by toxic concentrations of glutamate. Since cerebellar granule cells are susceptible to the neurotoxic effect of MPP$^+$, we determined whether the neuro-

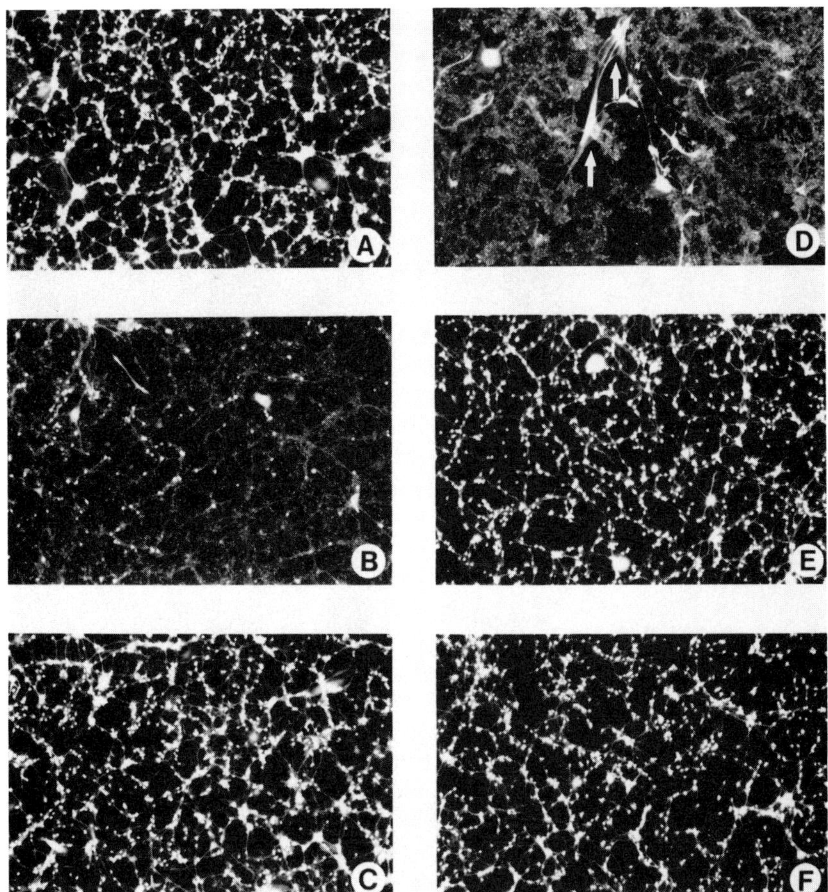

FIGURE 2. NMDA and glutamate protect cerebellar granule cells against MPP^+ toxicity. Preincubation of cerebellar granule cells at DIV 8 with either NMDA (100 μM) or glutamate (5 μM) was followed by exposure to MPP^+ (50 μM) for 120 hrs as described in the text. Fluorescein diacetate staining of cerebellar granule cells was carried out on DIV 13. Photomicrographs were made under UV microscopy (100×) and are of representative fields from a single experiment repeated at least 3 times with identical results. **A:** Untreated culture; **B:** culture following 120 h exposure to MPP^+ (50 μM); **C:** culture preincubated with NMDA (100 μM) for 60 min at DIV 8 followed by MPP^+ (50 μM) for 120 h; **D:** culture preincubated with MK-801 (1 μM) 5 min prior to the addition of NMDA (100 μM) and 65 min prior to media exchange with sister culture media containing MPP^+ (50 μM) for 120 h. **E:** culture at DIV 8 after exposure to glutamate (5 μM) for 60 min; **F:** culture preincubated with glutamate (5 μM) as in **(E)** followed by media exchange and exposure to MPP^+ (50 μM) for 120 h. Neither preincubation with NMDA (100 μM) (data not shown) or glutamate (5 μM) **(E)** alone for the indicated times affected neuronal viability. Note the marked toxicity **(B)** induced by MPP^+ (50 μM) which is blocked by preincubation with either NMDA **(C)** or glutamate **(F)**. MK-801 (1 μM) blocks the neuroprotective effects of NMDA **(D)**. *Arrows indicate astrocytes.*

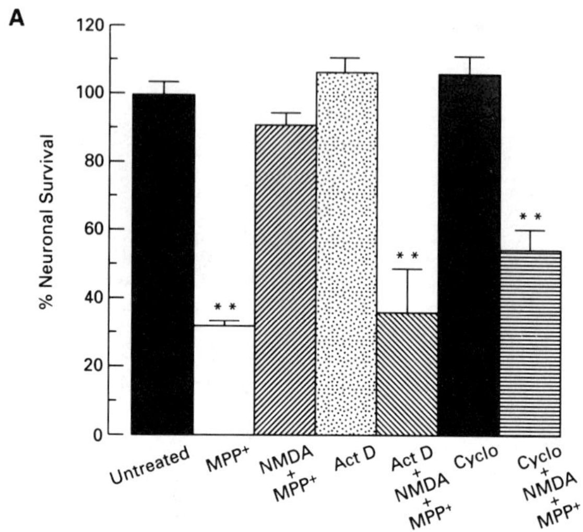

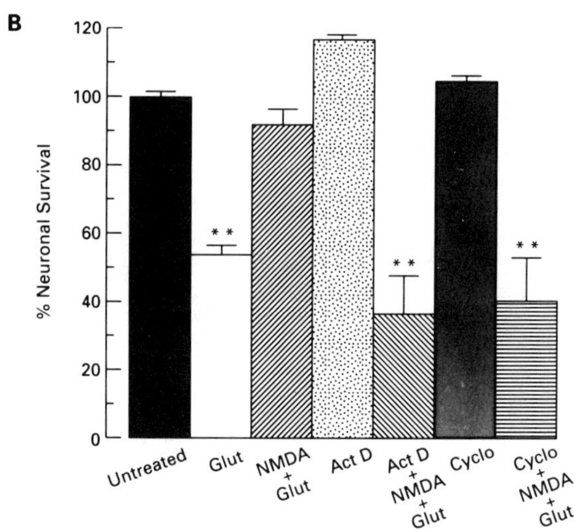

FIGURE 3. Cycloheximide and actinomycin D block the neuroprotective effects of NMDA against both MPP$^+$ **(A)** and glutamate **(B)** toxicity. **A:** Cultured cerebellar granule cells were exposed to NMDA (100 μM) for 60 min in the presence or absence of either cycloheximide (1 μg/ml) or actinomycin D (0.1 μg/ml). These concentrations of cycloheximide and actinomycin D were found in preliminary experiments to have no effect on granule cell viability when incubated for 60 min. Following preincubation, the media was removed and replaced with sister culture media containing MPP$^+$ (50 μM). Neuronal viability was measured 120 h later with fluorescein diacetate as described in FIGURE 2 and the text. **B:** Cerebellar granule

protective effects of subtoxic concentrations of NMDA (≤ 100 μM) or glutamate (≤ 10 μM) would extend to MPP$^+$, a neurotoxin which acts via an NMDA receptor-independent mechanism.[8] Pretreatment of the culture neurons with subtoxic concentrations of either NMDA or glutamate almost completely antagonizes the neurotoxic effect of MPP$^+$ (50 μM), a concentration which alone results in $\geq 75\%$ cell death (FIG. 2). The neuroprotective effect of NMDA against MPP$^+$ toxicity is concentration- and time-dependent (data not shown).

Coincubation of cerebellar granule cells with either the protein synthesis inhibitor cycloheximide or the RNA synthesis inhibitor actinomycin D along with NMDA completely blocked the NMDA-induced neuroprotection against MPP$^+$ (FIG. 3). Glutamate (50 μM) exposure kills approximately 50% of the granule cells within 24 hours whereas pretreatment with NMDA for 60 min almost completely prevents the toxicity induced by glutamate. Neuroprotection induced by NMDA against glutamate toxicity is almost completely prevented by coincubation with actinomycin D and cycloheximide (FIG. 3).

Our results demonstrate that subtoxic concentrations of NMDA or glutamate can induce a robust neuroprotective state in cerebellar granule cells against two mechanistically distinct neurotoxins. Moreover, NMDA receptor antagonists block NMDA-induced neuroprotection against MPP$^+$ toxicity. Thus, NMDA receptors can mediate *either* neurotoxicity or neuroprotection, depending upon the concentration of agonist. Presumably, glutamate differentially modulates cellular responses acting via NMDA receptors, most likely as a function of the degree of NMDA receptor activation. Neuroprotection by NMDA was not observed against glutamate or MPP$^+$ toxicity in cortical or mesencephalic cultures respectively (F. Finiels-Marlier, A. Marini, and S. M. Paul, unpublished data).

Since activation of NMDA receptors leads to calcium influx via NMDA receptor-operated cation channels, it seems likely that the level of intracellular calcium $[Ca^{2+}]_i$ may play an important role in initiating the neuroprotective state. Moreover, under depolarizing conditions, micromolar concentrations of NMDA have been reported to elevate $[Ca^{2+}]_i$ in cultured cerebellar granule cells.[10] Furthermore, we have recently compared the effects of glutamate in increasing $[Ca^{2+}]_i$ in cerebellar granule cells before and after preincubation with NMDA. Following a 60 min preincubation with NMDA (100 μM), the glutamate-induced elevation of $[Ca^{2+}]_i$ measured by microfluorimetry using the calcium-sensitive indicator fura-2, was

---

cells were preincubated with NMDA (100 μM) in the presence or absence of either cycloheximide (1.0 μg/ml) or actinomycin D (0.1 μg/ml) as in **(A)**. Following 60 min preincubation, the media was exchanged with sister culture media containing glutamate (50 μM). This concentration of glutamate has been previously shown in our laboratory to kill approximately 50% of granule cells when measured 24 h later. % Neuronal survival was determined as in FIG. 2. Values represent the mean % survival $\pm$ SEM and are from 2 separate experiments each performed in triplicate. **$p < 0.01$ compared to untreated control or compared to respective actinomycin D alone or cycloheximide alone controls using Student t-test. All other groups are not significantly different from untreated control. Note that actinomycin D and cycloheximide completely block the neuroprotective effect of NMDA against both MPP$^+$ and glutamate toxicity. The concentrations of cycloheximide (1 μg/ml) and actinomycin D (0.1 μg/ml) used in our experiments reduced [^{3}H]uridine and [^{3}H]leucine incorporation into RNA and protein by 85% and 80% respectively.

$$\% \text{ Neuronal survival} = \frac{\text{surviving neurons/LPF field in treatment condition}}{\text{surviving neurons/LPF in untreated cultures}} \times 100$$

identical to that observed in cells not exposed to NMDA (A. Marini, Y. Ueda, C. June, and S. M. Paul, in preparation). Low levels of intracellular calcium induced by subtoxic glutamate concentrations may activate other second and/or third messenger systems. For example, low NMDA concentrations have been shown to induce the transcription of the nuclear early inducible gene *c-fos* in cerebellar granule cells.[11] However, *c-fos* has also been observed to be induced in neurons where NMDA fails to confer neuroprotection, suggesting that *c-fos* may be a necessary but insufficient response for the neuroprotective actions of NMDA in cerebellar granule cells.[12]

Our observation that the neuroprotective state induced by NMDA and glutamate is blocked by either a RNA or protein synthesis inhibitor strongly suggest that NMDA and glutamate can induce the receptor-mediated expression of a neuroprotective protein(s). The neuroprotective effects of NMDA reported here may be related to the neurotrophic actions of NMDA reported in cerebellar granule cells by Balazs *et al.*[13] The trophic effects of NMDA on cerebellar granule cells occur when the latter are cultured in low (nondepolarizing) concentrations of potassium and are not observed when cerebellar granule cells are maintained, as was the case in our experiments, in high (depolarizing) potassium concentrations. It is conceivable that the mechanism underlying the neuroprotective and neurotrophic actions of NMDA are similar.

In summary, low (subtoxic) concentrations of NMDA and/or glutamate protect against subsequent exposure to MPP$^+$ or glutamate and the neuroprotective effect is completely blocked by NMDA receptor antagonists, demonstrating a role for NMDA receptors in inducing the neuroprotective state. The neuroprotection conferred by NMDA against MPP$^+$ toxicity is time- and concentration-dependent and is completely prevented by either an RNA or protein synthesis inhibitor. These data demonstrate that activation of NMDA receptors in cerebellar granule cells can result in either neurotoxicity or a generalized neuroprotective state. Since the neuroprotective effects of glutamate and NMDA require new RNA and protein synthesis, it appears that NMDA receptor activation in cerebellar granule cells induces the expression of a neuroprotective protein(s). The cloning of the genes responsible for the NMDA receptor-mediated neuroprotective state could result in novel strategies for protecting vulnerable populations of neurons.

REFERENCES

1. Choi, D. W. 1988. Glutamate neurotoxicity and diseases of the nervous system. Neuron **1:** 623–634.
2. Rothman, S. M. & J. W. Olney. 1987. Excitotoxicity and the NMDA receptor. Trends Neurosci. **10:** 299–302.
3. Watkins, J. C. & R. H. Evans. 1981. Excitatory amino acids transmitters. Annu. Rev. Pharmacol. Toxicol. **21:** 165–204.
4. Burgoyne, R. D. & M. A. Cambray-Deakin. 1988. The cellular neurobiology of neuronal development: the cerebellar granule cell. Brain Res. Rev. **13:** 77–101.
5. Schramm, M., S. Eimerl & E. Costa. 1990. Serum and depolarizing agents cause acute neurotoxicity in cultured cerebellar granule cells: Role of the glutamate receptor responsive to *N*-methyl-D-aspartate. Proc. Natl. Acad. Sci. USA **87:** 1193–1197.
6. Marini, A. M., J. P. Schwartz & I. J. Kopin. 1989. The neurotoxicity of 1-methyl-4-phenylpyridinium in cultured cerebellar granule cells. J. Neurosci. **9**(10): 3665–3672.
7. Kopin, I. J. & S. P. Markey. 1988. MPTP toxicity: Implications for research in Parkinson's disease. Ann. Rev. Neurosci. **11:** 81–96.
8. Marini, A. & A. Novelli. DL-threo-3-hydroxyasparte reduces NMDA receptor activation by glutamate in cultured neurons. Eur. J. Pharmacol. **194:** 131–132.

9. CHUANG, D. M., X. M. GAO & S. M. PAUL. 1992. *N*-methyl-D-aspartate exposure blocks glutamate toxicity in cultured cerebellar granule cells. Mol. Pharmacol **42:** 210–216.

10. BURGOYNE, R. D., I. A. PEARCE & M. CAMBRAY-DEAKIN. 1988. *N*-methyl-D-aspartate raises cytosolic calcium concentration in rat cerebellar granule cells in culture. Neurosci Lett. **91:** 47–52.

11. MANEV, H., E. COSTA, J. T. WROBLEWSKI & A. GUIDOTTI. 1990. Abusive stimulation of excitatory amino acid receptors: a strategy to limit neurotoxicity. FASEB J. **4:** 2789–2797.

12. SAGAR, S. M., F. R. SHARP & T. CURRAN. 1988. Expression of c-fos protein in brain: Metabolic mapping at the cellular level. Science **240:** 1328–1331.

13. BALAZS, R., N. HACK & O. S. JORGENSEN. 1990. *N*-methyl-D-aspartate promotes the survival of cerebellar granule cells in culture. Neuroscience **37:** 251–258.

Neurotoxic Effect of Okadaic Acid, A Seafood-related Toxin, on Cultured Cerebellar Neurons[a]

MARÍA TERESA FERNÁNDEZ,[b] VLADIMIR ZITKO,[c]
SANTIAGO GASCÓN,[b] ANGELES TORREBLANCA,[b] AND
ANTONELLO NOVELLI[b,d]

*bDepartamento de Biología Funcional
Area de Bioquímica y Biología Molecular
Facultad de Medicina, Universidad de Oviedo
33006 Oviedo, Spain*

*cMarine Chemistry Division, Biological Station
St. Andrews, N.B. E0G2X0, Canada*

INTRODUCTION

Okadaic acid (OKA) is a polyether compound of a C_{38} fatty acid produced by certain marine dinoflagellates which accumulates by filter feeding in the digestive gland of molluscs and marine sponges, such as *Halichondria okadaii* from which OKA was first isolated. It is well known to be the cause of human diarrhetic shellfish poisoning following ingestion of contaminated cultured mussels and scallops.[1] The biochemical properties of OKA have been recently reviewed.[2] Thus, this toxin has been found to be a potent tumor promoter acting through a mechanism different from that of TPA (12-0-tetradecanoyl-phorbol-13-acetate)-type tumor promoters, and it has been identified as a potent specific inhibitor of the serine/threonine protein phosphatases 1 and 2A (PP1, PP2A) *in vitro*. In intact cells, OKA produces a great increase in phosphorylation of several proteins (myosin light chain, elongation factor 2, acetyl CoA carboxylase, tyrosine hydroxilase) and modulates a variety of cellular functions such as smooth muscle contraction, fatty acid biosynthesis, protein synthesis, and cathecholamine synthesis and secretion. Calcium influx through voltage-sensitive calcium channels (VSCC) may be increased by OKA treatment,[3–5] although opposite effects of OKA have been reported on calcium dependent phenomena such as neurotransmitter release.[6,7] OKA does not appear to alter only VSCC. Recent data obtained in hyppocampal neurons in culture have indicated that OKA may increase the ionic influx through the ionotropic NON-NMDA type of excitatory amino acid (EAA) receptors possibly by inhibiting PP1 and PP2A activity.[8] EAA receptors and VSCC may be responsible for neuronal degeneration.[9–11] PP1 and PP2A may also be involved in the formation of the β amyloid protein present in the senile plaques of Alzheimer's disease,[12] as well as in the phosphorylation of the microtubule associated protein tau, another important protein in Alzheimer's disease.[13] Two recent studies de-

[a] This work was supported by the University of Oviedo, Grant DF90/1659 and by the Spanish Comisión Interministerial de Ciencia y tecnología, Grant SAL91-0613.

[d] Author to whom correspondence and reprint requests should be sent.

scribed the neurotoxic effects of OKA,[14,15] considering either the appearance of hyperphosphorylated tau and neurodegeneration following microinjections of OKA in rodent brain,[15] or the possible involvement of VSCC and EAA receptor in the neurotoxic effects of OKA in neuronal cultures.[14]

In this article we present further evidence suggesting that OKA is a potent neurotoxin for rat cerebellar neurons in primary culture and produce neurotoxicity through mechanisms that do not appear to involve either EAA receptors or VSCC.

MATERIALS AND METHODS

Cell Culture

Primary cultures of rat cerebellar neurons were prepared as described.[16] Briefly, cerebella from 8-day-old pups were dissected, cells were dissociated and suspended in basal Eagle's medium with 25 mM KCl, 2 mM glutamine, 100 μg/ml gentamycin and 10% fetal calf serum. Cells were seeded on poly-L-lysine coated (5 μg/ml) 35 mm dishes at 2.5 $\times$ 10^5 cells/cm^2 and incubated at 37°C in a 5% CO_2, 95% humidity atmosphere. Cytosine arabinoside (10 μM) was added after 20–24 h of culture to inhibit the replication of nonneuronal cells. Cerebellar neurons were kept alive for more than 30 days in culture (DIC) by replenishing the growth medium with glucose every 4 days and compensating for lost amounts of water due to evaporation.[17]

Neurotoxicology

Cultures were used for neurotoxicological studies between 5–20 DIC as indicated. Drugs were added in the growth medium for 24 or 48 hours. Then, the growth medium was removed and cultures were incubated for 5 min with 1 ml incubation buffer containing 154 mM NaCl, 5.6 mM KCl, 5.6 mM glucose, 8.6 mM Hepes, 1 mM $MgCl_2$, 2.3 mM $CaCl_2$, pH 7.4, to which the vital stain fluorescein diacetate (5 μg/ml) was added. Dead neurons did not retain any fluorescein diacetate and their nucleus could be stained in red by 1 min exposure to 50 μg/ml ethidium bromide.[14,16,17] Photographs of randomly selected culture fields were taken, and neurons were counted. The percentage of dead neurons, relative to their total number, was calculated.

Data Presentation and Analysis

Results are presented as indicated in each figure. Statistical analysis has been performed by Student *t*-test.

Materials

Okadaic acid was kindly provided by Dr. H. Fujiki (National Cancer Center Research Institute, Tokyo, Japan); (+)-10,11-dihydro-5-methyl-5H-dibenzo-[a,d]-cyclohepten-5,10-imine hydrogen maleate (MK-801), verapamil (VER) and nifedipine (NIF) were a generous gift from Dr. G. J. Kaczarowski (Merck Sharp and

TABLE 1. Neurotoxicity by Okadaic Acid and Excitatory Amino Acids in Cerebellar Granule Cells in Primary Culture

Drug	Swelling-Darkening	Neurite Degeneration	% Dead 24 h	% Dead 48 h
None	−	−	2	2
OKA 5 nM	−	+ + +	30	85
GLU 40 μM	+ +	+ +	80	80
DOM 20 μM	+ +	+ +	80	80

Neuronal cultures at 19 days in culture were exposed to the drugs at the indicated concentration in the growth medium. In order to detect early signs of swelling and darkening of the cell body,[16] cultures were observed by phase contrast microscopy from 10 min up to two hours.[17] The percentage of dead neurons, as well as neurite degeneration, was then quantified by staining the culture with fluorescein diacetate and ethidium bromide as described in the methods. Values reported are the mean of 6–8 determinations. Standard deviation was approx. 15% of the mean.

Dohme Laboratories, NJ, USA); D(−)-2-Amino-5-phosphovaleric acid (APV) was purchased from Cambridge Research Biochemicals; 6-cyano-7-nitroquinoxaline-2,3-dione (CNQX) was purchased from Tocris Neuramin. Domoic acid was purchased from Diagnostic Chemical Limited, Charlottetown, P.E.I., Canada. All other drugs were from Sigma.

RESULTS

Cerebellar neurons at 19 DIC were exposed to a neurotoxic concentration of OKA (5 nM) in the growth medium.[14] Signs of neurotoxicity, such as darkening and swelling of the cell bodies, degeneration of the neurites, and cell death, were timed as they developed (TABLE 1). For comparison, cultures were also exposed to two EAA receptor agonists, such as glutamate (GLU) for the NMDA receptor type[9,16,20] and domoate (DOM) for the NON-NMDA.[9,18–20] In cerebellar cultures, EAAs are known to produce a fast (~10 min) darkening and swelling of the cell bodies, followed first by the loss of capability to stain for fluorescein diacetate and then by neuronal degeneration.[16,17] Neurotoxicity by OKA was not characterized by any fast darkening/swelling of the neurons, which remained unaltered for up to 16 hours, when degeneration of neuronal network started to become evident.[14] After 24 hours exposure, OKA led to a complete degeneration of neuronal network, while ~70% of the neuronal cell bodies were still able to stain for fluorescein diacetate, and therefore they were considered alive under this criterion, as reported before.[14] After 48 hours exposure to OKA most of the neuronal bodies had degenerated (TABLE 1). The concentration producing 50% neurotoxicity (NTC$_{50}$) shifted from ~7.5 nM at 24 h, to ~1.8 nM at 48 h. Neurotoxicity by EAA did not change with exposure time longer than 24 hours (TABLE 1). The neurodegenerative effect of OKA was not reversible. Withdrawal of OKA (2.5 nM) after 24 h culture exposure did not reduce the extent of neuronal damage after 48 h, as compared to cultures where OKA was not withdrawn (data not shown).

The neurotoxic effect of OKA was quantified in neurons at different DIC. Neurotoxicity by OKA changed with the age of the culture (TABLE 2), although the neurotoxicity pattern described above did not. Following 24 h exposure to OKA, maximum neurotoxicity was observed in neurons at 9 DIC, when OKA NTC_{50} was ~1.5 nM. At 5 DIC, neurons presented lower sensitivity to OKA (NTC_{50} ~ 5 nM), than at 9 DIC. On the other hand, neurons at 19 DIC appeared to be much less sensitive to the toxin (NTC_{50} ~ 7.5 nM). As reported for comparison in TABLE 2, sensitivity of the neurons to the excitotoxic effects of both GLU and DOM did increase with time in culture until it stabilized at ~12 DIC for GLU and ~10 DIC for DOM.

The majority of cerebellar neurons in culture are glutamatergic granule cells which may release EAAs, such as glutamate, upon depolarization-induced calcium entry through VSCC.[21,22] We have explored the possibility that neurotoxicity by OKA could involve VSCC and endogenous EAA release. Incubation of the neurons for 48 hours in growth medium containing a depolarizing concentration of KCl (60 mM), resulted in a significant increase in neurotoxicity (FIG. 1). This effect was antagonized by VSCC antagonists such as the dihydropiridine nifedipine (NIF, 1 μM) and the phenilalkylamine verapamil (VER, 10 μM). VER was much more potent in blocking KCl-induced toxicity than NIF, in agreement with previous evidence showing that VER, but not NIF, completely blocks $^{45}Ca^{2+}$ uptake in cultured cerebellar neurons.[22] KCL-induced neurotoxicity was prevented also by antagonists of the excitatory aminoacids receptors, such as the NMDA receptor antagonist APV (1 mM)[9] or the noncompetitive glutamate antagonist MK-801 (1 μM), acting at the NMDA receptor channel,[9] indicating that neurotoxicity by KCl was mediated through the release of endogenous excitatory aminoacids acting at the NMDA receptor. The NON-NMDA receptor antagonist CNQX (50 μM),[9] partially prevented from KCl-induced neurotoxicity (FIG. 1), possibly because of its antagonism of glycine action at the NMDA receptor.[9] Neuronal survival in OKA-treated cultures was not significantly increased either by NIF or VER (FIG. 1). Moreover, both NMDA and NON-NMDA receptor antagonists failed to protect from OKA neurotoxicity (FIG. 1).

In order to demonstrate any toxicologically relevant effect of OKA on NON-NMDA receptors, we exposed 19 DIC cultures to OKA (1 nM) for a total of 48 h, of which 24 h were of preincubation before the addition of DOM (5 μM). In these conditions, OKA, which produced minimal network damage,[14] failed to potentiate the action of DOM (FIG. 2).

TABLE 2. Changes in Neurotoxicity by Okadaic Acid with Neuronal Time in Culture as Compared to Excitatory Amino Acids

	Concentration Producing 50% Neurotoxicity (NTC_{50})		
Drug	5 DIC	9 DIC	19 DIC
OKA	5 nM	1.5 nM	7.5 nM
GLU	>1000 μM	50 μM	13 μM
DOM	> 50 μM	10 μM	8 μM

Values were determined after 24 h exposure to the drugs. Each value has been calculated from a concentration-dependent neurotoxicity curve with 6 points, which has been repeated at least twice. Standard deviation was approx. 15% of the mean.

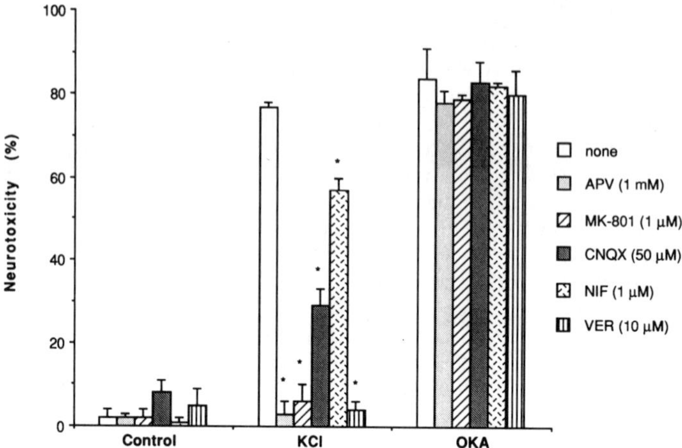

FIGURE 1. Pharmacology of neurotoxicity by okadaic acid and by KCl-induced depolarization. KCl (60 mM) and OKA (5 nM) alone and in combination with each of the indicated drugs were added to 19 DIC cerebellar neurons, and neurotoxicity was determined 48 h later as described in the methods. Values represent the mean ± SD (n = 6 − 8). *P < 0.01 vs KCl.

OKA is known to increase the level of protein phosphorylation by inhibiting PP1 and PP2A. We compared the neurotoxic effects of OKA (5 nM) with that of protein kinase C (PKC) activators, such as TPA (100 nM). As shown in FIGURE 3, 48 h exposure to TPA did not affect neuronal viability or morphology. In the same experiment, 24 h exposure to TPA (100 nM) protected from neurotoxicity by EAAs (data not shown), proving an effect on PKC.[23] The role of cAMP-dependent protein kinase (PKA) in neurotoxicity was also tested. As shown in

FIGURE 2. Okadaic acid does not potentiate domoate neurotoxicity. Neuronal cultures at 19 DIC were exposed to OKA for a total of 48 h, of which 24 h were of preincubation before the addition of DOM. Values represent the mean ± SD (n = 4).

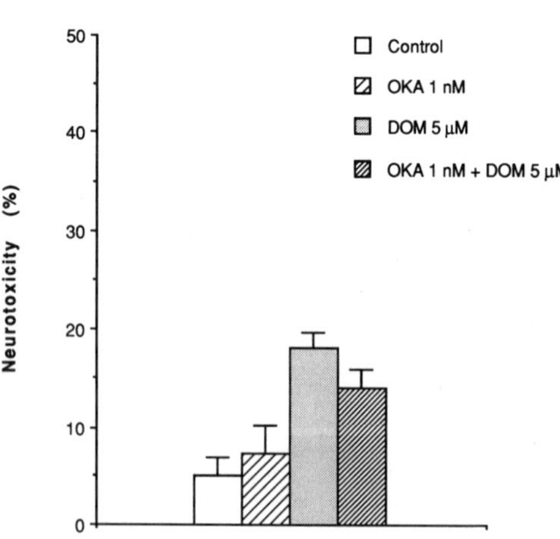

FIGURE 3, forskolin, a direct activator of adenylate cyclase, did not promote any neurotoxic effect. OKA (1-5 mM) toxicity was not potentiated in the presence of either TPA or forskolin (data not shown).

We also investigated whether the stimulation by neurotoxic concentrations of OKA could affect the intracellular levels of second messengers, such as cGMP or cAMP. As shown in FIGURE 4A, OKA did not significantly increase intracellular levels of cGMP which were substantially elevated by DOM. Similarly, no changes in intracellular levels of cAMP were detected during the 30 min following exposure to OKA, while forskolin produced a substantial increase in cAMP intracellular levels (FIG. 4B).

DISCUSSION

We used primary cultures of cerebellar neurons, a system that has been well characterized developmentally, biochemically, and electrophysiologically,[21,24-26] and is widely used for the study of EAA receptors.[16,17,20,23,27,28] Our results indicate

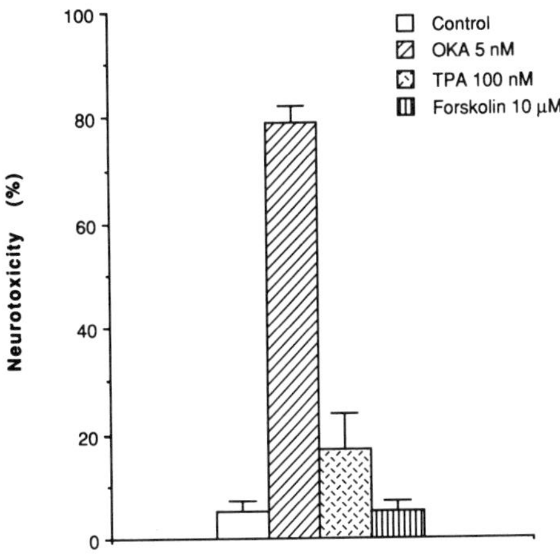

FIGURE 3. The neurotoxic effect of okadaic acid is not mimicked by TPA nor by forskolin. Neuronal cultures at 19 DIC were exposed to either OKA or TPA or forskolin for a total of 48 h. Values represent the mean ± SD (n = 4).

that neurotoxicity by OKA involves morphological changes different from those induced by EAA. Thus, OKA, at concentrations as low as 0.5 nM,[14] produces a neurotoxicity pattern characterized by a slow desintegration of neurites, followed by visible swelling of cell bodies, and later by cellular death. No fast swelling and darkening of the cell bodies was detected.

Neurons at 9 DIC showed maximum sensitivity to the toxic effects of 24 h exposure to OKA, as compared to 5 DIC and 19 DIC old neurons. Several authors have reported substantial developmentally related changes in morphology, microscopical structure, biochemistry, electrophysiology and physiology of cerebellar neurons in primary culture.[21,24-26] Some of the observed changes were calcium-mediated phenomena,[21,24,26] and an increase in the calcium influx through VSCC has been described during the *in vitro* differentiation of these neurons[22] together with the development of a calcium-dependent release of endogenous EAAs following neuronal depolarization,[21] and the development of a sensitivity to the neurotoxic effects of EAAs, as shown in TABLE 2. Despite previous evidence suggesting a role for VSCC in neurodegeneration,[10,11] our finding that the two NMDA receptor antagonists APV and MK-801, fully protected from KCl-induced neurotoxicity in the absence of VSCC antagonists, suggests that Ca^{2+} influx through VSCC, alone is not sufficient to promote toxicity in cerebellar neurons. Moreover, since OKA neurotoxicity cannot be antagonized by VSCC antagonists, the possibility that a potentiation of Ca^{2+} currents through VSCC by OKA[3–5] may play a role in neurotoxicity is unlikely (FIG. 5).

The complete prevention of the neurotoxic effect of KCl by NMDA receptor antagonists, suggests that endogenous ligands for the NON-NMDA receptor capable of inducing neurotoxicity, if any, are unlikely to be released. Consequently, the reported increase in ionic permeability of the NON-NMDA receptor channel subsequent to exposure to OKA[8] may not be relevant for the neurotoxic effect of OKA (FIG. 5). Furthermore, OKA failed to potentiate DOM toxicity, and OKA neurotoxicity was not prevented nor reduced by either NMDA or NON-NMDA receptor antagonists, excluding a role for EAA receptors in OKA neurotoxicity.

The increase in neurotoxicity by OKA in cultured cerebellar neurons between 5 and 9 DIC, appears to indicate that after approximately 1 week in culture, while neurons are undergoing a crucial step in their development,[21,24–26] a higher sensitivity towards the algal toxin is present. After 9 DIC, cerebellar neurons in culture may reach a steady-state in some of their functions (ref. 25 and Novelli et al., unpublished results), and become significantly more resistant to OKA. This

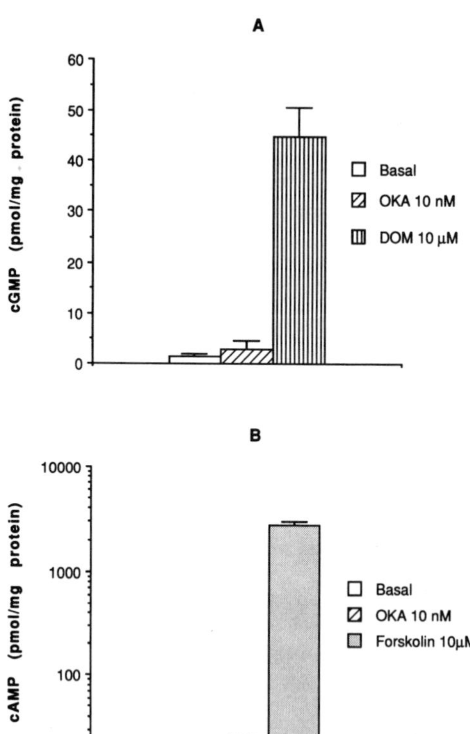

FIGURE 4. Okadaic acid effect on intracellular second messengers. A: Cultures were exposed to OKA for up to 30 min. The reported maximal cGMP increase was observed at 20 min and it was not statistically significative. cGMP increase by DOM was measured at 1 min. B: Cultures were exposed to OKA for 30 min. No increase above basal levels was detected at any time. cAMP increase by forskolin was measured at 5 min. Intracellular concentration of cGMP and cAMP were measured as described in the methods. OKA did not induce neurotoxicity during the incubation period. Data are reported as the mean ± SD (n = 3).

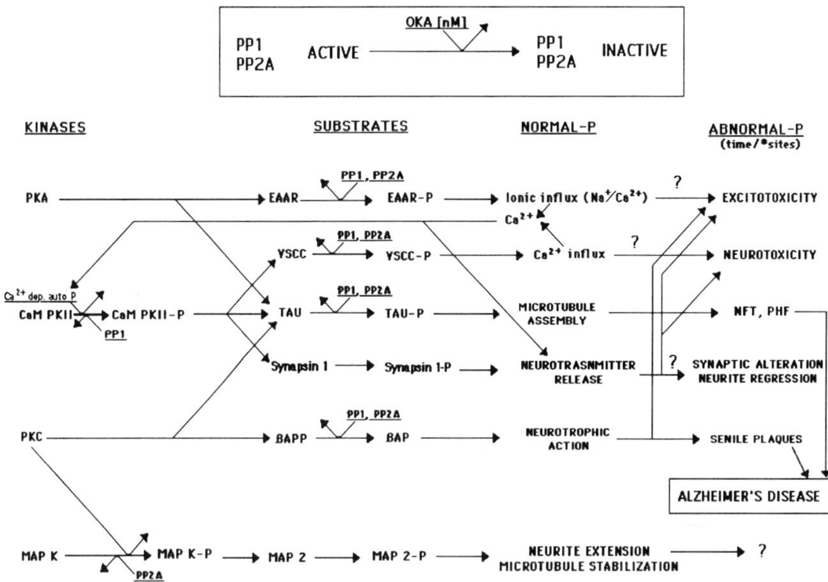

FIGURE 5. Neurochemical pathways affected by okadaic acid. Temptative scheme of the neurochemical pathways possibly affected by OKA as discussed in the text. Abnormal phosphorylation is conceived as an increase of either the % of time spent by the protein in the phosphorylated form, or the number of phosphorylated sites. EAAR = EAA receptors; NFT = neurofibrillary tangles; PHF = paired helical filaments; βAP = Alzheimer β/A4 amyloid protein; MAP K = MAP kinase.

may possibly occur through the slow down of biochemical pathways affected by OKA (FIG. 5). Thus, accordingly to our results, such resistance would be overwhelmed by longer exposures to the toxin. It is well documented that OKA is a potent inhibitor of PP1 and PP2A and therefore leads to a great increase in protein phosphorylation when added to intact cells.[2] The inhibition of PP1 and PP2A activity *in vitro* occurs at concentrations of OKA comparable to those we found to be neurotoxic.[2] Some of the proteins affected could be particularly important for neuronal functioning. In cerebellar neurons in culture OKA is capable of altering the equilibrium between the calcium-dependent and the calcium-independent forms of Ca^{2+}/calmodulin-dependent protein kinase II (CaM-K),[29] a process controlled by PP1. CaM-K appears to participate in the storage of synaptic weight.[30,31] Thus, OKA-mediated disruption of neuronal network might be reflecting changes in the phosphorylating equilibrium related to CaM-K activity, and consequently an alteration in synaptic transmission (FIG. 5).

For example synapsin I, one of the major synaptic vesicle-associated proteins, has been shown to control the vesicle ability for neurotransmitter release by binding to both synaptic vesicles and cytoskeletal-associated elements, and the affinity of the binding appears to be regulated by a phosphorylation-dephosphorylation mechanism in response to nerve impulses.[32] On the other hand, the microtubule-associated protein 2 (MAP2), which is increasingly phosphorylated in the presence of OKA,[33] has been suggested to be necessary for neuronal cells to undergo normal morphological differentiation including neurite extension and cessation of cell division[34] (FIG. 5). Another microtubule-associated protein, tau, appears to be abnormally phosphorylated in some neurodegenerative disorders such as Alzheimer's disease,[13] as well as in the brain of rodents microinjected with OKA.[15] Moreover, OKA has been recently shown to modulate the processing of Alzheimer β/A4 amyloid precursor protein (βAPP).[12] It may be worth noting that changes in the phosphorylation produced by OKA must possibly be directed toward a specific target since the tumor promoter TPA failed to either produce neurotoxicity or enhance OKA toxicity while it is known to phosphorylate several proteins in cerebellar neurons in culture[35] (FIG. 5). Furthermore, protein phosphorylation via c-AMP-dependent protein kinase does not appear to lead to neurodegeneration, as it can be inferred by the absence of both forskolin-induced toxicity and forskolin potentiation of OKA toxicity (FIG. 5). Thus, it is challenging to speculate about a possible use of algal toxins, such as OKA, for dilucidating the mechanisms leading to neuronal synaptic organization and pathological disorders, and therefore the neurotoxic effect of OKA should deserve further studies.

ACKNOWLEDGMENTS

We thank Dr. H. Fujiki for providing okadaic acid, and Dr. Kaczarowski for the gift of VSCC antagonists and MK-801.

REFERENCES

1. TACHIBANA, K., P. J. SCAUFER, Y. TSUKITANI, H. KIKUCHI, D. VAN ENGAN, J. CLARDY, Y. GOPICHAND & F. J. SCHMITZ. 1981. J. Am. Chem. Soc. **103:** 2469–2471.
2. COHEN, P., C. F. B. HOLMES & Y. TSUKITANI. 1990. TIBS **15:** 98–102.
3. KLUMPP, S., P. COHEN & J. E. SCHULTZ. 1990. EMBO J. **9:** 685–689.
4. HESCHELER, J., G. MIESKES, J. C. RÜEGG, A. TAKAI & W. TRAUTWEIN. Pflügers Arch. **412:** 248–252.
5. TOWNSEND, C., Y. WANG, K. FECHO, P. A. KOPLAS & R. L. ROSEMBERG. 1991. Soc. Neurosci. Abstracts **17:** 773, #310.4.
6. YANAGIHARA, N., Y. TOYOHIRA, Y. KODA, A. WADA & F. IZUMI. 1991. Biochem. Biophys. Res. Commun. **174:** 77–83.
7. ABDUL-GHANI, M., E. A. KRAVITZ, H. MEIRI & R. RAHAMINOFF. 1991. Proc. Natl. Acad. Sci. USA **88:** 1803–1807.
8. WANG, L. Y., M. W. SALTER & J. F. MacDONALD. 1991. Science **253:** 1132–1135.
9. COLLINGRIDGE, G. L. & R. A. J. LESTER. 1989. Pharmacol. Rev. **40:** 143–210.
10. CHOI, D. W. 1988. Trends Neurosci. **11:** 465–469.
11. WEISS, J. H., D. M. HARTLEY, J. KOH & D. W. CHOI. 1990. Science **247:** 1474–1476.
12. BUXBAUM, J. D., S. E. GANDY, P. CICCHETTI, E. EHRLICH, A. J. CZERNIK, R. P. FRACASSO, T. V. RAMABHADRAN, A. J. UNTERBECK & P. GREENGARD. 1990. Proc. Natl. Acad. Sci. USA **87:** 6003–6006.
13. BANCHER, C., I. GRUNDKE-IQBAL, K. IQBAL, V. A. FRIED, H. T. SMITH & H. M. WISNIEWSKI. 1991. Brain Res. **539:** 11–18.
14. FERNANDEZ, M. T., V. ZITKO, S. GASCON & A. NOVELLI. 1991. Life Sciences **49:** PL157–162.

15. KOWAL, N. W., M. F. BEAL, A. C. MCKEE & K. S. KOSIK. 1991. J. Cell Biol. **115** (3, Pt. 2): 385a, #2231.
16. NOVELLI, A., J. A. REILLY, P. G. LYSKO & R. C. HENNEBERRY. 1988. Brain Res. **451:** 205–212.
17. NOVELLI, A., J. KISPERT, A. REILLY & V. ZITKO. 1990. Canada Dis. Weekly Rep. **16** (S1): 83–89.
18. BETTLER, B., J. EGEBJERG, G. SHARMA, G. PECHT, I. HERMANS-BORGMEYER, C. MOLL, C. F. STEVENS & S. HEINEMANN. 1992. Neuron **8:** 257–265.
19. STEWART, G. R., C. F. ZORUMSKI, M. T. PRICE & J. W. OLNEY. 1990. Exp. Neurol. **110:** 127–138.
20. NOVELLI, A., J. KISPERT, M. T. FERNANDEZ-SANCHEZ, A. TORREBLANCA & V. ZITKO. 1992. Brain Res. **577:** 41–48.
21. GALLO, V., M. T. CIOTTI, A. COLETTI, F. ALOISI & G. LEVI. 1982. Proc. Natl. Acad. Sci. USA **79:** 7919–7923.
22. CARBONI, E. & W. J. WOJCIK. 1988. J. Neurochem. **50:** 1279–1286.
23. FAVARON, M., H. MANEV, R. SIMAN, M. BERTOLINO, A. M. SZEKELY, G. DEERAUS-QUIN, A. GUIDOTTI & E. COSTA. 1990. Proc. Natl. Acad. Sci. USA **87:** 1983–1987.
24. THOMAS, J. W., A. NOVELLI, J.-H. TAO-CHENG, R. C. HENNEBERRY, H. H. SMITH & C. BANNER. 1989. Mol. Brain Res. **6:** 47–54.
25. GALDZICKI, Z., F. LIN, O. MORAN, A. NOVELLI, G. PUIA & M. SCIANCALEPORE. 1991. Intern. J. Neurosci. **56:** 193–200.
26. NOVELLI, A. & R. C. HENNEBERRY. 1987. Dev. Brain Res. **34:** 307–310.
27. NICOLETTI, F., J. T. WROBLEWSKI, A. NOVELLI, H. ALHO, A. GUIDOTTI & E. COSTA. 1986. J. Neurosci. **6:** 1905–1911.
28. NOVELLI, A., F. NICOLETTI, J. T. WROBLEWSKI, H. ALHO, E. COSTA & A. GUIDOTTI. 1987. J. Neurosci. **7:** 40–47.
29. FOKUNAGA, K., D. P. RICH & T. R. SODERLING. 1989. J. Biol. Chem. **264:** 21830–21836.
30. SHIELDS, S. M., T. S. INGEBRITSEN & P. T. KELLY. 1985. J. Neurosci. **5:** 3414–3422.
31. LISMAN, J. 1989. Proc. Natl. Acad. Sci. USA **86:** 9574–9578.
32. BENFENATI, F., F. VALTORTA, & P. GREENGARD. 1991. Proc. Natl. Acad. Sci. USA **88:** 575–579.
33. GOTOH, Y., E. NISHIDA, & H. SAKAI. 1990. Eur. J. Biochem. **193:** 671–674.
34. DINSMORE, J. H. & F. SOLOMON. 1991. Cell **64:** 817–826.
35. SERAFIAN, T. & M. A. VERITY. 1993. Ann. N.Y. Acad. Sci. **679**. This volume.

Effects of ORG 2766, a Neurotrophic ACTH$_{4-9}$ Analogue, in Neuroblastoma Cells

R. MURRY,[a] J. A. McLANE,[b,d,e] AND G. GRUENER[c]

[a]*Graduate Neuroscience Program*
[b]*Department of Molecular and Cellular Biochemistry*
[c]*Department of Neurology*
Loyola University Stritch School of Medicine
Maywood, Illinois 60153

[d]*Rehabilitation Research and Development (151L)*
Edward Hines, Jr. DVA Hospital
Hines, Illinois 60141

INTRODUCTION

Damage to central or peripheral nervous tissue can result in profound motor, sensory and/or cognitive deficits. CNS tissue has a diminished capacity to recover from damage relative to PNS tissue. Clinical and basic neuroscientists are engaged in developing protocols to enhance/stimulate endogenous nerve tissue repair mechanisms. The cellular cytoskeleton is thought to play an integral role in these processes.

ORG 2766 is a tri-substituted ACTH analogue which retains the neurotrophic properties of endogenous ACTH, but has no hormonal activity. ORG 2766 has been shown to be effective in ameliorating the peripheral neuropathy which often develops as a consequence of chemotherapy;[1] speeds recovery following experimental nerve crush;[2] and hastens development of a compensatory mechanism in rats with striatal lesions.[3]

Initial studies are described here which are designed to begin elucidating possible cellular mechanisms of action of ORG 2766. An understanding of how this peptide stimulates regenerative processes is important in acquiring insight into the mechanisms underlying regeneration, per se, as well as leading to the development of more efficacious clinical strategies for the treatment of neural damage.

METHODS

Mouse neuroblastoma cells (Neuro2a) were cultured in MEM + 10% fetal bovine serum (FBS). Prior to experiments cells were plated in 35 mm tissue culture dishes containing media with 0.5% FBS. The reduced FBS content suspends cell proliferation and causes the cells to produce axon-like processes within 48 hours.

In experiments designed to evaluate the ability of ORG 2766 to protect differentiated cells from chronic treatments with toxic doses of spindle poisons or a Ca^{++}

[e] Address correspondence to Dr. Jerry A. McLane at the Hines DVA Hospital.

ionophore, cellular damage was quantitated by measuring the leakage of lactate dehydrogenase (LDH) activity into the culture media. LDH activity was assessed using a spectrophotometric analysis (Sigma Kit LD-L).

In order to assess treatment-induced alterations in protein synthesis cells were pulse-labelled for 60 min by adding 16 μCi of ^{35}S-Met (TRAN^{35}S-LABEL, ICN Biomedicals, Inc., 1180 Ci/mmole) in one milliliter of serum-free, methionine-deficient media. Total TCA precipitable protein in the cultures was determined by the method of Lowry,[4] and differences in the *de novo* protein synthesis calculated as a function of scintillation counts per μg protein.

The distribution of newly synthesized proteins among the cellular complement of proteins was examined by fractionating extracts of ^{35}S-Met-labeled cells by Laemmli SDS-PAGE[5] or O'Farrell 2-D PAGE.[6] An equal number of cells were extracted in each sample. Densitometer analyses of autoradiograms were completed using a Technology Resources, Inc. ImageMaster 2000 system.

TABLE 1. Effect of Drugs on LDH Release

Exposure Time (h)		Percent of Control LDH Activity		
Drug	Concentration	8	24	48
Cytochalasin D	10 μM	165	198	159
	100 nM	100	91	122
Colchicine	10 μM	191	130	107
	100 nM	109	116	121
Vincristine	10 μM	246	144	111
	100 nM	146	142	102
A23187	10 μM	164	169	151
	100 nM	132	122	102

RESULTS

The toxic substances tested (cytochalasin D, which depolymerizes microfilaments; vincristine sulfate, thought to destroy microtubule nucleation sites; colchicine, prevents microtubule elongation; A23187, a Ca^{++} ionophore) produced cell damage which resulted in leakage of LDH activity into the culture media (TABLE 1). Vincristine produced the greatest effect. ORG 2766 in concentrations between 10^{-12} and 10^{-6} M was able in many cases to reduce the leakage of LDH activity (TABLE 2). Additionally, ORG 2766 treatment alone was able to reduce the levels of LDH in the media in the absence of toxic insult.

The reduction of LDH release was not the result of a general ORG 2766-dependent inhibition of protein synthesis. ORG 2766 increased the incorporation of radiolabel into new cellular proteins (FIG. 1). The greatest increase was observed when cells were treated with 10^{-8} M ORG 2766. The ORG 2766 does not inhibit the activity of LDH (data not shown).

Analysis of newly synthesized polypeptides by SDS-PAGE showed that ORG 2766 treatment of cells increased incorporation of radiolabel into most bands by about 40%. Labeling of a 48–52 Kd polypeptide appeared to be markedly increased

TABLE 2. Effect of ORG 2766 on Drug-induced Release of LDH into Culture Media

t	Org 2766 [M]							
	10^{-13}	10^{-12}	10^{-11}	10^{-10}	10^{-9}	10^{-8}	10^{-7}	10^{-6}
10 μM cytochalasin D								
8	2% ↑	23% ↓ *	24% ↓ *	19% ↓ *	18% ↓ *	12% ↓ *	16% ↓ *	25% ↓ *
24	7% ↓ *	19% ↓ *	19% ↓ *	9% ↓ *	1% ↑	5% ↓	5% ↓	3% ↓
48	1% ↑	16% ↓ *	13% ↓ *	1% ↓	7% ↑ *	7% ↑ *	3% ↑	5% ↑
10 μM colchicine								
8	18% ↓ *	20% ↓ *	21% ↓ *	26% ↓ *	23% ↓ *	22% ↓ *	28% ↓ *	24% ↓ *
24	2% ↓	6% ↓	12% ↓ *	10% ↓ *	2% ↑	1% ↑	7% ↓	5% ↓
48	2% ↓	3% ↓	13% ↓ *	7% ↓	7% ↑	4% ↑	5% ↓	5% ↑
0.1 μM vincristine								
8	4% ↓	22% ↓ *	16% ↓ *	10% ↓ *	4% ↓	15% ↓ *	9% ↓	23% ↓ *
24	11% ↓ *	14% ↓ *	11% ↓ *	3% ↓	5% ↑	1% ↓	3% ↓	4% ↓
48	5% ↓	2% ↓	5% ↓	6% ↑	10% ↑ *	7% ↑ *	8% ↑ *	14% ↑ *
10 μM A23187								
8	10% ↓	7% ↓	3% ↓	24% ↓ *	11% ↓	1% ↓	3% ↓	21% ↓ *
24	8% ↓ *	1% ↑	3% ↑	22% ↓ *	2% ↓	13% ↑ *	13% ↑ *	3% ↓
48	8% ↓ *	0%	8% ↑ *	21% ↓ *	4% ↓	10% ↑ *	4% ↑	18% ↓ *
Org 2766 alone								
8	4% ↑	6% ↓	13% ↓ *	19% ↓ *	13% ↓ *	13% ↓ *	11% ↓	19% ↓ *
24	4% ↑	12% ↓ *	11% ↓ *	15% ↓ *	16% ↓ *	15% ↓ *	3% ↓	7% ↓
48	3% ↓	14% ↓ *	15% ↓ *	11% ↓ *	9% ↓ *	10% ↓ *	10% ↓ *	11% ↓ *

Values equal percent change and arrows indicate direction of change in LDH activity released into culture media.
 * Significantly different from Control at $\alpha = .05$ using a 1-way ANOVA with a Tukey HSD follow-up.

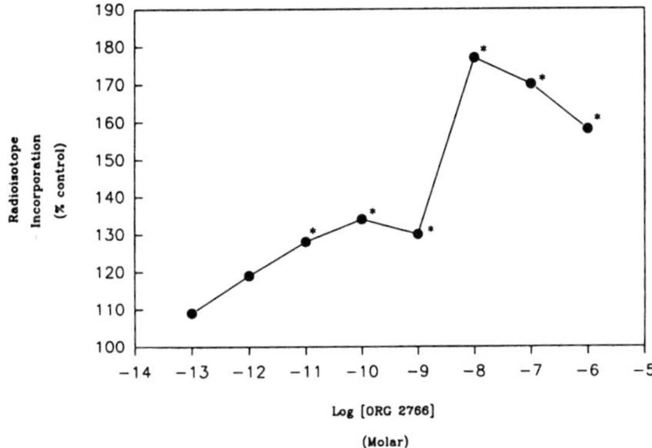

FIGURE 1. Effect of ORG 2766 on Neuro2a cell incorporation of ^{35}S-methionine. Cells differentiated for two days were exposed for 24 h to the doses of ORG 2766 indicated. The cells were then pulsed with ^{35}S-methionine for 1 h and the specific activity of the TCA pellets determined. $*p \leq 0.05$ vs. control by Student's *t*-test.

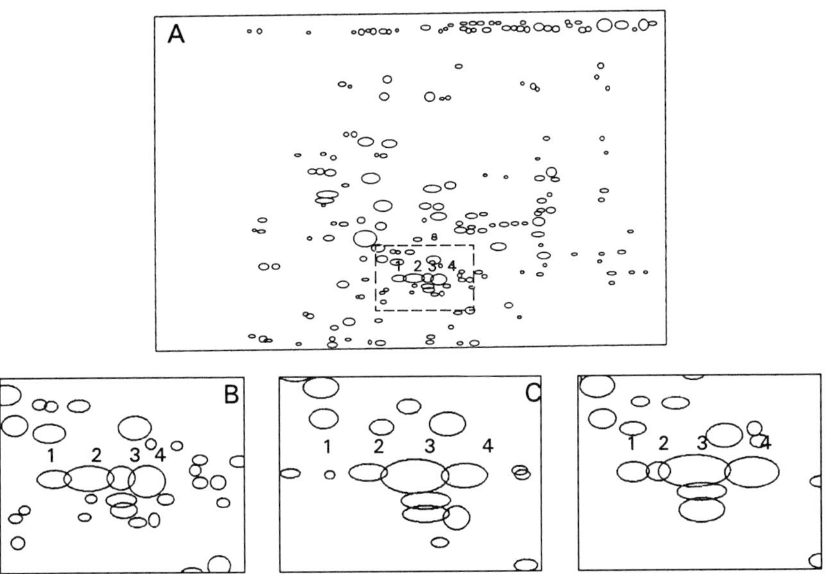

FIGURE 2. 2-D PAGE of ^{35}S-Met labeled cell extracts. Control cells and cells treated with 10^{-8} M ORG 2766 were incubated 1 h with isotope. Cells were then extracted in urea sample buffer in preparation for 2-D PAGE. **(A)** Densitometer trace of spots detected on a control gel. Box indicates area of gel enlarged below believed to include the actin family of polypeptides. The four members of this family of polypeptides are identified by the numbers 1-4. Enlarged sections of gels from control cells **(B)** and cells exposed to ORG 2766 for 1 h **(C)** and 4 h **(D)**.

above that level. A few bands showed increases less than 40%. 2-D Page analyses now in progress confirm that quantities of several polypeptides are affected by ORG 2766. In the example shown (FIG. 2 and TABLE 3), ORG 2766 may be altering the net charge on a polypeptide tentatively identified as actin. Western blot experiments are currently in progress to confirm the identity of this polypeptide family as actin and to quantitate the amount of protein in each charge species. Other polypeptides of interest, including cytoskeletal proteins, will also be identified and quantitated.

SUMMARY

Treatment of Neuro2a cells with drugs known to affect the integrity of microfilaments and microtubules, as well as with a calcium ionophore produced damage to the cellular membrane that was quantifiable by measuring the release of LDH into the culture medium. Concurrent exposure of the cells to ORG 2766 was found to modulate the release of LDH in a dose- and time-dependent fashion. ORG 2766 treatment was also able to reduce the basal release of LDH into the culture medium.

TABLE 3. Effect of ORG 2766 on the Charge Distribution among Members of a Polypeptide Family

Condition	Polypeptide Number	Distribution of Radiolabel (percent of total)			
		1	2	3	4
control		3.5	40.6	21.5	34.4
1 hour ORG		3.8	3.0	65.3	28.0
4 hour ORG		9.4	6.3	53.2	31.1

The ORG 2766-induced reduction in LDH release was not due to down-regulation of protein synthesis. The peptide produced significant increases in protein synthesis relative to control conditions at concentrations of 10^{-11} to 10^{-6} M with 10^{-8} M being an optimal dose. SDS-PAGE and 2-D PAGE analysis showed that *de novo* synthesis of most polypeptides was increased by about 40%. Additionally, a family of polypeptides tentatively identified as actins appear to undergo ORG 2766-dependent post translational charge modifications.

These data are consistent with the hypothesis that regulation of transcription and/or translation are mechanisms important to the neurotrophic actions of ORG 2766.

REFERENCES

1. MULLER, L., R. VAN DER HOOP, C. MOORER-VAN DELFT, W. GISPEN & E. ROUBOS. 1990. Morphological and electrophysiological study of the effects of cisplatin and ORG 2766 on rat ganglion neurons. Cancer Res. **50:** 2437–2442.
2. DEKKER, A. J. A. M., M. M. PRINCEN, H. DE NIJS, G. J. DE LEEDE & C. L. E. BROEKKAMP. 1987. Acceleration of recovery from sciatic nerve damage by the

ACTH(4-9) analog Org. 2766: Different routes of administration. Peptides **8:** 1057–1059.

3. ANTONAWICH, F. J. & F. L. STRAND. 1990. Alterations in rotational and open-field behavior following 6-OHDA lesioning of the substantia nigra and administration of Org 2766. Soc. Neurosci. Abst. **16:** 1157.

4. LOWRY, O. H., N. J. ROSENBROUGH, A. L. FARR & R. J. RANDALL. 1951. Protein measurement with the Folin phenol reagent. J. Biol. Chem. **193:** 265–275.

5. LAEMMLI, U. K. 1970. Cleavage of structural proteins during the assembly of the head of bacteriophage T4. Nature **227:** 680–685.

6. O'FARRELL, P. H. 1975. High resolution two-dimensional electrophoresis of proteins. J. Biol. Chem. **250:** 4007–4021.

Use of Neurite Outgrowth as an *in Vitro* Method of Assessing Neurotoxicity

ELIZABETH McFARLANE ABDULLA

Wellcome Research Laboratories
Beckenham, Kent, United Kingdom BR3 3BS

IAIN C. CAMPBELL

Institute of Psychiatry
Denmark Hill de Crespigny Park
London, United Kingdom SE5 8AF

INTRODUCTION

The differentiation of neurons in culture (seen as neurite outgrowth), provides a useful *in vitro* model for the assessment of neurotoxicity. Neurite outgrowth is a physiological process that is a general indicator of cellular well being—that is, one which will be affected by the widest possible spectrum of noxious agents. However, because, in biochemical terms, it is a multistage process, it also provides the opportunity to examine the specific effects of different groups of toxic substances and thus may eventually provide a new classification system for neurotoxic compounds.

Neurites are composed predominantly of microtubules and also contain actin and neurofilaments. Microtubules are composed of α- and β-tubulin and are inherently unstable; they will undergo catastrophic disassembly unless stabilized by the growing end's joining to unknown stabilizing factors. Microtubulin is stabilized by specific enzyme modification of tubulin, which acts as a signal for binding of microtubule associated proteins (MAPs). MAPs promote the process of nucleation, whereby tubulin polymerizes in a similar way to actin, with hydrolysis of GTP rather than ATP, as in actin polymerization.[3]

Neurite outgrowth is affected by a series of well defined extracellular events/substances including extracellular matrix (ECM) proteins and neural cell adhesion molecules, (N-CAM and N-cadherin) and nerve growth factor, (NGF). These extracellular signals are ultimately translated into changes in the neuronal cytoskeleton. Calpain activation, for instance, both modifies neurofilament proteins in axons to yield additional functional variants and degrades a variety of cytoskeletal proteins including neurofilaments, fodrin, and MAPs.[4]

METHODS

Mouse NB41A3 neuroblastoma cells were grown in HAM's F12 medium containing glutamine 20 mM, Flow 16-801-49, horse serum 7%, NBL S5212, and fetal calf serum 7%, NBL S102, (both heat inactivated), penicillin 500 IU/ml /streptomycin 500 μg/ml, Flow 16-700-49, and 2-mercaptoethanol 10-7 M, BDH 30415, nystatin, 50 units/ml, Sigma N1638. The medium used for the assay contained no fetal calf serum, no nystatin and *2% horse serum,* all other components were the same as the growing medium. The 96-well flat-bottom plates, costar 3595, were precoated first with poly-L-lysine,Sigma P5899, 0.1 mg/ml in 0.15 M borate buffer pH 8.3, 50 µl/well for 4 hours then washed twice with PBS, 100 µl/well and shaken for 20 minutes. The plates were then coated with laminin, Sigma L2020, 5 ng/ml PBS, 50 µl/well for 4 hours, immediately prior to use, then washed twice with PBS 100 µl/well and then shaken for 20 minutes. The cells were seeded at 1.6×10^5 cells/ml, 100 µl/well together with the test compounds in 100 µl/well and incubated for six days after which neurofilament proteins, 68 kD and 160 kD, were quantitated[5] using mouse monoclonal antineurofilament antibodies: L (68 kD) (ICN Code No. 69-703-1 clone NR4), M (160 kD) (ICN Code No. 69-704-1, NN18). Goat anti-mouse IgG horse radish peroxidase conjugate (Sigma A3682) was used together with a chromogenic substrate (TMB Sigma T3405), for quantitation of neurite outgrowth.

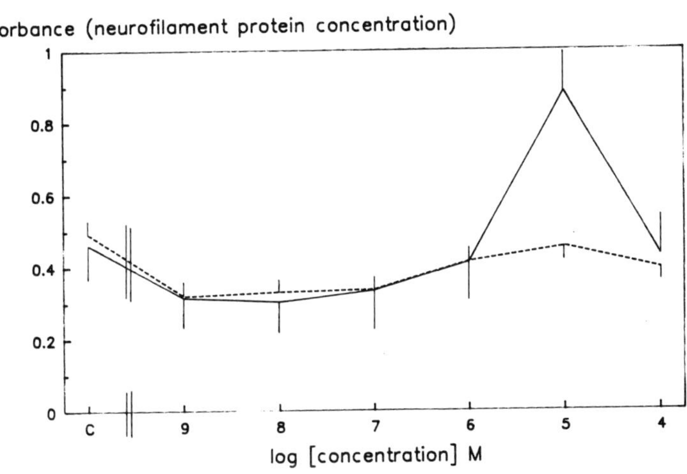

FIGURE 1. BMAA and kainate were incubated for 6 days with NB41A3 mouse neuroblastoma cells grown in a 96-well plate on poly-L-lysine/laminin-coated wells. The level of neurofilament protein 68 kD was estimated by an ELISA method using horseradish peroxidase anti-mouse conjugate incubated for 60 minutes with TMB substrate which gave a blue color and was read at 450 nm. L-BMAA ———, Kainate ------.

RESULTS AND DISCUSSION

Kainate and BMAA have a biphasic effect on both the 68 kD and the 160 kD neurofilament protein levels. At lower doses of (10^{-7} to 10^{-9} M), a decrease in the neurofilament proteins is seen, coinciding with a decrease in neurite outgrowth (seen by phase contrast microscopy). However, perhaps more interesting is the apparent increase in the neurofilament proteins seen at higher doses of the compounds, (10^{-6} to 10^{-5} M), particularly with BMAA. FIGURE 1 shows the results with the 68 kD neurofilament protein levels, for BMAA and kainate, where a parallel decrease is seen at 10^{-9} M. There is an apparent increase in neurofilament

68 kD protein levels at 10^{-5} M (which is more marked for BMAA). FIGURE 2 shows the 160 kD neurofilament protein levels following BMAA and kainate: at 10^{-9} M there is a dramatic decrease in levels, and at 10^{-6} to 10^{-5} M there is again an apparent rise (which is more marked for BMAA).

The exact mode of action of BMAA is unclear. It becomes cytotoxic to fetal mouse dissociated cortical neurons *in vitro* in the presence of bicarbonate, at $0.3–3 \times 10^{-3}$ M, after 1 day exposure,[6] perhaps through the formation of α-methyl carbamate, a putative glutamate analogue. The excitotoxicity of BMAA *in vitro* can be blocked by 2-amino-(5 or 7)-phosphonoheptanoic acid, (AP5 and AP7), indicating an action on N-methyl-D-aspartate (NMDA) receptors.[6] However, at lower concentrations (10^{-5} M), and after 1 day exposure, BMAA shows a selective excitotoxic action on NADPH-diaphorase-positive neurons, suggesting an action on non-NMDA receptors.[7] Thus, BMAA may act at more than one type of receptor.

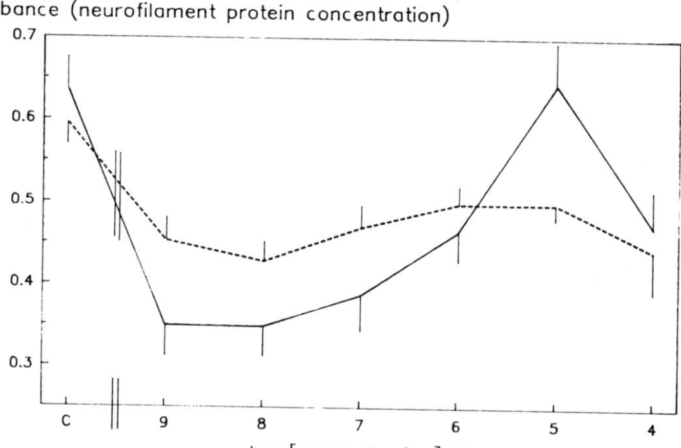

FIGURE 2. BMAA and kainate were incubated for 6 days with NB41A3 mouse neuroblastoma cells grown in a 96-well plate on poly-L-lysine/laminin-coated wells. The level of neurofilament protein 160 kD was estimated by an ELISA method using horseradish peroxidase anti-mouse conjugate incubated for 60 minues with TMB substrate which gave a blue color and was read at 450 nM. L-BMAA ——, Kainate ------.

There is a possible link between the effects of excitatory amino acids and proteins such as those seen during development, for example, fibroblast growth factor (FGF), which may protect against damage, or proteins reported to be involved in neurodegeneration, for example, β-amyloid, which may potentiate.[8]

Mattson *et al.*,[9] using 14-week human embryonic cerebral cortical neurons, showed developing susceptibility to glutamate toxicity, (acting at the NMDA and kainate type receptors), after culture for 30 days. They demonstrated that human cells had a better calcium-buffering capacity than rat cells and so resisted excitotoxic damage better. It is therefore likely that neuronal susceptibility to excitotoxic damage is dependent on the developmental stage and on the species.

The possible significance of the observations presented here is that the neuropathology of Guam disease has a high incidence of neurofibrillary tangles and thus the data showing the accumulation of neurofilament protein following BMAA exposure *in vitro* may directly mimic the *in vivo* situation.

SUMMARY

This work shows that the neurotoxic excitatory amino acids β-N-methylamino alanine, BMAA, and kainate, modulate neurite outgrowth; this was assessed by measuring the levels of two separate neurofilament proteins (68 kD and 160 kD), in a mouse neuroblastoma cell line, (NB41A3). BMAA has been proposed to be the exogenous excitotoxin in Guam disease or amyotrophic lateral sclerosis (ALS\ parkinsonian\ dementia; Guam ALS-PD).[1] Kainate is a glutamate analogue which causes excitotoxic damage associated with excessive entry of calcium into neurons.[2] The results show that at low doses (10^{-9} to 10^{-7} M) both BMAA and kainate decrease the concentration of the two neurofilament proteins. However at high doses (10^{-6} to 10^{-5} M) they cause an apparent accumulation of the neurofilament proteins; the effect is more marked with BMAA. These results support the continued development of an *in vitro* test for neurotoxicity based on neurite outgrowth.

ACKNOWLEDGMENTS

We acknowledge with thanks the efforts of Sofia Magnusson who participated in this study while on a visit from The University of Lund, Sweden.

REFERENCES

1. MELDRUM, B. & J. GARTHWAITE. 1990. Excitatory amino acid neurotoxicity and neurodegenerative disease. Trneds in Pharmacol. Sci. **11:** 379–387.
2. BERDKOWSKY, E., N. RIVEROS, S. SANCHEZ-ARMASS & F. ORREGO. 1983. Kainate, N-methyl-D-aspartate, and other excitatory amino acids increase calcium influx into rat brain cortex cells *in vitro*. Neurosci. Lett. **36:** 75–80.
3. ALBERTS, B., D. BRAY, J. LEWIS, M. RAFF, K. ROBERTS & J. D. WATSON, Eds. 1989. Molecular Biology of the Cell, 2nd Edition. Garland Publishing, Inc. New York & London.
4. NIXON, R. A., R. QUACKENBUSH & A. VITTO. 1986. Multiple calcium-activated neutral proteases (CNAP) in mouse retinal ganglion cell neurons; specificities for endogenous neuronal substrates and comparison to purified brain CNAP. J. Neurosci. **6:** 1252–1263.
5. DOHERTY, P., J. G. DICKSON, P. F. THOMAS & WALSH, F. S. 1984. Quantitative evaluation of neurite outgrowth in cultures of human foetal brain and dorsal root ganglion cell using an enzyme-linked immunoadsorbent assay for human neurofilament protein. J. Neurochem. **42**(4): 1116–1122.
6. WEISS, J. H. & D. W. CHOI. 1988. Beta-N-methylamino-L-alanine neurotoxicity: Requirement for bicarbonate as a co-factor. Science **241:** 973–975.
7. WEISS, J. H., J-Y. KOH & D. W. CHOI. 1989. Neurotoxicity of beta-N-methylamino-L-alanine (BMAA) and beta-N-oxalylamino-L-alanine (BOAA) on cultured cortical neurons. Brain Res. **497:** 64–71.
8. MATTSON, M. P., B. CHENG, D. DAVIS, K. BRYANT, I. LIEBERBURG & R. E. RYDEL. 1992. Beta-amyloid peptides destabilize calcium homeostasis and render human cortical neurons vulnerable to excitotoxicity. J. Neurosci. **12**(2): 376–389.
9. MATTSON, M. P., B. RYCHLIK, J. S. YOU & J. E. SISKIN. 1991. Sensitivity of cultured human embryonic cerebral cortical neurons to excitatory amino acid-induced calcium influx and neurotoxicity. Brain Res. **542:** 97–106.

Preliminary Observations on the *in Vitro* Toxicity of *N*-Butylbenzenesulfonamide: A Newly Discovered Neurotoxin

V. R. NERURKAR,[a] I. WAKAYAMA, T. ROWE,
R. YANAGIHARA, AND R. M. GARRUTO

Laboratory of Central Nervous System Studies
National Institute of Neurological Disorders and Stroke
National Institutes of Health
Bethesda, Maryland 20892

We have previously shown that *N*-butylbenzenesulfonamide (NBBS), a plasticizing agent used in the production of plastic resins and in the synthesis of agricultural herbicides, produces a dose-dependent, progressive spastic myelopathy characterized by neuroaxonal degeneration in New Zealand white rabbits.[1,2] The neurotoxicity of NBBS was discovered serendipitously when control rabbits developed a progressive spastic myelopathy, when inoculated once monthly with 0.9% saline solution stored continuously in a plastic filter flask for more than 18 months.[2] Later, we discovered that over time NBBS had leached out from the plastic container into the saline solution.

The environmental distribution and the sources and biological effects of NBBS are largely unknown. During routine analysis of herbicides in ground water and drinking water from Pavia, Italy, an unidentified substance later characterized as NBBS was found.[3] A study on the sources and movement of organic chemicals in the Delaware River also found NBBS in the water.[4] *In vivo* studies in rats, mice, rabbits and guinea pigs indicate that NBBS, at varying concentrations (lethal and threshold) and by different routes of exposure, usually targets the hematopoietic system.[5] The presence of benzene rings in the structure of the NBBS molecule is consistent with the bone marrow being a possible target organ, but hematologic abnormalities were not detected in our *in vivo* studies on rabbits inoculated intraperitoneally with NBBS.[2]

Using conventional assays for cell viability (trypan blue dye exclusion and lactate dehydrogenase [LDH]) and assays for cell growth and function (^{3}H-thymidine incorporation and immunostaining), we report the effects of varying concentrations of NBBS on C6 glioma and Neuro-2a cells (American Type Culture Collection, Rockville, MD), two continuous cell lines of glial and neuronal origin, respectively.

Micromolar (μM) concentrations of NBBS inhibited cell growth (FIG. 1) and produced morphological changes and altered cell function in these cell lines. A

---

[a] Author to whom correspondence and reprint requests should be addressed at Bldg. 376, NINDS, NCI-FCRDC, Frederick, Maryland 21702.

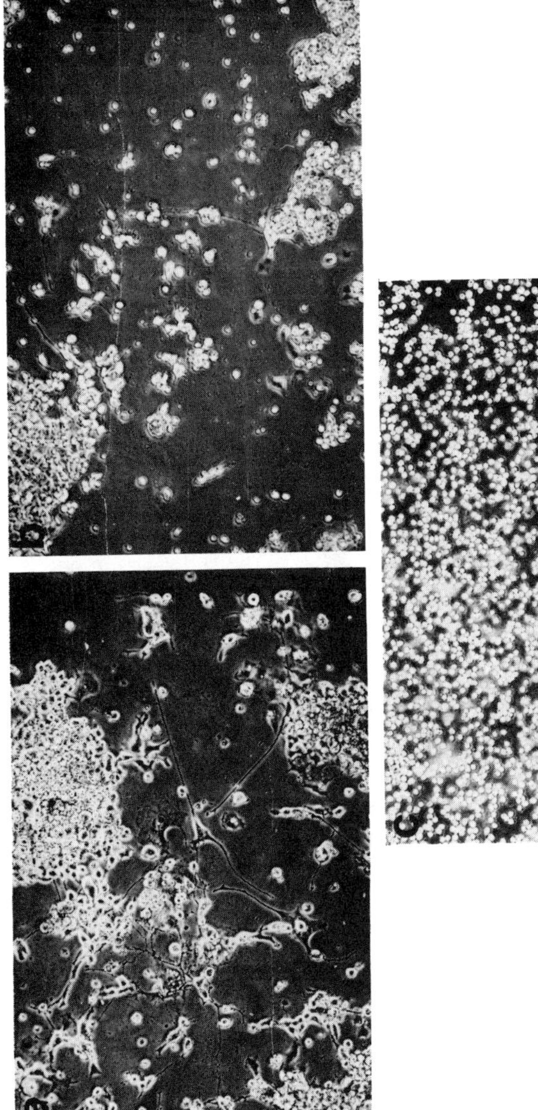

FIGURE 1. Effect of NBBS on Neuro-2a cells exposed to 10 μM and 100 μM of NBBS for 48 h. **(a)** Neurites of control cells with no NBBS were healthy and firmly attached to the substrate. Forty percent of cells subjected to **(b)** 10 μM NBBS, and 100% of cells exposed to **(c)** 100 μM NBBS had detached from the substrate, indicating cell death.

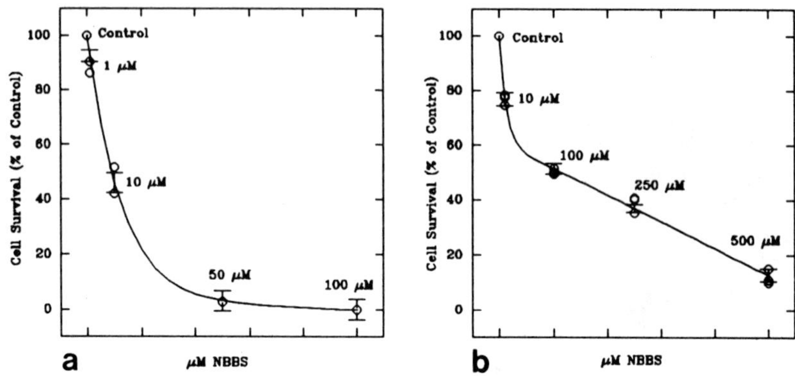

FIGURE 2. (a) Neuro-2a and (b) C6 glioma cells were plated at a density of 2×10^5 and 2.5×10^3 cells per well in 6-well and 12-well plates, respectively. After 24 h NBBS was added at varying concentrations from 10 μM to 500 μM for 72 h. Cells were counted for viability using the trypan blue dye-exclusion method. Results are expressed as percent of control and presented as mean $\pm$ SD of triplicate determinations. After 24 h at 50 μM NBBS, 30% of Neuro-2a cells started to detach from the substrate (data not shown) and at 72 h 90% of the cells were detached. Neuro-2a cells exhibited 50% cell death following exposure to 10 μM NBBS at 72 h. By contrast, 100 μM NBBS was required to produce 50% cell death in C6 glioma cells at 72 h. At 500 μM NBBS no Neuro-2a cells and only 10% C6 glioma cells survived the 72-h exposure.

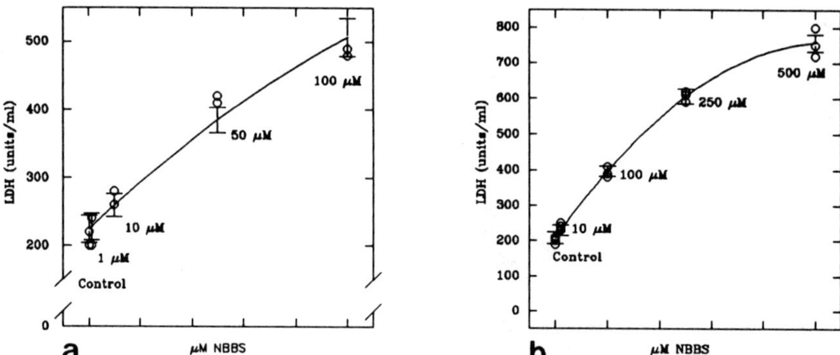

FIGURE 3. Release of lactate dehydrogenase (LDH), an indicator of cell death, was assessed by measuring LDH levels in the medium, using the Sigma LD assay kit, catalog #340-LD (Sigma Chemical Co., St. Louis, MO). (a) Neuro-2a and (b) C6 glioma cells, plated at a density of 2×10^5 and 2.5×10^3 cells per well in 6-well and 12-well plates, respectively, were subjected to varying concentrations of NBBS, ranging from 10 μM to 500 μM, for 72 h. Results are expressed as LDH units/ml and presented as mean $\pm$ SD of triplicate determinations. There was a positive correlation between increasing concentrations of NBBS and LDH released in the culture medium by both cell lines.

lower concentration of NBBS was required to inhibit DNA synthesis in Neuro-2a cells (10 μM) than in C6 glioma cells (100 μM), suggesting that neuronal cells are more sensitive than glial cells to NBBS toxicity (FIGS. 2 and 3).

The effect of NBBS on DNA synthesis in C6 glioma cells occurred as early as 24 h after exposure to a concentration of 10 μM as shown by an 18% inhibition of thymidine incorporation, with 30% inhibition at 72 h. At an NBBS concentration of 250 μM, DNA synthesis was strikingly inhibited (70%) at 72 h (FIG. 4). C6

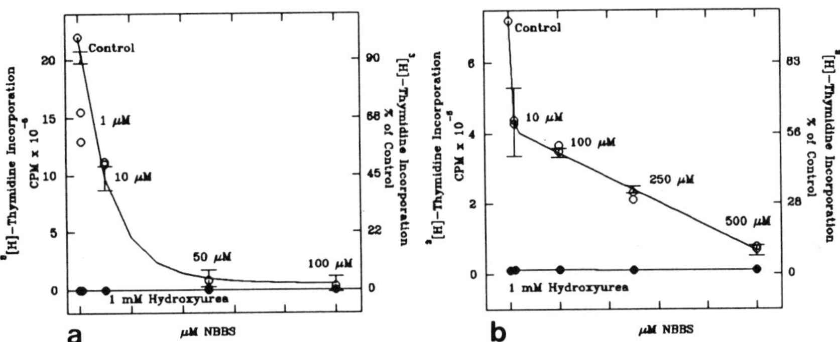

FIGURE 4. ³[H]-thymidine incorporation in **(a)** Neuro-2a and **(b)** C6 glioma cells, plated at a density of 2×10^5 and 2.5×10^3 cells per well in 6-well and 12-well plates, respectively, exposed for 72 h to varying concentrations of NBBS ranging from 10 μM to 500 μM. ³[H]-thymidine, at a concentration of 5 μCi/ml (Neuro-2a) and 2 μCi/ml (C6 glioma), was added to each well and incubation was continued for 4 h. Cells were washed once with ice-cold phosphate buffered saline, incubated on ice with 10% trichloroacetic acid (TCA) for 10 min, washed successively with ice-cold 10% TCA and 95% ethanol, solubilized with 1 ml 0.3 N sodium hydroxide/1% sodium dodecyl sulfate for 2 h at 37°C, transferred to 10 ml of scintillation fluid (Aquasure, Du Pont NEN, Wilmington, DE) and counted in a scintillation counter (Beckman Instruments Inc., Palo Alto, CA). Results are expressed as cpm $\times 10^{-5}$ and presented as mean $\pm$ SD of quadruplicate determinations and the experiment was repeated twice. In Neuro-2a cells, DNA synthesis was inhibited 70% at 20 μM NBBS. By contrast, 250 μM NBBS was required to produce 70% inhibition of DNA synthesis in C6 glioma cells, indicating a cell type-specific neurotoxicity of NBBS. Thymidine incorporation by subconfluent, actively growing C6 glioma cells was affected more than confluent cell monolayers. The addition of 1 mM hydroxyurea completely inhibited DNA synthesis.

glioma cells exposed to 100 μM and 250 μM NBBS exhibited markedly reduced or absent immunoreactivity with antibodies against glial fibrillary acidic protein (FIG. 5) and S-100 protein (FIG. 6), while Neuro-2a cells subjected to 1 μM and 10 μM NBBS showed significantly less staining for the 160 kDa neurofilament subunit protein (FIG. 7).

Our study demonstrates that NBBS is toxic to cells of neuronal and glial origin *in vitro*. Cells of neuronal origin are ten times more sensitive to NBBS than cells of glial origin, indicating a cell type-specific toxicity of NBBS, which support our earlier chronic *in vivo* studies in rabbits.[1,2] Studies are currently underway to evaluate the effects of NBBS on primary neuronal cell cultures.[6] Additional epide-

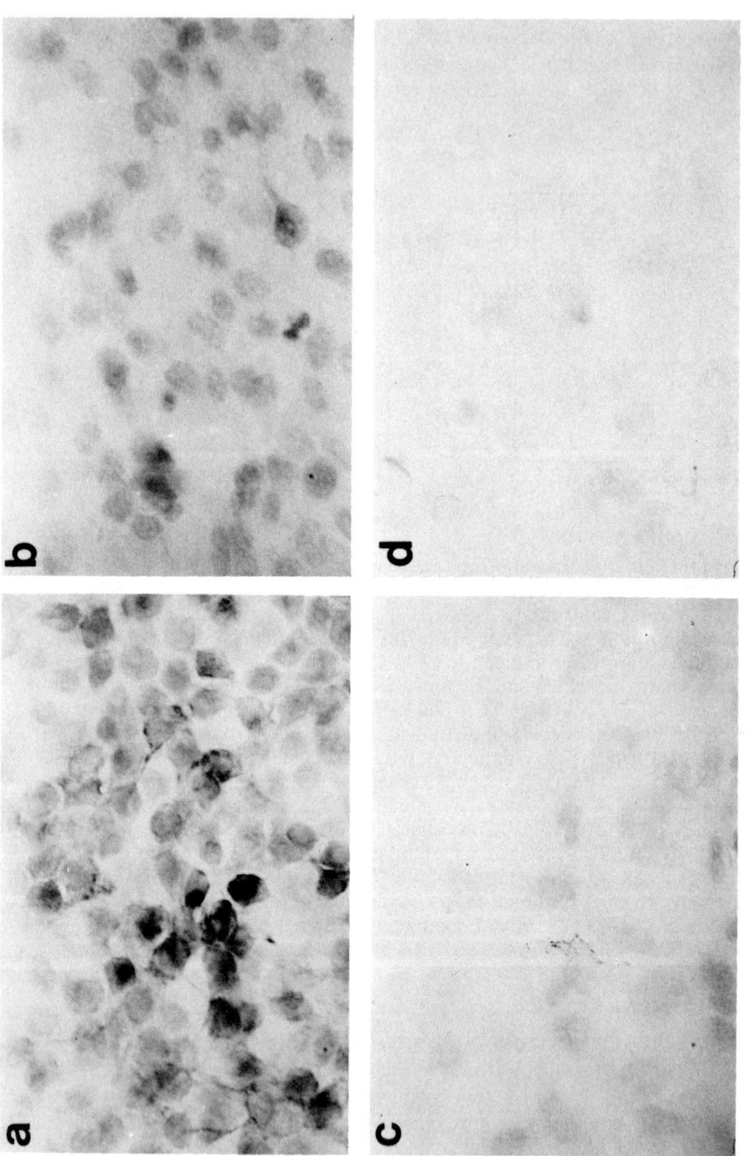

FIGURE 5. C6 glioma cells, exposed to various concentrations of NBBS for 72 h, were stained by the avidin-biotin peroxidase technique (Vectastain ABC kit, Vector Labs., Burlingame, CA) using a mouse monoclonal antibody against glial fibrillary acidic protein (GFAP) (1:100 dilution, Sigma Chemical Co., St. Louis, MO). C6 glioma (a) control cells showed robust immunoreactivity, while cells exposed to (b) 10 μM, (c) 100 μM and (d) 250 μM NBBS showed markedly reduced immunoreactivity, indicating inhibition of GFAP synthesis. Original magnification, × 250.

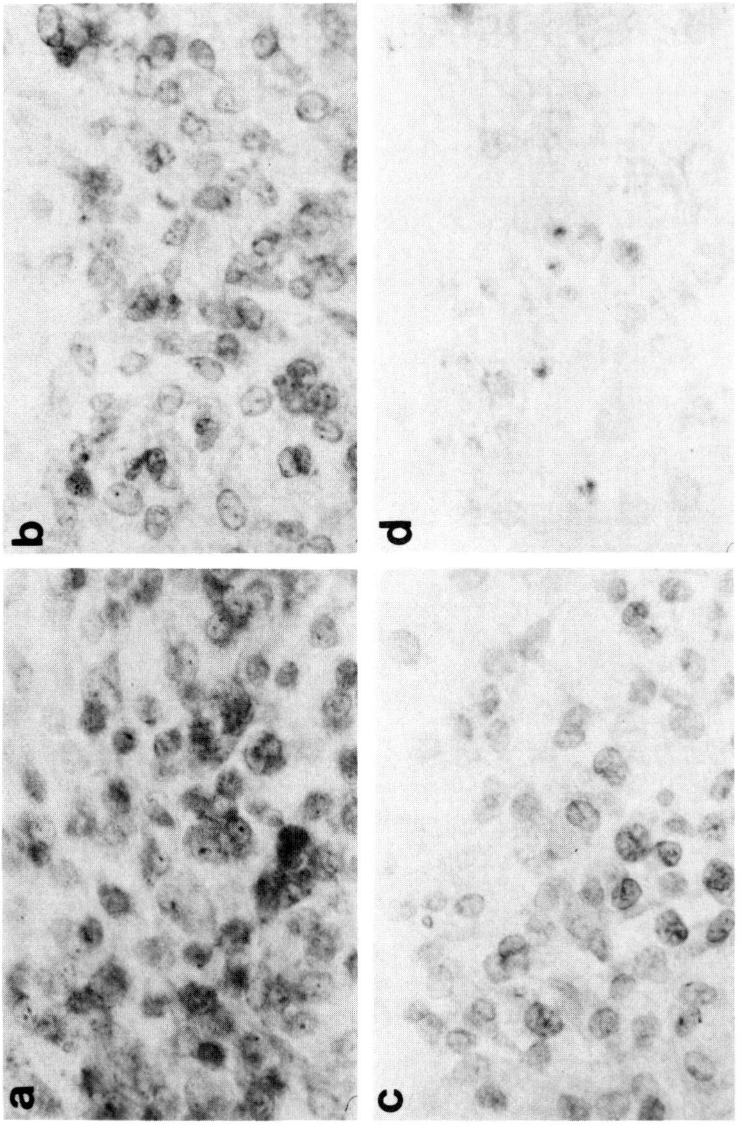

FIGURE 6. C6 glioma cells, exposed to various concentrations of NBBS for 72 h, were stained by the avidin-biotin peroxidase technique (Vectastain ABC kit), using a mouse monoclonal antibody against S-100 protein (1:100 dilution, Chemicon Int. Inc., Temecula, CA). C6 glioma (**a**) control cells showed robust immunoreactivity with anti S-100 protein, while cells exposed to (**b**) 10 μM, (**c**) 100 μM and (**d**) 250 μM NBBS showed progressively less immunostaining, demonstrating a general inhibition of S-100 protein synthesis. Original magnification, $\times$ 250.

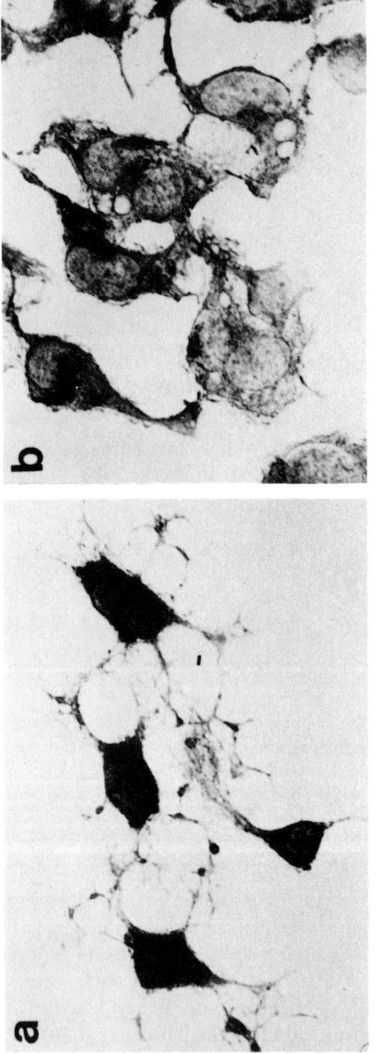

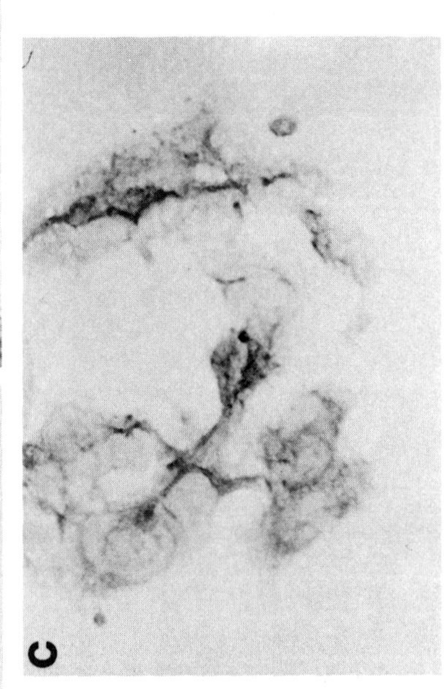

FIGURE 7. Neuro-2a cells, exposed to various concentrations of NBBS for 72 h, were stained by the avidin-biotin peroxidase technique (Vectastain ABC kit), using a mouse monoclonal antibody against the 160 kDa neurofilament protein subunit (1:40 dilution, Sigma Chemical Co.). **(a)** Control cells showed striking immunoreactivity in perikarya and neurites, while cells exposed to **(b)** 1 μM and **(c)** 10 μM NBBS exhibited markedly reduced immunoreactivity, indicating altered synthesis of neurofilament protein. Original magnification, $\times$ 250.

miological and experimental studies are needed to determine both the magnitude of exposure and the degree of NBBS neurotoxicity in humans and other mammals.

ACKNOWLEDGMENTS

We thank Mr. Matthew Fivash, Data Management Services, Inc., NCI-FCRDC, Frederick, Maryland for the statistical analysis.

REFERENCES

1. STRONG, M. J., R. M. GARRUTO, A. V. WOLFF, R. YANAGIHARA, S. M. CHOU & S. D. FOX. 1990. *N*-butylbenzenesulfonamide, a novel neurotoxic plasticising agent. Lancet **336:** 640.
2. STRONG, M. J., R. M. GARRUTO, A. V. WOLFF, S. M. CHOU, S. D. FOX & R. YANAGIHARA. 1991. *N*-butylbenzenesulfonamide: a neurotoxic plasticizer inducing a spastic myelopathy in rabbits. Acta Neuropathol. **81:** 235–241.
3. BRAMBILLA, A., L. BROGLIA & G. NIDASIO. 1991. *N*-butylbenzenesulfonamide in drinking water. Boll. Chim. Igien. **42:** 779–785.
4. SHELDON, L. S. & R. A. HITES. 1979. Sources and movement of organic chemicals in the Delaware River. Environ. Sci. Technol. **13:** 574–579.
5. BAZAROVA, L. A. & N. V. MIGUKINA. 1979. Evaluation of the toxicity and safety of benzenesulfonic acid butylamide. Toksikol. Nov. Prom. Khim. Veshshestv. **15:** 110–116.
6. WAKAYAMA, I., V. R. NERURKAR & R. M. GARRUTO. 1992. *N*-butylbenzenesulfonamide toxicity in primary neuronal cultures. Soc. Neurosci. Abst. **18:** 1606.

Heat Shock Proteins Used to Show that Haloperidol Prevents Neuronal Injury Produced by Ketamine, MK801, and Phencyclidine[a]

FRANK R. SHARP, MICHAEL BUTMAN, SHU WANG,
JARI KOISTINAHO, STEVEN H. GRAHAM,
STEPHEN M. SAGAR, PAUL BERGER,
AND FRANK M. LONGO

Departments of Neurology and Psychiatry
University of California at San Francisco
San Francisco, California 94117

Department of Veterans Affairs Medical Center
4150 Clement Street
San Francisco, California 94121

We and others have suggested that induction of the hsp70 gene is an extremely sensitive indicator of injury to the nervous system. Although hsp70 is not normally expressed in rat brain, hsp70 mRNA and HSP72 protein are induced following injury produced by global ischemia,[1,2] focal ischemia,[3] focal injections of excitotoxins,[3] and status epilepticus produced by kainic acid[3] and flurothyl.[4] Moreover, HSP72 protein is induced almost exclusively in neurons following global ischemia, excitotoxin injections, and status epilepticus, conditions that are known to primarily cause neuronal death without affecting glia. Following infarction, however, there is HSP72 induction in endothelial cells in the core of the infarct, and HSP72 induction in neurons and glial cells in the penumbra.[5,6]

Since it has been suggested that denatured proteins are the stimulus for induction of the hsp70 gene, and because Olney *et al.* had reported that phencyclidine (PCP), ketamine, and MK801 produced vacuoles in injured cingulate neurons,[7] we have examined the question of whether these noncompetitive N-methyl-D-asparate (NMDA) antagonists induce the hsp70 gene in brain. Once we showed that PCP, and related drugs induced the HSP72 protein in vacuolated neurons in the cingulate cortex,[8] we then showed that antipsychotic medications prevented the neuronal injury produced by the psychomimetics PCP, ketamine, and MK801.

Rats were administered PCP, ketamine, and MK801 i.p. Induction of HSP72 protein was examined 6 h to 14 days later. HSP72 protein was visualized immunocytochemically using the avidin-biotin technique described previously.[8] HSP72 was not detected in normal rat brain. Following administration of PCP, ketamine, and MK801, HSP72 protein was detected by 8 h, was maximal at 24 to 48 h, and disappeared between 7 and 14 days. HSP72 was induced only in neurons and localized to the cytoplasm of the dendrites, cell body, and axons of neurons only.

[a] Work presented in this paper was supported by NINCDS RO128167 grant entitled "Markers of Neural Injury."

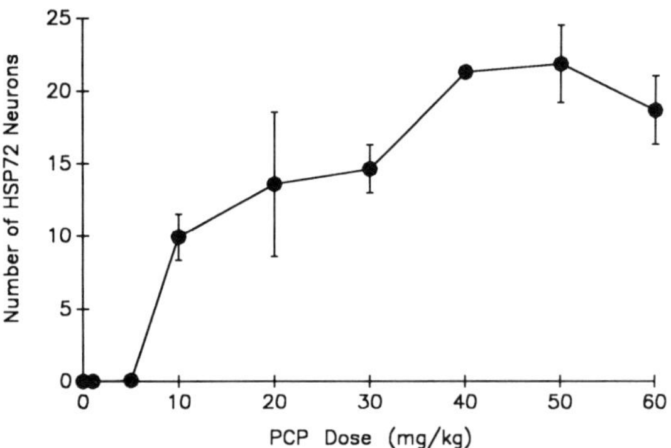

FIGURE 1. The number ($\pm$ SEM/0.0441 mm^2) of HSP72 immunoreactive neurons in layer 3 of granular posterior cingulate cortex is plotted for adult rats given various doses of phencyclidine (PCP) (0-60 mg/kg) intraperitoneally 24 h previously.

HSP72 was clearly localized to vacuolated, injured neurons when viewed under the electron microscope. MK801 induced HSP72 in doses of 0.1 mg/kg to at least 5 mg/kg; ketamine induced HSP72 in doses of 40 mg/kg up to at least 100 mg/kg; and PCP induced HSP72 in doses of 10 mg/kg to at least 60 mg/kg (see FIG. 1). MK801 and ketamine induced HSP72 in layer 2, 3 and 5 neurons in the posterior cingulate cortex and retrosplenial cortex of 30 day and older rats. PCP induced HSP72 in layer 2, 3 and 5 neurons in posterior cingulate and retrosplenial cortex; in layer 2, 3, 5, and 6 neurons in necortex; in layer 3 neurons in piriform cortex; and in neurons in several nuclei in the amygdala.

Because the major side effect of ketamine, MK801 and PCP is psychosis and because PCP is known to act at both NMDA and sigma receptors, we tested whether sigma receptor antagonists prevented the neuronal injury. Therefore, the sigma antagonists haloperidol and rimcazole were administered one hour prior to administration of 30 mg/kg of PCP, a dose which markedly induces HSP72 in many neurons throughout the rat brain. As shown in FIGURE 2, haloperidol produced a dose-dependent blockade of HSP72 induction normally produced by PCP. A 5 mg/kg dose of haloperidol totally prevented the HSP72 induction in neurons normally injured by PCP. Similarly, rimcazole also prevented injury produced by PCP, though at a higher dose (not shown).

Since haloperidol and rimcazole are both known to act at sigma receptors, and

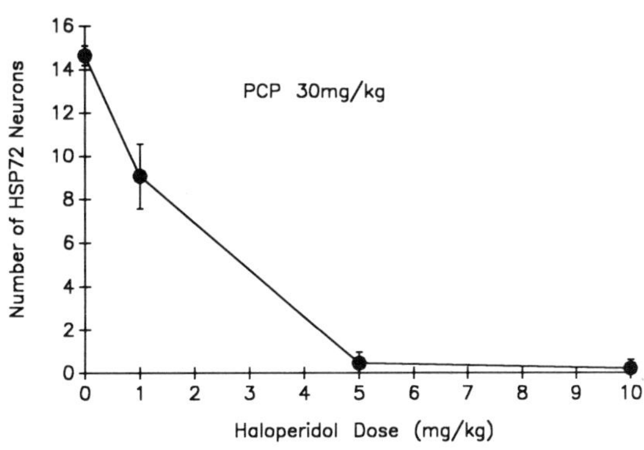

FIGURE 2. The number ($\pm$ SEM/0.0441 mm^2) of HSP72 immunoreactive neurons in layer 3 of granular posterior cingulate cortex is plotted for adult rats given PCP (30 mg/kg) intraperitoneally 24 hours previously. These subjects had had haloperidol administered intraperitoneally in various doses (0-10 mg/kg) one hour prior to administration of the Phencyclidine (PCP).

rimcazole has little effect on dopamine receptors, we have proposed that sigma receptors mediate injury following PCP, ketamine, and MK801 administration. How blockade of NMDA receptors might lead to overactivation of sigma receptors and neuronal injury is not known. This data has important clinical implications since it suggests that administration of antipsychotic medications can prevent brain injury produced by psychomimetic compounds like PCP, ketamine, MK801 and others. Moreover, it is possible that in a variety of psychotic states, such as occurs in schizophrenia, that endogenous or exogenous compounds might mediate neuronal injury at sigma or other receptors. If this were true, then antipsychotic medications might be decreasing psychosis by decreasing neuronal injury in these clinical situations.

REFERENCES

1. VASS, K., W. J. WELCH & T. S. NOWAK, JR. 1988. Localization of 70 kD stress protein induction in gerbil brain after ischemia. Acta Neuropathol. **77:** 128–135.
2. FERRIERO, D. M., H. Z. SOBERANO, R. P. SIMON & F. R. SHARP. 1990. Hypoxia-ischemia induces heat shock protein-like (HSP72) immunoreactivity in neonatal rat brain. Develop. Brain Res. **53:** 145–150.
3. GONZALEZ, M. F., K. SHIRAISHI, K. HISANAGA, S. M. SAGAR, M. MANDABACH & F. R. SHARP. 1989. Heat shock proteins as markers of neural injury. Mol. Brain Res. **6:** 93–100.
4. LOWENSTEIN D. H., R. P. SIMON & F. R. SHARP. 1990. The pattern of 72-kDa heat shock protein-like immunoreactivity in the rat following flurothyl-induced status epilepticus. Brain Res. **531:** 173–182.
5. GONZALEZ, M. F., D. LOWENSTEIN, K. HISANAGA, R. P. SIMON, S. M. SAGAR & F. R. SHARP. 1991. Induction of heat shock protein 72-kD like immunoreactivity in the hippocampal formation following transient global ischemia. Brain Res. Bull. **26:** 241–250.
6. SHARP, F. R., D. LOWENSTEIN, R. P. SIMON & K. HISANAGA. 1991. Heat shock protein HSP72 induction in cortical and striatal astrocytes and neurons following infarction. J. Cereb. Blood Flow Metab. **11:** 621–627.
7. OLNEY, J. W., J. LABRUYERE, G. WANG, D. F. WOZNIAK, M. T. PRICE & M. A. SESMA. 1991. NMDA antagonist neurotoxicity: Mechanism and prevention. Science **254:** 1515–1518.
8. SHARP, F. R., P. JASPER, J. HALL, L. NOBLE & S. M. SAGAR. 1991. MK-801 and ketamine induce heat shock protein HSP72 in injured neurons in posterior cingulate and retrosplenial cortex. Ann. Neurol. **30:** 801–809.

Light- and Electron-Microscopic Studies of Identified Septohippocampal Neurons Surviving Axotomy[a]

GARY M. PETERSON,[b,c] THOMAS NAUMANN,[c] AND
MICHAEL FROTSCHER[c]

*[b]Department of Anatomy & Cell Biology
East Carolina University School of Medicine
Greenville, North Carolina 27858-4354*

*[c]Anatomisches Institut
Universität Freiburg
D-7800 Freiburg, Germany*

A marked loss of neurons has been shown to occur in the medial septum (MS) and vertical limb of the diagonal band (vDB; collectively, MSDB) within two weeks following transection of the fimbria-fornix (FF). The neurons of the MSDB project to the hippocampal formation via the FF[1,2] and approximately half of these are cholinergic,[3,4] the other major population being GABAergic.[5,6] In this system, cell death after axotomy has been inferred from the disappearance of neurons stained for Nissl,[7] acetylcholinesterase[8] (AChE) and immunoreactivity for choline acetyltransferase[9] (ChAT) or glutamic acid decarboxylase (GAD).[6] Several studies have suggested that the degeneration of the cholinergic neurons results from the loss of contact with postsynaptic target cells which provide trophic support.[10–12] In support of this, it has been shown that loss of cholinergic neurons can be prevented by the exogenous application of nerve growth factor (NGF).[13–16] However, reduction in number of stained neurons does not necessarily indicate actual cell death. The loss of immunoreactivity may merely indicate alterations in gene expression,[17] and the reduction in numbers of Nissl-stained magnocellular neurons[7] may be the result of cell shrinkage rather than cell death.[18,19] To further study the possibility that axotomy does not cause neuronal death we have retrogradely labeled healthy neurons in the MSDB prior to FF transection and, using light and electron microscopy, examined the surviving neurons at various times after axotomy.

To retrogradely label healthy septohippocampal neurons, adult female Sprague-Dawley rats received stereotaxic injections of the fluorescent dye Fluoro-Gold (FG; 2%; 50 nl)[20] in the hilus of the dentate gyrus at 5 sites along its septotemporal axis. One week later the FF and overlying cortical tissue were bilaterally aspirated under visual guidance. Control animals received sham lesions. The animals were killed 3, 6, and 10 weeks after the FF transection and the brains were histologically processed for Nissl, ChAT-immunoreactivity, or visualization of FG and intracellular filling. The completeness of the axotomy was assessed by microscopic exami-

[a] Supported by the Alzheimer's Disease and Related Disorders Association (IIRG-88-059), the Alexander von Humboldt-Stiftung, and the Deutsche Forschungsgemeinschaft (Fr 620/1-5).

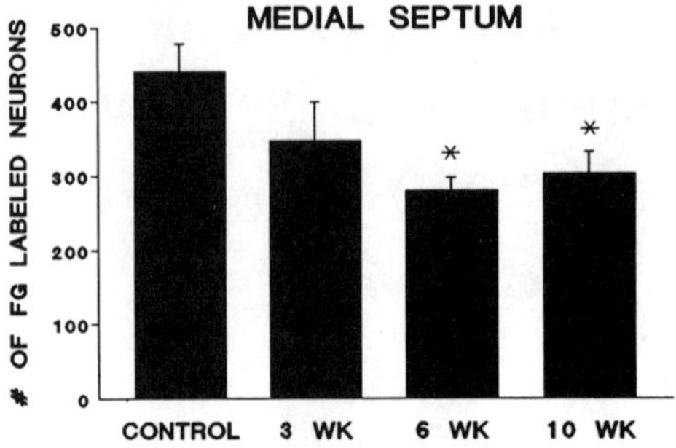

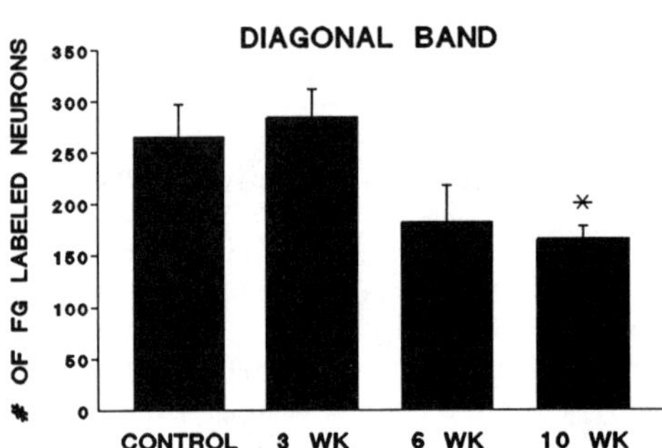

FIGURE 1. Mean (± SEM) number of FG-labeled neurons in the MS and vDB in control brains and in brains 3, 6, and 10 weeks after transection of the fimbria-fornix. (Reproduced from Peterson *et al.*[24] with permission from the publisher.)

nation of the lesion site and by loss of AChE staining in sections of the deafferented hippocampus. At the light microscopic level, numbers of FG- or ChAT-labeled neurons were counted at three levels of the MSDB which a previous study showed to have the greatest number of retrogradely labeled cells.[21] The somal area and diameter of FG-labeled cells were also measured. Data were analyzed using a one way ANOVA followed by individual Student's *t*-tests. For the EM analysis, retrogradely labeled septohippocampal neurons were visualized under a fluorescence microscope and were intracellularly injected with Lucifer Yellow (LY) to reveal the dendritic arbor of the cells.[22] Following photoconversion of LY to an electron dense product,[23] these identified septo-hippocampal neurons were further processed for electron microscopic analysis. Electron micrographs of retrogradely labeled, axotomized neurons were analyzed for the fine-structural preservation of cell body and dendrites, and for the presence of input synapses.

CELL COUNTS

Within the MS, the number of FG-labeled neurons was reduced by 21, 36 and 31% at each of the three survival times (FIG. 1). The decrease was not significantly different from controls 3 weeks after FF transection, but was at 6 and 10 weeks, and there were no significant differences between the three lesion groups.[24] Within the vDB, a slight increase of 7% was observed in the number of FG-labeled neurons three weeks after FF transection and this was followed by a decrease of 31 and 37% at 6 and 10 weeks (Fig. 1). Post-hoc tests showed that the number of cells after FF transection was significantly different from conrols only at 10 weeks.[24] In contrast, the numbers of ChAT-immunoreactive neurons in the MS was decreased by 83%, 80%, and 75% 3, 6, and 10 weeks after axotomy and by 13%, 43%, and 5% at the same time points in the vDB.[24] A comparison in the rate and degree of cell loss as indicated by different staining techniques is illustrated in Figure 2.

MORPHOMETRIC ANALYSIS

The surviving cells displayed a reduction in somal size (Fig. 3). Within the control MS, FG-labeled cells had a mean diameter of 18.4 ± 0.5 μm. Following transection, the surviving cells were reduced in diameter by 34%, 27% and 34% at the three time points. Within the vDB, FG-labeled neurons shrunk by 23%, 25%, and 29% from a mean diameter of 20.7 ± 0.8 μm in controls. Intracellular filling with LY[22,25] 10 weeks after FF transection revealed 3 classes of septohippo-campal neurons: a few cells (~10%) had apparently normal size and dendritic arbor,[26] a second group (~80%) had slightly shrunken somata and dendrites (Fig. 4a), and a third group (~10%) had severely shrunken somata, sometimes to a diameter of less than the 9 μm criterion used in the cell counting[24] and no dendrites at all.

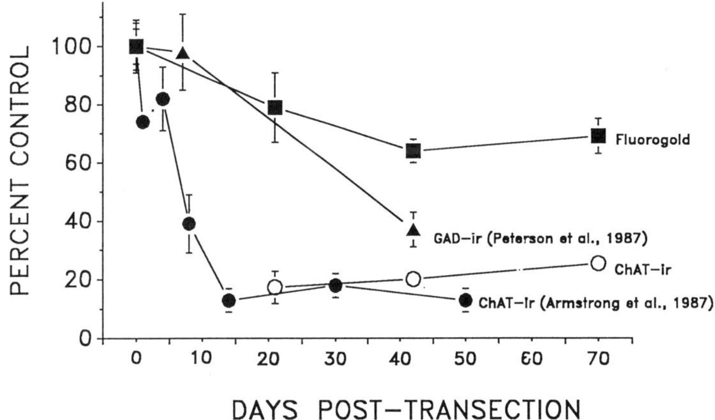

FIGURE 2. Comparison of the number of FG-labeled (■), GAD-immunoreactive (▲), and ChAT-immunoreactive (● and ○) over time following transection of the FF. Data are expressed as percentage of control. As indicated, the data for GAD-immunoreactive neurons are from ref. 6 and some of the data for ChAT-immunoreactive neurons (●) are from ref. 9. These data have been re-expressed as percent of control values. (Reproduced from Peterson *et al.*[24] with permission from the publisher.)

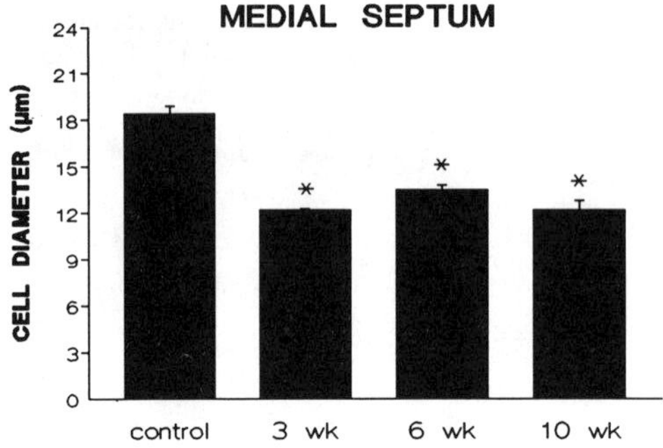

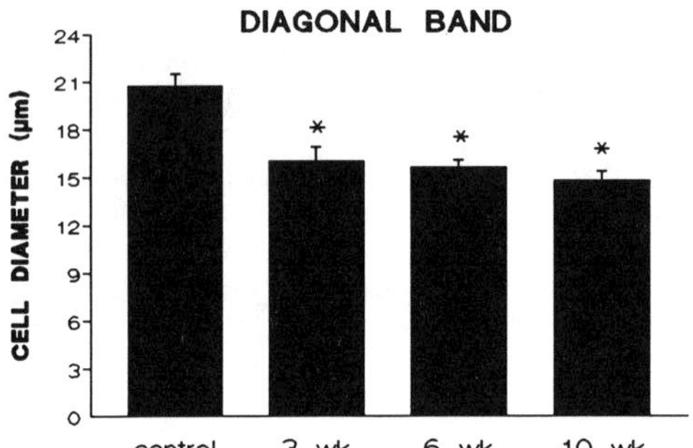

FIGURE 3. Mean (± SEM) diameter (long dimension) of FG-labeled neurons in the MS and vDB before and after axotomy. (Reproduced from Peterson *et al.*[24] with permission from the publisher.)

ULTRASTRUCTURAL ANALYSIS

Retrogradely labeled and intracellularly filled neurons were identified by the presence of electron-dense product throughout the cytoplasm and dark lysosome-like structures which indicate FG[27] (FIG. 4b,d). The ultrastructural morphology

FIGURE 4. A retrogradely labeled, axotomized, and intracellularly filled neuron in the medial septum 10 weeks after transection of the fimbria-fornix. **a:** Light micrograph showing the appearance of photoconverted LY and the presence of a reduced dendritic arbor. The arrow points to a blood vessel which can also be seen in **b**. **b:** Electron micrograph of the same cell. Note the presence of black lysosome-like bodies which are indicative of retrograde FG labeling throughout the cytoplasm, the dark, diffuse reaction product resulting from photoconversion of LY, and the infolded nucleus (Nc). The boxed region is shown at higher magnification in **d**. A retrogradely labeled cell which was not intracellularly filled can be seen at the top of the figure, between the bifurcating dendrites. **c:** A synapse of normal morphology on the soma of the cell shown in **a, b**. The asterisk indicates the presynaptic bouton and the white arrow identifies the postsynaptic thickening. **d:** The endoplasmic reticulum (ER) and a FG lysosome (*arrow*) from the boxed region in **b**, at higher magnification. (Reproduced from Peterson *et al.*[25] with permission from the publisher.)

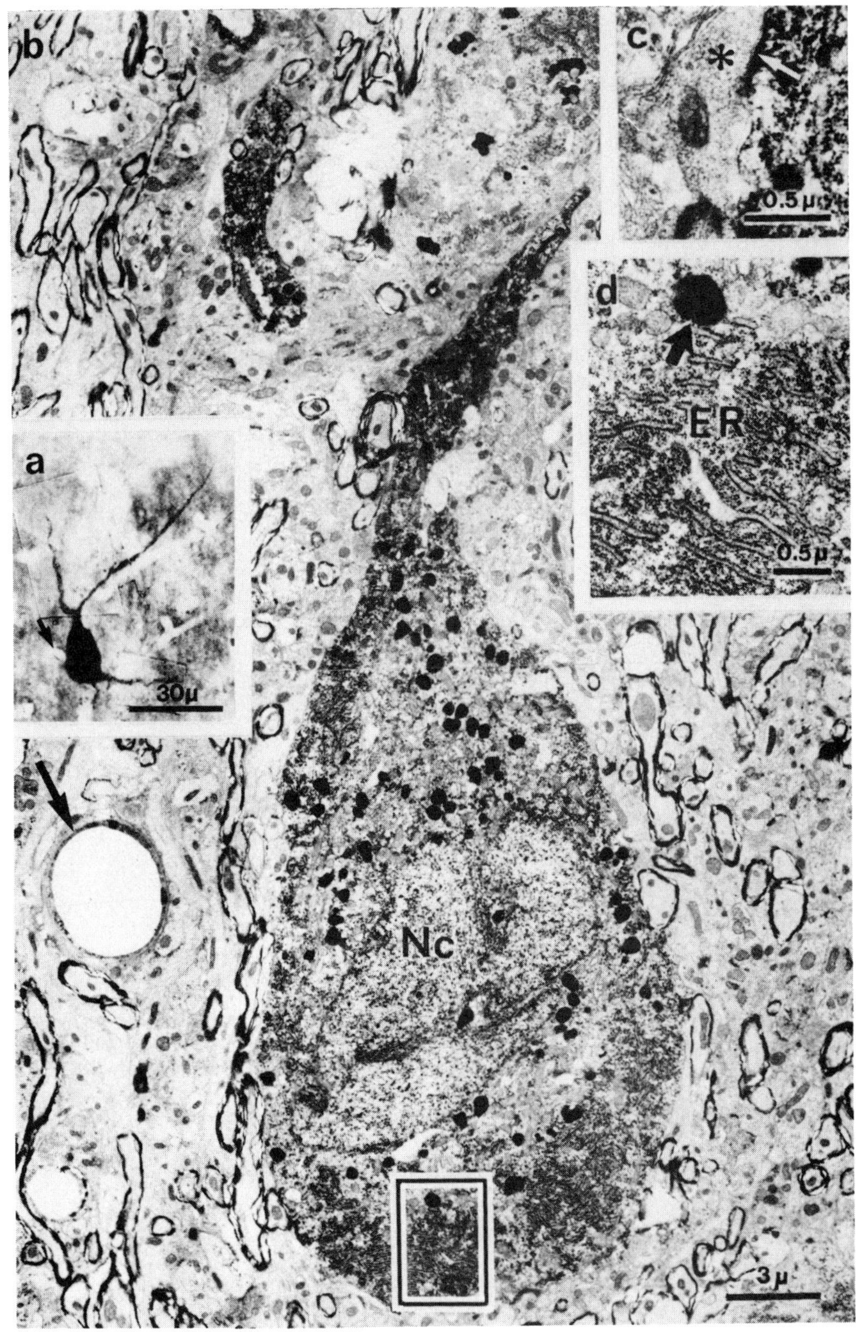
b
c
*
0.5 µ
d
ER
0.5 µ
a
30µ
Nc
3 µ

of all neurons examined was similar to one another and was similar to that described for ChAT-immunoreactive neurons in the MS.[28,29] Most of these neurons, including the severely shrunken ones, showed normal ultrastructural characteristics such as dense accumulations of rough endoplasmic reticulum (FIG. 4d) and intact axosomatic and axodendritic synapses (FIG. 4c).[25]

CONCLUSIONS

We conclude from these data that, following axotomy, septohippocampal neurons may become atrophic and shrink, but nevertheless remain alive and demonstrate both normal ultrastructure and input synapses. Several previous studies have indicated that ChAT- and GAD-immunoreactive neurons in the MS are lost within 2 to 6 weeks following transection of the FF;[6,9,13–16] however, in light of the present data, it appears that in many cases this loss is not due to neuronal death but rather to loss of immunocytochemically detectable transmitter-related enzymes such as ChAT and GAD. Thus, the main finding of this series of studies is that a large number of septohippocampal neurons survive axotomy although many are in an atrophic, shrunken state. These shrunken neurons would probably escape detection in light microscopic counts of Nissl-stained preparations.[7] Perhaps it is this group of shrunken cells which is re-activated by the delayed application of NGF.[30,31]

The survival of septohippocampal neurons for extended periods of time after axotomy leaves hope for pharmacological interference aimed at reactivating the expression of transmitter-related enzymes and axonal growth.

ACKNOWLEDGMENTS

The technical expertise of G. W. Lanford, I. Radke, A. Schneider and M. Winter is gratefully acknowledged.

REFERENCES

1. LEWIS, P. R. & C. C. D. SHUTE. 1967. The cholinergic limbic system: Projections to hippocampal formation, medial cortex, nuclei of the ascending cholinergic reticular system, and the subfornical organ and supra-optic crest. Brain **90:** 521–540.
2. SWANSON, L. W. & W. M. COWAN. 1979. The connections of the septal region in the rat. J. Comp. Neurol. **186:** 621–656.
3. AMARAL, D. G. & J. KURZ. 1985. An analysis of the origins of the cholinergic and noncholinergic septal projections to the hippocampal formation of the rat. J. Comp. Neurol. **240:** 37–59.
4. WAINER, B. H., A. I. LEVEY, D. B. RYE, M.-M. MESULAM & E. J. MUFSON. 1985. Cholinergic and non-cholinergic septohippocampal pathways. Neurosci. Lett. **54:** 45–52.
5. KÖHLER, C., V. CHAN-PALAY & J.-Y. WU. 1984. Septal neurons containing glutamic acid decarboxylase immunoreactivity project to the hippocampal region in the rat brain. Anat. Embryol. **169:** 41–44.
6. PETERSON, G. M., L. R. WILLIAMS, S. VARON & F. H. GAGE. 1987. Loss of GABAergic neurons in medial septum after fimbria-fornix transection. Neurosci. Lett. **76:** 140–144.
7. DAITZ, H. M. & T. P. S. POWELL. 1954. Studies on the connexions of the fornix system. J. Neurol. Neurosurg. Psychiat. **17:** 75–82.

8. GAGE, F. H., K. WICTORIN, W. FISHER, L. R. WILLIAMS, S. VARON & A. BJÖRKLUND. 1986. Retrograde cell changes in medial septum and diagonal band following fimbria-fornix transection: quantitative temporal analysis. Neuroscience **19:** 241–255.

9. ARMSTRONG, D. M., R. D. TERRY, R. M. DeTERESA, G. BRUCE, L. B. HERSH & F. H. GAGE. 1987. Response of septal cholinergic neurons to axotomy. J. Comp. Neurol. **264:** 421–436.

10. BARDE, Y.-A. 1990. Trophic factors and neuronal survival. Neuron **2:** 1525–1534.

11. KORSCHING, S., G. AUBURGER, R. HEUMANN, J. SCOTT & H. THOENEN. 1985. Levels of nerve growth factor and its mRNA in the central nervous system of the rat correlate with cholinergic innervation. EMBO J. **4:** 1389–1393.

12. SEILER, M. & M. SCHWAB. 1984. Specific retrograde transport of nerve growth factor (NGF) from neocortex to nucleus basalis in the rat. Brain Res. **300:** 33–39.

13. GAGE, F. H., D. M. ARMSTRONG, L. R. WILLIAMS & S. VARON. 1988. Morphological response of axotomized septal neurons to nerve growth factor. J. Comp. Neurol. **269:** 147–155.

14. HEFTI, F. 1986. Nerve growth factor promotes survival of septal cholinergic neurons after fimbrial transections. J. Neurosci. **6:** 2115–2162.

15. KROMER, L. F. 1987. Nerve growth factor treatment after brain injury prevents neuronal death. Science **235:** 214–216.

16. WILLIAMS, L. R., S. VARON, G. M. PETERSON, K. WICTORIN, W. FISCHER, A. BJÖRK-LUND & F. H. GAGE. 1986. Continuous infusion of nerve growth factor prevents basal forebrain neuronal death after fimbria fornix transection. Proc. Natl. Acad. Sci. USA **83:** 9231–9235.

17. LAMS, B. E., O. ISACSON & M. V. SOFRONIEW. 1988. Loss of transmitter-associated enzyme staining following axotomy does not indicate death of brainstem cholinergic neurons. Brain Res. **475:** 401–406.

18. PEARSON, R. C. A., M. V. SOFRONIEW, A. C. CUELLO, T. P. S. POWELL, F. ECKENSTEIN, M. M. ESIRI & G. K. WILCOCK. 1983. Persistence of cholinergic neurons in the basal nucleus in a brain with senile dementia of the Alzheimer's type demonstrated by immunohistochemical staining for choline acetyltransferase. Brain Res. **289:** 375–379.

19. SOFRONIEW, M. V., R. C. A. PEARSON, O. ISACSON & A. BJÖRKLUND. 1986. Experimental studies on the induction and prevention of retrograde degeneration of basal forebrain cholinergic neurons. Progr. Brain Res. **70:** 363–389.

20. SCHMUED, L. D. & J. H. FALLON. 1986. Fluoro-Gold: A new fluorescent retrograde axonal tracer with numerous unique properties. Brain Res. **377:** 147–154.

21. PETERSON, G. M. 1989. A quantitative analysis of the crossed septohippocampal projection in the rat brain. Anat. Embryol. **180:** 421–425.

22. BUHL, E. H., W. K. SCHWERDTFEGER & P. GERMROTH. 1990. Intracellular injections of neurons in fixed brain tissue combined with other neuroanatomical techniques at the light and electron microscopic level. *In* Handbook of Chemical Neuroanatomy. A. Björklund, T. Hökfelt, F. G. Wouterlood & A. N. van den Pol, Eds. Vol. 8: 273–304. Elsevier. Amsterdam.

23. MARANTO, A. R. 1982. Neuronal mapping: A photooxidation reaction makes Lucifer Yellow useful for electron microscopy. Science **217:** 953–955.

24. PETERSON, G. M., G. W. LANFORD & E. W. POWELL. 1990. Fate of septohippocampal neurons following fimbria-fornix transection: A time course analysis. Brain Res. Bull. **25:** 129–137.

25. PETERSON, G. M., T. NAUMANN & M. FROTSCHER. 1992. Identified septohippocampal neurons survive axotomy: A fine structural analysis in the rat. Neurosci. Lett. **138:** 81–85.

26. BRAUER, K., W. SCHOBER, L. WERNER, E. WINKELMANN, W. LUNGWITZ & F. HAJDU. 1988. Neurons in the basal forebrain complex of the rat: A Golgi study. J. Hirnforsch **29:** 43–71.

27. SCHMUED, L. C., K. KYRIAKIDIS, J. H. FALLON & C. E. RIBAK. 1989. Neurons containing retrogradely transported Fluoro-Gold exhibit a variety of lysosomal profiles: A combined brightfield, fluorescence, and electron microscopic study. J. Neurocytol. **18:** 333–343.

28. ARMSTRONG, D. M. 1986. Ultrastructural characterization of choline acetyltransferase-containing neurons in the basal forebrain of rat: Evidence for a cholinergic innervation of intracerebral blood vessels. J. Comp. Neurol. **250:** 81–92.
29. BIALOWAS, J. & M. FROTSCHER. 1987. Choline acetyltransferase-immunoreactive neurons and terminals in the rat septal complex: A combined light and electron microscopic study. J. Comp. Neurol. **259:** 298–307.
30. FISCHER, W. & A. BJÖRKLUND. 1991. Loss of AChE- and NGFr-labeling precedes neuronal death and axotomized septal-diagonal band neurons: Reversal by intraventricular NGF infusion. Exp. Neurol. **113:** 93–108.
31. HAGG, T., B. FASS-HOLMES, H. L. VAHLSING, M. MANTHORPE, J. M. CONNER & S. VARON. 1989. Nerve growth factor (NGF) reverses axotomy-induced decreases in choline acetyltransferase, NGF receptor and size of medial septum cholinergic neurons. Brain Res. **505:** 29–38.

The Effects of Intraseptal Brain-derived Neurotrophic Factor on Cognition in Rats with MS/DB Lesions

MARY ANN PELLEYMOUNTER[a] AND
MARY JANE CULLEN

Department of Neurobiology
Amgen, Inc.
1840 DeHavilland Drive
Thousand Oaks, California 91320

The distribution pattern of mRNA for brain-derived neurotrophic factor (BDNF) in the central nervous system coincides closely with the projection areas of the basal forebrain cholinergic system.[1,2] Signal strength for BDNF mRNA is particularly intense in the hippocampal formation,[1,2] which is the projection site for the septohippocampal component of the basal forebrain cholinergic system. The basal forebrain cholinergic system (particularly the septohippocampal component) has been extensively characterized as a biological substrate for memory. Lesions in the medial septal/diagonal band (MD/DB) area have been shown to produce deficits in several memory tasks, including the 8 arm radial maze,[3–5] the water maze,[6,7] active avoidance retention, and passive avoidance acquisition.[4] These lesions typically result in a loss of hippocampal choline acetyl transferase (ChAT) activity of 40–60%,[4–6] suggesting a partial destruction of MS/DB cell bodies and their corresponding hippocampal projections.

Since there is evidence that BDNF can act as a trophic factor for cholinergic neurons[8,9] and can be regulated by neuronal damage,[10,11] we hypothesized that instraseptal infusion of BDNF might enhance sprouting of septal neurons that survived MS/DB lesions. We further hypothesized that enhanced sprouting of these BDNF-treated surviving neurons might result in a reversal of the cognitive deficits that are typical of rats with MS/DB lesions. These hypotheses were tested by comparing the effects of intraseptal BDNF infusion in rats with MS/DB lesions on two forms of cognition: working memory and selective attention. In keeping with the spirit of the conference, these two forms of cognition could be viewed as functional "markers of neuronal degeneration or regeneration," since cognitive dysfunction or improvement has been shown to accompany the degeneration or regeneration of cholinergic terminals in the hippocampus.

Male Long-Evans rats (250–300 g) were used as subjects for the study. These animals were anesthetized with sodium pentobarbital (55 mg/kg; i.p.) and placed into a stereotaxic instrument with the skull at the level position. Lesions were made by passing direct currents (1.2 mA; 10 sec) through an electrode with a 1 mm uninsulated tip. Sham lesions were made by lowering the electrode without passing current. Coordinates for the lesions were: AP (+.48, +.48, +1.00 mm,

---

[a] Author to whom correspondence and reprint requests should be addressed.

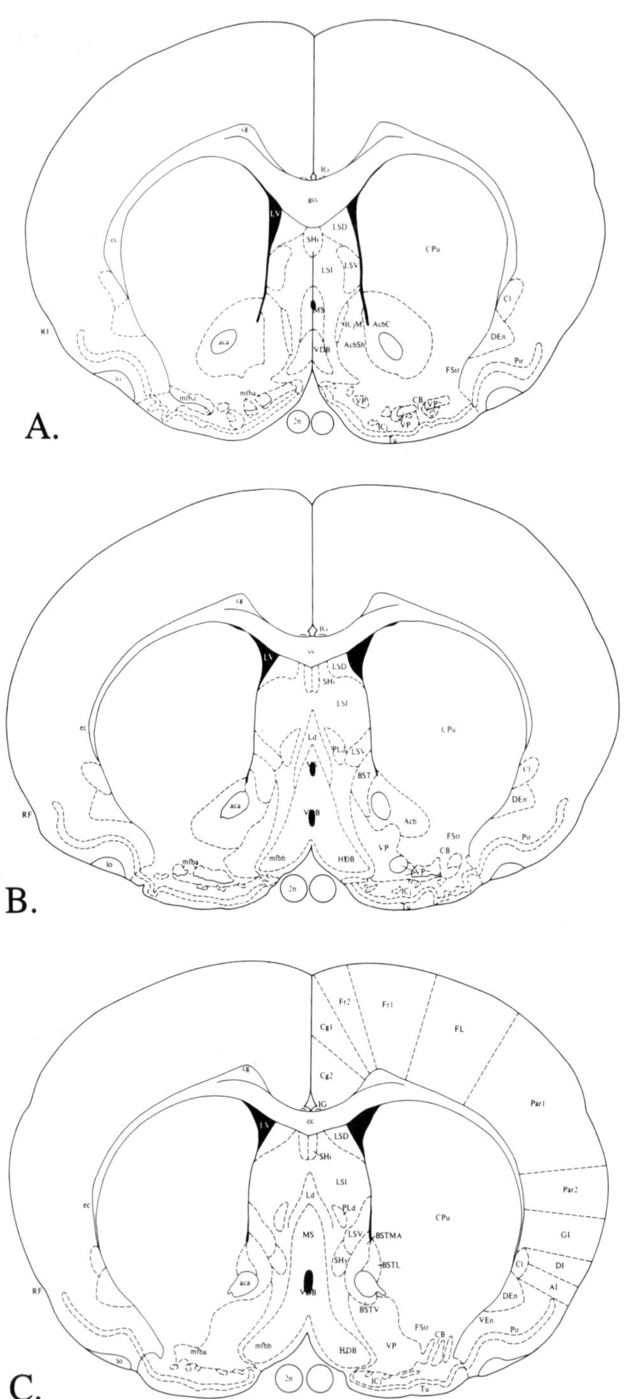

bregma); ML (0.0 for all three lesions); and DV (-5.8, -7.2, -6.2)[12]. See FIGURE 1, A and B for schematics of the lesion placements. Rats were allowed a three week recovery period, during which time they remained in their home cages. They were then trained on the 8 arm radial maze task for a period of 30 days.

The 8 arm radial maze is an octagonal "hub" surrounded by 8 arms that contain a depressed food cup at the end of each arm. The food cup cannot be seen from the center of the maze. Large, high contrast pictures and objects are stationary relative to the position of the maze throughout training. The object of training is to locate and consume all 8 food rewards without re-visiting any arm. The radial arm maze task was chosen because it requires a form of short term memory known as working memory, which has been shown to be dependent upon septo-hippocampal function.[13]

Radial arm maze training involved three stages: a restricted feeding regimen, habituation to the maze and training itself. The restricted feeding regimen was effected one week prior to radial arm maze training in order to motivate animals to locate the food rewards. This regimen was designed so that rats maintained 85% of their pre-training weight throughout training. The habituation phase was conducted on a one-arm version of the maze. Rats were placed onto the central "hub" area and allowed to search for randomly scattered Froot Loops on the hub and food cup areas. Each animal was allowed a maximum of ten minutes to go to the end of the arm and pick up a reward. These habituation trials (one/day) were conducted for three days. Habituation was necessary to avoid neophobic reactions to the maze. Training began on the day following the last habituation trial. All animals received one trial per day on the maze for a 30 day period. A trial began when a rat was placed into the center, or "hub" of the maze. The trial ended when the rat had either located all 8 food rewards, visited 16 arms or had remained on the maze for 10 min. Working memory errors were scored for each rat. A working memory error was defined as a repeated visit to an arm.

Statistical analysis of working memory errors for this 30-day training period showed that rats with MS/DB lesions were severely impaired in comparison to sham controls, as can be observed in FIGURE 2.[14] At the end of the thirty day training period, MS/DB and sham-lesion controls were further divided into two groups: VEH or BDNF. These animals were counterbalanced for working memory errors prior to pump implantation, so that an equal number of "slow" and "fast" learners were assigned to each BDNF or VEH group. Phosphate-buffered saline (pH 7.4) vehicle (VEH) or BDNF (6 μg/day) was infused into the medial septal area via an osmotic mini-pump.

Osmotic minipumps (Alzet 2002; 0.5 μl/hour) were implanted under pentobarbital anesthesia. The pump itself was implanted under the skin in the subscapular area of the neck, and was connected to a stainless steel cannula that was placed stereotaxically into the medial septal area (AP; $+0.2$, ML; 0.0, DV; -6.8).[12] Rats remained in their home cages during the 14-day period of BDNF infusion. Pumps were removed after this period, and rats were allowed an additional week to

---

FIGURE 1. This figure is a schematic showing the approximate placement of the MS/DB lesions, using the coordinates described above. **A** and **B** show placements of the lesions, and **C** shows placement of the cannula that delivered BDNF or VEH. (These schematics are from Paxinos & Watson, The Rat Brain in Stereotaxic Coordinates, 1982.[12])

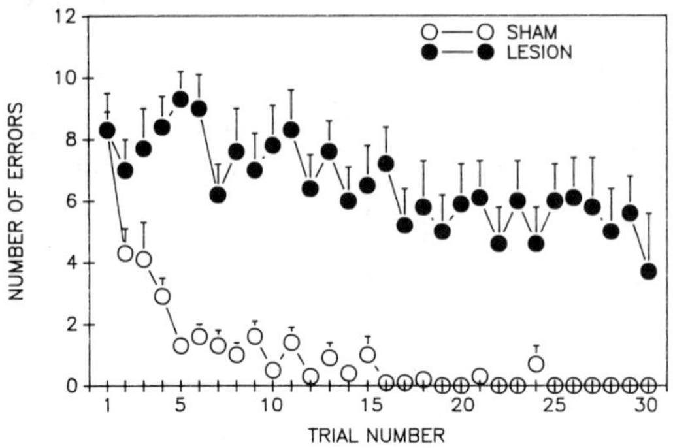

FIGURE 2. This figure illustrates mean number of working memory errors for sham-operated or MS/DB rats during the first 30 days of training. A working memory error is defined as a repeated visit to the same arm. Error bars represent standard error of the mean. (These data are from Pelleymounter & Cullen, 1992.[14])

remain in their home cages and to reach 85% of their post-BDNF body weight. Rats were then re-tested on the radial arm maze task for two weeks, using the original maze and room cues. As in original training, working memory errors were scored for each rat.

Statistical analysis of working memory errors for the second radial arm maze training session (after BDNF or VEH had been infused) indicated: 1) that MS/DB rats that were infused with VEH were still making significantly more working memory errors at the end of the second phase of training, and 2) that MS/DB rats that had received BDNF had improved their performance on the radial maze task to the point that they could not be distinguished from controls.[14] These data are illustrated in FIGURE 3.

Three weeks after radial arm maze training, all rats were tested on an overshadowing task. Overshadowing has been characterized as a selective attention task.[15,16] In overshadowing, rats are presented with a compound stimulus, where one stimulus has a very low intensity and the other a very high intensity. In this case, a dim light and a loud tone were used. Presentation of the compound stimulus is followed immediately by a footshock (.5 mA; 5 sec). Training comprises three such trials. Twenty-four hours later, rats are tested for lick suppression in response to the light alone; 48 hours later, they are tested with the tone. Normal rats will

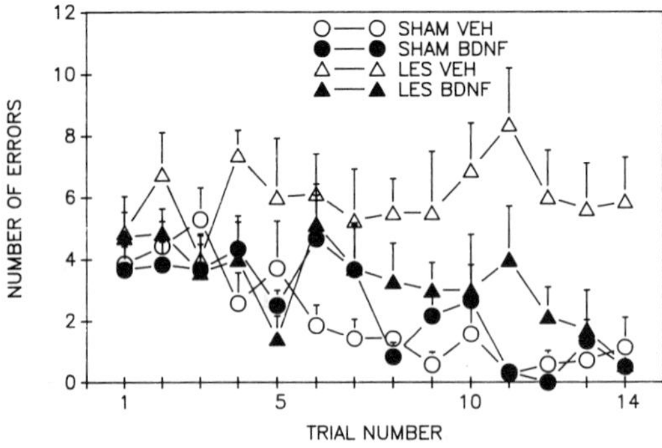

FIGURE 3. This figure shows the mean number of working memory errors for sham-operated or MS/DB rats treated with either VEH or BDNF during the second phase of radial arm maze training. Again, error bars reflect standard error of the mean. (These data are from Pelleymounter & Cullen, 1992.[14])

suppress licking in response to the tone or light if they associate it with shock. Typically, normal rats will show more suppression to the tone than to the light because they associated the stronger neutral stimulus (tone) with shock, essentially ignoring the weaker neutral stimulus.[15]

Animals were placed on a 23.5-h water deprivation schedule for three days in their home cages. They were then placed into the test cages and allowed to lick from a water spout for a 30 min period each day for five days to establish baseline drinking levels. After baseline was established training began. During training, the animal was placed into the test cage at the time it normally was allowed access to water, and was exposed to the simultaneous presentation of a light and tone for a period of 30 sec. Immediately following the compound stimulus presentation, a 0.5 mA, 5-sec footshock was delivered to the rat through the grid floor of the test cage. Rats were given three such training trials, with inter-trial intervals random (mean 67 sec; range 60–75 sec). Twenty-four hours later, all rats were again placed into the test cages, and presented with three 30-sec trials of light

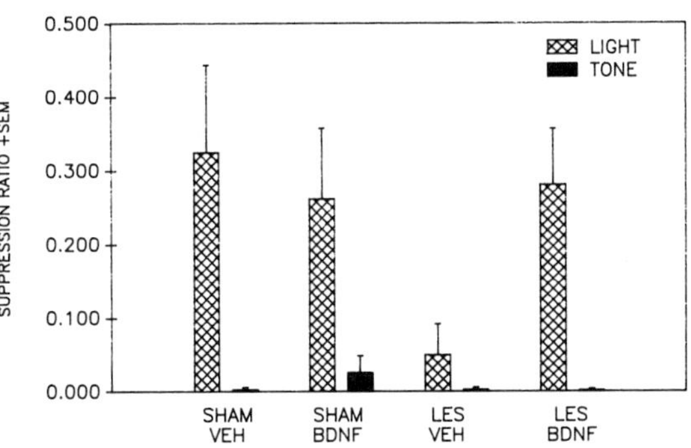

FIGURE 4. This figure shows suppression ratios in response to the light vs. tone test for MS/DB or sham rats treated with either VEH or BDNF. Lick suppression decreases as the suppression ratio increases, as described below. The overshadowing effect is defined as a significantly higher suppression ratio for light than for tone. Differential suppression to light vs. tone indicates that animals do not attend to the light components of the compound stimulus used for training, and therefore, do not associate it with footshock. (These data are from Pelleymounter & Cullen, 1992.[14])

alone. Inter-trial interval was random with the same mean and range as in training. As in training, number of licks were measured. Forty-eight hours later, all rats were presented with trials of the tone alone. Again, inter-trial intervals and lick measurements were the same as in the previous test trial. Lick suppression to the light versus the tone was compared for each group. Lick suppression was calculated as the ratio: number of licks during the middle stimulus presentation/number of licks during the middle stimulus presentation + number of licks during the last 30 sec of the preceeding intertrial interval.

Statistical analysis of the lick suppression ratio showed that rats with sham lesions suppressed to the tone significantly more than they did to the light, as did MS/DB rats that had been infused with intraseptal BDNF. MS/DB rats that had been infused with VEH, however, suppressed to the light stimulus more than any other group (suggesting that MS/DB rats showed less overshadowing).[14] These results are illustrated in FIGURE 4.

Our results suggested that rats with lesions of the medial septal area and nucleus of the horizontal limb of the diagonal band had severe working memory and selective attention deficits. The finding that MS/DB rats had a severe working memory impairment was not novel; it was in agreement with several other reports,[3,4,17] and concurred with the idea that the predominately cholinergic MS/DB projection system was important in working memory. Interestingly, the working memory impairment in these animals was associated with the use of a perseverative strategy to locate unvisited arms of the maze. Although the tendency to perseverate on one or two arms was common in all rats at the beginning of training, rats without lesions or those infused with BDNF began to use more flexible strategies with continued training. In contrast, those with MS/DB lesions and vehicle treatment were unable to adapt a more efficient strategy and continued to show perseverative behavior throughout training.

Our data also suggested that MS/DB lesions disrupted selective attention, as defined by overshadowing. Since overshadowing involves memory as well as attention, it is possible that MS/DB rats were impaired on overshadowing because the lesion disrupted storage of the information that tone or light predicted shock. This is doubtful for the following reasons: 1) MS/DB rats showed as much suppression to tone as sham controls even though suppression to tone was tested 48 h after training: this suggests that the lesion did not affect the strength of the tone-shock association. 2) MS/DB rats remembered the association between light and shock better than any other group, as can be seen by group comparisons of the suppression ratios. 3) Group differences occurred instead, in the response to light, where only the MS/DB rats treated with VEH appeared to associate light with shock. 4) BDNF improved performance in MS/DB rats by decreasing their suppression to light, rather than increasing suppression to the tone. For these reasons, it seems more probable that the impaired performance of MS/DB rats on the overshadowing task was due to a deficit in selective attention, rather than to one in memory. These data might also suggest that neurons affected by previous BDNF infusion "normalized" reactivity in MS/DB rats, allowing them to ignore competing extraneous or weak stimuli.

These preliminary data suggest that intraseptal infusion of BDNF improved the performance of MS/DB rats in both types of information processing tasks, despite the fact that cognitive testing was not begun until BDNF infusion had been discontinued. Although these data suggest that BDNF may have some effect on the plasticity of surviving MS/DB neurons, neuroanatomical and biochemial data are necessary to answer questions about the biological mechanism underlying these effects of BDNF. Immunohistochemical studies are currently underway in these same animals that will assess the integrity of the septohippocampal cholinergic system. Depending upon the results of these immunohistochemical studies, the long-lasting effects of BDNF on cognition in MS/DB rats could suggest an indication for the use of BDNF in neurodegenerative disorders involving cognition.

REFERENCES

1. HOFER, M., S. PAGLIUSI, A. HOHN, J. LEIBROCK & Y.-A. BARDE. 1990. Regional distribution of brain-derived neurotrophic factor mRNA in the adult mouse brain. EMBO J. **9:** 2459–2464.
2. PHILLIPS, H., J. HAINS, G. LARAMEE, A. ROSENTHAL & J. WINSLOW. 1990. Widespread expression of BDNF but not NT-3 by target areas of basal forebrain cholinergic neurons. Science **250:** 290–294.
3. CRUTCHER, K., R. KESNER & J. NOVAK. 1983. Medial septal lesions, radial arm maze

performance, and sympathetic sprouting: A study of recovery of function. Brain Res. **262:** 91–98.

4. HEPLER, D., G. WENK, B. CRIBBS, D. OLTON & COYLE. J. 1985. Memory impairments following basal forebrain lesions. Brain Res. **346:** 8–14.

5. PALLAGE, V., G. TONIOLO, B. WILL & F. HEFTI. 1986. Long-term effects of nerve growth factor and neural transplants on behavior of rats with medial septal lesions. Brain Res. **386:** 197–208.

6. HAGAN, J., J. SALAMONE, J. SIMPSON, S. IVERSEN & R. MORRIS. 1988. Place navigation in rats is impaired by lesions of medial septum and diagonal band but not nucleus basalis magnocellularis. Behav. Brain Res. **27:** 9–20.

7. RIEKKINEN, P., J. SIRVIO & RIEKKINEN, P. 1990. Similar memory impairments found in medial septal-vertical diagonal band of Broca and nucleus basalis lesioned rats: Are memory defects induced by nucleus basalis lesions related to the degree of non-specific subcortical cell loss? Behav. Brain Res. **37:** 81–88.

8. ALDERSON, R., A. ALTERMAN, Y.-A. BARDE & R. LINDSAY. 1990. Brain-derived neurotrophic factor increases survival and differentiated functions of rat septal cholinergic neurons in culture. Neuron **5:** 297–306.

9. KNUSEL, B., J. WINSLOW, A. ROSENTHAL, L. BURTON, D. SEID, K. NIKOLICS & F. HEFTI. 1991. Promotion of central cholinergic and dopaminergic neuron differentiation by brain-derived neurotrophic factor but not neurotrophin-3. Proc. Natl. Acad. Sci. USA **88:** 961–965.

10. CECCATELLI, S., P. ERNFORS, M. VILLAR, H. PERSSON & T. HÖKFELT. 1991. Expanded distribution of mRNA for nerve growth factor, brain-derived neurotrophic factor, and neurotrophin-3 in the rat brain after colchicine treatment. Proc. Natl. Acad. Sci. USA **88:** 10352–10356.

11. BALLARIN, M., P. ERNFORS, N. LINDEFORS & H. PERSSON. 1991. Hippocampal damage and kainic acid injection induce a rapid increase in mRNA for BDNF and NGF in the rat brain. Exper. Neurol. **114:** 35–43.

12. PAXINOS, G. & C. WATSON. 1982. The Rat Brain in Stereotaxic Coordinates. Academic Press. New York.

13. OLTON, D., J. BECKER & G. HANDLEMAN. 1979. Hippocampus, space and memory. Behav. Brain Sci. **2:** 313–365.

14. PELLEYMOUNTER, M. & M. CULLEN. The effects of intraseptal BDNF on cognition in rats with hippocampal nerve terminal degeneration. In preparation.

15. MACKONTOSH, N. 1976. Overshadowing and stimulus intensity. Animal Learn. Behav. **4:** 186–192.

16. MILES, C. & H. JENKINS. 1973. Overshadowing in operant conditioning as a function of discriminability. Learn. Motiv. **4:** 11–27.

17. KNOWLTON, B., G. WENK, D. OLTON & J. COYLE. 1985. Basal forebrain lesions produce a dissociation of trial-dependent and trial-independent memory performance. Brain Res. **345:** 315–321.

Developmental Differences in Neural Damage following Trimethyl-Tin as Demonstrated with GFAP Immunohistochemistry

STANLEY BARONE, JR.

ManTech Environmental Technology
Research Triangle Park, North Carolina 27709

INTRODUCTION

GFAP immunohistochemistry was used to anatomically localize the effects of a prototypical developmental neurotoxicant, trimethyl-tin (TMT), on the developing brain because an earlier report indicated that TMT altered brain development as evidenced by decrements in proteins linked to synaptogenesis and myelinogenesis as well as an increase in the glial fibrillary acidic protein, GFAP.[1] GFAP, the principal intermediate filament protein of astrocytes[2] is increased in response to injury of the central nervous system (CNS) and this injury-induced gliosis has been demonstrated after mechanical lesions,[3-6] chemical lesions (reviewed,[7] and neurodegenerative diseases of the CNS (reviewed).[8] The present study expands on neurochemical studies following acute dosing with TMT on PND 5[1] by providing more definitive neuroanatomical localization of neuronal damage and gliosis after different time points of exposure postnatally. Here neural damage resulting from developmental TMT administration was assessed indirectly by examining the astrocyte response to injury using GFAP immunohistochemistry. This GFAP data were compared to Nissl-stained sections which provides more direct evidence of neuron loss.

METHODS

Forty-eight Long-Evans rat pups, derived from 6 litters, served as subjects. Littes were culled to 8 pups per dam as previously described.[9] On PND 10 or PND 18, half of the pups in each litter (2 males and 2 females) were injected i.p. with TMT hydroxide (6 mg/kg) and half with saline (vehicle) as described previously.[9] Animals were killed on PND 12, 18, 20, and 25 by transcardial perfusion with chilled 4.0% buffered paraformaldehyde. After perfusion, the brains were removed and post-fixed in the same fixative for 1.5 h and subsequently transferred to 20% sucrose in phosphate-buffered saline (PBS) until sectioning. Frozen 40 μm sections were cut in the sagittal plane through the right hemisphere and collected in a serial series in PBS. One series of sections were Nissl-stained with (0.1%) cresyl violet and another series stained by immunohistochemistry for GFAP. Free floating sections were stained for GFAP IR by incubating in a rabbit anti-GFAP serum diluted 1:2000 (Dako, Carpenteria, CA) in PBS with 1% NGS and 0.5% Triton X-100 for 2 days at 4°C. After rinsing in PBS, sections were incubated in a biotinylated secondary antiserum followed by further rinsing and incubation in an avidin-biotin-peroxidase complex solution (ELITE ABC, Vector Labs, Burlingame, CA) as modified from Hsu *et al.*[10] The bound peroxidase complex was visualized with the chromagen, (0.05%) 3,3′-diaminobenzidine (Sigma, St. Louis, MO) in the presence of (0.003%) hydrogen peroxide. Sections were mounted on glass slides, and examined under the light microscope in a blind fashion as described previously.[9] Additional sections were processed in parallel under the same conditions as above except the primary antiserum was omitted. Under these parallel conditions without primary antisera, no immunoreactivity was observed.

RESULTS

TMT on Postnatal Day 10

Pups dosed on PND 10 with TMT and sacrificed PND 12, 18, 20, or 25 showed a marked gliosis in several regions of the brain in a time dependent fashion. Two days post-dosing (PND 12) with TMT there was a marked increase in GFAP immunoreactivity (IR) in the hippocampus, cingulate, amygdala, piriform, and entorhinal cortex (FIG. 1B,D). This increase in IR was usually restricted to cortical lamina and select anatomical regions, with the CA3 region of the dorsal hippocampus exhibiting the most dense IR. There was a similar pattern of GFAP IR in the hilus of the dorsal and ventral hippocampus located primarily subjacent to the granule cell layer and in the outer molecular layer (FIG. 1D,d and FIG. 2D). At one and two weeks post-dosing with TMT, the extent of GFAP IR was limited to the hippocampus and corpus callosum (FIG. 3B,b). Furthermore, there was an apparent septo-temporal gradient in GFAP IR, with the dorsal hippocampus exhibiting more extensive involvement of the CA cell fields than the ventral hippocampus (data not shown). There were no apparent sex differences seen in Nissl-stained or GFAP IR sections at any of the time points examined. In addition, the basal levels of GFAP IR in saline-treated control sections increased with age in all brain regions, except in the olfactory bulb and cerebellum in which basal levels were higher in controls on PND 12. The overt damage in the hippocampus was readily apparent with both a traditional histological stain for Nissl substance and GFAP IR. However, GFAP IR revealed areas of more subtle damage in the amygdala, piriform, and entorhinal cortex not apparent in Nissl-stained sections. These data indicate that GFAP immunohistochemistry may have some utility in localizing areas of damage in laminar and non-laminar structures.

TMT on Postnatal Day 18

Pups dosed on PND 18 with TMT and sacrificed 2 and 7 days post-dosing exhibited marked gliosis in similar brain regions compared to PND 10 exposure, but the time course of the reactive gliosis and apparent magnitude was qualitatively different from the earlier dose group (FIG. 4). Two days after dosing on PND 18, there was an increase in GFAP IR in the CA3 region and hilus of the hippocampus and a more diffuse increase in the other cortical regions (piriform and entorhinal cortex) relative to that seen 2 days following PND 10 dosing. However, the regional increases in GFAP IR 2 days post-dosing were not apparent by the overt loss of Nissl-stained neurons (data not shown). Although, by one week post-dosing there

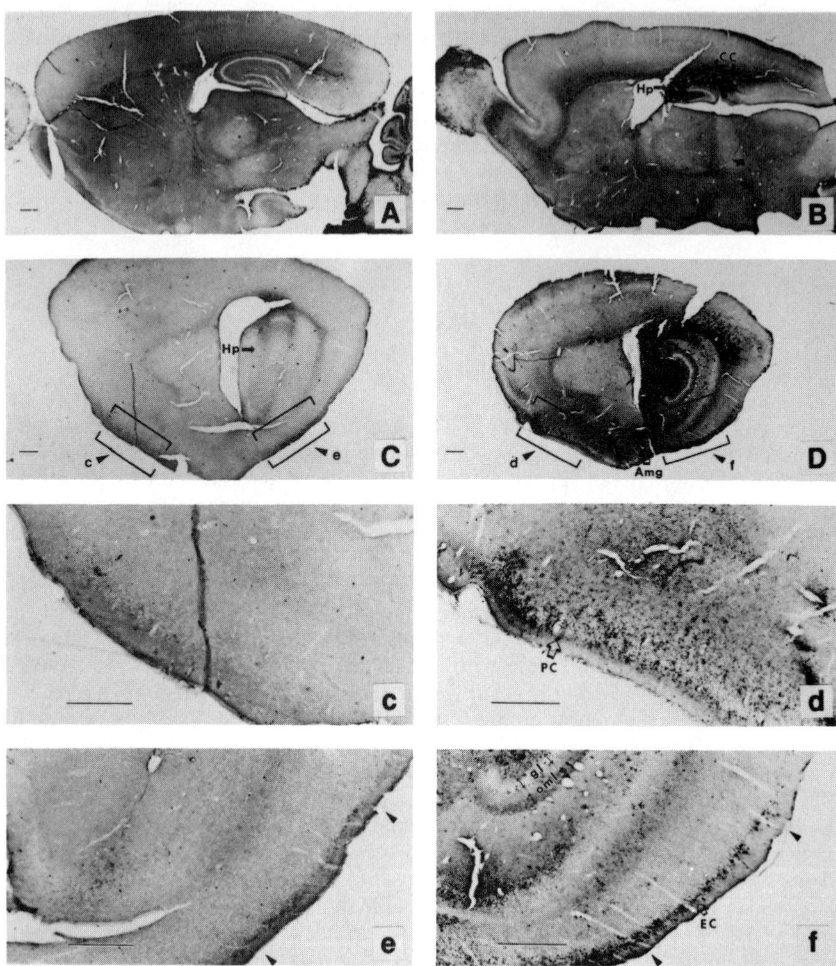

FIGURE 1. GFAP IR in sagittal sections from pups dosed on PND 10 and sacrificed on PND 12. Boxed regions with letters are shown in corresponding panels at higher magnification. Saline injected control is in left column **(A,C,c,e)** and TMT-injected pup in the right column **(B,D,d,f)**. Note the increase in GFAP IR in the amygdala (Amg), hippocampus (Hp) and corpus callosum (CC) of the TMT-treated rat **(B & D)**. Note the lack of GFAP IR in the granule cell layer (gl) and the increase in GFAP IR in the outer molecular layer (oml) of the dentate gyrus and in the hilar region (hl; **d,f**). *Arrowheads* **(e,f)** indicate corresponding regions of entorhinal cortex (EC) of vehicle and TMT treated pups respectively. Note significant increase in GFAP IR in the superficial layers of the piriform (PC) and entorhinal cortex (**d,f**; bar = 500 μm).

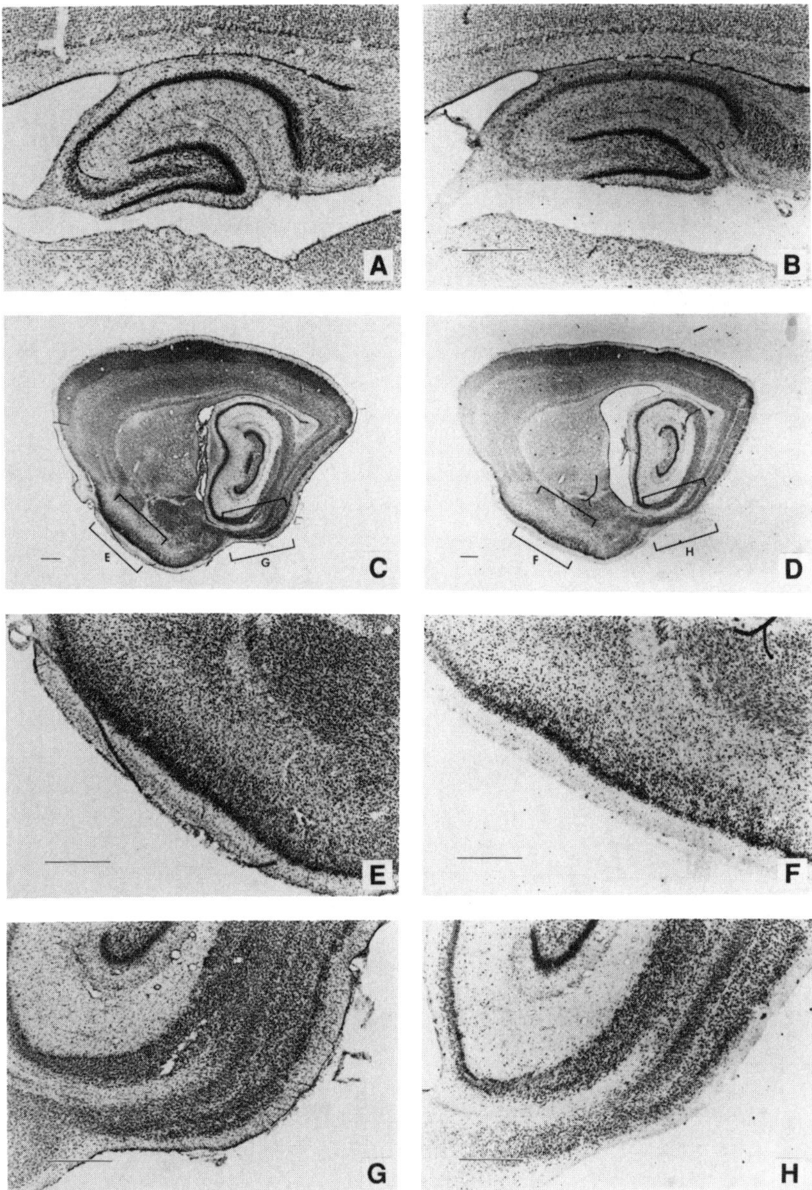

FIGURE 2. Nissl-stained sagittal sections from pups dosed on PND 10 and sacrificed on PND 12. Boxed regions with letters are shown in corresponding panels at higher magnification. Saline injected control is in left column **(A,C,E,G)** and TMT-injected pup in the right column **(B,D,F,H)**. Note the qualitative decrease in Nissl-stained neurons in the hippocampus of the TMT-treated rat **(B)**. Note the decrease in Nissl-stained neurons in the piriform and entorhinal cortex **(D,F,H**; bar = 500 μm).

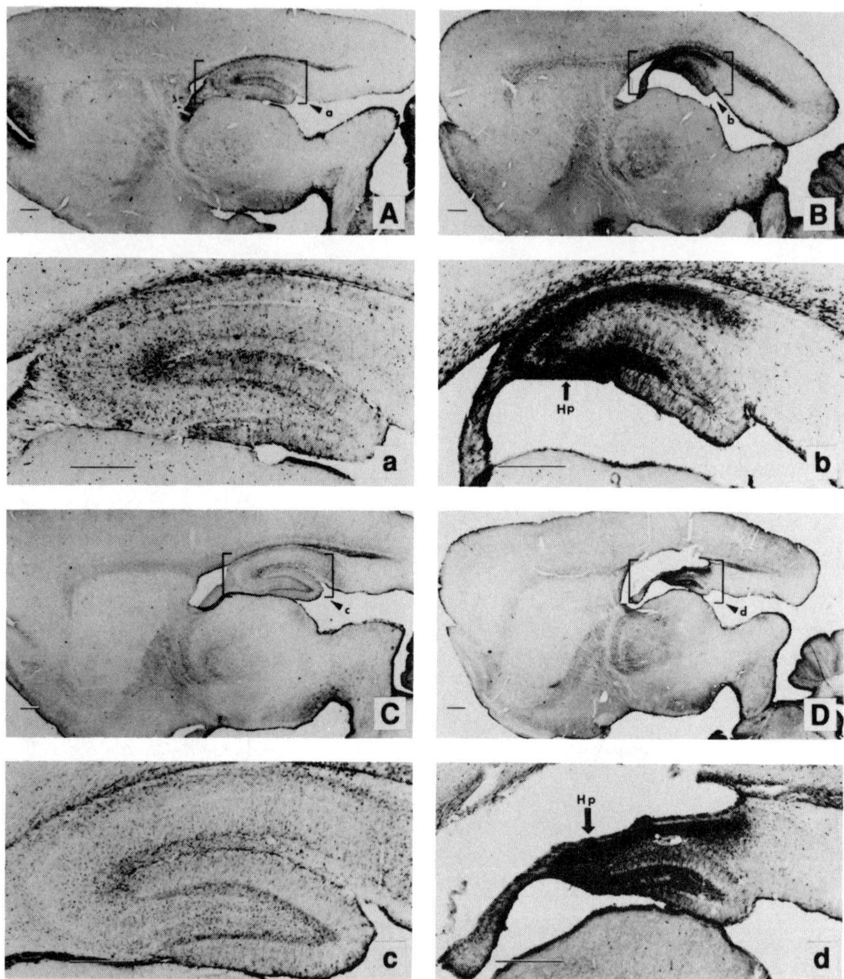

FIGURE 3. GFAP IR in sagittal sections from pups dosed on PND 10 and sacrificed on PND 18 **(A,a,B,b)** or PND 25 **(C,c,D,d)**. Boxed regions with letters are shown in corresponding panels at higher magnification. Saline injected control is in left column **(A,C,c,e)** and TMT-injected pup in the right column **(B,D,d,f)**. Other more lateral sagittal section are not shown because GFAP IR was limited to hippocampus alone. Note the persistent increase in GFAP IR in the hippocampus (Hp) of treated pups **(B,b,D,d**; bar = 500 μm).

was a marked increase in GFAP IR in the cingulate, piriform, entorhinal cortex and an apparent concomitant shrinkage of neuropil and cell loss in Nissl-stained sections in the same regions (FIGS. 5 and 6). The apparent increase in GFAP IR seen in the neocortex after dosing with TMT on PND 18 (FIG. 5B,g) was not apparent at any of the time points examined in the group dosed on PND 10 with TMT (FIG. 1). This increase in GFAP IR in the neocortex was limited principally

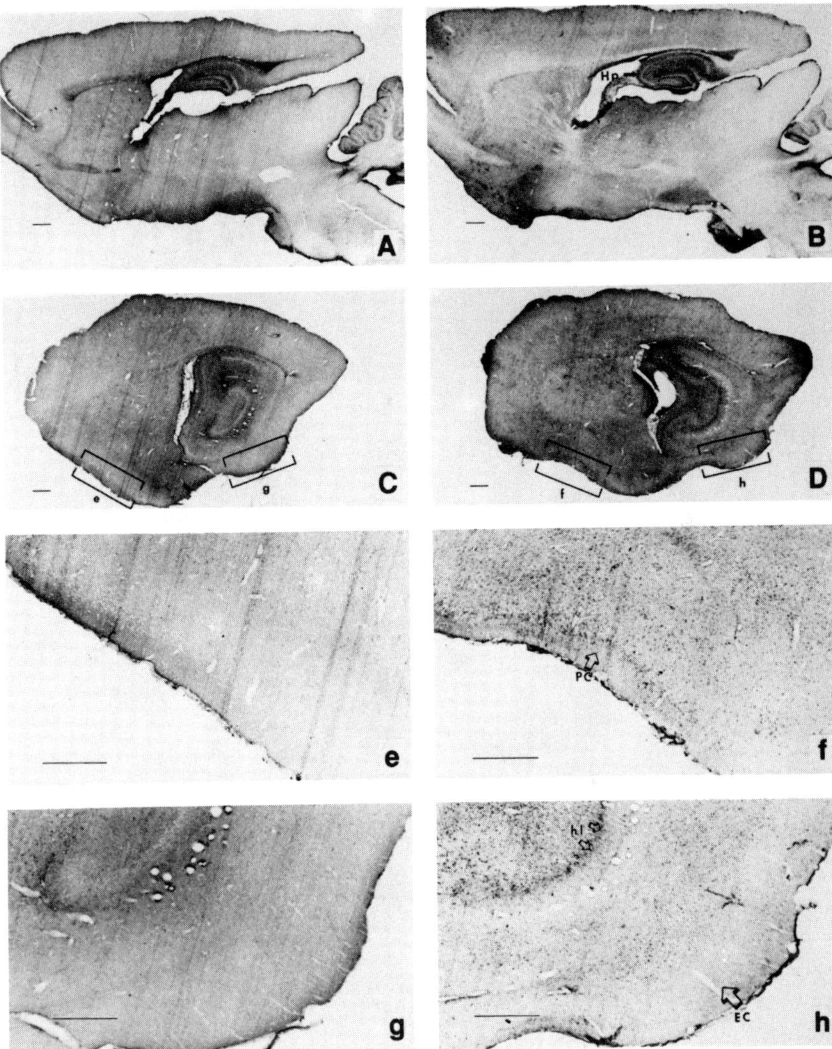

FIGURE 4. GFAP IR in sagittal sections from pups dosed on PND 18 and sacrificed on PND 20. Boxed regions with letters are shown in corresponding panels at higher magnification. Saline injected control is in left column (**A,C,e,g**) and TMT-injected pup on right (**B,D,f,h**). Note diffuse increase in GFAP IR in piriform (PC: **f**) and entorhinal cortex (EC; **h**) and in the hilar (hl) region of the hippocampus (**D,h**; bar = 500 μm).

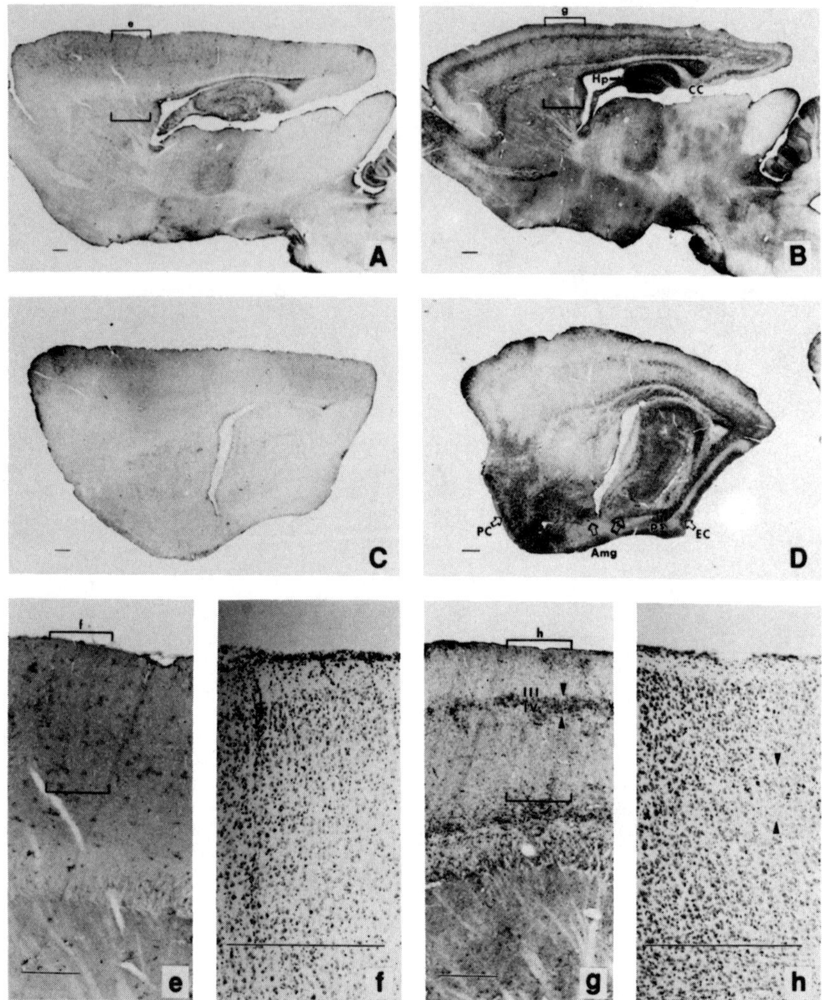

FIGURE 5. GFAP IR **(A,B,C,D,e,g)** and adjacent Nissl-stained **(f,h)** sagittal sections from pups dosed on PND 18 and sacrificed on PND 25. Boxed regions with letters are shown in corresponding panels at higher magnification. Saline injected control is in left column **(A,C,e,f)** and TMT-injected pup on right **(B,D,g,h)**. Note increase in GFAP IR in layer III/IV in the neocortex **(B,g)** and increase in the hippocampus (Hp; **B,D**), amygdala (Amg), piriform (PC), subiculum (S), presubiculum (PS) and layer II of the entorhinal cortex (EC; **D**). There was an apparent gliosis (see between arrows, **g,h**) and shrinkage of the neocortex with an increse in the packing density of Nissl-stained cells **(h)** as compared to control **(f;** bar = 500 μm).

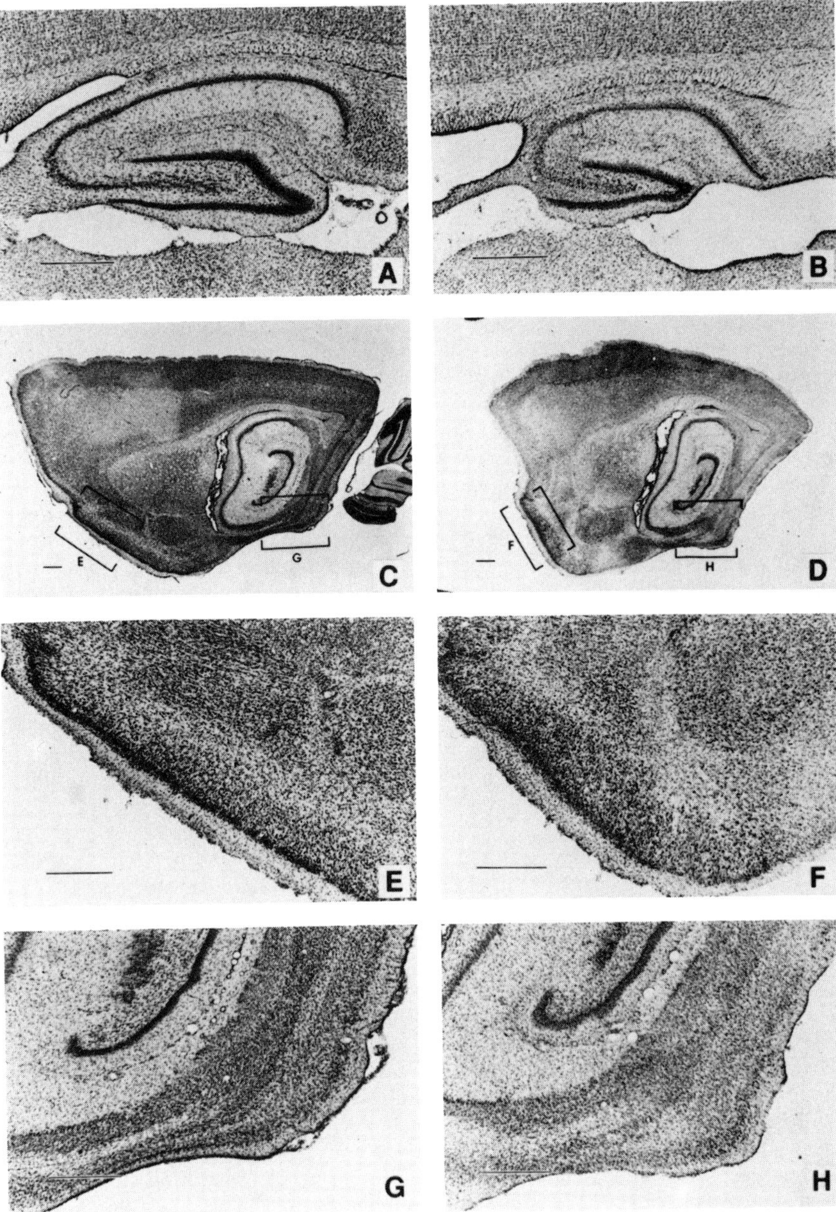

FIGURE 6. Nissl-stained sagittal sections from pups dosed on PND 18 and sacrificed on PND 25. Boxed regions with letters are shown in corresponding panels at higher magnification. Saline injected control is in left column **(A,C,E,G)** and TMT-injected pup on right **(B,D,F,H)**. Note the qualitative increase in Nissl-stained glia in the CA3 cell field **(B)** and hilus of the hippocampus **(H)**, and decrease in Nissl-stained neurons in the piriform, subiculum, presubiculum and layer II of the entorhinal cortex **(H**; bar = 500 μm).

to layers III and VI and in corresponding Nissl-stained sections there was shrinkage of the neuropil of all cortical layers and an apparent increase in the packing density of Nissl-stained neurons.

CONCLUSIONS

TMT produced severe degeneration and gliosis as shown by loss of Nissl-staining and increased GFAP immunoreactivity in several cortical regions with the earliest and most overt pathology apparent in the hippocampus. In general, similar brain regions were susceptible to the effects of acute postnatal dosing with TMT at two different time points. However, the magnitude and time course of gliosis differ dramatically between the two ages of exposure. Developmental susceptibility to TMT-induced damage of the hippocampus has been observed previously in mice[11] and rats.[1,12,13] The present study has further characterized the longitudinal and regional profile of damage following acute TMT exposure on the postnatal brain.

Several caveats to the immunohistochemical localization of GFAP need to be considered: 1) the fixation protocol employed can dramatically affect the antigenicity of the protein epitope localized immunohistochemically, 2) the use of free-floating versus slide-mounted tissue can decrease immunoreactivity, 3) the embedment of tissue in embedding media (i.e. paraffin) may decrease immunoreactivity, and most importantly, 4) the time course of tissue collection after the insult should include early time points (days) and later time points (weeks) depending on the nature of the damage. This is not a trivial task with respect to development because of possible different age-dependent susceptibilities of neural cell populations. However, consistent with previous data, the increases in GFAP IR after neonatal neurotoxicant administration indicate that reactive gliosis can be induced during a developmental period when gliogenesis is an ongoing process.[1] In addition, preliminary evidence suggests that gestational neurotoxic insults will induce astrogliosis.[14]

With the apparent early signs of damage and the possible increased susceptibility of pups dosed on PND 10 versus PND 18 is speculative, but the earlier onset of TMT-induced damage is consistent with data in which brain levels of tin were measured in neonates (PND 5)[15] and adults.[15,16] In this previous study, neonates reached a maximal brain tin concentration 8 h post exposure whereas adults did not reach similar levels until 24 h post exposure.[15] This supports the existence of age-dependent differences in the blood brain barrier permeability to an organotin species may exist.

The apparent gliosis in cortical layers III and IV in different regions of the neocortex which was observed 7 days following PND 18 dosing was consistent with both the astroglial response seen in neonatal mice[11] and the pattern of neurodegeneration observed in adult rats using silver degeneration techniques (cupric silver staining methods) after acute TMT exposure.[17] This apparent shrinkage with increased packing density may be attributed to somatodendritic shrinkage as observed at the ultrastructural level in other cortical regions after TMT exposure.[18] The regions in which gliosis and shrinkage were consistent between the different time points of TMT administration were the amygdala, hippocampus, piriform cingulate and entorhinal cortex. Although the apparent magnitude and onset of the glial response was different, the net results were indicative of pathology in several cortical regions.

SUMMARY

Long-Evans rat pups received intraperitoneal (i.p.) injections of trimethyl-tin (TMT) 6 mg/kg hydroxide or saline on postnatal day (PND) 10 or PND 18 and were sacrificed for immunohistochemical staining for glial fibrillary acidic protein (GFAP) on PND 12, 18, 20, or 25. After dosing with TMT on PND 10 there was a transient increase in GFAP immunoreactivity (IR) in the amygdala, piriform, and entorhinal cortex 2 days post-dosing (PND 12) and a persistent increase in GFAP IR in the hippocampus and cingulate cortex up to two weeks post-dosing. Following dosing with TMT on PND 18 there was a delayed (PND 25) increase in GFAP IR in the amygdala, hippocampus, cingulate, piriform, and entorhinal cortex. In addition, increases in GFAP IR were observed in the neocortex 7 days post-dosing, which was not observed following earlier postnatal dosing. The regions in which gliosis and loss of Nissl-staining were consistent for the different time points of TMT treatment were the amygdala, hippocampus, cingulate, piriform, and entorhinal cortex. The present findings indicate the GFAP immunohistochemistry can be used to reveal regional effects of developmental neurotoxicant exposure during early stages of development.

ACKNOWLEDGMENTS

The author is deeply grateful for the technical assistnce of Ms. Kim Oxendine, photographic assistance of Ms. Julia Davis and Ms. Kim Jones, and for the editorial comments of E. S. Goldey, G. M. Peterson and J. P. O'Callaghan. This manuscript has been reviewed by the Health Effects Research Laboratory, USEPA, and approved for publication. Data from this manuscript was presented in published form in *Neurotoxicology and Teratology,* in press.[9] Mention of trade names and commercial products does not constitute endorsement or recommendation for use.

REFERENCES

1. O'CALLAGHAN, J. P. & D. B. MILLER. 1989. Assessment of chemically-induced alterations in brain development using assays of neuron- and glia-localized proteins. Neurotoxicology **10:** 393–406.
2. ENG, L. F. 1985. Glial fibrillary acidic protein (GFAP): The major protein of glial intermediate filaments in differentiated astrocytes. J. Neuroimmunol. **8:** 203–214.
3. BIGNAMI, A. & D. DAHL. 1976. The astroglial response to stabbing. Immunofluorescence studies with antibodies to astrocyte-specific protein (GFA) in mammalian and submammalian vertebrates. Neuropathol. Appl. Neurobiol. **2:** 99–110.
4. AMADUCCI, L., K. I. FORNO & L. F. ENG. 1981. Glial fibrillary acidic protein in cryogenic lesions of the rat brain. Neurosci. Lett. **21:** 27–32.
5. EISENFELD, A. J., A. H. BUNT-MILAM & P. V. SARTHY. 1984. Mueller cell expression of glial fibrillary acidic protein after genetic and experimental photoreceptor degeneration in the rat retina. Invest. Ophthalmol. Vis. Sci. **25:** 1321–1328.
6. REIER, P. J. 1986. Gliosis following CNS injury: the anatomy of astrocytic scars and their influences on axonal elongation. *In* Astrocytes: Cell Biology and Pahtology of Astrocytes, Vol. 3: 263–324. S. Federoff & A. Vernadkis, Eds. Academic Press. Orlando, FL.
7. O'CALLAGHAN, J. P. 1988. Neurotypic and gliotypic proteins as biomarkers of neurotoxicity. Neurotoxicol. Teratol. **10:** 445–452.
8. ENG, L. F. 1988. Astrocytic response to injury. *In* Current issues in Neural Regeneration

Research. P. J. Reier, R. P. Bunge & F. J. Seil, Eds.: 247–255. Alan R. Liss. New York.

9. STANTON, M. & S. BARONE, JR. 1993. Neonatal exposure to TMT impairs retention of olfactory learning and increases GFAP immunoreactivity in hippocampus, piriform and entorhinal cortex. Neurotoxicol. Teratol. In press.

10. HSU, S.M., L. RAINE & H. FANGER. 1981. Use of avidin-biotin peroxidase complex (ABC) in immunoperoxidase techniques: A comparison between ABC and unlabeled antibody (PAP) procedures. J. Histochem. Cytochem. **29:** 577–580.

11. REUHL, K. R., E. A. SMALLRIDGE, L. W. CHANGE & B. A. MACKENZIE. 1983. Developmental effects of trimethyltin in the neonatal mouse. I. Light microscopic studies. Neurotoxicology **4:** 19–28.

12. CHANG, L. W. 1984. Hippocampal lesions induced by trimethyltin in the neonatal rat brain. Neurotoxicology **5:** 205–216.

13. CHANG, L. W. 1984. Trimethyltin induced hippocampal lesions at various neonatal ages. Bull. Environ. Contam. Toxicol. **33:** 295–301.

14. GOLDEY, E. S., M. E. STANTON, J. P. O'CALLAGHAN & K. M. CROFTON. 1992. Screening for developmental neurotoxicants: Possible alternatives to existing guidelines. Toxicologist **12**(1): 1362.

15. COOK, L. L., J. S. JACOBS & L. W. REITER. 1984. Tin distribution in adult and neonatal rat brain following exposures to triethyltin. Toxicol. Appl. Pharmacol. **73:** 564–568.

16. COOK, L. L., K. E. STINE & L. W. REITER. 1984. Tin distribution in adult rat tissues after exposure to trimethyl and triethyl tin. Toxicol. Appl. Pharmcol. **76:** 344–348.

17. BALABAN, C. D., J. P. O'CALLAGHAN & M. L. BILLINGSLEY. 1988. Trimethyltin induced neuronal damage in the rat: Comparative studies using silver degeneration stains, immunocytochemistry and immunoassay for neurotypic and gliotypic proteins. Neuroscience **26:** 337–361.

18. BOULDIN, T. W., N. D. GOINES, C. R. BAGNELL & M. R. KRIGMAN. 1981. Pathogenesis of trimethyltin neuronal toxicity. Am. J. Pathol. **97:** 237–249.

The Goldfish as a Drug Discovery Vehicle for Parkinson's Disease and Other Neurodegenerative Disorders

HARVEY B. POLLARD,[a] MARTENS ADEYEMO,[a]
KULDEEP DHARIWAL,[a] MARK LEVINE,[a]
HUNG CAOHUY,[a] SANFORD MARKEY,[b]
CAROL J. MARKEY,[b] AND MOUSSA B. H. YOUDIM[c]

[a]Laboratory of Cell Biology and Genetics
National Institute of Diabetes, Digestive and Kidney Diseases
National Institutes of Health
Bethesda, Maryland 20892

[b]Laboratory of Clinical Sciences
National Institute of Neurological Diseases
and Communicative Disorders
National Institutes of Health
Bethesda, Maryland 20892

[c]Department of Pharmacology and Rappaport Family Center
Technion Medical School
Haifa, Israel

INTRODUCTION

Neurodegenerative diseases such as Parkinson's Disease (PD) and Alzheimer's Disease (AD) are now recognized as among the most important challenges facing biomedical research. These diseases mostly affect a large fraction of the most aged in our society, and it has been predicted that by the beginning of the 21st century more centigenarians will be alive than were ever alive in the history of mankind. Humans lose dopamine neurons sustainedly as they age. It has been estimated that as many as 75% of persons may lose enough dopamine neurons to develop PD if they live long enough. By comparison, a larger percentage of persons may be at risk for AD, as the target cholinergic neurons all appear to be susceptible.

However, PD and AD affect some of the most primitive and sophisticated aspects of the central nervous system. The problem is that not only that the brain and its functions are not well understood, but that there are very few animal models of PD or AD upon which to base a phenomenological search for useful drugs. However, one attractive model for Parkinson's Disease is that provided by the neurotoxin MPTP (1-methyl-4-1,2,3,6-tetrahydropyridine). Inadvertant administration of MPTP to humans as a contaminant in a "designer" drug led to the discovery that it could cause PD-like symptoms in man[1] and lower primates.[2] However, MPTP effects with animals lower down on the evolutionary scale such as dogs,[3,4] cats,[5,6] rats,[7] and mice[8] were more difficult to detect and document.

The mechanism of MPTP action in primates involves oxidation by monoamine oxidase B (MAO-B) to the active toxin, MPP+.[9,10] This process seems to occur primarily in the glial cells. MPP+ then leaves the cell of origin and enters susceptible neurons in the substantia nigra and elsewhere through dopamine transporters. The immediate intracellular target for MPP+ is the mitochondrion, and reduction of ATP stores in the target cell leads to cell death. Cell death occurs because the loss of ATP leads to a decrease in the activity of the Na-K ATPase. Consequently, depolarization of the cell leads to sustained calcium entry through voltage-sensitive calcium channels, and it is the elevated intracellular calcium which administers the final blow to the target cell.

Authentic, idiopathic Parkinson's Disease in man is manifest by the loss of other transmitter systems in addition to dopamine.[11–13] However, the experiments with MPTP do seem to illustrate the intrinsic susceptibility to energetic compromise of the circuits controlling the Parkinson's Disease-related behavior. MPTP toxicity is thus a compelling model to use in searches for anti-Parkinson's Disease drugs. Indeed, L-deprenyl, an MAO-B inhibitor drug found to be useful in treating iodiopathic Parkinson's Disease,[14,15] also protects primates against MPTP toxicity.[16] However, primates present many difficulties for routine neurotoxicological studies, and a simpler vertebrate model has been long sought for use with MPTP as a paradigm for drug discovery of use in PD.

NEUROTOXICOLOGICAL STUDIES WITH THE GOLDFISH

Our recent experiences with the goldfish nervous system have led us to give a lot of consideration to this simpler vertebrate as a useful model for neurochemistry and behavior in higher organisms. Our first indication about the value of the goldfish for this purpose came from studies on omega-conotoxin.[17] Omega-conotoxin is a polypeptide toxin from the cone snail which causes death by directly blocking N-type calcium channels in the CNS of many vertebrate species. Monoclonal antibodies against omega-conotoxin proved to be protective when tested *in vivo* in both goldfish and rat. In the rat, intrathecal administration of both toxin and antibodies were necessary because of the blood brain barrier. However, In the goldfish, simple intraperitoneal injection was sufficient to elicit toxicity and protection since the goldfish has only a limited blood brain barrier.[18]

More recently we have extended our application of the goldfish model to the study of Parkinson's Disease by treating goldfish with MPTP.[19–21] We found that administration of as little as one injection of 20 mg/kg MPTP, i.p., led to a progressive and substantial reduction in the movement of the treated animals (TABLE 1). We were able to quantitate changes in movement by using the conventional Columbus Activity Meter. For this purpose we simply placed a goldfish in a transparent chamber containing water, and followed the sequential interruption of infrared light beams as the goldfish moved within the chamber. We also noted

TABLE 1. Influence of MPTP on Mobility of Goldfish

Condition	Mobility		
	TD, cm	RT, 5 min	V, cm/min
Control	698 ± 20	0.53 ± 0.03	157 ± 5
MPTP	125 ± 40	2.90 ± 0.08	59 ± 8

MPTP was administered at 50 mg/kg, i.p., and mobility assessed 72 hours post treatment. TD = total distance traveled; RT = total resting time; V = apparent velocity. Results for each condition are mean ± SEM (n = 10).

TABLE 2. Influence of MPTP on Dopamine (DA), Noradrenaline (NA) and MPP+ in Goldfish Brain

Condition	NA	DA	MPP+
	(pmol/mg protein)		(ng)
Control	71.2 ± 8.0	22.0 ± 4.8	0
MPTP	19.4 ± 1.7	3.9 ± 1.1	4.3 ± 0.8

MPTP was administered at 30 mg/kg, i.p., and changes assessed 8 days post treatment. Results for each condition are mean $\pm$ SEM (n = 6). (Summarized from ref. 21.)

that MPP$^+$ accumulated in the brain, and that both forebrain and midbrain regions accumulated the most. Using a sensitive HPLC method we also found that both noradrenaline and dopamine were reduced profoundly in all regions of the brain (TABLE 2).

Furthermore, MAO-A and MAO-B activities were apparent in the brain homogenates, and were differentially sensitive to clorgyline and L-deprenyl, respectively. As might be anticipated, both the non-selective MAO blocker, tranylcypromine, and the MAO-B selective blocker L-deprenyl were able to protect MPTP treated goldfish in terms of bradykinesia. Tranylcypromine also protected against loss of catecholamines. By contrast, clorgyline, an MAO-A -selective blocker, was without significant efficacy in protecting against bradykinesia.

DRUG DISCOVERY FOR NEUROPROTECTION USING THE GOLDFISH SYSTEM

Although briefly summarized here, our rather extensive study of the goldfish system and its response to the toxin MPTP has convinced us that, at least for Parkinson's Disease, the system has real advantages as a drug discovery vehicle. Perhaps foremost is the fact that goldfish respond to MPTP with a biochemical and behavioral syndrome having some qualitative similarity to that induced by MPTP in primates. By contrast, rats, and with some exceptions, mice, are extremely resistant to MPTP in terms of behavioral and neurochemical consequences. In fact, MPTP was once tested for toxicity on rodents, and found to be "safe."

In addition, at least one drug presently of use in humans, L-deprenyl, proved to be protective in the goldfish system. By contrast, a drug of no use in human PD, clorgyline, was of no value as a neuroprotective agent for the MPTP-goldfish system. Clearly, using the goldfish, L-deprenyl could have been detected in systematic screening, and clorgyline rejected. It is therefore reasonable to anticipate that additional candidate drugs might be detected through application of a goldfish "screen." and that efficacious compounds might then be reserved for further scrutiny in scarce primates.

REFERENCES

1. LANGSTON, J. W., P. BALLARD, J. W. TETRUD & I. IRWIN. 1983. Science **219:** 979–980.
2. BURNS, R. S., C. C. CHIUEH, S. P. MARKEY, M. H. EBERT, D. M. JACOBOWITZ & I. P. KOPIN. 1983. Proc. Natl. Acad. Sci. USA **80:** 4546–4550.

3. PARISI, J. E., & R. S. BURNS. 1986. *In* MPTP-A Neurotoxin Producing a Parkinsonian Syndrome. S. Markey, N. Castagnoli, A. J. Trevor & I. J. Kopin, Eds.: 141. Academic Press. New York.

4. JOHANNESSEN, J. N., C. C. CHIUEH, J. P. BACON, N. A. CARRICK, D. L. MURPHY, R. S. BURNS, B. K. WEISE, I. J. KOPIN & S. P. MARKEY. 1985. Soc. Neurosci. Abstracts **11**: 185.14.

5. SCHNEIDER, J. S. & C. H. MARKHAM. 1986. Brain Res. **373**: 258–267.

6. AMBROSIO, S., R. BLESA, G. M. MINTENIG, L. PALACIOS-ARAUS, N. MAHY & A. GUAL. 1988. Toxicol. Lett. **44**: 1–6.

7. CHIUEH, C. C., S. P. MARKEY, R. S. BURNS, J. N. JOHANNESSEN, D. M. JACOBOWITZ & I. J. KOPIN. 1984. Psychopharm Bull. **20**: 546–553.

8. HEIKKILA, R. E., A. HESS & R. DUVOISIN. 1984. Science **224**: 1451–1453.

9. JAVICH, J. A., R. J. D'AMATO, S. M. STRITTMATTER & S. H. SNYDER. 1985. Proc. Natl. Acad. Sci. USA **82**: 2173–2177.

10. FRITZ, R. R., C. W. ABELL, N. T. PATEL, W. GESSNER & A. BROSSI. 1985. FEBS. Lett. **186**: 224–228.

11. KOPP, N., L. DENOROY, M. THOMASI, N. GAY, G. CHAZOT & B. RENAUD. 1982. Acta Neuropathol. **56**: 17–21.

12. SCATTON, B., F. JAVOY-AGID, L. ROUQUIER, L. DUBOIS & Y. AGID. 1983. Brain Res. **275**: 321–328.

13. WOOTEN, G. F. 1987. *In* Handbook of Parkinson's Disease. W. C. Coller, Ed.: 237–251. Marcel Dekker. New York.

14. BIRKMEYER, W., J. KNOLL, P. REIDERER & M. B. H. YOUDIM. 1983. Mod. Problem. Psychopharm. **19**: 170–176.

15. BIRKMEYER, W., J. KNOLL, P. REIDERER, M. B. H. YOUDIM, V. HARS & J. MARTON. 1985. J. Neural Trans. **664**: 113–127.

16. COHEN, G., P. PASIK, B. COHEN, A. LEIST, C. MYTILLINEOU M. D. YAHR. 1984. Eur. J. Pharmac. **106**: 209–210.

17. ADEYEMO, O. M., S. SHAPIRA, D. TOMBACCINI, H. B. POLLARD, G. FEUERSTEIN & A-L. SIREN. 1991. Tox. Appl. Pharm. **108**: 489–496.

18. BRADBURY, M. 1979. The Concept of the Blood Brain Barrier. John Wiley and Sons. New York. pp. 301–319.

19. YOUDIM, M. B. H., K. DHARIWAL, M. LEVINE, C. J. MARKEY, S. MARKEY, O. M. ADEYEMO, H. CAOHUY & H. B. POLLARD. 1990. *In* Fourth International Amine Oxidases Workshop: Metabolic Aspects. Abstract book.

20. YOUDIM, M. B. H., K. DHARIWAL, M. LEVINE, C. J. MARKEY, S. MARKEY, O. M. ADEYEMO, H. CAOHUY & H. B. POLLARD. 1992. Neurochem. Int. **20**(Suppl.): 275S–278S.

21. POLLARD, H. P., K. DHARIWAL, O. M. ADEYEMO, C. J. MARKEY, H. CAOHUY, M. LEVINE, S. MARKEY & M. B. H. YOUDIM. 1992. FASEB J. **6**: 3108–3116.

The Interactions of MK-801 with the Amphetamine Analogues D-Methamphetamine (D-METH), 3,4-Methylenedioxymethamphetamine (D-MDMA) or D-Fenfluramine (D-FEN): Neural Damage and Neural Protection[a]

DIANE B. MILLER[b] AND JAMES P. O'CALLAGHAN

United States Environmental Protection Agency
Health Effects Research Laboratory
Research Triangle Park, North Carolina 27711

Recently there has been intense speculation concerning the neurotoxicity of certain of the amphetamine analogues, including MDMA and FEN (Ricaurte *et al.*[1]). Although depletion of a particular neurotransmitter may signify damage of that brain area (*e.g.*, Sonsolla *et al.*[2]) it is not always synonymous with CNS injury (see O'Callaghan *et al.*[3]). Many investigators utilize loss of neurotransmitter level and/or enzyme activity in a particular brain area as evidence for damage or degeneration in that area. Both MDMA and FEN can produce long-lasting neurotransmitter depletions in rodents, hence the conclusion they induce injury. Gliosis, however, is typically associated with the CNS injury induced by a variety of means (see O'Callaghan this volume for further discussion). Because injury to the mammalian nervous system provokes hypertrophy of astrocytes at the sites of damage the enhanced expression of the astrocyte-localized protein, glial fibrillary acidic protein (GFAP) can be used to define and explore chemically induced neurotoxicity (*e.g.*, O'Callaghan *et al.*[3]). Thus, in this work we used the level of GFAP in specific brain areas to determine the comparative neurotoxicity of the D isomers of METH, MDMA and FEN in the cortex, striatum and hippocampus of mice.

There is evidence that glutaminergic mechanisms may play a role in the CNS changes associated with exposure to the amphetamines (Sonsalla *et al.*[2,4]). Glutaminergic mechanisms have been implicated in a variety of forms of brain trauma and injury as well as the CNS alterations observed in Alzheimer's and Huntington's diseases. Further, it is suspected that hypoxia-ischemia and other forms of brain injury cause excess levels of excitatory amino acids and overstimulation of glutamate receptors with subsequent damage. Consequently, the blockade of glutamate receptors would be expected to have a protective effect and compounds with the

[a] This work was partially supported by Grant IAG ND-89-4 from the National Institute on Drug Abuse.

[b] Send correspondence regarding this manuscript to Diane B. Miller, Ph.D., U.S. EPA, NTD/HERL, MD-74B, RTP, NC 27711; (919) 541-4186.

ability to block these receptors are the focus of much research interest. Recent work has suggested a role for excitatory amino acids in the dopaminergic toxicity conferred by the amphetamine analogue, METH. Sonsalla and colleagues[2] determined that pretreatment with a non-specific blocker of NMDA receptors, MK-801, blocks that striatal depletion of dopamine and the loss of tyrosine hydroxylase activity caused by METH. Therefor, in addition to determining whether D-METH, D-MDMA, D-FEN induce CNS damage we also examined the role of glutaminergic overstimulation in the neurotoxicity of these compounds by using MK-801 as a pretreatment. We now report D-METH and D-MDMA, but not D-FEN, cause damage to mouse striatum that is prevented by pretreatment with MK-801.

METHODS

Species

C57B1/6 female mice, approx. 5 months of age (Jackson Labs, Bar Harbor, ME) (N = 6/gp) were used.

Dosing

The dosages of D-METH (10.0 mg/kg; Sigma Chemical Co.), D-MDMA (25.0 mg/kg; obtained through the Research Technology Branch of the National Institute on Drug Abuse from the Research Triangle Institute, Research Triangle Park, NC) and D-FEN (10.0 mg/kg; generously supplied by Servier of France), as well as the dosing regimen, were based on preliminary work in our laboratories (see O'Callaghan & Miller.[5] All amphetamine analogues were administered s.c. as the base every 2 h for a total of 4 injections. MK-801 (Research Biochemicals Inc., Natick, MA) pretreatment (1.0 mg/kg s.c. as the salt) occurred 0.5 h prior to the first and third injection of each of the substituted amphetamines; controls not receiving MK-801 were given saline on the same injection schedule.

Preparation of Tissue and Biochemical Assessment

Mice were killed 48 h following the final injection; 48 h allows a sufficient time post exposure to observe changes in the endpoints of interest (see O'Callaghan et al.[3]). The brain was removed; the striatum, hippocampus and cortex were free-hand dissected and frozen at $-70°C$ for later analysis of GFAP. A sandwich ELISA was used to determine the levels of GFAP in samples of brain sonified in hot 1% SDS (O'Callaghan[6]).

RESULTS

D-METH, D-MDMA or D-FEN did not alter GFAP levels in hippocampus or cortex (data not shown). However, D-METH and D-MDMA caused large and significant (214% and 225% over control, respectively) increases in striatal GFAP

(FIG. 1). MK-801 was able to substantially, although not completely, block the elevations in GFAP associated D-METH. GFAP elevations in striatum induced by D-MDMA were completely blocked by pretreatment with MK-801. In contrast, the treatment with D-FEN did not alter striatal levels of GFAP suggesting this particular analogue of amphetamine does not damage mouse striatum. MK-801, whether given alone or as a pretreatment to D-FEN, was without effect.

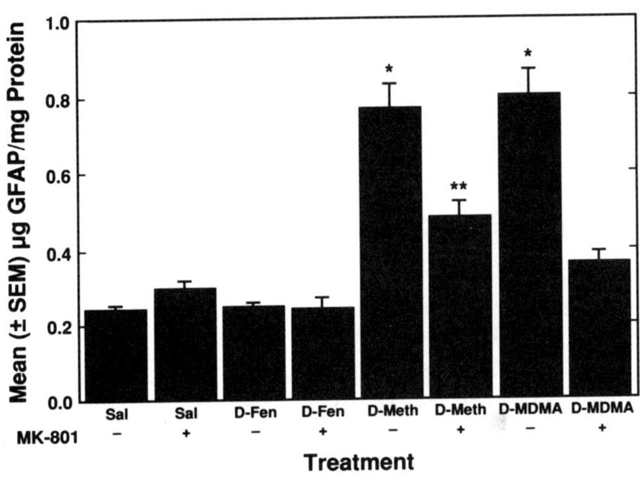

FIGURE 1. Effects of D-FEN (10 mg/kg), D-METH (10.0 mg/kg) and D-MDMA (25 mg/kg) alone and after pretreatment with MK-801 (1.0 mg/kg s.c. at 0.5 h prior to the first and third injection) on amount of GFAP in striatum of the C57B16/J female mouse at 48 h following the last of 4 injections given s.c. at 2 h intervals. Data were analyzed by analysis of variance followed by Duncan's multiple range test for mean comparisons. *significant difference from saline-treated and D-FEN treated animals, $p < .05$; **significant difference from same compound without MK-801 pretreatment, $p. < .05$.

DISCUSSION

Previous reports concerning the neurotoxicity of D-METH have utilized neurotransmitter depletion and loss of enzyme activity as a gauge of the degree of damage induced by this amphetamine analogue (Sonsolla *et al.*[2]). Here we present confirmatory evidence that, in the mouse, D-meth causes damage to striatum but not to hippocampus or striatum. The robust elevation in striatal GFAP following D-MDMA support the conclusion that this analogue, like D-METH, causes damage to the mouse striatum. Likewise the failure of D-FEN to induce GFAP elevations in any brain area examined suggest this agent does not cause injury. It could be considered that D-FEN is not as potent as D-MDMA and exposure to a higher dosage of D-FEN would result in neural damage. However, subsequent work in our laboratories has demonstrated that 25 mg/kg of D-FEN is without effect while both 10.0 and 25.0 mg/kg of D-MDMA cause robust increases in striatal but not hippocampal GFAP. While our data do not speak directly to the mechanism by which D-METH and D-MDMA are able to damage certain areas of CNS the blockade of their striatal neurotoxicity by MK-801 certainly suggests a role for excitatory amino acids in the production of injury in this brain area. The failure of MK-801 to completely block the damage in striatum induced by D-METH suggest that some portion of the injury may be mediated by other than glutaminergic overstimulation. Future work should determine if competitive and noncompetitive NMDA antagonists are equally effective in preventing this neural damage. Variables such as handling and body temperature have been shown to interact with many of the effects (*e.g.*, lethality; neurotransmitter depletion) engendered by the amphetamine analogues (Bowyer *et al.*[7] Schmidt *et al.*[8]). It has also been suggested that MK-801 produces some of its neuroprotection in cases of ischemia/hypoxia by reducing body temperature (*e.g.*, Bucan & Pulsinelli[9]). Consequently, the contribution of environmental variables to the neural damage induced by the amphetamine analogues, D-METH and D-MDMA should be the subject of future investigation.

REFERENCES

1. RICAURTE, G. A., M. E. MOLLIVER, M. B. MARTELLO, J. L. KATZ, M. A. WILSON & A. L. MARTELLO. 1991. Dexfenfluramine neurotoxicity in brains of non-human primates. Lancet **338:** 1487–88.
2. SONSALLA, P. K., W. J. NICKLAS & R. E. HEIKKILA. 1989. Role for excitatory amino acids in methamphetamine-induced nigrostriatal dopaminergic toxicity. Science **243:** 398–400.
3. O'CALLAGHAN, J. P., D. B. MILLER & J. F. REINHARD, JR. 1990. Characterization of the origins of astrocyte response to injury using the dopaminergic neurotoxicant, 1-methyl-4-phenyl-1,2,3,6-tetrahydropyridine. Brain Res. **521:** 73–80.
4. SONSALLA, P. K., D. E. RIORDAN & R. E. HEIKKILA. 1991. Competitive and noncompetitive antagonists at *N*-methyl-D-aspartate receptors protect against methamphetamine-induced dopaminergic damage in mice. J. Pharmacol. Exp. Ther. **256:** 506–512.
5. O'CALLAGHAN, J. P. & D. B. MILLER. 1992. Quantification of reactive gliosis as an approach to neurotoxicity assessment. *In* Assessing Neurotoxicity of Drugs of Abuse. L. Erinoff, Ed. National Institute on Drug Abuse Monograph. Washington, D.C. U.S. Government Printing Office. In press.
6. O'CALLAGHAN, J. P. 1991. Quantification of glial fibrillary acidic protein: Comparison of slot-immunobinding assays with a novel sandwich ELISA. Neurotoxicol. Teratol. **13:** 275–281.
7. BOWYER, J. F., A. W. TANK, G. D. NEWPORT, W. SLIKKLER, JR., S. F. ALI & R. R. HOLSON. 1992. The influence of environmental temperature on the transient effects of methamphetamine on dopamine levels and dopamine release in rat striatum. J. Pharmacol Exp. Ther. **260:** 817–824.
8. SCHMIDT, C. J., C. K. BLACK, G. M. ABBATE & V. L. TAYLOR. 1991. Methylenedioxymethamphetamine-induced hyperthermia and neurotoxicity are independently regulated by 5-HT2 receptors. Brain Res. **529:** 85–90.
9. BUCHAN, A. & W. A. PULSINELLI. 1990. Hypothermia but not the *n*-methyl-D-aspartate antagonist, MK-801, attenuates neuronal damage in gerbils subjected to transient global ischemia. J. Neurosci. **10:** 311–316.

Calpain Activity in Organophosphorus-induced Delayed Neuropathy (OPIDN): Effects of a Phenylalkylamine Calcium Channel Blocker[a]

HASSAN A. N. EL-FAWAL[b,d] AND MARION F. EHRICH[c]

[b]Institute of Environmental Medicine
New York University Medical Center
Tuxedo Park, New York 10987

[c]Virginia-Maryland Regional College of Veterinary Medicine
Blacksburg, Virginia 24061

Calpains (calcium-activated neutral proteases) are cysteine proteases which have been identified in numerous cell types.[1] Two isozymes of calpain have been identified and designated calpain I and calpain II, according to their requirement for either μM or mM concentration of calcium, respectively, for activation.[2] However, chicken tissues apparently contain only calpain II.[3] Studies of both the central and peripheral nervous system indicate that proteases, including calpains, may precipitate the breakdown of cytoskeletal elements in Wallerian degeneration,[1] Alzheimers Disease[4] and excitotoxicity.[5] This role of calpains in the pathophysiology of the nervous system is likely a consequence of increases in free cytosolic calcium.[6,7]

Organophosphorus compounds (OP) are widely used in agriculture and in industry as plasticizes or lubricant and hydraulic fluid additives. Some of these OPs, typified by tri-ortho cresyl phosphate (TOCP), produce an irreversible peripheral neuropathy one or two weeks following a single exposure.[8] This neuropathy is characterized by a flaccid paralysis with a "dying-back" Wallerian degeneration of peripheral nerves. A reliable biomarker of OPIDN has been identified, neuropathy target esterase (NTE), which appears to be predictive of an OP's potential for inducing OPIDN when significant inhibition (>70%) occurs. However, the role of NTE as the target for initiating OPIDN has not received universal acceptance.[8]

We have hypothesized that development of OPIDN may involve an increase in calcium influx with a subsequent activation of calpain and the precipitation of axonal cytoskeletal degeneration. Using White Leghorn hens, the accepted model of OPIDN,[8] we have previously shown that dihydropyridine (DHP) and phenylalkylamine calcium channel blockers could attenuate the development of clinical, electrophysiological and morphological deficits associated with OPIDN.[9,10] Furthermore, attenuation of the neuropathy by the DHP nifedipine was associated with preventing the increase in calpain activity.[11] Therefore, the present study was

[a] Supported at New York University by a Center Grant ES-00260 and in Virginia by Research Grant ES-3384, both from the U.S. Department of Health and Human Services.
[d] Author to whom correspondence should be addressed.

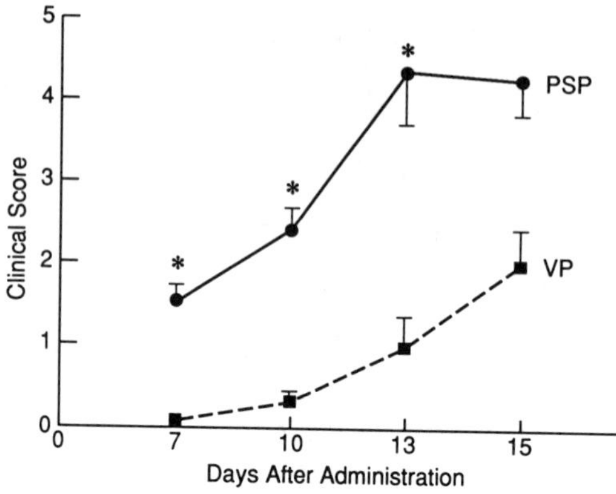

FIGURE 1. Development of clinical deficits in hens after administration of PSP or verapamil + PSP (X ± SE). 0 = normal; 1 = altered gait; 2 = difficulty walking and standing; 3 = severe ataxia; 4 = leg paralysis; 5 = leg and wing paralysis (* indicates significantly different from verapamil + PSP, Student's t-test; $p < 0.05$; n = 5).

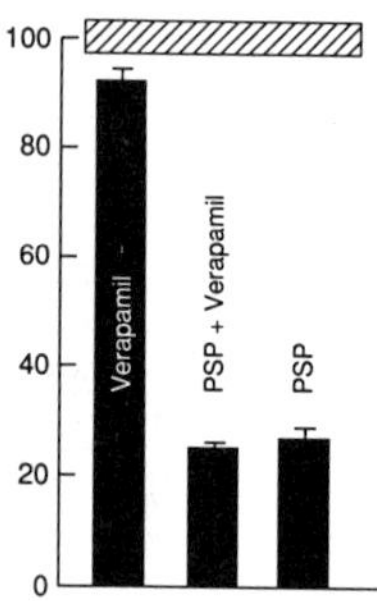

FIGURE 2. Brain NTE activity as percentage of control (23.8 ± 0.7 nmol/min/mg protein) following administration of verapamil only, or at 72 hours after PSP (last day of verapamil treatment) (ANOVA, Newman-Keuls test for multiple comparisons, $p < 0.05$, n = 3–4).

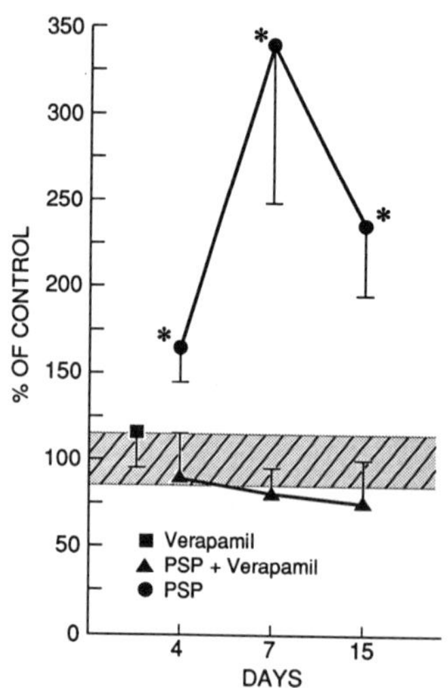

FIGURE 3. Calpain activity in sciatic nerve as percentage of control (20 ± 3 absorbance units at 440 nm/30 min/μg protein) following treatment with verapamil only and at 4, 7 and 15 days following PSP treatment (ANOVA, Newman-Keuls test for multiple comparisons, $p < 0.05$, n = 4–10).

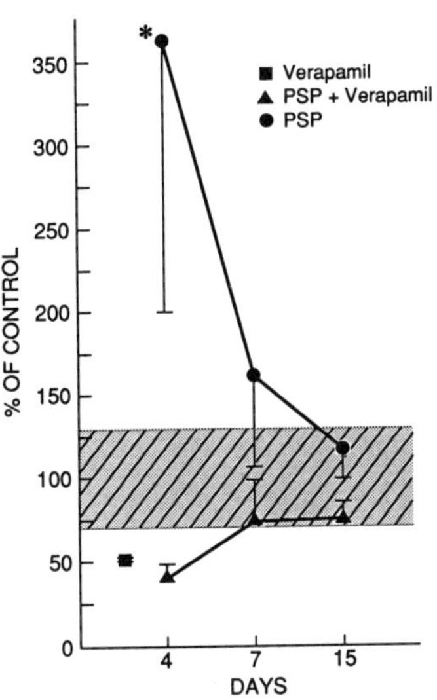

FIGURE 4. Calpain activity in gastrocnemius muscle as percentage of control (218 ± 63 absorbance units at 440 nm/30 min/μg protein) following treatment with verapamil only and at 4, 7, and 15 days following PSP treatment (ANOVA, Newman-Keuls test for multiple comparisons, $p < 0.05$, n = 4–10).

performed to assess whether a phenylalkylamine, verapamil, may also attenuate neuropathy by influencing calpain activity.

Adult White Leghorn hens were given intramuscular injections of verapamil (7 mg/kg) for 4 days, with a single dose of phenyl saligenin phosphate (PSP, 2.5 mg/kg), an active congener of TOCP, administered on the second day of verapamil treatment. The activity of partially purified calpain was determined spectrophotometrically[11] in sciatic nerve and gastrocnemius muscle of hens 4, 7, and 15 days after PSP administration. Verapamil treatment significantly attenuated the development of PSP-induced clinical deficits (FIG. 1). However, this did not appear to rely on the competitive protection of brain NTE as reported for other modifiers

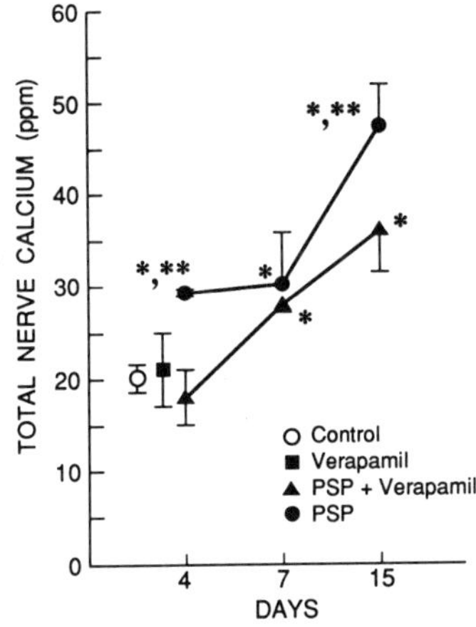

FIGURE 5. Total calcium in nitric-perchloric acid digests of sciatic nerve (determined by atomic absorbtion at 422.7 nm against a calcium carbonate standard) of controls, verapamil only, and at 4, 7, and 15 days following PSP (* significantly different from controls: ** significantly different from verapamil + PSP; ANOVA, Dunnett's test for multiple comparisons, $p < 0.05$, n = 4–5).

of OPIDN (*e.g.*, phenyl methyl sulfonyl fluoride, some carbamates[8]), since NTE was equally inhibited whether hens did or did not receive verapamil (FIG. 2). Treatment with verapamil prevented the PSP-induced increase in calpain activity in sciatic nerve and gastrocnemium muscle of hens (FIGS. 3 and 4). The early

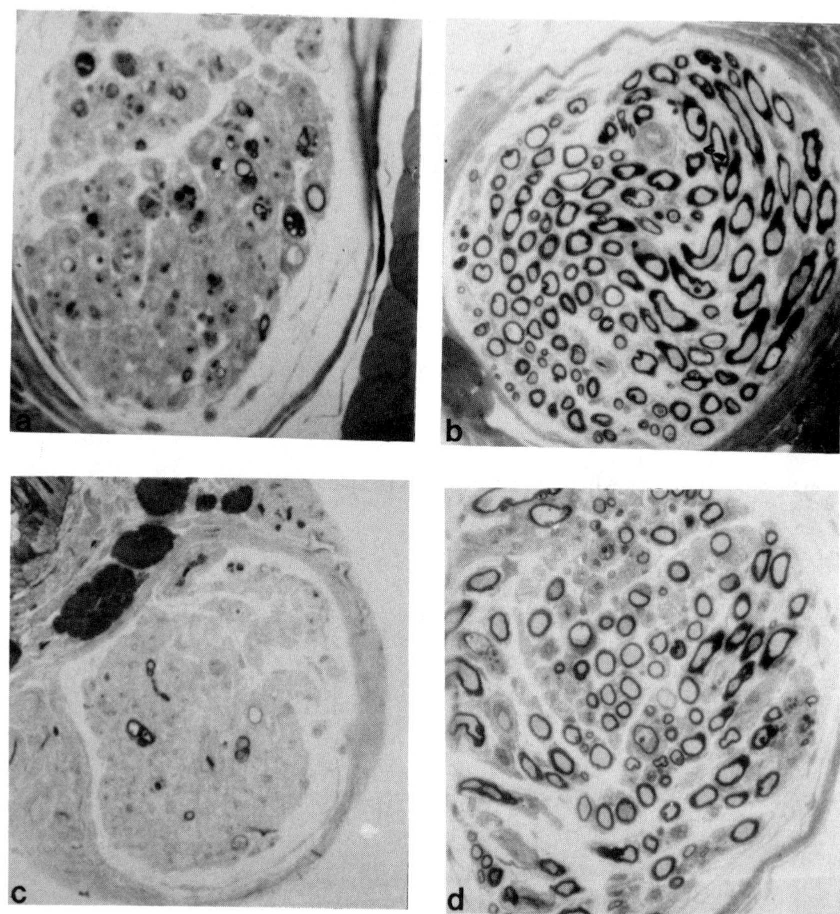

FIGURE 6. Distal level of biventer cervicis nerve from hens at 7 **(a, b)** and 15 **(c, d)** days after PSP administration. Nerves from hens given only PSP have early lesions indicative of Wallerian degeneration **(a)** which increased in severity to show the widespread loss of myelinated fibers and empty Schwann cell tubes **(c)**. The degenerative process appears to be less severe and widespread in nerves of hens treated with verapamil + PSP **(b, d)**. Toluidine blue-safranin stain; magnification: ×200.

increase in muscle calpain activity, in hens given only PSP, followed by recovery may indicate a transient myopathy associated with some OPs.[12] Total nerve calcium, while not differentiating between sequestered or free calcium (that capable of activating calpain), indicated an earlier significant increase in calcium following treatment with PSP alone (FIG. 5). This was greater than the increase in nerves from hens receiving verapamil and PSP, which showed a delayed increase. Histological evaluation of the biventer cervicis nerve, a peripheral nerve shown to be sensitive to OPIDN,[13] supported the clinical and biochemical evidence that verapamil does protect against the development of neuropathy (FIG. 6). This is consistent with our earlier reports on the protection by calcium channel blockers of neuromuscular function during OPIDN.[9,10]

The results of this and earlier studies suggest that increases in intracellular calcium, possibly mediated by increased calcium influx through the L-type calcium channel, which is blocked by both DHP and phenylalkylamines, may play a role in the development of OPIDN. Elevation in cytosolic free calcium following exposure of cells to neuropathy-inducing OPs has been reported.[14] Calcium influx through the DHP channel is of particular interest since it has been linked to calpain activation during long-term potentiation and excitotoxicity.[15,16] That increased influx through a channel occurs in OPIDN may be indicated by the diminished effeciveness of DHP blockers in attenuating OPIDN when given after an OP rather than before.[10] This, however does not preclude the invovlement of calcium release from intracellular stores or other cellular calcium homeostatic mechanisms in the development of neuropathy. Specifically, elevation of axoplasmic calcium may produce lesions of Wallerian degeneration during OPIDN by the activation of calpain,[11] in addition to other calcium-dependent mechanisms, such as calmodulin kinase II.[8] The extent to which calcium channel activation and calpain activity may participate in the development of neuropathies, including neurotoxicant-induced neuropathy, need to be further investigated.

REFERENCES

1. SCHLAEPFER, W. W. & U. P. ZIMMERMAN. 1985. Ann. N.Y. Acad. Sci. **455:** 552–562.
2. GOLL, D. E., W. C. KLEESE, A. OKITANI, T. KUMAMOTO, J. KONG & H. KAPPRELL. 1990. *In* Intracellular Calcium-Dependent Proteolysis. R. L. Mellgren & T. Murachi, Eds.: 3–24. CRC Press. Boca Raton, FL.
3. OHNO, S., Y. EMORI, S. IMAJOH, H. KAWASAKI, M. KISARAGI & K. SUZUKI. 1984. Nature **312:** 566–570.
4. NIXON, R. A. & A. M. CATALDO. 1993. Ann. N.Y. Acad. Sci. **679:**. This volume.
5. ROBERTS-LEWIS, J. M. & R. SIMAN. 1993. Ann. N.Y. Acad. Sci. **679:**. This volume.
6. MATTSON, M. P., R. E. RYDEL, I. LIEBERBURG & V. SMITH-SWINTOSKY. 1993. Ann. N.Y. Acad. Sci. **679:**. This volume.
7. GIBBONS, S. J., J. R. BRORSON, D. BLEAKMAN, P. S. CHARD & R. J. MILLER. 1993. Ann. N.Y. Acad. Sci. **679:**. This volume.
8. ABOU-DONIA, M. B. & D. M. LAPADULA. 1990. Annu. Rev. Pharmacol. Toxicol. **30:** 405–440.
9. EL-FAWAL, H. A. N., B. S. JORTNER & M. EHRICH. 1989. Toxicol. Appl. Pharmacol. **97:** 500–511.
10. EL-FAWAL, H. A. N., B. S. JORTNER & M. EHRICH. 1990. Neurotoxicol. **11:** 573–592.
11. EL-FAWAL, H. A. N., L. CORRELL, L. GAY & M. EHRICH. 1990. Toxicol. Appl. Pharmacol. **103:** 133–142.
12. TOTH, L., S. KARSCU, M. POBERAI & G. SAVAY. 1983. Acta Histochem. **72:** 72–75.
13. DYER, K. R., H. A. N. EL-FAWAL & M. EHRICH. 1991. Neurotoxicol. **12:** 687–696.
14. NOSTRANDT, A. & M. EHRICH. 1990. Toxicologist **10:** 107.
15. LYNCH, G. & M. BAUDRY. 1984. Science **224:** 1057–1063.
16. SIMAN, R., J. C. NOSZEK & C. KEGERISE. 1989. J. Neurosci. **9:** 1579–1590.

Tirilazad Mesylate Attenuates the Accumulation of Neutrophils in Ischemic Gerbil Brain

LAWRENCE R. WILLIAMS[a] AND JO A. OOSTVEEN

CNS Diseases Research
The Upjohn Company
Kalamazoo, Michigan 49001

INTRODUCTION

Transient unilateral carotid occlusion (UCO) in the Mongolian gerbil, *Meriones unguiculatus,* results in severe unilateral focal cerebral ischemia to the ipsilateral hemisphere in a subpopulation of animals.[1,2] After 24 hours of reperfusion the damaging effect of the ischemia and reperfusion is dramatic and can be quantified by counting cresyl violet-positive, neuron-like profiles that survive in the CA1 region of the hippocampus and the lateral cerebral cortex.[1,2] We are interested in studying the progress of neuronal death in this model using other histochemical techniques to better understand the molecular mechanisms mediating neuronal death and the mechanisms of action of the cytoprotective compound, tirilazad mesylate (U-74006F).[3] A major goal of these studies is to identify a reliable predict-ive marker of neuronal injury and death.

CYTOCHROME OXIDASE HISTOCHEMISTRY

In beginning experiments, we examined the usefulness of cytochrome oxidase (CO) histochemistry, a marker of mitochondrial viability,[4] to identify regions of the ischemic hemisphere affected by the UCO. The subpopulation of gerbils susceptible to UCO was identified by ophthalmoscopic criteria.[2] After 3 hours of UCO and 24 hours of reperfusion, brains were collected and 50 μm sections were stained for cytochrome oxidase,[4] myeloperoxidase, and with cresyl violet.

After 24 hours of reperfusion, the neuronal death in the ischemic hemisphere is very apparent as indicated by the loss of cresyl violet staining across the hemisphere (FIG. 1A). There is a similar decrease in CO staining intensity (FIG. 1B). The CO reaction product is not localized to neuronal or glial cell bodies within the brain parenchyma, but is diffusely localized throughout the neuropil. Some regional concentration differences are apparent, *e.g.*, across the strata of the hippocampus (FIG. 1B). Semi-quantitative analysis of CO intensity by computer-assisted image analysis may provide a useful marker of neuronal degeneration and cytoprotection in this model of focal cerebral ischemia.

However, a unique population of CO-positive cells was found in the ischemic

[a] Present address for correspondence: Lawrence R. Williams, Ph.D., Neurobiology, 5-1-A-238, AMGEN, 1840 De Havilland Dr., Thousand Oaks, CA 91320. Tel.: (805) 447-1049; FAX: (805) 499-1140.

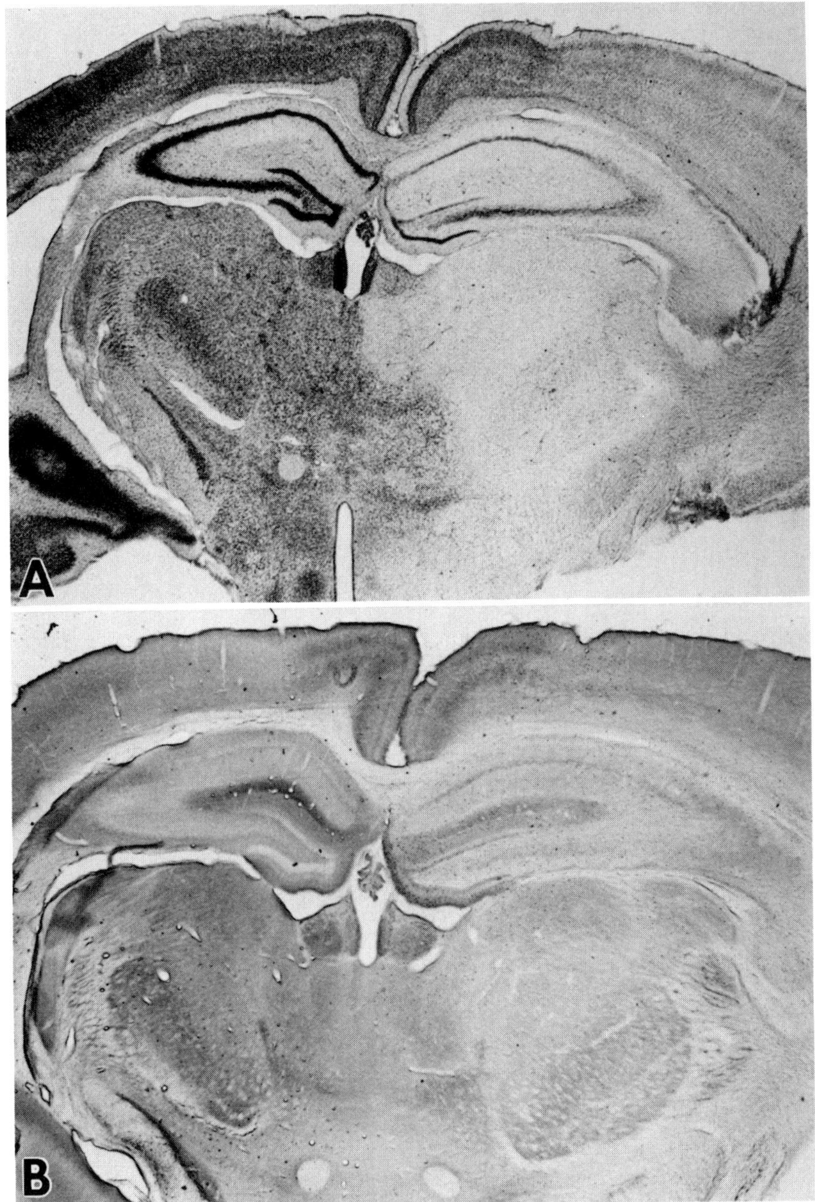

FIGURE 1. The damage to the ipsilateral hemisphere is illustrated after 24 h of reperfusion following 3 h UCO. The loss of neurons and glia is apparent in cresyl violet-stained sections **(A)**. The loss of CO activity is also obvious in sections stained with CO histochemistry **(B)**.

hemisphere and only in the ischemic hemisphere (FIG. 2). Staining of adjacent sections with the neutrophil-specific marker, myeloperoxidase, confirmed that these cells were neutrophils that had migrated into the brain parenchyma over the course of reperfusion (FIG. 2A).

NEUTROPHILS AND ISCHEMIA-REPERFUSION INJURY

The role of neutrophils in cerebral reperfusion injury is not well defined.[5,6] In other ischemia models, treatment of animals with anti-neutrophil antiserum to eliminate neutrophil involvement in the reperfusion injury results in increased postischemic blood flow, reduced edema formation, and a reduction in infarct size.[7,8] The discovery of the involvement of neutrophils in the gerbil UCO model motivated our continued experiments to investigate the role that neutrophils play in the reperfusion injury to the ischemic hemisphere, and to identify a possible action of tirilazad mesylate on neutrophil behavior.

EFFECT OF TIRILAZAD ON NEUTROPHIL ACCUMULATION

Animals were prepared as described previously, were pre-treated 10 min prior to occlusion of the right common carotid artery with vehicle (0.05N HCl) or tirilazad mesylate (U-74006F) at 10 mg/kg i.p., and dosed again immediately following reperfusion of the artery. At 12 hours and 24 hours of reperfusion, the animals were sacrificed and the brains prepared for histologic evaluation. Analysis of neuronal survival in the CA1 region of the hippocampus was made using a Viability Index score, where cresyl violet-stained sections were blindly evaluated and scored from 0 to 4, based on the percentage of apparently damaged tissue, $i.e.$, 0 = normal, and 4 = $>75\%$ damage. The number of neutrophils was obtained by counting CO-positive cells in a calibrated strip across the hippocampus; data are expressed as the number of neutrophils per mm^2. Statistical significance was determined using Student's t-test.

FIGURE 3 illustrates the quantitative data comparing the accumulation of neutrophils within the hippocampus with the degree of neuronal death in the CA1 region in control and tirilazad-treated animals. In the vehicle-treated gerbils, there is a progressive accumulation of neutrophils from 12 h to 24 h reperfusion and an increase in the Viability Index as evidence of progressive neuronal death. In the tirilazad-treated animals, there is a significant reduction in the number of neutrophils in the hippocampus at both time points, 76% and 64%, respectively. The reduction in neutrophils correlates with a significant reduction in the Viability Index by 35% and 24%, respectively, indicating cytoprotection of the neurons.

There is clearly a participation of neutrophils in the reperfusion sequelae in the gerbil UCO model of transient focal cerebral ischemia. However, it is not known whether the neutrophils play an active destructive role in the reperfusion injury as is known to occur in other tissues, or if the neutrophils are passive responders to the damaged neuropil and participate as scavengers of dead tissue. Experiments are now in progress to determine if depletion of systemic neutrophils results in neuronal cytoprotection. The effects of tirilazad on neutrophil accumulation and neuronal survival suggest an active role of neutrophils in the reperfusion injury and an action of tirilazad on neutrophil behavior.

Tirilazad mesylate was developed as a potent antioxidant and inhibitor of

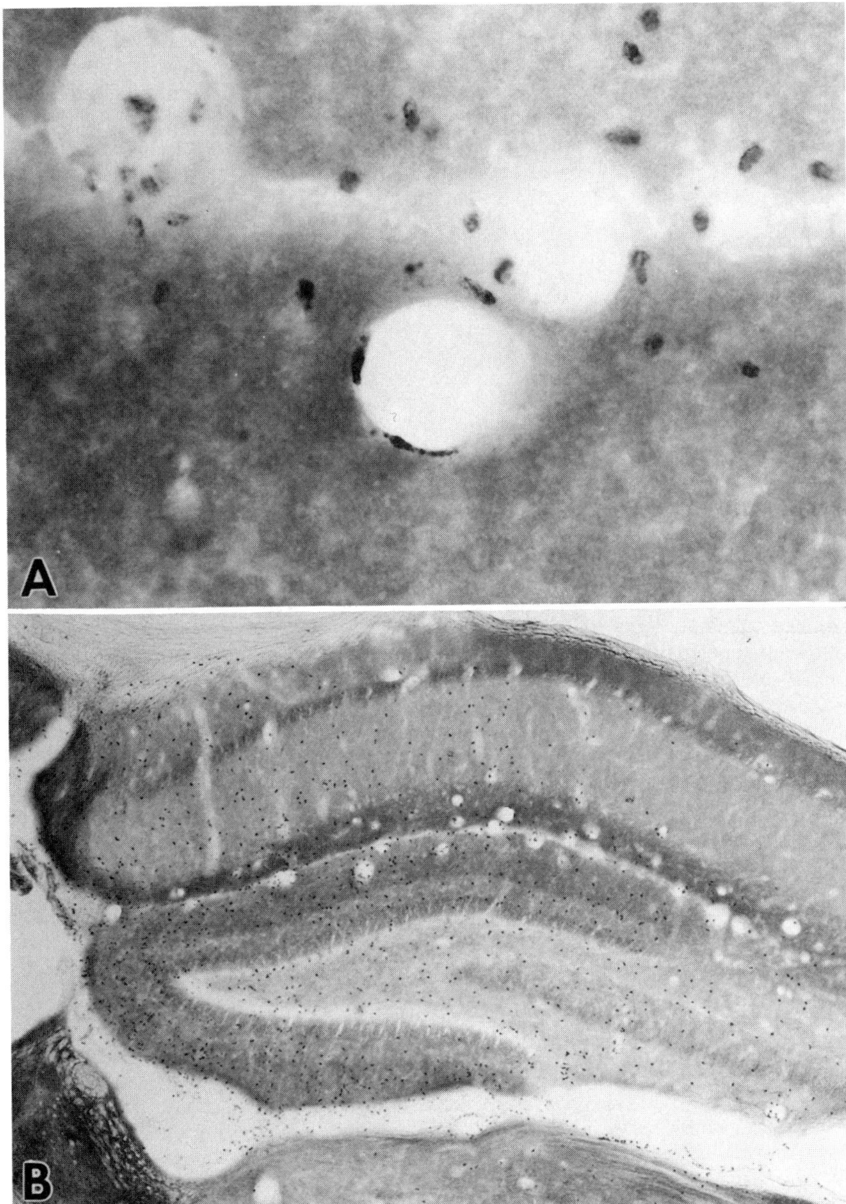

FIGURE 2. The neutrophil involvement in reperfusion injury is illustrated. After 4 h of reperfusion, CO-positive neutrophils are observed adhering to the cerebral vasculature and diapedesing through the endothelium into brain parenchyma (**A**). After 24 h reperfusion, there is a large accumulation of neutrophils within the parenchyma; the accumulation in hippocampus is illustrated in **B**.

iron-catalyzed lipid peroxidation.[3] Following trauma and ischemia, the drug is hypothesized to scavenge free radicals and inhibit free radical-initiated peroxidative damage thus limiting the secondary injury to brain parenchyma. Tirilazad may very likely have its first site of action at the vascular endothelium, and scavenge superoxide radicals produced by reoxygenated endothelial cells.[9] Local quenching of superoxide production would reduce expression of adhesive glycoproteins[10,11] the adherence of neutrophils, and result in reduced accumulation of neutrophils within the brain parenchyma, and limited destruction of neuronal tissue.

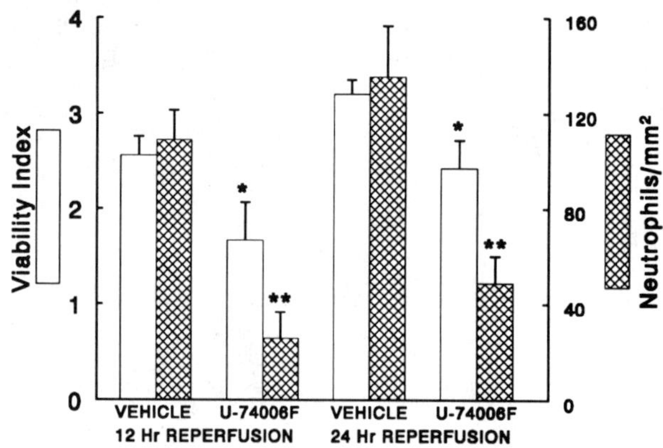

FIGURE 3. The correlation of neutrophil accumulation and neuronal viability is illustrated at both 12 hours (vehicle n = 16, tirilazad n = 5), and 24 hours of reperfusion (vehicle n = 10, tirilazad n = 12) for both vehicle-treated and tirilazad-treated animals. There is a significant reduction in neutrophils and a significant increase in neuronal survival, *i.e.*, decreased Viability Index score, in the drug-treated groups at both time points.

REFERENCES

1. HALL, E. D., K. E. PAZARA & J. M. BRAUGHLER. 1988. 21-Aminosteroid lipid peroxidation inhibitor U-74006F protects against cerebral ischemia in gerbils. Stroke **19:** 997–1002.
2. OOSTVEEN, J. A., K. TIMBY & L. R. WILLIAMS. 1992. Prediction of focal cerebral ischemia by ophthalmoscopic observation of retinal perfusion following unilateral carotid occlusion in the mongolian gerbil. Stroke **23:** 1588–1593.
3. HALL, E. D. 1990. Lazaroids: Efficacy and anti-oxidant mechanism in experimental cerebral ischemia. *In* Pharmacology of Cerebral Ischemia. J. Krieglstein & H. Oberpichler, Eds.: 343–350. Wissenschaftliche Verlagsgesellschaft. Stuttgart.
4. WONG-REILLY, M. 1979. Changes in the visual system of monocularly sutured or enucleated cats demonstrable with cytochrome oxidase histochemistry. Brain Res. **171:** 11–28.
5. KOCHANEK, P. M., E. M. NEMOTO, R. W. EVANS & R. J. SCHOETTLE. 1990. Polymorphonuclear leukocytes, platelets, and lipid mediators in the pathogenesis of ischemic and traumatic central nervous system injury. *In* Lipid Mediators in Ischemic Brain

Damage and Experimental Epilepsy. New Trends Lipid Mediators Res. N.G. Bazan, Ed.: 220–240. Karger. Basel.

6. HALLENBECK, J. M. & A. J. DUTKA. 1990. Background review and current concepts of reperfusion injury. Arch. Neurol. **47:** 1245–1254.

7. GRØGAARD, B., L. SCHÜRER, B. GERDIN & K. E. ARFORS. 1989. Delayed hypoperfusion after incomplete forebrain ischemia in the rat. The role of polymorphonuclear leukocytes. J. Cereb. Blood Flow Metab. **9:** 500–505.

8. SHIGA, Y., J. ONODERA, K. KOGURE, Y. YAMASAKI, Y. YASHIMA, H. SYOZUHARA & F. SENDO. 1991. Neutrophil as a mediator of ischemic edema formation in the brain. Neurosci. Lett. **125:** 110–112.

9. LUM, H., D. A. BARR, J. R. SHAFFER, R. J. GORDON, A. M. EZRIN & A. B. MALIK. 1992. Reoxygenation of endothelial cells increases permeability by oxidant-dependent mechanisms. Circ. Res. **70:** 991–998.

10. SUZUKI, M., M. B. GRISHAM & D. N. GRANGER. 1991. Leukocyte-endothelial cell adhesive interactions: Role of xanthine oxidase-derived oxidants. J. Leukocyte Biol. **50:** 488–494.

11. PATEL, K. D., G. A. ZIMMERMAN, S. M. PRESCOTT, R. P. McEVER & T. M. McINTYRE. 1991. Oxygen radicals induce human endothelial cells to express GMP-140 and bind neutrophils. J. Cell Biol. **112:** 749–759.

Detection of Early Axonal Degeneration in the Mammalian Central Nervous System by Magnetization Transfer Techniques in Magnetic Resonance Imaging[a]

FRANK J. LEXA,[b,d] ROBERT I. GROSSMAN,[b] AND
ALAN C. ROSENQUIST[c]

[b]Neuroradiology Section, Department of Radiology
Hospital of the University of Pennsylvania
[c]Department of Neuroscience, School of Medicine
University of Pennsylvania
Philadelphia, Pennsylvania 19104

INTRODUCTION

Wallerian degeneration is the response of a distal axonal segment to damage to the cell body and/or the proximal axon. First described by Waller in 1850,[1] this represents a fundamental response to injury in both the central and peripheral nervous system. It is a complex process encompassing several phases,[2-4] beginning with axonal collapse and physical destruction of myelin, followed by chemical degradation and removal of myelin lipid with edema and cellular proliferation, and ending with fibrosis and volume loss.

Magnetic resonance (MR) imaging has revolutionized noninvasive imaging of the central nervous system during the past decade, providing a truly remarkable window for understanding pathologic conditions which affect the brain. It has many advantages over computed tomography (CT) scanning but in particular it is far superior for detection of diseases of white matter such as multiple sclerosis. Nevertheless, conventional MR appears relatively insensitive to the early changes of Wallerian degeneration in both human clinical reports and animal models (reviewed in ref. 5).

Magnetization transfer represents a relatively new application of MR imaging technology that may be able to provide this ability. This method was initially developed[6] for quantitatively measuring the rate of magnetization exchange between two chemical moieties. This is achieved by selectively saturating one of the two exchanging species by radiofrequency irradiation. Chemical exchange of saturated protons with unaffected spins then occurs. These techniques have been adapted for imaging *in vivo*[7,8] and have the potential to generate novel forms of

[a] This work was supported by the American Society of Neuroradiology through a Basic Science Fellowship Award for 1991–1992 to F.J.L. and by NIH Grants NS 29029 to R.I.G. and EY 02654 to A.C.R. This paper is a shortened version of a longer manuscript to be published by Am. J. Neuroradiol.[5]

[d] Address all correspondence to Dr. Lexa at the above address; Tel.: (215)662-3064 or 662-4000 (page operator); FAX: (215)662-3283.

MR contrast in living tissue. This investigation tested the hypothesis of whether or not magnetization transfer rate measurement can be a useful probe for detecting changes of axonal degeneration in a well-understood animal model.

MATERIALS AND METHODS

Neurologically normal (including visual perimetry) adult cats were used for this study. Magnetization transfer rate measurement was performed at 1.5 Tesla (Signa, General Electric, Milwaukee, WI, USA). A headholder of synthetic polymer was designed for compatability with the MR scanner in order to maintain the animal's head in the Horsely-Clark anatomic plane. Gradient imaging with TR/TE/flip angle of 106 milliseconds/6 milliseconds /12 degrees was performed both with and without a saturation pulse to create a magnetization transfer effect. Region of interest measurements were performed at a workstation on archived cases in a consensus fashion by a neuroanatomist and a neuroradiologist of brain structures with and without the saturation pulse. Magnetization transfer was calculated as:

$$\frac{\text{(Signal intensity pre-saturation)} - \text{(Signal intensity post-sat)}}{\text{Signal intensity pre-saturation}} \times 100\%$$

[Formula 1]

The first phase of this investigation involved measuring normal magnetization transfer rates in various gray and white matter structures of the brain in five normal cats. This confirmed that reliable, highly reproducible magnetization transfer values could be obtained. The next phase investigated the changes which occur during Wallerian degeneration. Unilateral aspiration of the visual cortex in the cat was performed using standard neurosurgical techniques guided by standard visual cortical maps.[9] Post-operative magnetization transfer imaging was performed serially. FIGURE 1 shows a representative pair of coronal images. Measurements were made of the lateral geniculate nucleus, thalamo-cortical white matter tracts (projections which interconnect the LGN and the visual cortex) and more remote white matter tracts. Comparison to pre-operative values and to the control side was performed:

Change in MTR = MTR of lesioned side-MTR of control side   **[Formula 2]**

Tissue was processed for light and electron microscopy using standard techniques, details provided in reference 5.

RESULTS

During the first two weeks there is a statistically significant *increase* in MTR relative to the control hemisphere within the white matter connections between the lateral geniculate nucleus (LGN) and the visual cortex ($p < .02$) at a time when no effects are visually detectable on spin-echo images. At this time no significant changes are appreciated on light microscopy either; however, early changes of Wallerian degeneration were confirmed at 8 and 11 days by elecron microscopy. Between 16 and 28 days, the change in MTR reverses to a decrease in MTR in both the thalamo-cortical white matter ($p < 0.01$) and LGN ($p < 0.05$). Anatomically remote white mater tracts remained stable, without significant change in MTR relative to baseline control values.

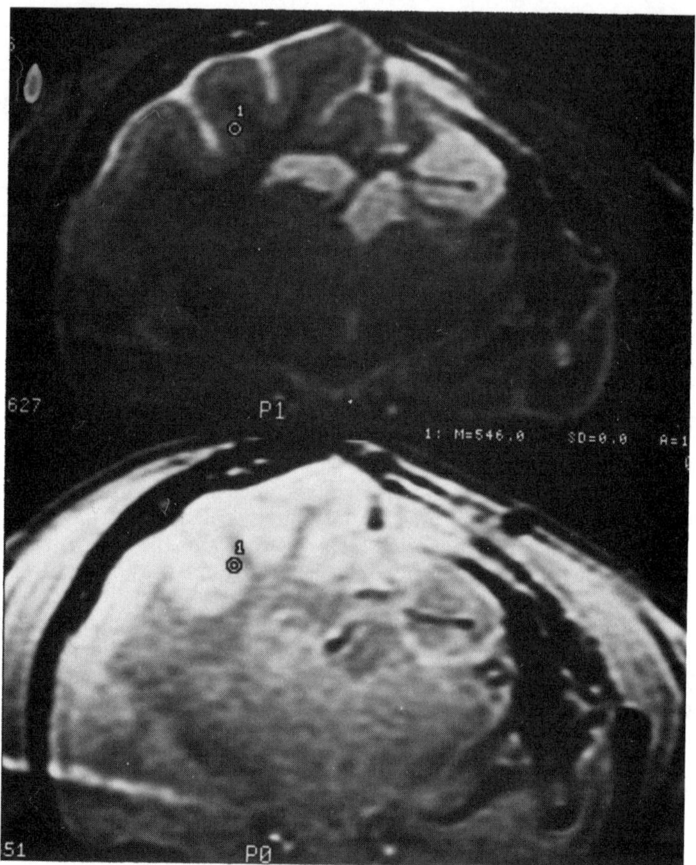

FIGURE 1. Pair of coronal images from an animal after unilateral aspiration of the visual cortex. TR/TE/flip angle = 106/6/12. The upper image has had a saturation pulse applied, the lower did not. Note the improved grey white differentiation with the saturation pulse. The region of interest marker has been placed in the cortical grey matter of the control hemisphere.

DISCUSSION

This study demonstrates several important points. First, magnetization transfer values can be obtained *in vivo* in the mammalian CNS in a highly reproducible fashion, with histologic correlation. Second, magnetization transfer appears to be able to detect changes of axonal injury at a time as early as the first week after the occurrence of a lesion. This is prior to detection with conventional spin-echo techniques implying that magnetization transfer may be able to provide novel forms of contrast. This may therefore prove useful for the detection of subtle forms of white matter disese which elude conventional techniques. Third, there were at least two detectable phases occurring during the first month of degeneration: first an early rise in MTR during the first two weeks, with a later fall during the third and fourth week.

The histochemical processes which underlie these observations are of critical importance. Previous work in this model system and others can provide plausible explanations for the observed drop in MTR. Magnetization transfer is probably a component of T2 relaxation in conventional spin-echo imaging. The observation of lengthening of T2 seen clinically late in degenerating human CNS may reflect in part the reduction in magnetization transfer which occurs during the later stages of Wallerian degeneration.

The earlier rise in MTR, however, was unexpected and may reflect several processes. First, we speculate that the increase in MTR may reflect an increase in exchange sites between bound and free protons from the increase in intracellular macromolecular concentration. This is reflected by the increase in axoplasmic density seen on electron microscopy during the first phase of degeneration due to increases in cytoplasmic protein concentration. Second, an increase in the availability of exchange sites could occur with disorganization of the myelin sheath and opening of Schmidt-Lantermann incisures. This would also increase the opportunity for magnetization transfer to occur and lead to an increase in the detectable MTR effect.

CONCLUSIONS

There is an early reproducible rise in MTR, preceding detectable changes on spin-echo imaging, which occurs within the first week of axonal degeneration. Early changes of axonal degeneration were noted on electron microscopy, confirming the ability of magnetic resonance techniques to noninvasively detect axonal degeneration as early as the first week after injury.

MTR measuremens that compare degenerating white matter tracts to normal white matter demonstrate a later fall in measureable MTR, which correlates with the second stage of Wallerian degeneration and appears to continue during the third stage.

Effects are greatest in the white matter pathways which connect the visual cortex with the geniculate with both an early rise and then a later fall. The lateral geniculate shows a definite decrease in MTR during the later phase with a suggestion that there may be an early rise at this site as well. More remote fiber pathways, which would not be expected to undergo large scale degeneration from this type of lesion, did not show statistically significant changes in MTR.

REFERENCES

1. WALLER, A. V. 1850. Experiments on the section of the glossopharyngeal and hypoglossal nerves of the frog, and observations of the alterations produced thereby in the structure of the primitive fibres. Philos. Trans. R. Soc. Lond. **140:** 423–429.

2. ROSSITER, R. J. 1961. The chemistry of wallerian degeneration. *In* Chemical Pathology of the Nervous System. J. Folch-Pi, Ed.: 207–227. New York. Pergamon Press.

3. WEBSTER, H., F. DE. 1964. The relationship between Schmidt-Lanterman insicures and myelin segmentation during Wallerian degeneration. Ann. N.Y. Acad. Sci. **122:** 29–41.

4. DANIEL, P. M. & S. J. STRICH. 1969. Histological observations on Wallerian degeneration in the spinal cord of the baboon, Papio papio. Acta Neuropathol. (Berlin) **12:** 314–328.

5. LEXA, F. J., R. I. GROSSMAN & A. C. ROSENQUIST. 1993. Wallerian degeneration in the feline visual system: Characterization by magnetization transfer rate with histopathologic correlation. Am. J. Neuroradiol. In press.

6. FORSEN, S. & R. A. HOFFMAN. 1963. Study of moderately rapid chemical exchange reactions by means of nuclear magnetic double resonance. J. Chem. Phys. **39:** 2892–2901.

7. WOLFF, S. D. & R. S. BALABAN. 1989. Magnetization transfer contrast (MTC) and tissue water proton relaxation in vivo. Magn. Reson. Med. **10:** 135–144.

8. ENG, J., T. L. CECKLER & R. S. BALABAN. 1991. Quantitative 1H magnetization transfer imaging in vivo. Magn. Reson. Med. **17:** 304–314.

9. ROSENQUIST, A. C. 1985. Connections of visual cortical areas in the cat. *In* Cerebral Cortex. A. Peters & E. G. Jones, Eds.: 81–117. New York. Plenum.

Silver Staining Methods:
Their Role in Detecting Neurotoxicity

ROBERT C. SWITZER III

Department of Pathology
University of Tennessee Medical Center
Knoxville, Tennessee 37920

Neuroscience Associates
10915 Lake Ridge Drive
Knoxville, Tennessee 37922

The ultimate neuronal injury is the death of the neuron, and the best marker of this event is the degenerative debris associated with the disintegration of the neuron. Detection of neuronal death deserves the highest priority in assessing neurotoxicity,[1] since in mammals new neurons cannot be created to replace those that die, (except, of course, for the olfactory receptor neurons).

As can be seen from the other reports in this volume, there are numerous specific probes which have been developed to detect changes that take place in neurons following a given level of perturbation. Some of these occur in succession to one another forming a sequence, the length or duration of which may be dependent on the nature and degree of perturbation or insult to the system. If the insult causes damage, transcription for molecular entities associated with repair will occur. In spite of these cellular responses the form and/or degree of insult may overwhelm the cell beyond recovery resulting in its death and disintegration. FIGURE 1 depicts levels of such sequences.

The particular form of an insult that ultimately causes the cell to die can be expected to determine the premortem sequence of changes that take place. Death by mitochondrial poisoning, blockage of protein synthesis (*e.g.*, puromycin, cycloheximide), blockage of transcription from DNA (*e.g.*, actinomycin-D) or ion channel blockers, to suggest but a few, can result in different sequences of chemical changes that can be markers of a particular route to death. Clearly, the "Holy Grail" of markers of irreversible neuronal injury is that which is present only when the cell will subsequently die.

Changes in cells other than neurons constitute indirect markers of neuronal injury and death. For example, proliferation of glia (gliosis) at the site of damage and increased synthesis of the astrocyte-specific protein, glialfibrillic acid protein (GFAP) have been commonly used as evidence of neurotoxic effects. Often, the occurrence of either of these is coincident with the destruction of neural elements. However there are also examples of increased GFAP expression not attended by degeneration of neural elements.[2]

DETECTION OF DAMAGE TO NEURAL ELEMENTS

Classical histopathologic methods stain various components of an injured or dying cell differently than in a normal cell. Using the hematoxylin and eosin (H&E) staining method the term "red and dead" is an apt expression applied to the appearance of the cytoplasm in a cell that has just died, and "pink" if it is atrophic and near death. If such cells are not coalesced and part of a massive lesion but instead make up a dispersed population among normal-appearing cells, detection is difficult since it requires microscopic examination at high magnifications. These

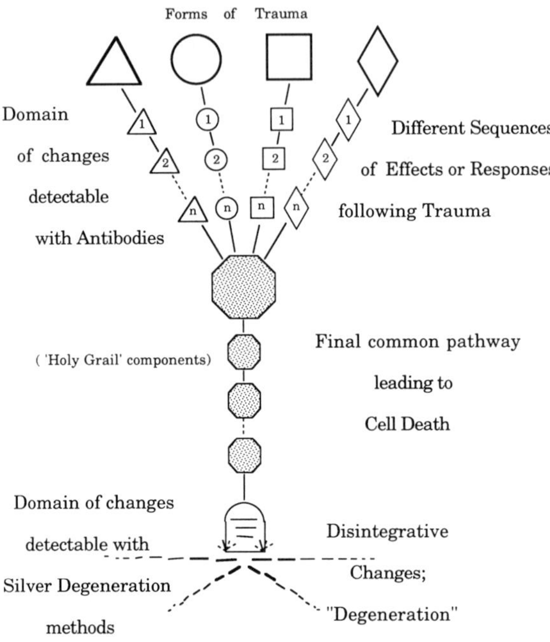

FIGURE 1. Schematic of potentially neurotoxic biochemical changes that follow different forms of trauma. The spectrum of neurotoxic effects encompasses a broad range of changes in a cell that can culminate in its death. Depending on the form of insult, a different sequence of effects may ensue, all of which may be reversible. In the extreme, any given insult or trauma (represented by the geometric forms at the top) can result in the death of the cell even though it may occur by different sequences (the strings of small, numbered geometric forms). All of these, however, can progress and converge (on the stippled cricle, a 'point of no return') to traverse a final common path of changes (small stippled circles) resulting in cell death. Antibodies probes have been developed against different proteins (*e.g.*, triangle-2 or diamond-1) that are constituents of the sequence of biochemical changes that follow a particular form of insult. Unless an antibody is directed against a component along the 'final common path' to cell death, the presence of immunoreactivity of proteins in the earlier sequences does not necessarily mean cell death. Since it is unlikely that even a polyspecific antibody could be raised against the amorphous disintegrative debris of a degenerated cell, the silver-degeneration stains currently remain the best probe to mark this endpoint of neurotoxicity.

classical methods also are incapable of revealing little, if anything, about the demise of synaptic terminals, dendrites and axons (especially unmyelinated axons). Furthermore, the brain is a mosaic of different neuronal types (>600!), each with its own vulnerability to types of insult, so that numerous levels of the brain must be examined to make an adequate sampling. The standard histopathologic stains are not well suited for this purpose.

Considerable advances were made possible in the detection of damage to cells with the advent of immunohistologic techniques and the discovery and development of antibodies against proteins expressed by cells when stimulated under extreme conditions. For example, the family of 'heat shock proteins'[3] and the c-fos proteins[4] are rapidly synthesized following certain stimuli or trauma. The domain in which application of antibodies has yielded the greatest benefits in neurotoxicologic research is depicted in FIGURE 1. With the intrinsic high specificity of antibodies, the trauma-induced sequences of biochemical change can be mapped. Such precision, however, poses a disadvantage for the use of any particular antibody as a general indicator of neurotoxicity. Unless the antibody is against a component of the "Holy Grail" sequence in FIGURE 1, the resulting pattern of immunoreactivity would be a very restricted, monochromatic view of neurotoxic effects. As of this time, antibodies have not been employed to probe the degenerative domain. The disintegrative debris of degenerating elements is probably too amorphous and of inconsistent composition for even a polyspecific antibody to be raised against these nondescript moieties.

There is, however, a set of histologic silver staining methods that have been empirically tailored to be degeneration specific (see Beltramino et al.[5] for an historic overview). In the hands of experimental neuroanatomists these methods were used to trace axon pathways in animals in which specific lesions had been made. During the days subsequent to the lesion, the axons of destroyed cell bodies underwent disintegrative degeneration. With appropriate pretreatment of sections of these brains, products of degeneration could be made to have a higher affinity for binding silver ions than normal, intact neural elements. Chemical reduction of the accumulated silver ions yielded black deposits marking the sites of degeneration. If stained early in the stages of degeneration, the intact morphology of a neuron was visible. With longer survival times the neural elements become fragmented (FIGS. 2 and 3).

These silver stained sections, with degeneration seen as black stained objects against a pale, unstained background (of normal unaffected neural components), provide a high "signal to noise ratio" of objects of interest, so that detection of degenerated entities is easily and efficiently accomplished.

ANTIBODIES VS. SILVER STAINS; A QUESTION OF SPECIFIC AND GENERAL STAINING

In these times of highly specific antibody probes, there appears to be some discomfort among many researchers in employing a given silver stain because it is not known exactly what is being stained. This is true not only for researchers in neurotoxicology but also for those investigating Alzheimer's disease. In this field there have also been significant advances in using antibodies for detecting and probing the neuritic plaques and neurons with tangles that are characteristic of this disease. Comparing the silver stains recently developed specifically for revealing these features[6] with the arsenal of antibodies against components of the lesions in AD, each of the antibodies appears to stain a subset of the features revealed by the silver methods. But even among the silver methods, there are those that "zero in" on a subset of the pathologic features (e.g., Gallyas' method revealing neurofibrillary tangles and neuropil threads[7]).

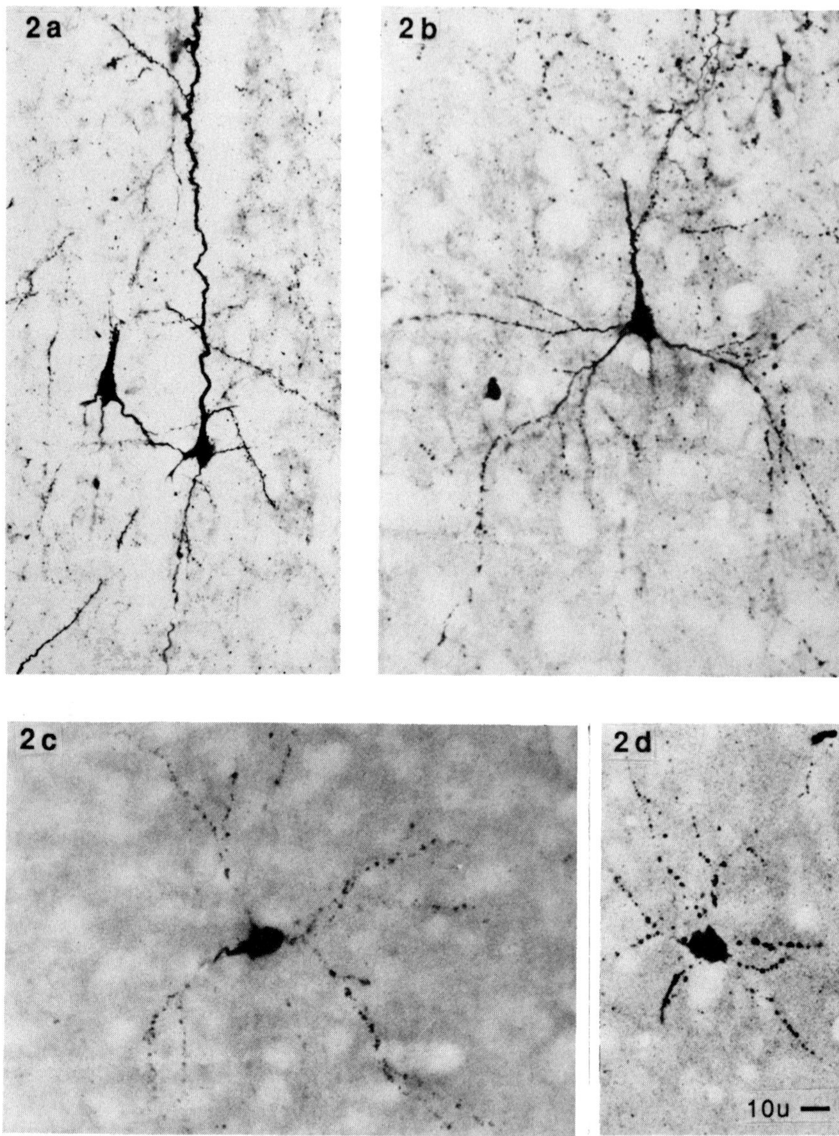

FIGURE 2. Silver impregnated neurons in different stages of degeneration (cupric silver method of de Olmos[9]). Shown in **a** is a cortical neuron on the periphery of a lesion 8 h prior to the sacrifice of the rat. All components are still intact, including dendritic spines. Note, however, the waviness of the dendrites and axons. The apical acendrite of the neurons to the left has been cut and is out of the plane of this section. A neuron in a more advanced state of degeneration is shown in **b**. There is fragmentation of the distal portions of the dendrites while the more proximal protions of the processes, including the axon (seen at the bottom of the cell body and slightly out of focus) are still intact. More extreme degrees of fragmentation are shown in **c** and **d**.

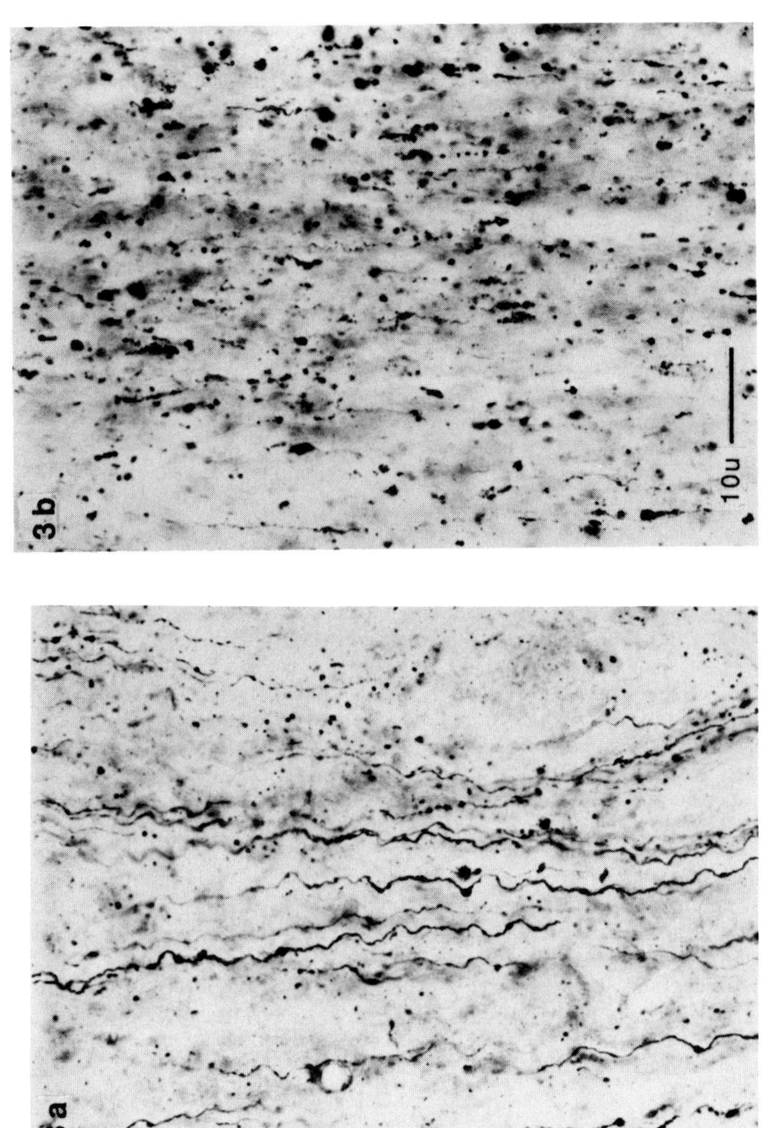

FIGURE 3. Silver impregnated axons in different stages of degeneration (cupric silver method of de Olmos[9]). In **a** axons are shown in the internal capsule near a lesion site in the cortex of a rat sacrificed three days after the lesion was made. The axons are mostly intact but display the same waviness as seen in the early stages of dendritic disintegration. **b** shows the debris of fragmented axons in the internal capsule of a rat dosed 70 days prior to sacrifice with the organophosphate, soman. While these examples show the appearance of axonal degeneration over a wide range of survival times, both of the stages shown here can also be observed in different brain areas of the same animal. The time course of degeneration is dependent on several factors, especially the kind of insult and the areas of the brain affected.

Such "directed staining" is also found among the silver methods for revealing degeneration. There are those that give an overall picture (Fink-Heimer method[8] and cupric silver methods of de Olmos[9,10]) and others that reveal a subset of degenerative features such as those of Gallyas.[11-13] In a series of innovative experiments, Gallyas demonstrated that silver impregnation of selective features could be directed by selecting an appropriate chemical treatment of tissue sections prior to exposure to silver, the particular composition of the silver solution and the kind of developer (reducing agent) employed.

For example, the cupric silver method and the Alzheimer's stain developed in this author's lab,[6] both employ a silver and pyridine mixture for initial silver impregnation and use formaldehyde as a reducing agent for development. The Alzheimer's stain does not reveal degenerated neural elements and the cupric silver method does not reveal the plaques and tangles in Alzheimer's tissue. In spite of the similarities of these two methods, the sequence of steps and exact composition of each step is crucial for determining the features that are revealed by the silver reaction.

Among the silver staining methods applied to neurotoxicology there is a subset of silver methods that has recently evolved that stain stressed neurons as early in their response to perturbation as do such markers as c-fos.[14,15] Since these methods stain a broad range of induced features in a perturbed cell and seem to be as sensitive as antibody probes,[5] this set of silver stains may provide powerful tools for identifying the cells most susceptible to a particular form of insult.

As indicated earlier, the specific protocol of a silver method dictates exactly which features will be stained. Unless these newer silver methods can be shown to stain cellular components that are expressed or present when the cell is in the stage of the 'final common path to cell death,' they will suffer from the same problem as the antibody probes for biochemical markers in that not all, and possibly not any, of the cells stained will necessarily die. In using these methods at times shortly after insult (<12 h), one must pose the question of: in how many of the stained cells is this a reversible change? By using longer intervals between insult and sacrifice and the appropriate method, the results of staining are more dichotomous. That is, disintegrated cells stain and intact cells do not.

The so-called silver degeneration methods are generally applied to sections from animals sacrificed 2–3 days after trauma. By this time, disintegration of neural elements has already begun. In some instances the disintegrative process has been observed to have occurred in less than 24 hours. To ensure that the silver-impregnated features are actually in a disintegrative state and not one from which there is recovery, the researcher must not only select the appropriate staining method but also a survival time after trauma that will allow enough time for the disintegrative process to take place.

Optimal survival times for observing degenerated states for different neural elements are as follows: synaptic terminals, 1–3 days (*e.g.*, FIG. 4); cell bodies and dendrites, 1–4 days; axons, 3–7 days (however, the debris of axons can still be impregnated months (FIG. 3b) to years after destruction of the axons (*e.g.*, see Grafe and Leonard[16]).

CONCLUSION

There are two primary missions in neurotoxicologic research: 1) to study mechanisms of known neurotoxins and, 2) to identify indicators or markers that will allow the detection of various endpoints of neurotoxicity and thereby provide a reliable means of screening. (To date, nearly all known neurotoxicants have been discovered through human incidents. Clearly, an aggressive screening program for neurotoxicants, comparable to that which screens for carcinogens, needs to be implemented.)

To study mechanisms, a set of highly specific probes are required with which the trauma-induced sequences, such as those depicted in FIGURE 1, can be dis-

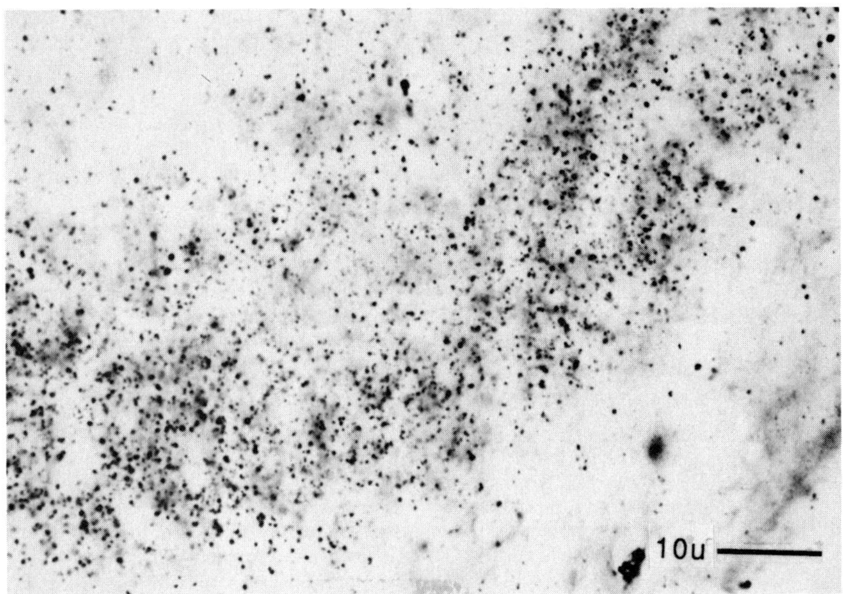

FIGURE 4. Silver impregnated degenerated synaptic terminals (cupric silver method of de Olmos[9]). The grains seen in this photo are degenerated synaptic boutons or terminals in layer 1b (the association band) of the olfactory cortex of a rat. A lesion had been made caudal to the site of this photograph 3 days before the rat was sacrificed. Such terminals typically can be seen as early as 1 day and for as long as 4–5 days following the lesion. For example, in the olfactory cortex of an opossum following a transection of its olfactory bulb, the degenerated synaptic terminals were prominently visible after 2 days of survival but were absent after 3 days. A new subset of neurotoxic effects is synaptic terminal degeneration without the concurrent death of the cell body as has been observed with MPTP in young but not old mice (Switzer, unpublished results).

sected. For this endeavor the antibody and associated *in situ* hybridization techniques are well suited.

To screen compounds for neurotoxicity, the tools must be sensitive to a broad range of changes as well as efficient in their application. The application of silver-degeneration stains is clearly best directed to the screening process to assess the end point of destruction of neurons and their components.[1] There are also benefits to be realized from their use in the study of mechanisms to provide an initial overview. Whether or not destruction has occurred and determining "where the trouble is" can provide the researcher with direction in deciding what probes to apply and where to look.

REFERENCES

1. SWITZER, R. C. 1991. Strategies for assessing neurotoxicity. Neurosci Biobehav. Rev. **15:** 89–93.
2. KHURGEL, M., R. C. SWITZER, G. C. TESKEY, A. E. SPILLER, R. J. RACINE & G. O. IVY. 1992. Absence of neuronal death in kindling: A study with the cupric silver degeneration stain. Soc. Neurosci. Abstr. **18:** 906.
3. LINDQUIST, S. 1986. The heat shock response. Ann. Rev. Biochem. **55:** 1151–1191.
4. SAGAR, S. M., F. R. SHARP & T. CURRAN. 1988. Expression of c-fos protein in brain: Metabolic mapping at the cellular level. Science **240:** 1328–1331.
5. BELTRAMINO, C. A., J. S. DE OLMOS, F. GALLYAS, L. HEIMER & L. ZABORSZKY. 1993. Silver staining as a tool for neurotoxic assessment. *In* Assessing neurotoxicity of drugs of abuse. L. Erinoff, Ed. National Institute of Drug Abuse Monograph. In press.
6. CAMPBELL, S. K., R. C. SWITZER III & T. L. MARTIN. 1987. Alzheimer's plaques and tangles: Control of silver staining through physical development. Soc. Neurosci. Abstr. **13:** 189.9.
7. GALLYAS, F. 1971. Silver staining of Alzheimer's neurofibrillary changes by means of physical development. Act. Morphol. Acad. Sci. Hung. **19:** 1–8.
8. FINK, R. P. & L. HEIMER. 1967. Two methods for selective silver impregnation of degeneration axons and their synaptic endings in the cnetral nervous system. Brain Res. **4:** 369–374.
9. DE OLMOS, J. S., S. O. E. EBBESSON & L. HEIMER. 1981. Silver methods for the impregnation of degenerating axoplasm. *In* Neuroanatomical Tract-Tracing Methods. L. Heimer & M. J. Robards, Eds.: 117–170, Plenum Press. New York.
10. CARLSEN, J. & J. S. DE OLMOS. 1981. Silver impregnation of degenerating neurons and their processes. A modified cupric-silver technique. Brain Res. **208:** 426–431.
11. GALLYAS, F., L. ZABORSZKY & J. R. WOLFF. 1980. Experiments on the mechanism of impregnation methods demonstrating axonal and terminal degeneration. Stain Tech. **55:** 281–290.
12. GALLYAS, F., J. R. WOLFF, H. BOTTCHER & L. ZABORSZKY. 1980. Selective demonstration of axonal degeneration. Stain Tech. **55:** 291–297.
13. GALLYAS, F., J. R. WOLFF, H. BOTTCHER & L. ZABORSZKY. 1980. A reliable and sensitive method to locate terminal degeneration and lysosomes in the CNS. Stain Tech. **55:** 299–306.
14. DE OLMOS, J. S., C. A. BELTRAMINO, M. E. SHAFFREY, N. K. KEOMAHATHAIO & J. A. JANE. 1992. Very early detection of ischemic neuronal degeneration in the CNS by an amino-cupric-silver technique. Anat. Rec. **232**(4): 26A.
15. VAN DEN POL, A. N. & F. GALLYAS. 1990. Trauma-induced Golgi-like staining of neurons: A new approach to neuronal organization and response to injury. J. Comp. Neurol. **296:** 654–673.
16. GRAFE, M. R. & C. M. LEONARD. 1981. Successful silver impregnation of degenerating axons after long survivals in the human brain. J. Neuropathol. Exp. Neurol. **39:** 555–574.

Elevation of Nerve Growth Factor Receptor-truncated in the Urine of Patients with Diabetic Neuropathy

ROBERT E. HRUSKA,[a,c] M. M. CHERTACK,[b]
AND D. KRAVIS[b]

[a]*Abbott Laboratories*
One Abbott Park Road
Abbott Park, Illinois 60064

[b]*64 Old Orchard Road*
Skokie, Illinois 60077

Nerve growth factor receptor (NGFR) is a cell surface receptor which binds nerve growth factor (NGF).[1] NGFR appears to be an important trophic compound associated with neuronal development and regeneration. For instance, NGFR levels on Schwann cells, measured immunohistochemically after nerve biopsy, are increased after rat sciatic nerve section[2] and in human peripheral neuropathies.[3,4] While it is not practical to perform multiple nerve biopsies to monitor trophic factor levels, the soluble, extracellular cleavage product of NGFR, termed NGFR-truncated (NGFR-t), is found in plasma and urine.[5] NGFR-t appears to correlate with NGFR since both urine levels and Schwann cell immunoreactivity are elevated after rat sciatic nerve section.[2,5] In order to measure NGFR-t in human specimens, specific monoclonal antibodies were produced and used to identify a developmental regulation of urinary NGFR-t levels.[6] In a separate study, the level of NGFR-t in the urine of ALS patients was found to be elevated.[7] Based on these reports, we proposed that the urinary levels of NGFR-t would be elevated in patients with neuropathy. We choose to study the most common form of peripheral neuropathy, namely diabetic neuropathy.

A sensitive assay was developed to quantitate the levels of NGFR-t in urine. A specific monoclonal antibody (XIF1) at a concentration of 0.5 μg/0.1 ml PBS was used to coat Nunc-Immuno plates for 2 h at room temperature. The coat solution was removed and the plate blocked with 1.5% BSA in PBS (0.2 ml) for one hour. After washing the plate with PBS, the specimen or standard was added after 1:1 dilution with 0.15 M PBS at pH 7.5 (0.1 ml). One hour later the plate was washed and monoclonal antibody IIIG5, coupled to alkaline phosphatase, was added (0.05 μg/0.1 ml Tris-buffered saline (TBS), 1.5% BSA, 1 mM Mg and 0.1 mM Zn). After 2 h the plate was washed with TBS and substrate added (0.1 ml p-nitrophenylphosphate in diethanolamine buffer, obtained from KPL). The absorbance was read at 405 nm.

The standard was affinity-purified from a cell line constructed to express the NGFR-t protein and it was used to quantitate the results. At the time of analysis, all urine specimens were diluted with a buffer (0.15 M PBS) to normalize the pH.

---

[c] Address correspondence to Robert E. Hruska, Ph.D., Department 90J, Building AP20, Abbott Laboratories, One Abbott Park Road, Abbott Park, IL 60064-3500.

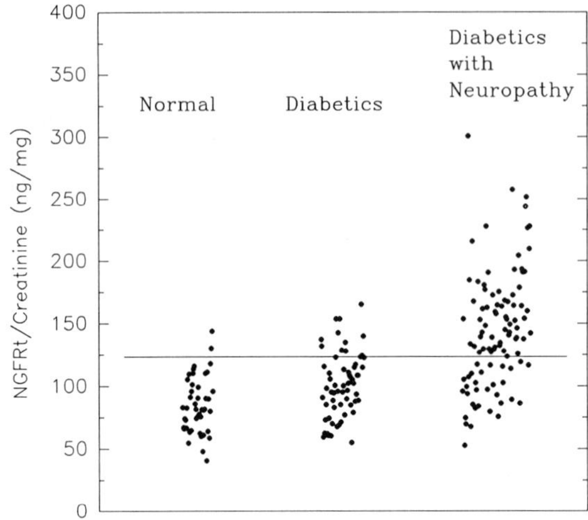

FIGURE 1. Scatter plots of the levels of NGFR-t/creatinine in normals (N = 45), diabetics (N = 61), and diabetics with neuropathy (N = 98). The horizontal line at about 125 ng/mg is set at 2 standard deviations above the mean of the normal group.

NGFR-t in urine specimens was stable at room temperature for at least 2 days and after at least 3 freeze-thaw cycles. The specimens were routinely frozen within 8 hours of collection. All urine specimens were tested for creatinine levels by TDx automated procedure[8] and for microalbumin by the method of Neuman and Cohen.[9] Urine specimens were collected from normal volunteers, from patients with Type I and Type II diabetes without peripheral neuropathy, and from patients with either Type I or Type II diabetes with neuropathy.

NGFR-t, corrected for creatinine, was elevated in patients with neuropathy. Using a limit set at two standard deviations above the normal mean concentration, 67% of the patients with neuropathy have elevated levels (FIG. 1). When the results are analyzed by each group (TABLE 1), NGFR-t/creatinine values are

TABLE 1. The Levels of NGFR-t in Various Groups of Normals or Patients

Group	N	Age (years)	NGFR-t/Creatinine (ng/mg)
Normal Male	18	39 ± 9	85.5 ± 20.3
Normal Female	27	35 ± 9	84.1 ± 24.0
Type I DM Male	33	36 ± 12	95.4 ± 27.9
Type I DM Female	9	35 ± 7	106.9 ± 18.0[a]
Type II DM Male	11	57 ± 14	96.1 ± 18.5
Type II DM Female	8	64 ± 13	123.6 ± 22.4[a]
Type I DM/Neuropathy Male	26	50 ± 12	123.0 ± 54.2[b]
Type I DM/Neuropathy Female	13	59 ± 14	153.8 ± 35.1[c]
Type II DM/Neuropathy Male	39	64 ± 12	139.8 ± 34.7[b]
Type II DM/Neuropathy Female	20	66 ± 10	173.6 ± 45.8[c]

DM = Diabetes Mellitus; All values are the mean ± the standard deviation.
[a] $p < 0.02$ compared to the normal female group.
[b] $p < 0.02$ compared to the normal male group or the respective male DM Type.
[c] $p < 0.01$ compared to the normal female group or the respective female DM Type.

equivalent in normal males and females and in male patients with only diabetes. Both groups of females with diabetes have moderately elevated values. The females with the highest levels of NGFR-t/creatinine are described as overweight, over the age of 60, and depressed about their clinical condition. While the groups are not completely age-matched, no other age-related changes were evident. Of the patients with neuropathy, all groups clearly have elevated levels when compared to either the normal group or the respective sex and DM Type groups.

If the levels of NGFR-t are reported without correction for creatinine, the NGFR-t values range from 30 to 300 ng/ml with no difference between any of the groups. The measurement of microalbumin did not correlate with either NGFR-t or creatinine levels. Correction of NGFR-t for microalbumin did not provide any discrimination between the groups.

This is the first report of elevated NGFR-t/creatinine levels in patients with diabetic neuropathy. The elevation occurs in both males and females and in both Type I and Type II diabetes and is not affected by proteinuria, as measured by microalbuminuria. The increase in urinary NGFR-t may be related to the increase in NGFR found on Schwann cells in patients with neuropathy.[3,4] The increase in NGFR on Schwann cells may lead to an increase in NGFR available for cleavage or an increase in the turnover of NGFR, eventually resulting in an increase in NGFR-t in the urine. The NGFR-t levels may be informative in the evaluation and monitoring of diabetic neuropathy.

REFERENCES

1. STACH, R. W. & J. R. PEREZ-POLO. 1987. Binding of nerve growth factor to its receptor. J. Neurosci. Res. **17:** 1–10.
2. TANIUCHI, M., H. B. CLARK & E. M. JOHNSON, JR. 1986. Induction of nerve growth factor receptor in Schwann cells after axotomy. Proc. Natl. Acad. Sci. USA **83:** 4094–4098.
3. SCARPINI, E., S. BERETTA, A. H. ROSS, M. MOGGIO, S. JANN, D. PLEASURE & G. SCARLATO. 1989. Rapid quantitative immunohistochemical assessment of human peripheral neuropathies using a monoclonal antibody against nerve growth factor receptor. J. Neurol. **236:** 439–444.
4. SOBUE, G., T. YASUDA, T. MITSUMA, A. H. ROSS & D. PLEASURE. 1988. Expression of nerve growth factor in human peripheral neuropathies. Ann. Neurol. **24:** 64–72.
5. DISTEFANO, P. S. & E. M. JOHNSON, JR. 1988. Identification of a truncated form of the nerve growth factor receptor. Proc. Natl. Acad. Sci. USA **85:** 270–274.
6. DISTEFANO, P. S., M. CLAGETT-DAME, D. M. CHELSEA & R. LOY. 1991. Developmental regulation of human truncated nerve growth factor receptor. Ann. Neurol. **29:** 13–20.
7. FESTOFF, B. W., A. ROZIER, V. MEININGER, D. HANTAI & P. S. DISTEFANO. 1992. Correlation of truncated urinary nerve growth factor receptor (NGF-Rt) with disease progression in Amyotrophic Lateral Sclerosis (ALS). Neurology **42:** 456.
8. ROBIN, B. 1985. Assay for creatinine in serum, plasma, or urine on the TDx analyzer. Clin. Chem. **6:** 970.
9. NEUMAN, R. G. & M. P. COHEN. 1989. Improved competitive enzyme-linked immunoassay (ELISA) for albuminuria. Clin. Chim. Acta **179:** 229–238.

Oxidative Damage in Double-stranded Genomic DNA as Measured by GC/MS Assay of a Thymine Glycol Derivative[a]

S. P. MARKEY, C. J. MARKEY, AND T.-C. L. WANG

Section on Analytical Biochemistry
Laboratory of Clinical Science
National Institute of Mental Health
Bethesda, Maryland 20892

INTRODUCTION

We have sought to define a substance to serve as a marker of neuronal injury and indicate the presence of oxidative damage to DNA. Ordinarily, damaged DNA bases are efficiently repaired by a family of highly conserved enzymes found in all organisms. It has been postulated that the accumulation of unrepaired oxidative damage to nuclear or mitochondrial neuronal DNA bases could be involved in disorders of aging such as Parkinson's and Alzheimer's diseases (reviewed comprehensively by Friedberg[1]). Unrepaired damage could result if enzymatic repair capacity were to be overwhelmed by oxidative stresses of environmental or drug origin. Damage to the gene regions coding for repair enzymes would effect the ability of a cell to survive over time. Most of the reported methods for assessing DNA repair deficiencies require the use of dividing cells in culture. However, the measurement of damage to DNA in non-dividing cells requires an alternative strategy, such as the measurement of DNA breaks or cross-links. We have chosen to develop a physicochemical method for directly measuring thymine glycol, one product of hydroxyl radical attack on thymine in DNA (see FIG. 1). A sensitive and specific gas chromatographic-mass spectrometric (GC/MS) assay of thymine glycol has been the object of these studies.

There have been several published assays for quantifying thymine glycol in DNA, using radiochemical, immunoassay or chromatographic procedures.[2–5] These have been successful in measuring the oxidative damage in solutions of DNA exposed to various chemical or radiochemical agents, but have not permitted the detection of damage to DNA *in vivo* or in cultured cells, except when cells have been pre-labeled with radioactive thymine so that radioactive 'dihydrothymines' are released.[6–8] The goal of the present research is to define methods which can be applied to DNA isolated from human tissues, or the detection of thymine glycol released into media by repair enzymes in cultured cells. Toward this objective, a radiochemical method developed by Schellenberg and Shaeffer[9] has been modified. Thymine glycol in double-stranded, genomic DNA can be converted quantitatively to 2-methylglyceric methyl ester by base hydrolysis, sodium borohy-

[a] We wish to thank the Alzheimer's Disease and Related Disorders Association for providing grant support (PRG-91-104).

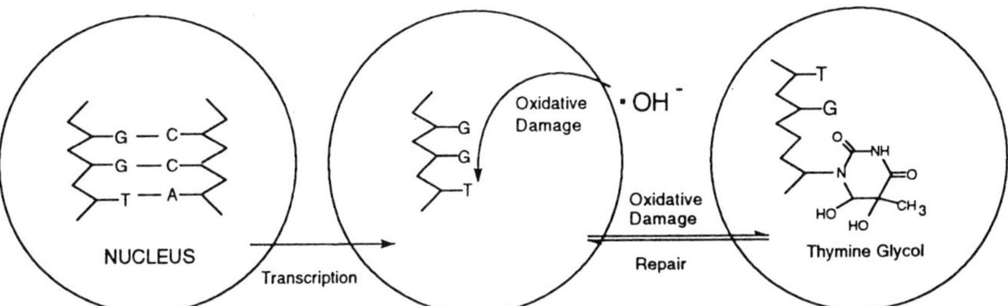

FIGURE 1. Thymine glycol production by free radical attack is usually repaired enzymatically.

dride (or borodeuteride, for added specificity) reduction, and methanolysis, as shown in SCHEME 1.

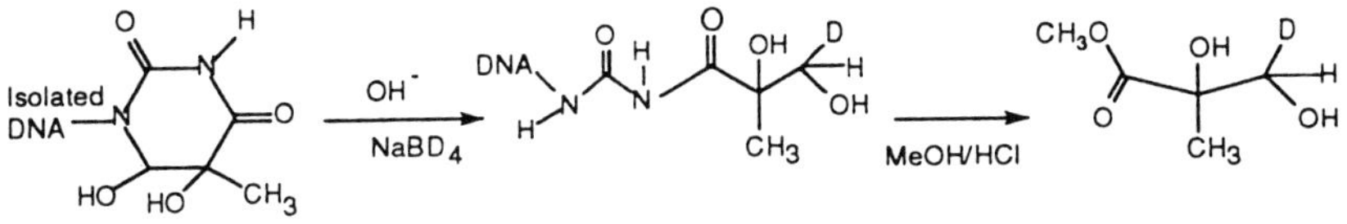

SCHEME 1

The result is that one molecule of a unique and characteristic structure, containing a single deuterium atom when borodeuteride is used, and with a low molecular weight is released from a complex polymer for every molecule of oxidized thymine in DNA. This simplifies the analytical task considerably, and the detection of 2-methylglyceric methyl ester can be significantly improved by chemical derivitization to enhance its gas phase stability and its mass spectrometric properties. Multiple derivatization schemes have been tried, and the most satisfactory results have been obtained with formation of a di-(tertiarybutyl-dimethylsilyl) ether for quantification (SCHEME 2).

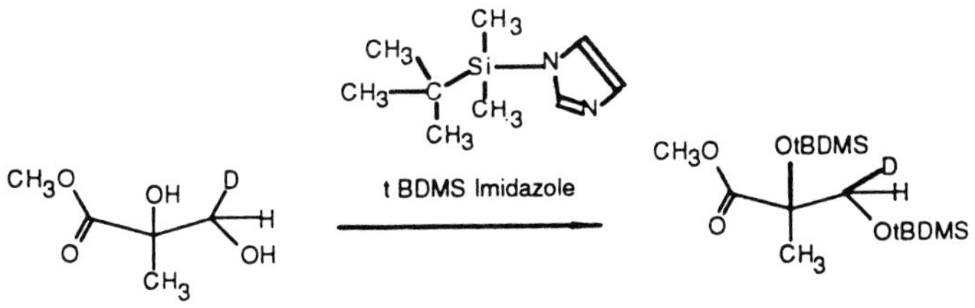

SCHEME 2

The progress of these investigations is summarized in the following, but the methods are continuously being improved with the goal of quantifying thymine glycol in 1–10 μg of DNA in order to apply the assay to small sections of tissue or cultured cells.

EXPERIMENTAL METHODS

Procedure

A solution of the internal standard (d$_1$-thymine glycol, 16 ng/10 μL) is added to each tube. Then DNA (0.5–2 mg in 50–100 μL water) or thymine glycol quantitative standards (0.1-to-25 ng) are added, and 100 μL of NaBD$_4$ (10 mM) in 0.2 M NaOH (prewashed with CH$_2$Cl$_2$ and stored in non-glass containers) is added next, and the mixture is heated for 1 hour at 37°C. All solutions are prepared fresh prior to use. The reaction is quenched with 100 μL of 6 M HCl and dried in a vacuum desiccator. Anhydrous methanolic/HCl (200 μL, 0.5 M) is added, vortexed, and heated for 30 min at 70°C. The samples are dried in a vacuum desiccator or under nitrogen. For the sperm DNA samples, the 2-methylglyceric methyl ester was separated from the bulk of the solid residue using hot ethyl acetate washes (2 × 0.5 mL), transferred to clean tubes, and dried under nitrogen.

The dried residue was derivatized with 100 μL of t-butyldimethylsilyl imidazole reagent (prepared from 150 mg t-butyldimethylsilyl chloride, 170 mg imidazole in 1 mL acetonitrile, washed five times with equal volumes of heptane) and heated at 70°C for 30 min. The products are partitioned between 100 μL heptane/decane (90/10) and 100 μL water, and the organic phase is removed after freezing the tube with dry ice. The organic extracts in autosampler vial inserts are concentrated in vacuo to approximately 20–25 μL.

GC/MS

Mass spectrometric analyses (GC/EI/MS, or PCI/MS/MS or EI/MS/MS) were performed on a Finigan TSQ70 mass spectrometer equipped with a Varian 3400 gas chromatograph. A 15 meter, 0.25 mm i.d., 0.25 μ DB-225 column was programmed from 110°C (1 minute) to 220°C (1 minute) at 35°C/minute, followed by a 40°C/minute ramp to 240°C. The 2-methylglyceric methyl ester di-(tBDMS) ether elutes at approximately 2 min 45 sec, and is characterized by intense M-57 ions at m/z 306 (d$_1$), or 310 (d$_5$) as shown in FIGURE 2. A standard curve showing the assay linearity from 50 pg to 5 ng is shown in FIGURE 3.

CONCLUSIONS

This thymine glycol assay meets several important criteria necessary to demonstrate that it is a valid and precise method. First, the generation of consistent linear standard curves for crystalline thymine glycol over the range from 50 pg to 25 ng indicates the assay validity for homogeneous solutions. Second, we have applied this assay to a variety of test substances (pure nucleotides, poly A, poly dA-poly dT) in order to demonstrate that only thymine-containing materials can contribute to the measurement of thymine glycol. Analyses have not been influenced by the presence of deoxyglucose, phosphate, or other DNA bases. Third, we have obtained consistent and reproducible values for the determination of ng

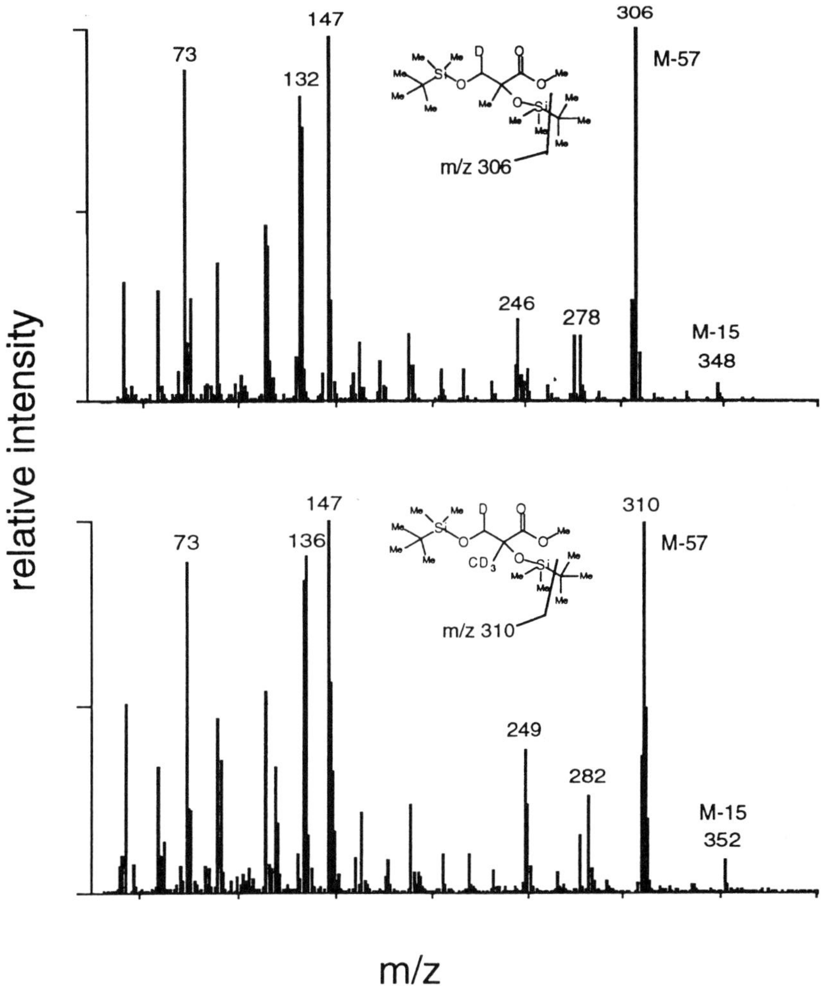

FIGURE 2. Mass spectra of d_1 (upper)- and d_5 (lower)-methyl-2-methylglycerate-di(tBDMS) resulting from the sodium borodeuteride reduction of d_0- and d_4-thymine glycol. The prominent ions at m/z 306 and 310 that result from the characteristic loss of a tertiary butyl radical are used for selected ion monitoring. Note that there are several other major ions which are structure specific (m/z 132, 246, 278, 348) and retain 3 or 4 deuterium ions in the internal standard spectrum (m/z 136, 249, 282, and 352) and can be used for structure confirmation. However, chemical background at these specific m/z values precluded their use for quantitative purposes.

of thymine glycol per mg of DNA over a range of DNA concentrations (0.5–2 mg). These values (0.378 ± 0.07 ng/thymine glycol/mg herring sperm DNA; 0.335 ± 0.071 for salmon sperm DNA) correspond to 3–4 thymine glycol residues per million thymine bases. Because these determinations were performed upon commercially obtained DNAs, the significance of these low levels cannot be addressed until measurements have been repeated with freshly isolated DNA.

The precision of repeated measurements of herring sperm DNAs exposed to varying oxidative stresses, and the direct correlation of these measures with strand breakage as measured by gel chromatography (studies performed in collaboration with Dr. L. Daniel, NCI) provides independent verification of the thymine glycol assay. Usually it is possible to use mass spectrometric isotope dilution assays as definitive and accurate benchmark measurements. However, because the deuter-

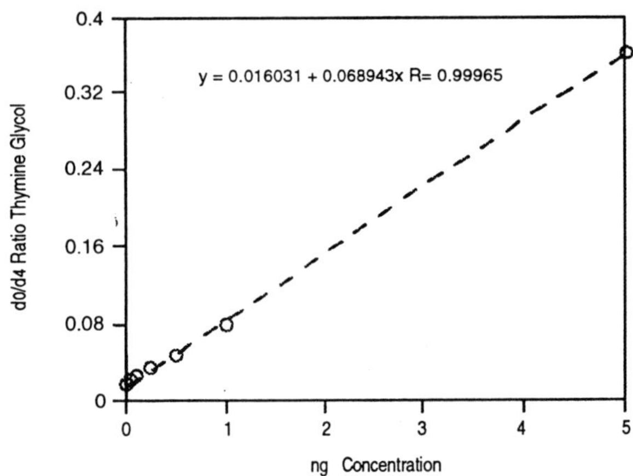

FIGURE 3. Standard curve resulting from the analysis of known concentrations of d_0-thymine glycol in the presence of a constant amount of d_4-thymine glycol internal standard. The d_0/d_4 ratio is measured by comparing the signal intensities at m/z 306 and 310, derived from the d_1 and d_5 2-methylglyceric acid derivative spectra shown in FIGURE 2.

ated thymine glycol internal standard is a monomer and cannot be fully equilibrated with double-stranded DNA, this is not a conventional mass spectrometric isotope dilution assay. The recovery of hydrolyzed and reduced 2-methylglyceric methyl ester is a precise measure of thymine glycol content for any given assay, but the accuracy of the measure awaits verification by an independent methodology.

REFERENCES

1. FRIEDBERG, E. C. 1984. DNA Repair. W. H. Freeman & Co. New York.
2. CATHCART, R., E. SCHWIERS, R. L. SAUL & B. N. AMES. 1984. Thymine glycol and thymidine glycol in human and rat urine: A possible assay for oxidative DNA damage. Proc. Natl. Acad. Sci. USA **81:** 5633–5637.
3. HUBBARD, K., H. HUANG, M. F. LASPIA, H. IDE, B. F. ERLANGER & S. S. WALLACE.

1989. Immunochemical quantitation of thymine glycol in oxidized and X-irradiated DNA. Radiat. Res. **118:** 257–268.

4. SHARMA, M., H. C. BOX & D. J. KELMAN. 1990. Fluorescence postlabeling assay of *cis*-thymidine glycol monophosphate in X-irradiated calf-thymus DNA. Chem. Biol. Interact. **74:** 107–17.

5. WEST, G. J., I. W.-L. WEST & J. F. WARD. 1982. Radioimmunoassay of a thymine glycol. **90:** 595–608.

6. LEWIS, J. G. & D. O. ADAMS. 1985. Induction of 5,6-ring-saturated thymine bases in NIH-3T3 cells by phorbol ester-stimulated macrophages: role of reactive oxygen intermediates. Cancer Res. **45:** 1270–1275.

7. LEWIS, J. G., T. HAMILTON & D. O. ADAMS. 1986. The effect of macrophage development on the release oxygen intermediates and lipid oxidation products, and their ability to induce oxidative DNA damage in mammalian cells. Carcinogenesis **7:** 813–8.

8. LEWIS, J. G. & D. O. ADAMS. 1987. Inflammation, oxidative DNA damage, and carcinogenesis. Environ. Health Perspect. **76:** 19–27.

9. SCHELLENBERG, K. A. & J. SHAEFFER. 1986. Formation of methyl ester of 2-methylglyceric acid from thymine glycol residues: a convenient new method for determining radiation damage to DNA. **25:** 1479–1482.

Free Radical and Lipid Peroxidation in Manganese-induced Neuronal Cell Injury

A. Y. SUN,[a] W. L. YANG, AND H. D. KIM

Department of Pharmacology
University of Missouri
Columbia, Missouri 65212

INTRODUCTION

Manganese (Mn) in trace amounts is essential in human nutrition. This metal ion is found in several enzyme systems (*e.g.*, pyruvate carboxylase and superoxide dismutase) and is involved in carbohydrate and lipid metabolism, although the biochemical basis for its involvement remains to be elucidated.[1,2]

Exposure of mammals to excessive amounts of Mn has been shown to cause a toxic effect. There is an extensive literature on Mn toxicity in humans due to chronic inhalation of high concentrations of airborne Mn from Mn mines, steel mills, and chemical industries. The principal organ affected by Mn toxicity is the brain, and acute Mn intoxication is characterized by disorientation, memory impairment, acute anxiety, and hallucination.[3] The biochemical lesions underlying the Mn pathology are not understood. Chronic Mn intoxication can cause permanent degenerative damage in the nigrostriatal system. Autopsy finding of low dopamine levels, morphologic lesions and the extrapyramidal signs suggest that this type of abnormality is similar to Parkinson's disease.[4] Studies with monkey and rodents given chronic administration of $MnCl_2$ have also demonstrated the depletion of dopamine in the striatum.[5] Cotzias[6] pointed out that the pathogenesis of Mn may be related to its ability to undergo changes in oxidation states. Similar to other transition metal ions, Mn^{2+} may be involved in neuronal degeneration owing to its ability to participate in the toxic free radical reaction.[7] A parallel situation may be found in Parkinson's disease which is thought to be associated with peroxidative stress.[8] Under these conditions, H_2O_2 formed during metabolism of dopamine may lead to the formation of hydroxyl radical through the Fenton type reaction in the presence of Mn^{2+}.

Since PC-12 cells are widely used as a model for catecholaminergic neurons, this cell line was used to study the effect of Mn on lipid peroxidation and cell death. The cell model will allow further investigation of the mechanisms involved in the Mn toxicity.

---

[a] Author to whom correspondence should be addressed.

MATERIALS AND METHODS

Cell Culture and Maintenance

PC-12 cells were grown routinely in 35 cm^2 plastic tissue culture dishes at 37°C under an atmosphere of 5% CO_2/95% air in Dulbecco's modified Eagle's medium (DME medium) containing 10% horse serum, 5% fetal calf serum and 50 units/ml penicillin.

Measurements of Lactate Dehydrogenase Release

Cytotoxicity was estimated by measuring the leakage of lactate dehydrogenase (LDH) from the cells into the medium using the procedure described by Bergmeyer and Brent.[9]

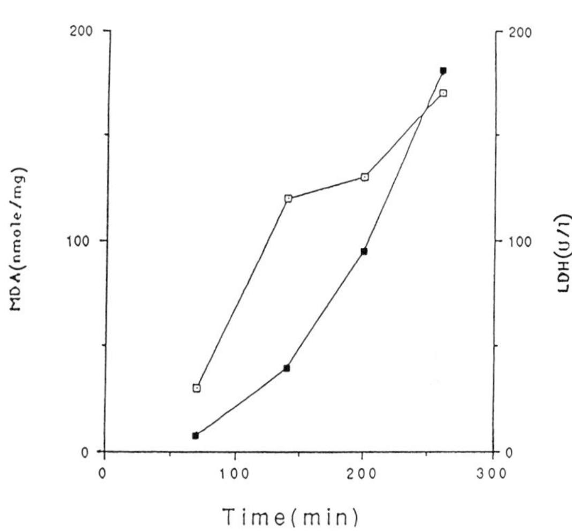

FIGURE 1. Time course of lipid peroxidation and LDH release in PC-12 cell culture after the addition of $MnCl_2$ and tyrosine. The conditions for cell culture were described in the text. $MnCl_2$ (10^{-4} M) and tyrosine (10^{-4} M) were added to the culture medium simultaneously and, at different time intervals, 1 ml of medium was pipetted out for LDH assay and 1 ml of medium including suspended cells was used for lipid peroxidation analysis. Open squares represent the amount of malonyldialdehyde (MDA) formed at each time point. The values of LDH release are shown by black squares. Each point was obtained from the average of three determinations.

Lipid Peroxidation Assay

Malondialdehyde (MDA) formed as a product of lipid peroxidation was estimated by the thiobarbituric acid test.[10]

RESULTS

Mn, Free Radicals, Lipid Peroxidation and Cell Death

Since oxygen free radicals have been suggested to be a causative factor for degeneration of the dopaminergic nigrostriatal cells,[8] our focus here is on the involvement of dopamine metabolism in manganese neurotoxicity. Previously, we reported that both Fe^{2+} and Mn^{2+} ions can catalyze the formation of hydroxyl free radical in the presence of dopamine and purified MAO.[11] Similar results have been reported by Yim *et al.*[12] It is reasonable to conclude that in dopaminergic neurons where dopamine is actively synthesized, high amounts of Fe^{2+} or Mn^{2+} may potentiate the lipid peroxidation processes leading to cell death. FIGURE 1 shows the time course of lipid peroxidation and the release of intracellular lactic dehydrogenase (LDH) by PC-12 cell culture grown in the presence of $MnCl_2$ (0.1 mM) and tyrosine (0.1 mM). Both lipid peroxidation and LDH release increased with time of epxosure to Mn^{2+} and tyrosine. It appears that lipid peroxidation has taken place in the early phase of incubation and this event is followed by cell death as indicated by the release of LDH. These results suggest that lipid peroxidation may have an important role in cell degeneration and cell death.

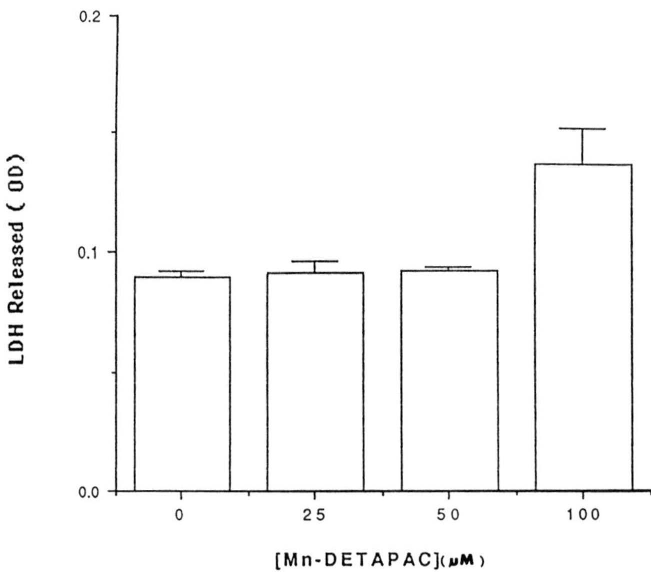

FIGURE 2. LDH released after Mn^{2+} treatment. Conditions for Mn^{2+} and tyrosine treatment are similar to those described in FIGURE 1 except that the treatment was terminated 24 h later. Different concentrations of $MnCl_2$ in equimolar concentration of diethylenetriamine-pentaacetic acid (DETAPAC) was added to initiate the treatment in the presence of 10^{-4} M tyrosine. Values are means ± SD of triplicate determinations.

It appears that in the presence of tyrosine, the enhanced cell death in PC-12 cells is dependent on the concentration of Mn^{2+}. At 10^{-4} M, Mn^{2+} increased cell death by 35% (FIG. 2). However, in the absence of added tyrosine, no increase in cell death was detected during 24 h of culture even after 10^{-4} M Mn was added to the medium (data not shown).

Possible Involvement of MAO

It is possible that tyrosine serves as a precursor for the synthesis of dopamine, which in turn serves as the substrate for the MAO reaction.

Subsequently, this reaction may lead to the generation of hydroxyl free radicals. However, direct addition of dopamine and its catechol-derivatives, such as L-DOPA, can also cause auto-oxidation, especially in the presence of heavy metal ions. Although auto-oxidation of dopamine was implicated to take place *in vivo* under pathological conditions,[13,14] the oxidative deamination catalyzed by MAO could also play an important role in the pathogenesis of Parkinson's disease. Since 2-*o*-methyldopamine (Mt) dose not undergo auto-oxidation, it is an ideal substrate for studying the role of MAO in oxidative stress. We have shown that Mt alone did not cause an increase in lipid peroxidation as compared with control (FIG. 3A). However, Mn at 0.1 mM added to the medium containing Mt resulted in an increase in lipid peroxidation (FIG. 3A) as well as cell death as indicated by the increase in LDH release (FIG. 3B). We have also used pargyline, a general MAO inhibitor, and superoxide dismutase (SOD) to see whether MAO is involved in the oxidative damage to the cell. As shown in FIGURE 3C and D, both SOD and pargyline prevent the further increase in lipid peroxidation in the presence of Mn and Mt. Interestingly, neither of these agents could significantly prevent cell death.

DISCUSSION

Metabolism of monoamines may be associated with an increased production of H_2O_2 and increased oxidative damage of the monoamine system.[15] Studies in our laboratory not only demonstrated the formation of hydroxyl free radical in the presence of Mn^{2+} and MAO system,[11] but also showed that addition of Mn^{2+} to PC-12 cells resulted in lipid peroxidation and cell death (FIG. 1). It is possible that hydroxyl radical is produced through a Haber-Weiss reaction in the presence of heavy metal ions, such as Fe^{2+}, Mn^{2+} and Cu^{2+}, and this reaction is catalyzed by MAO.[16] Since O_2^- is the first intermediate produced by MAO, the inhibitory effect of SOD and pargyline on lipid peroxidation further supports the role of MAO in oxidative damage (FIG. 3C). However, in the same experiment, we were not able to relate the protective effect of SOD and pargyline to the reduction of cell death (FIG. 3D). Consequently, it is possible that Mn causes other cellular damage besides the lipid peroxidation process. Our earlier study had indicated that subchronic treatment of rats with Mn^{2+} (80 mg/day for 8 days) resulted in alterations of the liver mitochondrial respiratory activity and oxidative phosphorylation.[17] The decrease in oxidative phosphorylation may lead to energy failure, loss of ion homeostasis and cell death. The possibility of energy failure and alteration of ion homeostasis in the Mn-induced neuronal degeneration and cell death is an area of intensive research in our laboratories.

Iron, manganese and copper are enriched in some brain regions such as the hypothalamus and basal ganglia.[4] Manganese has been also shown to accumulate in the basal ganglia region, especially when administered a high Mn^{2+} and low Ca^{2+} diet.[18] Excess amounts of Mn^{2+} can be taken in through contaminated water or exposure to Mn dust in mining and industrial settings, and to the fungicide Maneb[19] or manganese carbonyl compounds used as an antiknocking agent in gasoline.[4] Thus, possibility exists that life-long exposure to these agents may lead to accumulation of Mn^{2+} in these brain regions causing neurologic symptoms similar to those in Parkinson's disease.

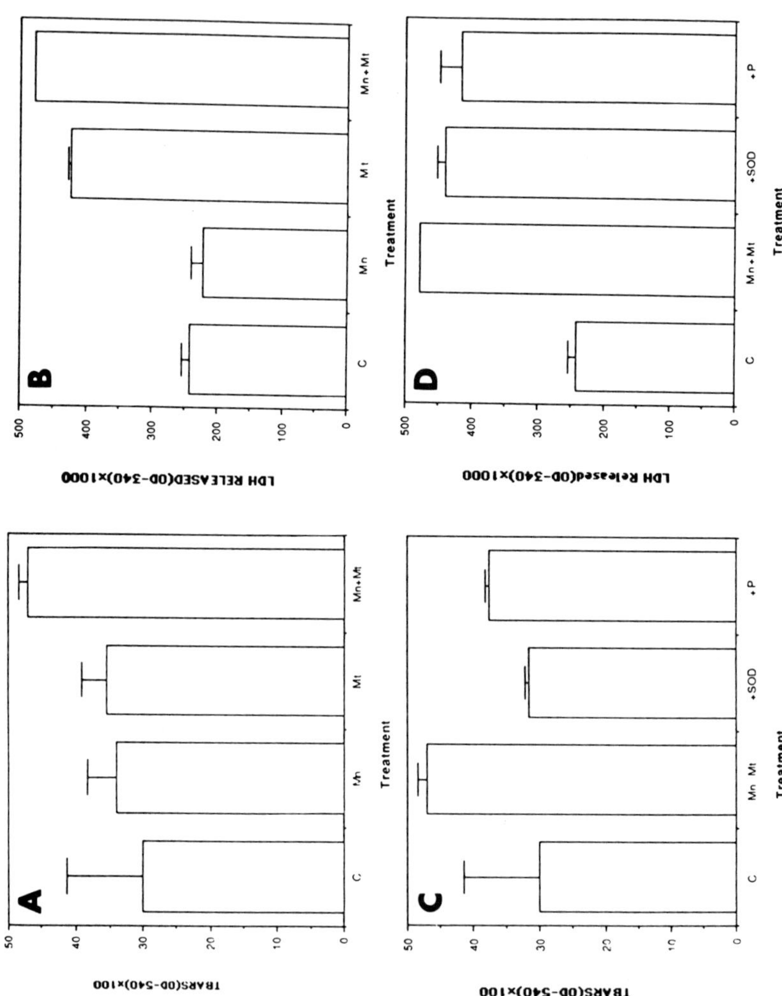

FIGURE 3. The involvement of MAO in manganese toxicity. Cells were treated with a MAO substrate, 3-o-methyl dopamine (Mt, 1 mM), and/or MnCl$_2$-DETAPAC (Mn, 10^{-4} M). Superoxide dismutase (SOD, 150 units/ml) and pargyline (P, 10^{-4} M) were also added, where indicated, at the same time with the (Mn + Mt) treatment. TBARS formed and LDH released were determined as described 24 h after the treatment. Each column represents mean ± SD of three determinations.

REFERENCES

1. HURLEY, L. S. 1980. Manganese. *In* Current Topics in Nutrition and Disease. A. S. Prasad, Ed., Vol. 6: 369–378. A. R. Liss, Inc. New York.
2. KEEN, C. L., B. LONNERDAL & L. S. HURLEY. 1984. Manganese. *In* Biochemistry of the Essential Ultra Trace Elements. E. Frieden, Ed.: 89–132. Plenum Press. New York.
3. DONALDSON, J. & A. BARBEAU. 1985. Manganese neurotoxicity: Possible clues to the etiology of human brain disorders. *In* Metal Ions in Neurology and Psychiatry. S. Gabay, H. Harris & B. T. Ho, Eds.: 259–285. Alan R. Liss, Inc. New York.
4. DONALDSON, J., D. McGREGOR & F. LaBELLA. 1982. Manganese neurotoxicity: A model for free radical mediated neurodegeneration. Can. J. Physiol. Pharmacol. **60:** 1398–1405.
5. CHANDRA, S. V., R. S. SRIVASTAVA & G. S. SHUKLA. 1979. Regional distribution of metals and biogenic amines in the brain of monkeys exposed to manganese. Toxicol. Lett. **4:** 189–192.
6. COTZIAS, G. C. 1958. Manganese in health and disease. Physiol. Rev. **38:** 503–532.
7. DONALDSON, J. 1981. The pathophysiology of trace metal: Neurotransmitter interaction in the CNS. Trends Pharmacol. Sci. **2:** 75–78.
8. COHEN, G. 1990. Monoamine oxidase and oxidative sress at dopaminergic synapse. J. Neural. Transm. **32**(Suppl.): 229–238.
9. BERGMEYER, H. U. & E. BRENT. 1974. UV-assay with pyruvate and NADH. *In* Methods of Enzymatic Analysis. H. U. Bergmeyer, Ed.: 574–579. Academic Press. New York.
10. BLOOM, R. J. & W. W. WESTERFIELD. 1971. The thiobarbituric acid reaction in relation to fatty liver. Arch. Biochem. Biophys. **145:** 669–675.
11. OLDFIELD, F. F., D. L. COWAN & A. Y. SUN. 1990. Possible involvement of some environmental toxin in Parkinson's disease: Free radical production. Free Radical Biol. Med. **9**(Suppl. 1): 41.
12. YIM, M. B., B. S. BERLETT, P. B. CLOCK & E. R. STADTMAN. 1990. Manganese (II)-bicarbonate-mediated catalytic activity for hydrogen peroxide dismutation and amino acid oxidation: Detection of free radical intermediates. Proc. Natl. Acad. Sci. USA **87:** 394–398.
13. FORNSTEDT, B., A. BRUN, E. ROSENGREN & A. CARLSSON. 1989. The apparent autooxidation rate of catechols in dopamine-rich regions of human brain increases with the degree of depigmentation of substantia nigra. J. Neural Transm. (Park. Dis. Dement. Sec.) **1:** 279–295.
14. YOUDIM, M. B. H., D. BEN-SHACHAR, G. ESHEL, J. P. M. FRIBERG & P. RIDERER. 1991. Protection from 6-hydroxydopamine-induced nigrostriatal dopamine lesion by the iron chelator deferoxamine mesalate: implications of increase in iron in Parkinson's disease. *In* International Workshop Berlin Parkinson's Disease. U. K. Rinne, T. Nagatsu & R. Harowski, Eds.: 26–36. Medicom Europe. Bussum, the Netherlands.
15. SPINA, M. B. & G. COHEN. 1989. Dopamine turnover and glutathione oxidation: Implication for Parkinson's disease. Proc. Natl. Acad. Sci. USA **86:** 1398–1400.
16. COHEN, G. 1986. Monoamine oxidase, hydrogen peroxide and Parkinson's disease. Adv. Neurol. **45:** 119–125.
17. SUN, A. Y., B. P. CHANG, V. CORPUS, G. SMITH, C. MARIENFELD & C. MIDDLETON. 1981. Effect of dietary manganese on the respiratory activity of liver mitochondria. Trace Substances Environ. Health **15:** 144–153.
18. MURPHY, V. A., K. C. WADHWANI, Q. R. SMITH & S. I. RAPOPORT. 1991. Suturable transport of manganese (II) across the rat blood-brain barrier. J. Neurochem. **57:** 948–954.
19. FERRAZ, H. B., P. H. F. BERTOLUECI, J. S. PEREIRA, J. G. C. LIMA & L. A. F. ANDRADE. 1988. Chronic exposure to the fungicide maneb may produce symptoms and signs of CNS manganese intoxication. Neurology **38:** 550–553.

Glutathione Disulfide (GSSG) as a Marker of Oxidative Injury to Brain Mitochondria[a]

PETER WERNER AND GERALD COHEN[b]

Graduate School in Biomedical Sciences (Biochemistry)
Department of Neurology and Center for Neurobiology
Mount Sinai School of Medicine
New York, New York 10029

INTRODUCTION

Monoamine oxidase (MAO) is localized to the outer mitochondrial membrane, where it exists in two isoforms, MAO-A and MAO-B. MAO-A and -B differ in their affinity for substrates and inhibitors, but both perform the identical oxidative deamination of neurotransmitter amines, producing hydrogen peroxide (H_2O_2) as one of the products (1). H_2O_2 is potentially toxic. However the H_2O_2 is detoxified by GSH peroxidase, resulting in the oxidation of 2 molecules GSH to form one of GSSG (2). H_2O_2 can also be decomposed by catalase.

$$\text{monoamine} + O_2 + H_2O \rightarrow \text{aldehyde} + H_2O_2 + NH_3 \tag{1}$$

$$2\,GSH + H_2O_2 \rightarrow GSSG + 2\,H_2O \tag{2}$$

The presence within mitochondria of GSH peroxidase and GSSG reductase, the two major enzymes dealing with detoxification of hydroperoxides within cells, is well documented.[1] Mitochondrial GSH peroxidase accounts for up to 26% of the total cellular content in rat liver.[2] Catalase in liver is mainly peroxisome-bound[3] and mitochondria appear not to contain catalase.[4] The involvement of H_2O_2 production by MAO as a toxicologic factor in Parkinson's disease has long been suspected, and there is mounting evidence for increased turnover of dopamine (DA) accompanied by oxidative stress in Parkinson's disease.[5–7]

In previously published experiments,[8] we observed that incubation of mouse liver mitochondria with benzylamine (an artificial MAO-B substrate) resulted in an increase in intramitochondrial GSSG, indicating a vulnerability of liver mitochondria towards H_2O_2 produced by MAO. Here we show that brain mitochondria respond in a similar fashion to MAO-induced oxidative stress with either benzylamine or DA as substrate, thereby making mitochondria in brain a target for oxidative injury when monoamine turnover is increased. The accumulation of

[a] Research reported in this paper was supported by Grant NS-28937 from the U.S. Public Health Service to G.C. Peter Werner was supported by a grant-in-aid from the Gottlieb Daimler and Karl Benz Foundation (Germany).

[b] Address correspondence to: Dr. Gerald Cohen, Box 1137, Department of Neurology and Center for Neurobiology, Mount Sinai School of Medicine, New York, N.Y. 10029; Tel.: (212)241-7312; FAX: (212)348-1310.

GSSG serves as a marker for changes in redox status and the presence of an oxidative stress.

METHODS

Mitochondria from brain and liver were prepared at 0–4°C essentially as described by Clark and Nicklas.[9] The buffer used for isolation of mitochondria and for subsequent incubation consisted of 0.225 M mannitol, 0.075 M sucrose and 1 mM EGTA, buffered with 5 mM MOPS at pH 7.4. Incubations were done at 30°C, 10 minutes, and approximately 150 oscillations/min., and they were terminated by the addition of 50 μL 4.0 M perchloric acid. Assays for GSSG were conducted with the Tietze[10] method, as modified by Slivka et al.[11] and further adapted for a plate reader (Werner and Cohen, in preparation). Protein was determined according to Lowry et al.[12]

RESULTS AND DISCUSSION

Experiments with Mouse Liver Mitochondria

In prior studies,[8] we observed a buildup of GSSG in mouse liver mitochondria during the oxidative deamination of the MAO-B substrate benzylamine. Added catalase did not prevent the rise in GSSG. Therefore, it appears that mitochondrial GSH peroxidase (and GSSG reductase) bear major responsibility for overcoming the oxidative stress that accompanies turnover of MAO substrates.

When mitochondria were separated from the incubation medium by centrifugation through a dibutylphthalate oil layer, no GSSG was detected in the medium (the supernatant). Previous studies by Olafsdottir and Reed[13] with t-butylhydroperoxide used in place of H_2O_2 showed that the GSSG that formed was similarly retained by the mitochondria. However, in intact liver perfused with benzylamine, some of the formed GSSG is released from the cells and effluxes from the organ,[14,15] suggesting that either part of the H_2O_2 is detoxified by GSH peroxidase in the cytosol and then extruded from the cell, or that GSSG leaks from the mitochondria into the cytosol.

Benzylamine is a selective substrate for MAO-B.[16] Addition of deprenyl (20 μM), a widely used selective inhibitor of MAO-B,[16] completely suppressed the rise in GSSG.[8] Clorgyline (20 μM), a selective MAO-A inhibitor,[16] was ineffective. These observations verify that the rise in GSSG is derived from the oxidative deamination of benzylamine by MAO-B. In additional experiments, DA (100 μM) evoked a GSSG rise of 21.2 ± 8.2 ng/mg protein under similar experimental conditions ($p < 0.02$). In Parkinson's disease, the turnover of DA is increased.[7] Therefore, the GSH peroxidase/GSSG reductase system should be especially important in this brain disorder.

Experiments with Rat Brain Mitochondria

More recent experiments have evaluated the response of rat brain mitochondria to incubation with MAO substrates. FIGURE 1 depicts the results from 4 experiments conducted in triplicate. As in the experiments with mouse liver mitochondria, incubation of rat brain mitochondria with DA resulted in a large rise in GSSG. These data illustrate the fact that the GSSG rise evoked by an artificial MAO-B substrate (benzylamine) with mouse liver mitochondria is not exclusive for that organ or substrate. The fact that incubation with DA significantly increased the GSSG content of brain mitochondria means that mitochondria in dopaminergic neurons are a potential target of MAO-induced oxidative stress in Parkinson's disease. Our observations on GSSG accumulation are in concordance with observations by Sandri et al.,[17] who reported loss of GSH on incubation of brain mitochondria with MAO substrates.

Under identical experimental conditions with 100 μM DA, mouse liver mitochondria responded with a much smaller rise in GSSG (106 ng/mg) compared to the rise observed for brain mitochondria shown in FIGURE 1 (391 ng/mg protein). The greater sensitivity of brain mitochondria indicates that brain is more susceptible to damage by the oxidative stress that accompanies increased DA turnover. It is not possible to compare directly the results with mouse liver reported here with that described earlier because different experimental conditions were used.

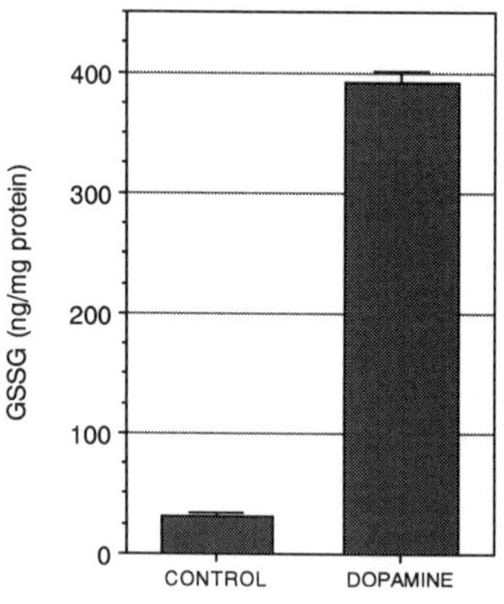

FIGURE 1. Rise in mitochondrial GSSG after incubation of rat brain mitochondria with dopamine. Rat brain mitochondria (1 mg protein/500 μL) were incubated for 10 min at 30°C with and without 100 μM dopamine. Results are the mean ± SEM from 4 experiments conducted in triplicate.

In addition to differences in time of incubation (5 vs. 10 min) and temperature (25°C vs. 30°C) for the previously published and new experiments, respectively, we have found that factors such as the oscillation speed of the shaker and concentration of mitochondria can affect the results.

Because DA is a mixed MAO-A/MAO-B substrate, additional experiments were performed with selective inhibitors for the two isoforms of MAO. Clorgyline and deprenyl were used as selective inhibitors of MAO-A and MAO-B, respectively. The MAO inhibitors (20 μM) were added at zero time along with the MAO substrate. The results shown in FIGURE 2 indicate that each inhibitor produced partial inhibition of the rise in GSSG. Clorgyline was the more effective inhibitor of GSSG accumulation. Neither clorgyline nor deprenyl altered the GSSG levels by themselves in the absence of added DA. In a single experiment (not shown in FIG.), deprenyl and clorgyline were added together in order to simultaneously inhibit both MAO-A and MAO-B. The presence of both inhibitors dropped the GSSG level from 112.4 ± 25.6 ng/mg for clorgyline by itself to 43.4 ± 3.1 ng/mg for clorgyline and deprenyl combined. The data are consistent with oxidation of DA by both MAO-A and MAO-B by brain mitochondria. Since the substrate and

FIGURE 2. Effect of selective MAO-A and MAO-B inhibitors on the rise in mitochondrial GSSG during incubation of rat brain mitochondria with 100 μM dopamine. Brain mitochondria (1 mg protein/500 μL) were incubated for 10 min at 30°C with 100 μM dopamine with and without deprenyl (20 μM, selective MAO-B inhibitor) or clorgyline (20 μM, selective MAO-A inhibitor). Results are the mean ± SEM from 2 experiments conducted in triplicate.

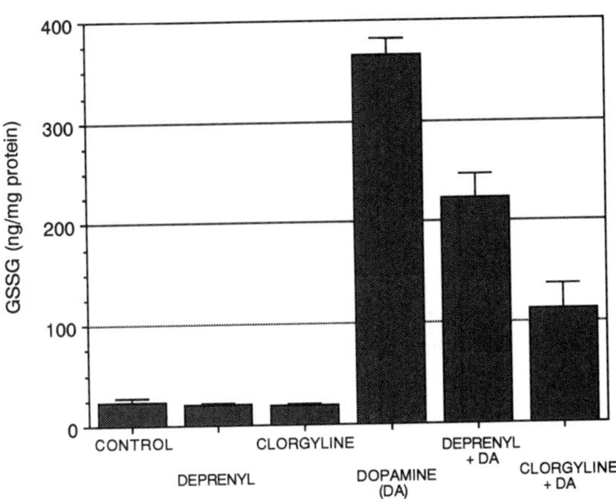

MAO inhibitors, which were added together, compete for the active site of MAO, the small residual rise in GSSG in the presence of both inhibitors can probably be attributed to formation of a small amount of GSSG before MAO was completely inhibited.

In additional experiments, the transfer of reduction equivalents from mitochondrial metabolism to GSSG reductase was evaluated. To achieve this, succinate or pyruvate was added; metabolism of these substrates provides NADH, which yields NADPH via the mitochondrial transhydrogenase reaction (3). The NADPH is required by GSSG reductase for conversion of GSSG to 2 GSH (4), which lowers the amount of GSSG in the mitochondria. Results are shown in TABLE 1.

$$\text{NADH} + \text{NADP} \rightarrow \text{NAD} + \text{NADPH} \tag{3}$$

$$\text{GSSG} + \text{NADPH} + \text{H}^+ \rightarrow 2\ \text{GSH} + 2\ \text{NADP}^+ \tag{4}$$

TABLE 1. Effect of Added Succinate or Pyruvate on Mitochondrial GSSG Accumulation with Benzylamine Substrate

	GSSG Accumulation	
Additions	Control	Benzylamine
	% Benzylamine Alone (± SEM)	
None	6.1 ± 1.2	100.0 ± 1.5
1 mM succinate	2.7 ± 1.5	70.0 ± 1.9*
1 mM pyruvate	2.2 ± 1.4	67.1 ± 1.4*
20 μM CCCP	3.2 ± 1.7	108.9 ± 3.0**
succinate + CCCP	2.9 ± 1.5	99.2 ± 5.1
pyruvate + CCCP	1.2 ± 2.4	87.0 ± 1.7*

Benzylamine (200 μM) was added to rat brain mitochondria. Other additions are as indicated in the table. Results are pooled from three experiments conducted in triplicate (N = 9). To facilitate comparisons, the GSSG levels are expressed as a % of the samples treated with benzylamine alone. The absolute amount of GSSG formed in samples incubated with benzylamine alone was 665 ± 10 ng/mg protein. Statistical assessment was performed with a 2-tailed t-test. * $p < 0.001$ and ** $p < 0.01$ compared to benzylamine alone.

The absolute amount of GSSG formed in TABLE 1 (see Table legend) was higher than that shown previously in FIGURES 1 and 2 with DA as substrate. A major reason for this is that the concentration of benzylamine used in TABLE 1 (200 μM) was double that used for DA in FIGURES 1 and 2 (100 μM). An additional factor is a differential response between benzylamine and DA as noted in the experiments with mouse liver mitochondria, cited above. The GSSG levels for control samples in the absence of benzylamine were all very low compared to that observed after 10 min. incubation with 200 μM benzylamine. Succinate and pyruvate each suppressed the GSSG level to 67.1–70.0% of that observed during incubation with benzylamine by itself. Therefore, substrates for NADH/NADPH generation in mitochondria effectively diminish GSSG levels during oxidative deamination of benzylamine MAO-B.

CCCP (carbonyl cyanide m-chlorophenylhydrazone), an uncoupler of mito-chondrial respiratory control, was also used in these experiments to investigate the effect of competition by the respiratory chain for the NADH reduction equivalents. CCCP was present from the start in a final concentration of 20 μM in order to stimulate the mitochondrial respiratory chain, thus consuming NADH in a futile attempt to maintain the potential of the inner membrane. CCCP alone had very little effect on the accumulation of GSSG during incubation with benzylamine. However, when CCCP was combined with succinate, the GSSG level was restored to that observed with benzylamine by itself (*viz.*, 99.2% of control). CCCP also lessened to a large extent the protective effect of pyruvate, although suppression of the GSSG buildup by pyruvate was still evident.

One possible reason why pyruvate or succinate might protect is that the stimula-tion of oxygen consumption could limit the activity of MAO, which requires oxygen. However, addition of CCCP is well known to dramatically enhance oxygen consumption by mitochondria. Since CCCP did not further enhance the protective effects of succinate and pyruvate, but reversed them instead, we conclude that the suppressive effects of these respiratory chain substrates cannot be attributed to a limitation in oxygen availability for MAO activity.

The current results with brain mitochondria cast an interesting light on the current clinical trial with the MAO-B inhibitor deprenyl as an agent that might slow the progression of Parkinson's disease. Clear evidence of benefit in terms of delay in the onset of disability necessitating intervention with L-dopa therapy was evident in early results from the trial[6] ($p < 10^{-10}$). Although the mechanism for the delay is not yet established, protection from damage by H_2O_2 at dopaminergic synapses could play a prominent role, as originally proposed in the design of the trial.[18] Since both MAO-A and MAO-B can deaminate DA, and current evidence indicates that MAO-A is the predominant isoform in DA neurons in primate brain,[19] additionally clinical trials of MAO-A inhibitors are clearly warranted.

REFERENCES

1. REED, D. J. 1990. Glutathione: Toxicological implications. Annu. Rev. Pharmacol. Toxicol. **30:** 603–631.
2. FLOHE, L. & W. SCHLEGEL. 1971. Glutathion-Peroxidase, IV. Intrazellulare Verteiling des Glutathion-Peroxidase-Systems in der Rattenleber. Hoppe-Seyler's Z. Physiol. Chemie **352:** 1401–1410.
3. DEDUVE, C. & P. BAUDHUIN. 1966. Peroxisomes (microbodies and related particles). Physiol. Rev. **46:** 323–357.
4. LEIGHTON, F., B. POOLE, H. BEAUFAY, P. BAUDHUIN, J. W. COFFEY, S. FOWLER & C. DEDUVE. 1968. The large-scale separation of peroxisomes, mitochondria, and

lysosomes from the livers of rats injected with triton WR-1339. J. Cell. Biol. **37:** 482–513.

5. SPINA, M. B. & G. COHEN. 1989. Dopamine turnover and glutathione oxidation: implications for Parkinson disease. Proc. Natl. Acad. Sci. USA **86:** 1398–1400.

6. Parkinson Study Group. 1989. Effect of deprenyl on the progression of disability in early Parkinson's disease, New Engl. J. Med. **321:** 1364–1371.

7. HORNYKIEWICZ, O. & S. J. KISH. 1986. Biochemical pathophysiology of Parkinson's disease. Adv. Neurol. **45:** 19–34.

8. WERNER, P. & G. COHEN. 1991. Intramitochondrial formation of oxidized glutathione during the oxidation of benzylamine by monoamine oxidase. FEBS Lett. **280:** 44–46.

9. CLARK, J. & W. J. NICKLAS. 1970. The metabolism of rat brain mitochondria. J. Biol. Chem. **245:** 4724–4731.

10. TIETZE, F. 1969. Enzymic method for quantitative determination of nanogram amounts of total and oxidized glutathione: applications to mammalian blood and other tissues. Anal. Biochem. **27:** 502–522.

11. SLIVKA, A., M. B. SPINA & G. COHEN. 1987. Reduced and oxidized glutathione in human and monkey brain, Neurosci. Lett. **74:** 112–118.

12. LOWRY, O. J., N. J. ROSEBROUGH, A. L. FARR & R. J. RANDALL. 1951. Protein measurement with the Folin phenol reagent. J. Biol. Chem. **193:** 265–275.

13. OLAFSDOTTIR, K. & D. J. REED. 1988. Retention of oxidized glutathione by isolated rat liver mitochondria during hydroperoxide treatment. Biochim. Biophys. Acta **964:** 377–382.

14. SIES, H., G. M. BARTOLI, R. F. BURK & C. WAYDHAS. 1978. Glutathione efflux from perfused liver after phenobarbital treatment, during drug oxidations, and in selenium deficiency. Eur. J. Biochem. **89:** 113–118.

15. OSHINO, N. & B. CHANCE. 1977. Properties of glutathione release observed during reduction of organic hydroperoxide, demethylation of aminopyrine and oxidation of some substances in perfused rat liver, and their implications for the physiological function of catalase. Biochem. J. **162:** 509–525.

16. FOWLER, C. J. & K. F. TIPTON. 1984. On the substrate specificities of the two forms of monoamine oxidase. J. Pharm. Pharmacol. **36:** 111–115.

17. SANDRI, G., E. PANFILI & L. ERNSTER. 1990. Hydrogen peroxide production by monoamine oxidase in isolated rat-brain mitochondria: Its effect on glutathione levels and Ca^{2+} efflux. Biochim. Biophys. Acta Gen. Subj. **1035:** 300–305.

18. PARKINSON STUDY GROUP. 1989. DATATOP: A multicenter controlled clinical trial in early Parkinson's disease. Arch. Neurol. **46:** 1052–1060.

19. WESTLUND, K. N., R. M. DENNEY, L. M. KORCHERSPERGER, R. M. ROSE, & C. W. ABELL. 1985. Distinct monoamine oxidase A and B populations in primate brain. Science **230:** 181–183.

Hydroxyl Free Radical (·OH) Formation Reflected by Salicylate Hydroxylation and Neuromelanin

In Vivo Markers for Oxidant Injury of Nigral Neurons

C. C. CHIUEH,[a] D. L. MURPHY, H. MIYAKE, K. LANG,[b]
P. K. TULSI,[b] AND S.-J. HUANG

Laboratory of Clinical Science
National Institute of Mental Health
National Institutes of Health Clinical Center 10/Rm 3D-41
Bethesda, Maryland 20892

INTRODUCTION

The 1-methyl-4-phenyl-1,2,3,6-tetrahydropyridine (MPTP)-induced animal model of parkinsonism appears to be an ideal model for studying Parkinson's disease. It has been demonstrated that MPTP causes a selective retrograde degeneration of nigral neurons and thus the parkinsonian syndrome in monkeys.[1-3] Prior studies have shown that the 1-methyl-4-phenylpyridinium metabolite of MPTP (MPP$^+$) causes a sustained biphasic dopamine overflow from the striatum,[4,5] which may last for hours in rodents and for days in pigmented animal species (dog, monkey, and human). Moreover, dopamine overflow elicited by MPP$^+$ appears to be a voltage-sensitive and calcium-dependent exocytotic process.[6] Therefore, we proposed that MPTP analogues may promote a site-specific formation of oxygen free radicals primarily through nonenzymatic dopamine autoxidation[7] in the basal ganglia where high levels of iron and dopamine are present.

In theory, metal-catalyzed dopamine autoxidation may lead to the formation of not only semiquinone anion radicals but also reactive oxygen species.[8-10] The putamen and the caudate nucleus are the brain regions most likely to generate cytotoxic free radicals by virtue of their high levels of dopamine, oxygen, and iron.[11] However it has been extremely difficult to assess the generation of short-lived oxygen free radicals in the central nervous system *in vivo*. For this purpose, a salicylate hydroxylation trapping procedure[12] was modified[13] and used to detect *in vivo* generation of ·OH free radicals in the striatum elicited by MPTP analogues.[14,15]

[a] Author to whom correspondence should be addressed; Tel.: (301) 496-9820; FAX: (301) 402-0188.

[b] Ms. K. Lang and Ms. P. Tulsi were supported by FAES summer student research grants.

FIGURE 1. Generation of ·OH free radicals assayed by salicylate hydroxylation *in vitro*: 6-hydroxydopamine versus dopamine. Sodium salicylate (1 mM) was added to freshly prepared 1 mM dopamine (DA) and 6-hydroxydopamine (6-OHDA) in pH 7 Ringer's solution. The ·OH products of salicylate (*i.e.*, catechol, 2,3-DHBA and 2,5-DHBA) were separated by an HPLC-EC procedure. The results depict the ·OH adducts of salicylate generated by 1 nmol of DA and 6-OHDA in the presence of 50 μM Fe^{2+}.

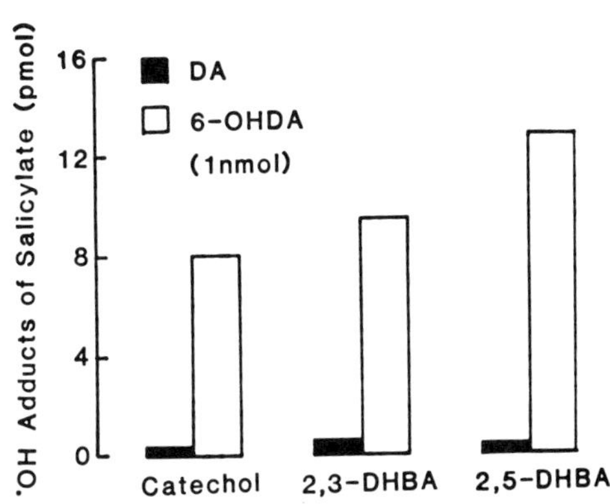

RESULTS AND DISCUSSION

Dopamine Melanin: In Vivo *Marker of Oxidant Damage Elicited by ·OH in A9 Substantia Nigra Compacta Neurons*

It has been shown that neurotoxicity elicited by 6-hydroxydopamine can be suppressed by oxygen free radical scavengers.[16] The present data demonstrates that 6-hydroxydopamine is nonenzymatically oxidized to generate ·OH free radicals in the presence of Fe^{2+} and oxygen. The amount of ·OH produced by Fe^{2+}-catalyzed autoxidation of dopamine is approximately 5% of that of 6-hydroxydopamine (FIG. 1). This *in vitro* result confirms that the autoxidation of dopamine leads to conversion of O_2 to O_2^-· and H_2O_2. H_2O_2 is then catalyzed by Fe^{2+} but not Fe^{3+} to generate ·OH through the Fenton reaction.

Dopamine autoxidation also leads to formation of melanin pigments. It is known that the formation of neuromelanin pigments and the accumulation of nonhemin iron in the A9 zona compacta neurons of the substantia nigra are age-dependent. The formation of dopamine-melanin is blocked completely by adding ·OH scavengers (sodium salicylate and salicylic acid, TABLE 1). Thus dopamine, oxygen and iron promote ·OH generation and neuromelanin formation in the A9 nigral neurons. Therefore, it is reasonable to suggest that the

TABLE 1. Blockade of Iron-catalyzed Dopamine Melanin Formation After Scavenging ·OH Radicals by Salicylate

Dopamine + Fe^{2+} + O_2	Melanin Formation (relative optical density, 450 nm)
Ringer's solution	0.841 ± 0.031
Salicyclic acid	0.012 ± 0.001*
Sodium salicylate	0.039 ± 0.002*

Melanin formation elicited by dopamine (5 mM), Fe^{2+} (50 μM) in pH 7 oxygenated Ringer's solution were measured by a spectrometer equipped with a 96-well microplate scanner. The formation and/or polymerization of dopamine-melanin was completely blocked by adding salicylate (5 mM) to the solution (*$p < 0.05$, Student's *t*-test, N = 3).

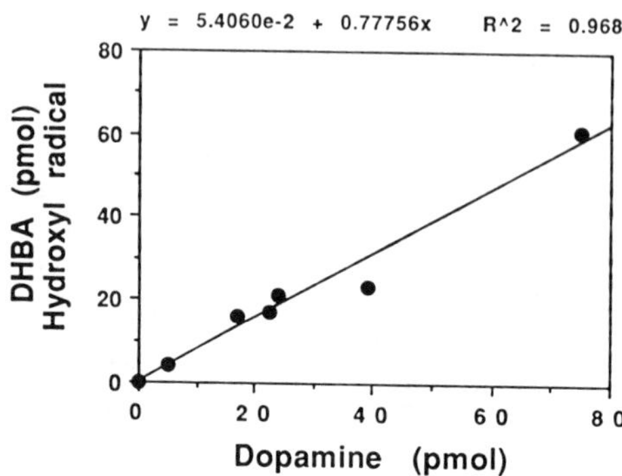

FIGURE 2. Positive linear correlation between dopamine overflow and ·OH generation elicited by MPP$^+$ in the striatum *in vivo*. The intracranial microdialysis procedure was modified for measuring dopamine release and ·OH radical formation in the striatum of anesthetized rats. MPP$^+$ (0 to 150 nmol) was infused through the microdialysis probe for 15 min to evoke a sustained dopamine overflow which lasts for more than two hours. ·OH radicals formed during dopamine overflow elicited by MPP$^+$ were trapped by salicylate and assayed by an HPLC-EC. The results show total formation of 2,3- and 2,5-DHBA above that of background in the strial dialysate collected during the period of dopamine overflow elicited by MPP$^+$ *in vivo*.

neuromelanin pigments in the A9 nigral neurons are valid *in vivo* markers for oxidant stress elicited by cytotoxic ·OH radicals generated via dopamine autoxidation.

In Vivo *·OH Generation in the Striatum Elicited by MPP$^+$: Evidence for Dopamine Involvement*

Perfusion of MPP$^+$, through a microdialysis probe, into the caudate nucleus of anesthetized rats causes a sustained, voltage-regulated (tetrodotoxin-sensitive), and calcium-dependent (nimodipine- and EDTA-sensitive) release of dopamine.[6] MPP$^+$ also causes a dose-dependent increase in ·OH generation[13] during and after the sustained dopamine efflux *in vivo* (FIG. 2). Owing to a unique accumulation pattern of nonhemin iron, the formation of ·OH elicited by MPP$^+$ through dopamine autoxidation occurs primarily in the A9 nigrostriatal rather than the A10 mesolimbic dopaminergic neurons. Furthermore, the formation of ·OH free radicals reflected by salicylate hydroxylation elicited by MPP$^+$ in the striatum appears to be greater than that generated during ischemia.[7]

MPDP$^+$ (1-methyl-4-phenyl-2,3-dihydropyridinium ion), the putative precursor of MPP$^+$, is as effective as MPP$^+$ in producing both dopamine overflow and ·OH formation.[14] Owing to its weak dopamine releasing action, MPTP does not significantly increase the formation of ·OH. However, 2'-methyl MPTP, a more potent MPTP analogue, increases dopamine overflow, thus leading to an increased ·OH generation; these effects can be suppressed by pretreatment with monoamine oxidase inhibitors.[15] These results indicate that the enhanced ·OH formation elicited by MPTP analogues is dopamine dependent. It further suggests that some of the released dopamine is nonenzymatically oxidized to not only ·OH free radicals but also semiquinone anion radicals in the iron-rich basal ganglia. This hypothesis is strengthened by the fact that NSD-

1015 blocks dopamine synthesis/turnover and thus MPTP-induced dopamine toxicity.[20]

Consequence of Enhanced ·OH Formation in Basal Ganglia: Melanin Pigmentation, Calcium Overload, and Retrograde Nigral Injury

The formation of dopamine-melanin pigments in the cell body of the A9 nigral neurons may be the outcome of a lifetime accumulation of ·OH-induced oxidant stress elicited by dopamine, oxygen, and iron. In fact, heavily melanized midbrain dopaminergic neurons are more vulnderable to degeneration in Parkinson's disease.[17] ·OH free radicals are very reactive; they may attack the lipid bilayer of cell membranes, open calcium ion channels, and also promote oxidant injury at the site of formation when formed near and/or inside A9 dopaminergic nerve terminals. This notion is supported by our present and earlier[18] results in which MPDP$^+$ and MPP$^+$, but not MPTP, generate cytotoxic free radicals and thus produce calcium overload and nigral loss. Furthermore, calcium overload triggers the activation of proteases, causes a cascade of potassium overflow (in preparation), and possibly increases the release of excitatory amino acids. The consequence of oxidative stress produced by an acute increase in the formation of cytotoxic ·OH in the iron-rich striatum is the "selective retrograde degeneration" of the A9 nigrostriatal dopaminergic neurons following MPTP administration.[1–3]

·OH Model of Parkinson's Disease and Dopaminergic Neuroprotection Perspectives

The present data[7,13–15] demonstrate that the formation of cytotoxic free radicals is significantly increased in the striatum following the administration of MPP$^+$, MPDP$^+$ and the 2'-methyl analogue of MPTP. The effects of 2'-methyl MPTP are suppressed by a combined pretreatment with clorgyline and deprenyl.[15] After overwhelming antioxidant defense mechanisms, enhanced ·OH formation in the iron-rich striatum produced by toxic pyridinium metabolites of MPTP analogues can lead to retrograde degeneration of the pigmented A9 nigrostriatal neurons. Enhanced ·OH formation through iron-catalyzed dopamine autoxidation thus may be the novel possible neurotoxic mechanism underlying selective nigrostriatal degeneration produced by MPTP analogues.[7]

These results lead to an interesting working hypothesis that oxidant stress elicited by reactive oxygen species generated by metal-catalyzed dopamine autoxidation may be the common neurodegenerative process involved in selective nigro-

TABLE 2. Evidence for Involvement of Dopamine Autoxidation and Oxygen Free Radicals in Nigrostriatal Degeneration

Nigrostriatal Degeneration: Free Radical Involvement via Dopamine Autoxidation
Idiopathic Parkinson's Disease—Fornstedt *et al.*, 1989
Animal Model of Parkinson's Disease
• 6-Hydroxydopamine–Cohen *et al.*, 1974
• Mn^{2+} Intoxication–Graham, 1984
• MPTP Analogues–Chiueh *et al.*, 1992; Obata and Chiueh, 1992

striatal degeneration in Parkinson's disease produced by environmental neurotoxins such as manganese[8,9] and compounds related to 6-hydroxydopamine[16,19] as well as MPTP[7,8,13–15] (TABLE 2). By investigating pathophysiological roles of ·OH free radicals in the central nervous system, researchers may be able to answer some of clinical questions concerning the use of neuroprotective agents (i.e., deprenyl, nimodipine, pergolide and lazaroid) to halt or treat progressive neurodegenerative brain disorders.

REFERENCES

1. BURNS, R. S., C. C. CHIUEH, S. P. MARKEY, M. H. EBERT, D. M. JOCOBOWITZ & I. J. KOPIN. 1983. A primate model of parkinsonism: Selective destruction of dopaminergic neurons in the pars compacta of the substantia nigra by N-methyl-4-phenyl-1,2,3,6-tetrahydropyridine. Proc. Natl. Acad. Sci. USA **80:** 4546–4550.

2. CHIUEH, C. C., S. P. MARKEY, R. S. BURNS, J. N. JOHANNESSEN & I. J. KOPIN. 1984. Neurochemical and behavioral effects of 1-methyl-4-phenyl-1,2,3,6-tetrahydropyridine in rat, guinea pig and monkey. Psychopharmacol. Bull. **20:** 548–553.

3. HERKENHAM, M., M. D. LITTLE, K. BANKIEWICZ, S.-C. YANG, S. P. MARKEY & J. N. JOHANNESSEN. 1991. Selective retention of MPP$^+$ within the monoaminergic systems of the primate brain following MPTP administration. An *in vivo* autoradiographic study. Neuroscience **40:** 133–158.

4. ROLLEMA H., W. G. KUHR, G. KRANENBORG, J. DE VRIES & C. VAN DEN BERG. 1988. MPP$^+$-induced efflux of dopamine and lactate from rat striatum have similar time courses as shown by *in vivo* brain dialysis. J. Pharmacol. Exp. Ther. **245:** 858–866.

5. MIYAKE, H. & C. C. CHIUEH. 1989. Effects of MPP$^+$ on the release of serotonin and 5-hydroxyindoleacetic acid from rat striatum *in vivo*. Eur. J. Pharmacol. **166:** 49–55.

6. CHIUEH, C. C. & S.-J. HUANG. 1991. MPP$^+$: A novel voltage-regulated ion channel activator for dihydropyridine-sensitive L-type calcium channels on nigrostriatal dopaminergic terminals. Posters Neurosci. **1:** 37–41.

7. CHIUEH, C. C., H. MIYAKE & M. T. PENG. 1993. Role of dopamine autoxidation, hydroxyl radical generation and calcium overload in underlying mechanisms involved in MPTP-induced parkinsonism. Adv. Neurol. **60:** 251–258.

8. POIRIER, J., J. DONALDSON & A. BARBEAU. 1985. The specific vulnerability of the substantia nigra to MPTP is related to the presence of transition metals. Biochem. Biophys. Res. Commun. **128:** 25–33.

9. GRAHAM, D. G. 1984. Catecholamine toxicity: A proposal for the molecular pathogenesis of manganese neurotoxicity and Parkinson's disease. Neurotoxicology **5:** 83–96.

10. FORNSTEDT, B., A. BRUN, E. ROSENGREN & A. CARLSSON. 1989. The apparent autoxidation rate of catechols in dopamine-rich regions of human brains increases with the degree of depigmentation of substantia nigra. J. Neural Transm. (P-D sect) **1:** 279–295.

11. HALLGREN, B. & P. SOURANDER. 1958. The effect of age on the non-haemin iron in the human brain. J. Neurochem. **3:** 41–51.

12. FLOYD, R. A., J. WATSON & P. K. WONG. 1984. Sensitive assay of hydroxyl free radical formation utilizing high pressure liquid chromatography with electrochemical detection of phenol and salicylate hydroxylation products. J. Biochem. Biophys. Methods **10:** 221–235.

13. CHIUEH, C. C., G. KRISHNA, P. TULSI, T. OBATA, K. LANG, S.-J. HUANG & D. L. MURPHY. 1992. Intracranial microdialysis of salicylate to detect hydroxyl radical generation through dopamine autoxidation in the caudate nucleus: effects of MPP$^+$ Free Radic. Biol. Med. **13:** 581–583.

14. OBATA, T. & C. C. CHIUEH. 1992. *In vivo* trapping of free radicals in the striatum utilizing intracranial microdialysis perfusion of salicylate: effects of MPTP, MPDP$^+$ and MPP$^+$. J. Neural Transm. **89:** 139–145.

15. CHIUEH, C. C., S.-J. HUANG & D. L. MURPHY. 1992. Enhanced hydroxyl radical generation by 2'-methyl analog of MPTP: Suppression by clorgyline and deprenyl. Synapse **11:** 346–348.

16. COHEN, G. 1988. Oxygen radicals and Parkinson's disease. *In* Oxygen Radicals and Tissue Injury. B. Halliwell, Ed.: 130–135. FASEB. Bethesda, MD.

17. HIRSCH, E., A. M. GRAYBIEL & Y. A. AGID. 1988. Melanized dopaminergic neurons are differentially susceptible to degeneration in Parkinson's disease. Nature (London) **334:** 345–348.

18. SUN, C. J., J. N. JOHANNESSEN, W. GESSNER, I. NAMURA, W. SINGHANIYOM, A. BROSSI & C. C. CHIUEH. 1988. Neurotoxic damage to the nigrostriatal system in rats following intranigral administration of MPDP$^+$ and MPP$^+$. J. Neural Transm. **74:** 75–86.

19. COHEN, G., R. E. HEIKKILA & D. MacNAMEE. 1974. The generation of hydrogen peroxide, superoxide radical and hydroxyl radical by 6-hydroxydopamine, dialuric acid and related cytotoxic agents. J. Biol. Chem. **249:** 2447–2452.

20. CHIUEH, C. C., J. N. JOHANNESSEN, J. L. SUN, J. P. BACON & S. P. MARKEY. 1986. Reversible Neurotoxicity of MPTP in the nigrostriatal dopaminergic system of mice. *In* MPTP: A Neurotoxin Producing a Parkinsonian Syndrome. S. P. Markey, N. Castagnoli, Jr., A. J. Trevor & I. J. Kopin, Eds.: 473–479. Academic Press. Orlando, FL.

Manganese Transport and Na/K/Cl Cotransport in PC-12 Cells[a]

H. D. KIM,[b] G. Y. SUN,[c] AND A. Y. SUN[b]

bDepartment of Pharmacology
cDepartment of Biochemistry
University of Missouri, School of Medicine
Columbia, Missouri 65212

INTRODUCTION

Manganese is an essential trace metal which is both absorbed and excreted by the alimentary tract. Manganese is present in minute amounts in various regions of the brain. It is known that manganese deficiency, while rare in humans, enhances the susceptibility to seizures.[1] In a number of species, manganese deficiency during the postnatal period elicits a congenital irreversible ataxia.[2] By contrast, manganese toxicity has been extensively documented.[2,3] The initial damage in early manganese toxicity appears to result from a biochemical defect in the metabolism of neurotransmitters, including dopamine, serotonin, and γ-amino-*n*-butyric acid.[2,3] With progression of manganese toxicity, histopathological lesions, not unlike those of Parkinson's disease, appear in the brain, causing a permanent neurological disorder.[2,3]

Manganese is transported across the blood-brain barrier by a saturable process.[4] Astrocytes also take up manganese by a specific high affinity transport system.[5] An interesting feature of the tissue distribution of manganese is that glial cells, but not neuronal cells, concentrate manganese an order of magnitude higher than can be accounted for by a simple passive diffusion.[5] Of the intracellular organelles, mitochondria are the primary site within which manganese is stored.[2]

In this communication, we report the results of our investigation on the mechanism by which manganese enters PC-12 cells, and the subsequent effects of intracellular manganese on other ion transport processes.

MATERIALS AND METHODS

Cell Culture

PC-12 cells were grown in 35 mm plastic tissue culture dishes under an atmosphere of 5% CO_2/95% air in Dulbecco's Modified Eagle's Medium containing 10% horse serum, 5% fetal calf serum, and 50 units/ml penicillin.

Manganese Transport

Cells grown to confluency were washed with a balanced salt solution composed of (mM): 5 KCl, 143 NaCl, 1 $CaCl_2$, 1.2 $MgSO_4$, 10 glucose, 15 HEPES-Tris

[a] This work was supported in part by National Institutes of Health grants DK33456 to H.D.K. and AA02054 to A.Y.S.

buffer, pH 7.45 and 0.1% BSA. The cells were maintained in this medium for 20 min at room temperature. To initiate manganese influx, the preincubation buffer was replaced by the same balanced salt solution except that it contained various manganese concentrations, as indicated in the legends to the figures, and ^{54}MnCl$_2$ (2 μCi/ml). At frequent intervals, the influx was terminated by removing the flux medium and washing the cells with cold 165 mM NaCl. The cells attached to the dish were digested with 1 M NaOH and then used for protein assay[6] and the determination of radioactive manganese in a TM Analytic gamma counter. Manganese efflux was measured after preloading the PC-12 cells with 100 μM manganese plus ^{54}MnCl$_2$ (3 μCi/ml) for 3 h in the same balanced salt solution used for the influx measurement. Cells were then washed and 3.3 ml of the same medium lacking manganese or containing 10 μM manganese was added. The appearance of ^{54}Mn in the supernatant was monitored with time. At the end of the efflux measurement, the solution used to wash the cells and the cell pellets were saved for the determination of total radioactivity associated with the cells.

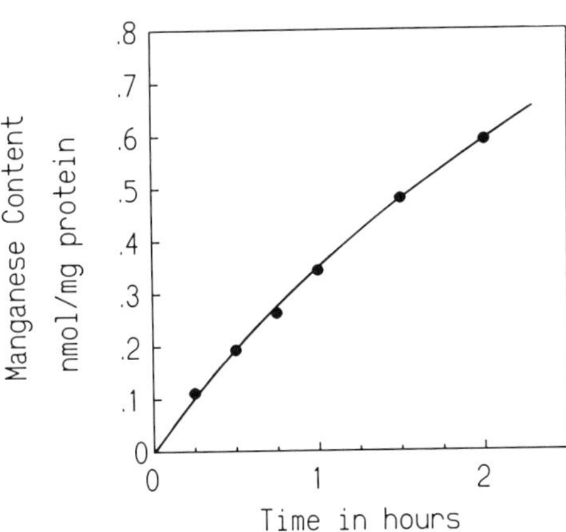

FIGURE 1. Manganese uptake by PC-12 cells. PC-12 cells were incubated in the presence of 10 μM manganese and ^{54}MnCl$_2$ (2 μCi/ml). At frequent intervals, cells were washed and solubilized with 1 M NaOH for the determination of ^{54}Mn and protein. Data shown are a representative result of two experiments, each determined in duplicate.

Na/K/Cl Cotransport

K influx was measured using ^{86}Rb as the K congener as described previously.[7] K influx was initiated by adding ^{86}Rb (1–2 μCi/ml) and the flux buffer composed of (mM): 143 NaCl or 147 *N*-methyl-D-glucamine (NMG) chloride, 4 KCl, 1 potassium phosphate, 1.2 MgSO$_4$, 1 CaCl$_2$, 10 glucose, 1 ouabain, 15 HEPES-Tris buffer, pH 7.45, and 0.1% BSA. At the end of a 20-min flux, cells were washed three times with ice cold 0.165 M NaCl and ^{86}Rb was extracted as described elsewhere.[6]

RESULTS

FIGURE 1 shows a time course of manganese uptake by PC-12 cells, which were incubated in the presence of manganese at a concentration of 10 μM. It is evident that PC-12 cells have a robust capacity to take up manganese. Manganese uptake is linear during the first 15–30 min but the rate becomes curvilinear over a 2-h period.

The capacity of PC-12 cells to release manganese is depicted in FIGURE 2, in which PC-12 cells were preloaded with external manganese at a concentration of 100 μM for 3 h at room temperature. Under these conditions, the intracellular manganese content amounted to approximately 3.7 nmol/mg protein. The release of manganese was monitored by measuring the appearance of ^{54}Mn into the medium containing no manganese or 10 μM manganese. Manganese efflux is linear up to 1 h but slows down significantly with time. Thus, as with the manganese uptake capacity, PC-12 cells unload the accumulated manganese effectively. However, at the end of the 3-h efflux period, PC-12 cells still retained nearly half of the preloaded manganese. There appears to be a small discernible effect of external manganese on manganese efflux in that manganese efflux tends to be slightly faster with manganese than without.

FIGURE 3 illustrates the results of manganese uptake kinetics. In this series of experiments, manganese uptake was measured for a period of 15 min in the presence of various manganese concentrations. Manganese uptake kinetics can

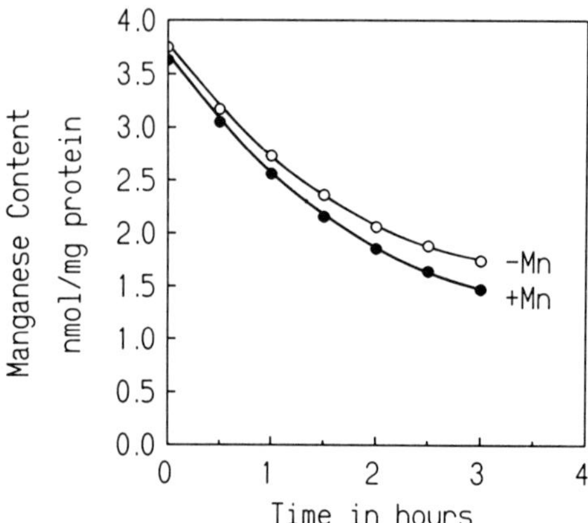

FIGURE 2. Efflux of manganese from PC-12 cells. PC-12 cells were preloaded with 100 μM manganese and ^{54}MnCl$_2$ (3 μCi/ml) for 3 h at room temperature. After preloading, flux medium containing 10 μM or no manganese was added and the appearance of radioactivity was monitored. Data shown are a representative result of three experiments, each determined in triplicate.

be described by a small saturable and a nonsaturable component. The nonsaturable component was determined by linear regression of manganese uptake rates above 20 μM manganese. The nonsaturable component had a rate constant of 1.27 $\times$ 10^{-3}/sec which was calculated by multiplying 0.0286 nmol/mg protein $\times$ h $\times$ μM and mg protein/6.23 μl cell water. To determine the saturable component, the nonsaturable component was subtracted from its total manganese influx. The K_m for manganese was 8.41 $\pm$ 4.3 μM (mean $\pm$ SE, n = 3) and V_{max} was 0.42 $\pm$ 0.9 nmol/mg $\times$ h. The saturable component, which implies the movement of manganese through a transport carrier, may explain the small stimulation of manganese efflux by the external manganese.

TABLE 1 summarizes the effects of a variety of agents on the manganese influx. All five divalent cations tested inhibited to a varying degree the manganese uptake. This contrasts with the findings reported for astrocytes in which cobalt, zinc, and lead had no effect[5] and for glial cells, where copper was found to acivate the manganese uptake.[8] On the other hand, calcium channel blockers and adenosine agonists were without effect.

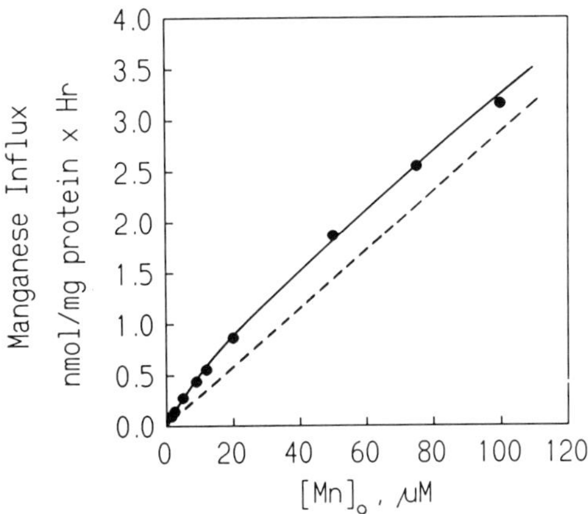

FIGURE 3. Manganese uptake kinetics. The experimental conditions were the same as in FIGURE 1 except that manganese was varied from 1.5 μM to 100 μM. The dotted line represents linear regression of influx rates above 20 μM manganese. Data shown are a representative result of three experiments, each determined in triplicate.

To determine the effects on intracellularly accumulated manganese cellular function, we examined the influence of manganese on K influx. Of the total K influx which was measured using ^{86}Rb as the K congener, nearly one third of the K transport pathway is accounted for by active K influx (data not shown). Moreover, nearly half of the total K influx is accounted for by Na/K/Cl cotransport which was deduced by the Na dependence and bumetanide sensitivity (data not shown). It was found that manganese had no effect on active K influx. However, intracellular manganese elicits an activation of the Na/K/Cl cotransport pathway as shown in FIGURE 4. It is evident that the Na/K/Cl cotransport activity is progressively increased as the intracellular manganese concentrations were raised. However, it is not known whether manganese regulates the cotransporter directly or indirectly through second messengers or ion channels.

TABLE 1. Manganese Uptake by PC-12 Cells

	nmol/mg Protein × Hour
Control	0.34 ± 0.03
100 μM CdCl$_2$	0.14 ± 0.00
100 μM NiCl$_2$	0.19 ± 0.02
100 μM CoCl$_2$	0.13 ± 0.01
100 μM CuSO$_4$	0.23 ± 0.02
100 μM ZnSO$_4$	0.09 ± 0.01
5 μM nifedipine	0.32 ± 0.02
2 μM bradykinin	0.31 ± 0.00
15 μM verapamil	0.31 ± 0.02
100 μM N[6]-cyclohexyladenosine	0.30 ± 0.02
100 μM 5′-(N-ethylcarboxamido)-adenosine	0.33 ± 0.01

PC-12 cells were preincubated for 20 min, then manganese influx was measured in the presence of 10 μM manganese for 1 h at room temperature. Agents listed in the table were present during the preincubation and flux period. Mean ± SE, n = 3.

DISCUSSION

In the companion article of this series, we used PC-12 cells, which have widely been regarded as a model for catecholaminergic neurons, to study the influence of manganese on lipid peroxidation and cell death. In this paper, we examined the manganese transport and subsequent effects of the accumulated manganese on other ion transport systems in PC-12 cells.

As stated earlier, manganese is transported by a saturable process across the blood-brain barrier and in astrocytes. In ferret red blood cells, manganese can be transported through the Na/Ca exchanger.[9] However, Murphy et al.[4] reported that except for the cerebral cortex in which manganese movement is mediated by a saturable process, hippocampus and six other regions of the brain exhibit both saturable and nonsaturable components of manganese transport. The K_m values for manganese vary widely depending on the type of brain cells

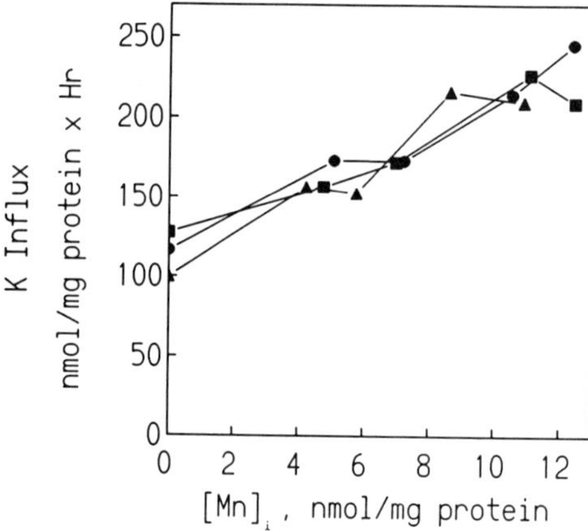

FIGURE 4. Activation of Na/K/Cl cotransport by intracellular manganese in PC-12 cells. To raise intracellular manganese content, which was determined by ^{54}Mn, PC-12 cells were incubated with 0.5 mM manganese for 30, 60, 120, and 180 minutes. K influx was measured after loading the cells with 0.5 mM manganese under identical conditions except lacking ^{54}MnCl$_2$ and washing cells free of manganese. Data shown are results of three experiments, each determined in duplicate. Each experiment is represented by a different symbol.

ranging from 0.3 μM in astrocytes[5] to 18 μM in glial cells.[8] The K_m value determined in PC-12 cells falls within this range. It is more difficult to compare the V_{max} values in these cells since the units used for estimating the cell mass were not always consistent. PC-12 cells and other brain cells having both saturable and nonsaturable manganese transport kinetics would be unable to limit the intracellular manganese content in response to increasing external manganese concentrations. To put it another way, the barrier function with respect to manganese of the plasma membranes of these cells is, in a sense, less competent in that excessive exposure of manganese causes correspondingly high levels of intracellular manganese. Indeed, the intracellular manganese levels measured in FIGURE 3 are several-fold higher than the calculated manganese levels assuming a simple passive distribution of manganese across the plasma membrane.

Our findings show that PC-12 cells possess the Na/K/Cl cotransport pathway which is stimulated by manganese. In ferret red cells, the cotransport is stimulated by magnesium.[10] During manganese loading and the flux measurements, both calcium and magnesium were present which was intended to ensure the attachment of PC-12 cells to the plastic dishes. Thus, it is possible that the basal levels of cotransport measured in PC-12 cells are already stimulated by magnesium. In any case, the ease with which PC-12 cells accumulate manganese suggests its potential role in the regulation of cotransport. We are currently evaluating the hypothesis that a prolonged exposure to trace amounts of manganese leads to an aberration of a selective ion transport system causing neuronal damage.

ACKNOWLEDGMENTS

The authors are grateful to Ms. Jane Burnett for technical assistance and to Ms. Judy Richey for assistance in the preparation of the manuscript.

REFERENCES

1. Prohaska, J. R. 1987. Functions of trace elements in brain metabolism. Physiol. Rev. **67:** 858–901.
2. Keen, C. L., B. Lönnerdal & L. S. Hurley. 1984. Manganese. *In* Biochemistry of the Essential Ultratrace Elements. E. Frieden, Ed. Vol. 3: 89–132. Plenum Press. New York.
3. Seth, P. K. & S. V. Chandra. Neurotoxic effects of manganese. 1988. *In* Metal Neurotoxicity. S. C. Bondy & K. N. Prasad, Eds.: 19–33, CRC Press. Boca Raton, FL.
4. Murphy, V. A., K. C. Wadhwani, Q. R. Smith & S. I. Rapoport. 1991. Saturable transport of manganese (II) across the rat blood-brain barrier. J. Neurochem. **57:** 948–954.
5. Aschner, M., M. Gannon & H. K. Kimelberg. 1992. Manganese uptake and efflux in cultured rat astrocytes. J. Neurochem. **58:** 730–735.
6. Lowry, O. H., N. J. Rosenbrough, A. L. Farr & R. J. Randall. 1951. Protein measurement with the folin phenol reagent. J. Biol. Chem. **193:** 265–275.
7. Kim, H. D., Y. Tsai, C. C. Franklin & J. T. Turner. 1988. Characterization of $Na^+/K^+/Cl^-$ cotransport in cultured HT29 human colonic adenocarcinoma cells. Biochim. Biophys. Acta **946:** 397–404.
8. Wedler, F. C., B. W. Ley & A. A. Grippo. 1989. Manganese (II) dynamics and distribution in glial cells cultured from chick cerebral cortex. Neurochem. Res. **14:** 1129–1135.
9. Frame, M. D. S. & M. A. Milanick. 1991. Mn and Cd transport by the Na-Ca exchanger of ferret red blood cells. Am. J. Physiol. **261:** C467–C475.
10. Flatman, P. W. The effects of magnesium on potassium transport in ferret red cells. 1988. J. Physiol. **397:** 471–487.

Effects of Focal Cerebral Ischemia on Expression and Activity of Inositol 1,4,5-Trisphosphate 3-Kinase in Rat Cortex[a]

G. Y. SUN,[b] T-A. LIN,[b] P. WIXOM,[c] AND R. T. ZOELLER[d]

[b]Department of Biochemistry
[c]Department of Pharmacology
[d]Department of Anatomy and Neurobiology
University of Missouri
Columbia, Missouri 65212

T-N. LIN, Y. Y. HE, AND C. Y. HSU

Division of Restoratory Neurology
Baylor College of Medicine
Houston, Texas 77030

INTRODUCTION

Prolonged cerebral ischemia due to cerebrovascular occlusion (stroke) has been shown to give rise to changes in cellular and metabolic processes leading to neuronal cell death.[1] Although there are indications that perturbation of neuronal Ca^{2+} homeostasis due to stimulation of the glutamate receptor may play an important role in the ischemia-induced neuronal cell death,[2] the exact mechanism underlying this process is not well understood. The primary emphasis of this study is on the metabolism of $Ins(1,4,5)P_3$, a second messenger that is responsible for mobilization of intracellular Ca^{2+} stores.[3] Since this second messenger plays an important role in regulating Ca^{2+} homeostasis within the neurons,[4] perturbation of its metabolism due to prolonged ischemic insult may lead to changes underlying neuronal cell death.

Besides binding to its intracellular receptor,[5] $Ins(1,4,5)P_3$ in cell is regulated by a 5-phosphatase and a 3-kinase.[6] The 5-phosphatase converts $Ins(1,4,5)P_3$ to $Ins(1,4)P_2$ and subsequently $Ins(4)P$. The 3-kinase is responsible for the synthesis of $Ins(1,3,4,5)P_4$, a compound which can also mobilize Ca^{2+} from an unknown source.[7] The $Ins(1,3,4,5)P_4$ is subsequently hydrolyzed to $Ins(1)P$. In this study, the effects of cerebral ischemia on these enzymes were examined utilizing a rat model of focal ischemia induced by temporary occlusion of the middle cerebral artery (MCA) together with the common carotid arteries.[8,9] This model has been shown to produce predictable focal cerebral infarcts depending on the time duration of ligation.[8,9] Previous studies have indicated that the ischemic insult led to a rapid breakdown of poly-phosphoinositides in the ischemic MCA cortex,[10] suggesting that $Ins(1,4,5)P_3$ is released during the initial phase of the ischemic insult.

[a] This research project was supported in part by USPHS research grant NS30178 from NINDS.

EXPERIMENTAL

Using the procedures described by Lee *et al*[11] and Heacock *et al.*,[12] assay of the activity of the 3-kinase and 5-phosphatase in brain tissue revealed obvious regional differences. High levels of the 3-kinase activity are found in the hippocampus, whereas activity of the 5-phosphatase is highest in the cerebellum (FIG. 1). When activities of these enzymes were assayed with respect to time of MCA occlusion, there was a time-dependent decrease in the 3-kinase activity in the right (ischemic) MCA cortex but activity in the left MCA cortex was not altered appreciably[13] (FIG. 2). Under similar conditions, there was a slight increase in the 5-phosphatase activity in the right MCA cortex but this change was not dependent

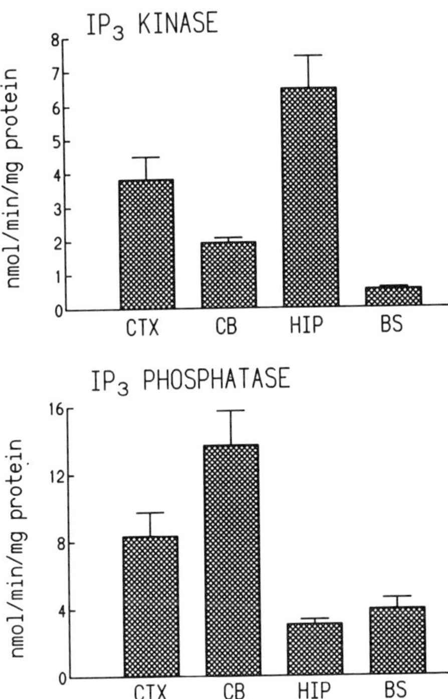

FIGURE 1. Activity of Ins(1,4,5)P$_3$ 3-kinase and 5-phosphatase in different regions of mouse brain. See reference 13 for details of enzyme assay procedure. IP$_3$ 3-kinase activity is expressed as nmol of IP$_4$ formed per min per mg protein and the 5-phosphatase activity is expressed as nmol of IP$_2$ and IP$_1$ formed per min per mg protein. **Abbreviations:** CTX, cerebral cortex; CB, cerebellum; HIP, hippocampus; BS, brain stem.

on the time of the ischemic insult. The ischemia-induced decrease in the 3-kinase activity was irreversible, as shown in FIGURE 3. In fact, there was a further decline in enzyme activity around 6 h after recirculation. By 24 h after a 60 min insult, a time when 90% of animals affected would have developed obvious focal infarcts, activity of the 3-kinase in the right MCA was practically abolished, whereas activity of the 5-phosphatase remained unchanged (FIG. 3).

The initial decrease in Ins(1,4,5)P$_3$ 3-kinase activity during the ischemic insult is not entirely surprising since this enzyme is susceptible to limited proteolysis by neutral calcium proteases such as calpain.[13] Furthermore, the purified enzyme[14] also shows several putative phosphorylation sites for cAMP-dependent protein

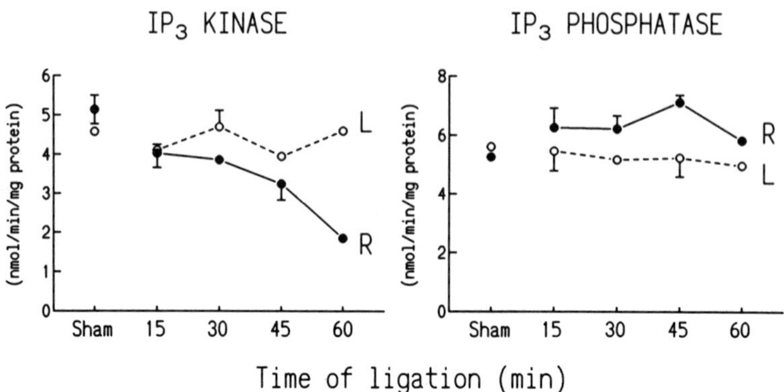

FIGURE 2. Activity of Ins(1,4,5)P$_3$ 3-kinase and 5-phosphatase in left (L, *open circle*) and right (R, *closed circle*) rat MCA cortex with respect to time of ischemic insult. Sham-operated controls are tissues from rats that were subjected to the same surgical procedures but without occlusion of the arteries. See reference 13 for details of the enzyme assay procedure. (Data reproduced from reference 13 with permission from Academic Press.)

kinase, protein kinase C, and Ca^{2+}/calmodulin-dependent protein kinase II. Thus, modification of enzyme activity may be affected by any one of these factors. Nevertheless, the second decline in enzyme activity during the reperfusion period further suggests that additional damage to the enzyme has occurred.

Experiments were carried out to determine whether the second phase of decrease in 3-kinase activity is related to a change in the mRNA expression encoding

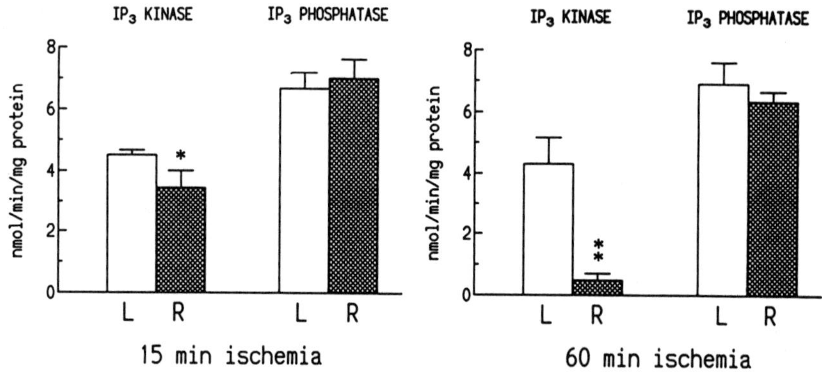

FIGURE 3. Activity of Ins(1,4,5)P$_3$ 3-kinase and 5-phosphatase in left (L) and right (R) MCA cortex with 24 h reperfusion after a 15 min or a 60 min ischemic insult. Values are mean ± SD from 4 brains. Statistical analysis based on Student's *t*-test indicates significant differences comparing the right (ischemic) MCA cortex to that on the left side, *$p < 0.05$; **$p < 0.005$. (Data reproduced from reference 13 with permission from Academic Press.)

this enzyme protein. Two oligomer probes similar to those described by Mailleux *et al.*[15] were synthesized for hybridization studies. Analysis of the levels of mRNA by Northern blot hybridization of labeled probes with total RNA isolated from rat brain cortex indicated a single band in the autoradiogram. Levels of Ins(1,4,5)P$_3$ 3-kinase mRNA in the left and right cortices were examined at various times after a 90 min ischemic insult. There was no obvious change in mRNA levels until 18 h after the ischemic insult and by 3 days, mRNA in the right cortex was almost abolished (FIG. 4). In most experiments, a β-actin probe was used for normalizing the amount of RNA applied to the gel. However, an induction of the mRNA for this protein was observed at 18 h and 3 days after the ischemic insult. Thus, the decrease in levels of mRNA for Ins(1,4,5)P$_3$ 3-kinase was marked by a concomitant increase in the levels of β-actin.

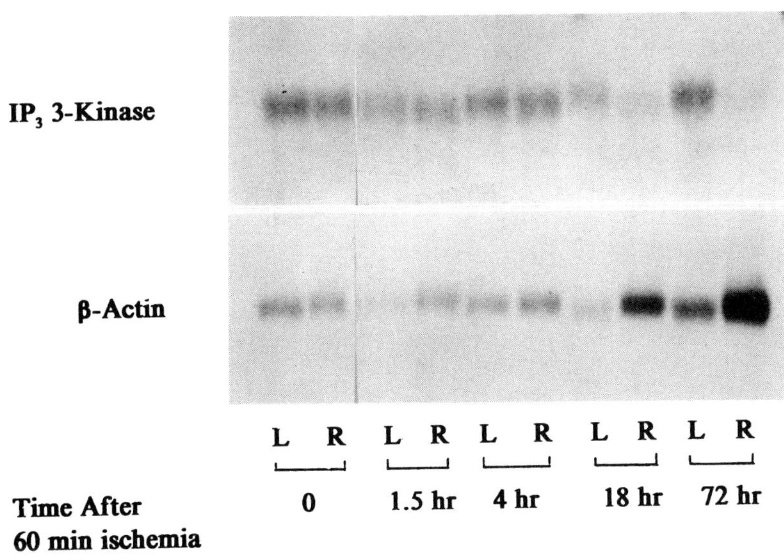

FIGURE 4. Northern blot analysis of the mRNA expression of Ins(1,4,5)P$_3$ 3-kinase in the left and right cortices of Long Evans rats at different times after a 90 min MCA occlusion. Each lane of the gel contained @ 20 μg RNA from brain cortex. Total RNA was blotted to membranes (GeneScreen, NEN) which were sequentially hybridized with ^{32}P-labeled probes for Ins(1,4,5)P$_3$ 3-kinase and β-actin.

In situ hybridization of frozen brain coronal sections was used to examine the 3-kinase mRNA in different brain regions after the ischemic insult. In agreement with the results of Mailleux *et al.*,[14] high levels of the Ins(1,4,5)P$_3$ 3-kinase mRNA were found in the hippocampus and in the dentate gyrus (FIG. 5). There was no change in mRNA expression in the right MCA cortex after 60 min of ischemic insult. However, a small but discernable increase in message could be observed in the right MCA cortex at 8 h after the insult. By 24 h after a 60 min of ischemic insult, the right MCA cortex was almost devoid of mRNA. Interestingly, the decrease in message was confined mainly to the neocortical area whereas the hippocampus was not affected (FIG. 5).

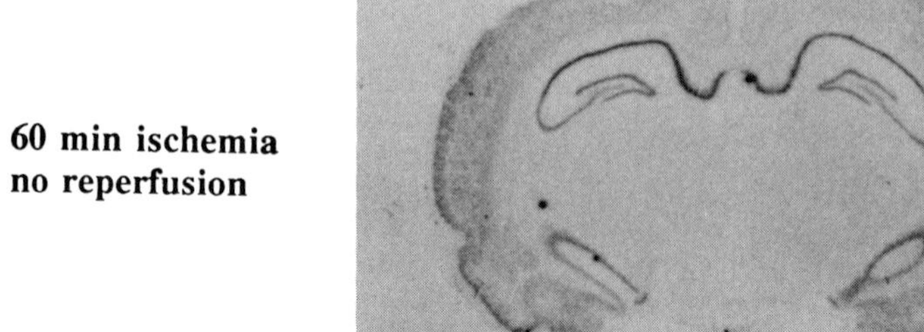

**60 min ischemia
no reperfusion**

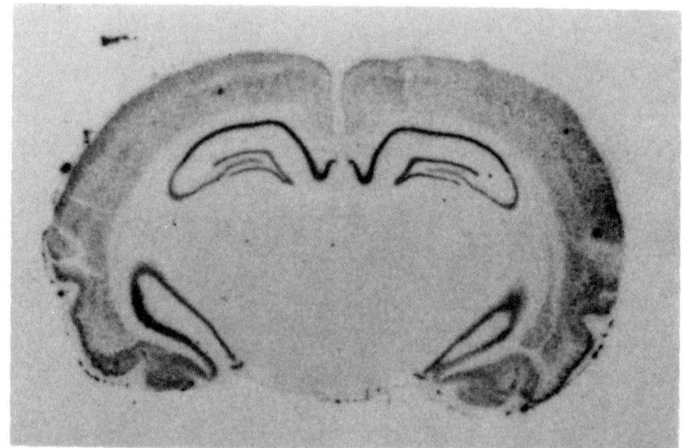

**60 min ischemia
8 hr reperfusion**

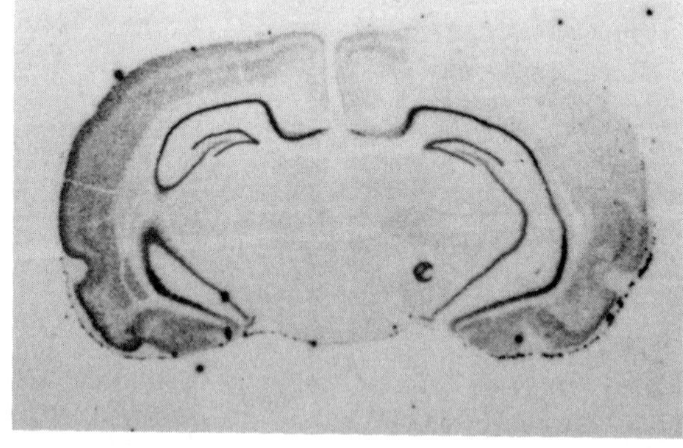

**60 min ischemia
24 hr reperfusion**

FIGURE 5. *In situ* hybridization of rat brain coronal sections demonstrating the expression of Ins(1,4,5)P$_3$ 3-kinase mRNA at 0, 8 and 24 h after 60 min ischemic insult.

SUMMARY

Results from this study clearly indicate that $Ins(1,4,5)P_3$ 3-kinase is a target enzyme of cerebral ischemia insult. This enzyme is responsible for removal of $Ins(1,4,5)P_3$ which, in turn, plays an important role in the maintenance of intracellular Ca^{2+} homeostasis. Not only did a time-dependent decrease in enzyme activity occur due to the focal cerebral ischemic insult, but there was also a second phase for the decline in enzyme activity around 6 h after the insult. Examination of the mRNA for the 3-kinase in frozen brain sections suggested an increase in message at a time (around 8 h) prior to development of tissue infarct. Since the initial decline in enzyme activity during ligation correlated well with the time for development of an infarct, assay of this enzyme could be used as a biochemical marker of cerebral ischemic insult.

REFERENCES

1. SIESJO, B. K. 1988. Historical overview. Calcium, ischemia, and death of brain cells. Ann. N.Y. Acad. Sci. **522:** 638–661.
2. CHOI, D. W. 1988. Calcium-mediated neurotoxicity: Relationship to specific channel types and role in ischemic damage. TINS **11:** 465–469.
3. BERRIDGE, M. J. 1987. Inositol trisphosphate and diacylglycerol: Two interacting second messengers. Ann. Rev. Biochem. **56:** 159–193.
4. NAHORSKI, S. R. 1988. Inositol polyphosphates and neuronal calcium homeostasis. Trends Neurosci. **11:** 444–448.
5. MIGNERY, G. A., C. L. NEWTON, B. T. ARCHER & T. C. SUDHOF. 1990. Structure and expression of the rat inositol 1,4,5-trisphosphate receptor. J. Biol. Chem. **265:** 12679–12685.
6. ERNEUX, C. & K. TAKAZAWA. 1991. Intracellular control of inositol phosphates by their metabolizing enzymes. TINS **12:** 174–176.
7. BERRIDGE, M. J. & R. IRVINE. 1989. Inositol phosphates and cell signalling. Nature **341:** 197–205.
8. CHEN, S. T., C. Y. HSU, E. L. HOGAN, H. MARICQ AND J. P. BALENTINE. 1986. A model of focal ischemic stroke in the rat: Reproducible extensive cortical infarction. Stroke **17:** 738–743.
9. LIU, T. H., J. S. BECKMAN, B. A. FREEMAN, E. L. HOGAN & C. Y. HSU. 1989. Polyethylene-glyco-conjugated superoxide dismutase and catalase reduce ischemic brain injury. Am. J. Physiol. **256:** H589–H593.
10. LIN, T-N., T. H. LIU, Y. XU, C. Y. HSU & G. Y. SUN. 1990. Effect of focal ischemia on poly-phosphoinositide breakdown in rat cortex. Stroke **22:** 495–498.
11. LEE, S. Y., S. S. SIM, J. W. KIM, K. H. MOON, J. H. KIM & S. G. RHEE. 1990. Purification and Properties of D-myo-inositol 1,4,5-trisphosphate 3-kinase from rat brain. J. Biol. Chem. **265:** 9434–9440.
12. HEACOCK, A., E. SEQUIN, & B. AGRANOFF. 1990. Developmental and regional studies of the metabolism of inositol 1,4,5-trisphosphate in rat brain. J. Neurochem. **54:** 1405–1411.
13. LIN, T-A., T-N. LIN, Y. Y. HE, C. Y. HSU & G. Y. SUN. 1992. Effects of focal cerebral ischemia on inositol 1,4,5-trisphosphate 3-kinase and 5-phosphatase activities in rat cortex. Biochem. Biophys. Res. Commun. **184:** 871–877.
14. JOHANSON, R. A., C. A. HANSON & J. R. WILLIAMSON. 1988. Purification of D-myoinositol 1,4,5-trisphosphate 3-kinase from rat brain. J. Biol. Chem. **263:** 7465–7471.
15. MAILLEUX, P., K. TAKAZAWA, C. ERNEUX & J. J. VANDERHAEGHEN. 1991. Inositol 1,4,5-trisphosphate 3-kinase mRNA: High levels in the rat hippocampal CA1 pyramidal and dentate gyrus granule cells and in cerebellar purkinje cells. J. Neurochem. **56:** 345–347.

The Neuronal Cytoskeleton
in Disorders of Late Onset
and Slow Progression

MICHAEL J. STRONG,[a,b] IKURO WAKAYAMA,[c]
AND RALPH M. GARRUTO[c,d]

[b]Department of Clinical Neurological Sciences
The University of Western Ontario
London, Ontario, Canada

[c]The National Institute of Neurological Disorders and Stroke
The National Institutes of Health
Bethesda, Maryland 20892

Within the last decade, we have gained significant insights into the role of the neuronal cytoskeleton in neurodegenerative disorders of late onset and slow progression, including amyotrophic lateral sclerosis (ALS), Alzheimer's disease and Parkinson's disease. While these disorders differ significantly in their clinical manifestations, each reflects the degeneration of specific neuronal populations, often accompanied by the induction of a variety of intraneuronal inclusions. There is mounting evidence of a disturbance in the regulation of neuronal cytoskeletal protein metabolism underlying several of these disorders. Understanding the cellular and molecular mechanisms giving rise to these inclusions in both naturally occurring and experimental disease states will provide an understanding of the pathogenesis of these disorders with an ultimate goal aimed at intervention.

AMYOTROPHIC LATERAL SCLEROSIS

Among adult onset neurodegenerative disorders, ALS is perhaps the best understood in that the neuropathology is well-defined and several natural and experimental models exist that provide insights into the pathophysiology of the disease process. Three clinically indistinguishable variants are recognized—classical sporadic, familial, and western Pacific. Classical sporadic ALS is an age-dependent neurodegenerative process with little worldwide variability in incidence rates of 1.0–1.8/100,000 population, although increasing incidence rates disproportionate to the rate of aging of the population have been observed.[1,2] The disease manifests as a uniformly fatal muscular wasting and weakness while sparing intellect, oculomotor, and sensory modalities.

The neuropathological hallmark of all ALS variants is a topographically specific loss of descending supraspinal motor pathways and lower motor neurons. Amongst the earliest neuropathological findings are the presence of abnormal

[a] M. J. Strong is supported by a Medical Research Council of Canada Scholarship.
[d] Address correspondence to: Ralph M. Garruto, Ph.D., Bldg. 36, Rm. 5B-21, NINDS, NIH, Bethesda, Maryland 20892.

numbers of inracytoplasmic inclusions and neuroaxonal swellings, consisting of inerwoven skeins or parallel arrays of morphologically normal phosphorylated neurofilament within degenerating motor neurons.[3–5] This immunohistochemical observation has been taken to indicate a fundamental abnormality in the process of neurofilament phosphorylation in the induction of ALS.

In addition to neurofilamentous inclusions, hyaline inclusions,[6] lipofuscin, Lewy body-like inclusions,[7,8] and Bunina bodies have been observed. The latter 2–5 μm diameter conglomerates consist of homogenous electron-dense material with a rim of ribosomal particles that may reflect a condensation of the larger hyaline inclusions.[3] Although the majority of these intracytoplasmic inclusions are ubiquitin-conjugated, diffuse ubiquitin immunoreactivity[7] and skeins of ubiquitin-immunoreactive material are also observed within motor neurons,[4] suggesting that ubiquitin-conjugated fibril accumulation may be an early feature of ALS. While this phenomenon is not unique to ALS, it does suggest either an ineffective ATP-dependent nonlysosomal proteolytic degradation or a resistance of the cytoskeletal protein to this pathway.

The dramatic decline in incidence in the once hyperendemic western Pacific foci of ALS has provided an insight into the role of environmental factors in the pathogenesis of ALS.[9] The demonstration of a 20 year latency period prior to disease onset in Chamorro migrants from Guam[10] and in Filipino migrants to Guam[11] and the failure to find evidence for a genetic or infectious etiology[12] suggests that the western Pacific variant of ALS was an environmentally induced and place-specific disease phenomenon, associated with abnormally low calcium and magnesium levels and high levels of bioavailable aluminum in garden soil and drinking water. Coupled with observations of abnormalities in vitamin D and calcium metabolism,[13] radiographic and densitometric decreases in bone mass,[14] and the finding of intraneuronal co-localization of calcium, aluminum and silicon within degenerating neurons in patients with Guamanian ALS and parkinsonism-dementia,[15] a working hypothesis has been put forth that chronic dietary deficiencies associated with the Guam environment induce a form of secondary hyperparathyroidism accompanied by enhanced gastrointestinal absorption of bioavailable aluminum.[9] This hypothesis has been supported by the experimental induction of neuropathological lesions reminiscent of those seen in human ALS and in non-human primates (cynomolgus monkeys and macaques) chronically fed a hypocalcemic, aluminum-supplemented diet.[16,17]

ALZHEIMER'S DISEASE

Similar to ALS, Alzheimer's disease (AD), the most common adult onset neurodegenerative disorder, also demonstrates age-specific incidence rates with estimates of 17–30% of the population at age 80 clinically affected.[18] The cerebral cortex of patients with Alzheimer's disease demonstrates widespread and significant changes when compared to normal aged individuals, including neurofibrillary tangles, neuropil threads, and senile plaques. Although each of these lesions can be seen in other neurodegenerative diseases and to some extent in normal aged individuals, their combination and numbers are the classical hallmark of Alzheimer's disease. Moreover, the presence and severity of dementia has been correlated with senile plaque density,[19] neurofibrillary tangle density,[20] loss of neurons,[21] and the extent of neuropil threads.[22]

In Alzheimer's disease, cell death is preceded by the development of dystrophic changes, notably neurofibrillary pathology, in at least a subset of neurons. These cytoskeletal abnormalities, first recognized histochemically as neurofibrillary tangles, are made of paired helical filaments in which aberrantly phosphorylated form of a cytoskeletal protein, the microtubule-associated protein tau, is a major component.[23,24] Monoclonal antibodies produced against Alzheimer's disease brain homogenates[25] have been shown to recognize aberrantly phosphorylated tau protein. Additionally, aberrantly phosphorylated tau protein accumulates within neurons prior to the development of neurofibrillary tangles.[26]

Neurites displaying abnormal morphology—dystrophic neurites—constitute a major feature of Alzheimer's disease. While many of these originate from aberrant sprouting, it has not been proven that this is the case for all dystrophic neurites. The abnormal neurites of Alzheimer's disease form two distinct subsets. One of these, neuropil threads, consists of randomly oriented tau-immunoreactive processes, probably derived from dendrites of tangle-bearing neurons.[27] The second type of dystrophic neurites are arranged in clusters around amyloid deposits, forming classic plaques. These senile plaque neurites express a variety of markers, including tau protein.[28] While the latter may indicate that dendrites are incorporated in plaques, other neurites in these structures express axonally transported proteins, such as the synaptic vesicle protein synaptophysin, chromogranin A,[29] a soluble protein of dense core synaptic vesicles, and amyloid β-precursor protein.[30]

EXPERIMENTAL MODELING

It remains unresolved whether the genesis of neurofilamentous inclusions in ALS or neurofibrillary tangles in Alzheimer's disease is dependent solely on aberrant phosphorylation of cytoskeletal proteins, or is a consequence of the aggregation of normal cytoskeletal proteins which are then secondarily phosphorylated. While an experimental model that recapitulates the ultrastructural features of Alzheimer's disease does not exist, both the topographic selectivity and morphological characteristics of neurofilamentous inclusions in spinal motor neurons in ALS can be mimicked by *in vivo* and *in vitro* models of aluminum neurotoxicity.[31-34]

In contrast to conventional acute models of aluminum neurotoxicity that are accompanied by an acute fulminant encephalopathy marked by seizuring, quadraparesis and death (10 to 14 days post inoculation) with diffuse, nonspecific neuronal degeneration and suppression of gene transcription that is not known to occur in ALS,[35,36] chronic sublethal inoculums of aluminum chloride induce a slowly progressive motor neuron degeneration. In this "chronic" model, repeated intracisternal inoculations of low dose (100 μg) $AlCl_3$ once monthly in young adult New Zealand white rabbits (age 8–9 wks) leads to the development of a spastic myelopathy[33] and the formation of neurofilamentous inclusions in spinal motor neurons and select brainstem nuclei. These inclusions have a spectrum of immunoreactivity with monoclonal antibodies against phosphorylated and nonphosphorylated epitopes of neurofilament subunit proteins—reminiscent of the immunohistochemical studies of ALS reported by Schmidt *et al.*[5] Regardless of the phosphorylation state, all inclusions consist of interwoven skeins of morphologically identical 10 nm intermediate filaments. *In vitro* observations suggest that the preferential involvement of motor neurons in this chronic model reflects their specific threshold to aluminum neurotoxicity.[32]

Finally, we are in the process of exploring new natural experimental models of chronic neurodegeneration in fish from aicd rain lakes that are relevant to the neuronal injury and degeneration observed in chronic experimental aluminum intoxication and in human disorders of late onset and slow progression. While it is known that aluminum is the main toxicant leading to fish extinction in areas where acid rain has leached metal from minerals in the soil,[37] with the main target organ being the gill structure, the nervous system of these fish has not been previously examined. We have now demonstrated that the central nervous system of fish from aluminum-rich lakes develop neuropathological changes such as chromatolysis, perikaryal and neuritic inclusions, and plaque-like structures consisting of aggregated cytoskeletal proteins including neurofilament and microtubule associated protein tau.[38] By histochemical staining with solochrome azurine, we found widespread aluminum deposition in fresh unfixed cryocut olfactory epithelium of all fish from aluminum-rich lakes. In one fish, we also found diffuse, but clear aluminum staining inside the olfactory bulb.

In summary, a major lesson from our long-term studies of the cellular and molecular mechanisms of neuronal degeneration in Alzheimer's disease, ALS and parkinsonism in the western Pacific, and in our chronic *in vivo* and *in vitro* experimental studies of neuronal degeneration is that it is crucial to avoid premature conclusions from simplistic study designs and experimental protocols regarding the relevance of environmental agents in the etiology of neurodegenerative disorders of long latency and slow progression. Many researchers are now concentrating their efforts on questions of aluminum bioavailability and mechanisms of pathogenesis and on the development of new experimental models in an attempt to move us away (at least temporarily) from the controversy and emotion surrounding aluminum as an etiological factor in human neurodegenerative disorders towards testable hypotheses regarding aluminum intoxication that may ultimately bring us nearer to solutions that have evaded us for decades.

REFERENCES

1. DURRLEMAN, S. & A. ALPEROVITCH. 1989. Increasing trend of ALS in France and elsewhere: Are the changes real? Neurology **39:** 768–773.
2. LILIENFELD, D. E., J. EHLAND, P. J. LANDRIGAN, E. CHAN, J. GODBOLD, G. MARSH & D. P. PERL. 1989. Rising mortality from motoneuron disease in the USA, 1962–84. Lancet (April 1): 710–712.
3. CHOU, S. M. 1979. Pathognomy of intraneuronal inclusions in ALS. *In* Amyotrophic Lateral Sclerosis. Y. Tsubaki & T. Toyokura, Eds.: 135–176. University of Tokyo Press, Tokyo.
4. LEIGH, P. & M. SWASH. 1991. Cytoskeletal pathology in motor neuron diseases. *In* Advances in Neurology, Amyotrophic Lateral Sclerosis and Other Motor Neuron Diseases. L. P. Rowland, Ed.: 115–124. Raven Press Ltd. New York.
5. SCHMIDT, M. L., M. J. CARDEN, V. M.-Y. LEE & J. Q. TROJANOWSKI. 1987. Phosphate dependent and independent neurofilament epitopes in the axonal swellings of patients with motor neuron disease and controls. Lab. Invest. **56:** 282–294.
6. HIRANO, A. 1991. Cytopathology of amyotrophic lateral sclerosis. *In* Advances in Neurology, Amyotrophic Lateral Sclerosis and Other Motor Neuron Disorders. L. P. Rowland, Ed.: 91–101. Raven Press Ltd. New York.
7. MURAYAMA, S., H. MORI, Y. IHARA, W. BOULDIN, K. SUZUKI & M. TOMONAGA. 1990. Immunocytochemical and ultrastructural studies of lower motor neurons in amyotrophic lateral sclerosis. Ann. Neurol. **27:** 137–148.
8. WAKAYAMA, I. 1992. Morphometry of spinal motor neurons in amyotrophic lateral sclerosis with special reference to chromatolysis and intracytoplasmic inclusion bodies. Brain Res. **586:** 12–18.
9. GARRUTO, R. M. 1991. Pacific paradigms of environmentally-induced neurological

disorders: Clinical, epidemiological and molecular perspectives. Neurotoxicology **12:** 347–377.

10. GARRUTO, R. M., D. C. GAJDUSEK & K.-M. CHEN. 1980. Amyotrophic lateral sclerosis among Chamorro migrants from Guam. Ann. Neurol. **8:** 612–619.

11. GARRUTO, R. M., D. C. GAJDUSEK & K.-M. CHEN. 1981. Amyotrophic lateral sclerosis and parkinsonism-dementia among Filipino migrants to Guam. Ann. Neurol. **10:** 341–350.

12. GIBBS, C. J., JR. & D. C. GAJDUSEK. 1982. An update of long-term in vivo and in vitro studies designed to identify a virus as the cause of amyotrophic lateral sclerosis, parkinsonism dementia, and Parkinson's disease. *In* Human Motor Neuron Diseases. L. P. Rowland, Ed.: 343–353. Raven Press. New York.

13. YANAGIHARA, R., R. M. GARRUTO, D. C. GAJDUSEK, A. TOMITA, T. UCHIKAWA, Y. KONAGAYA, K.-M. CHEN, I. SOBUE, C. C. PLATO & C. J. GIBBS, JR. 1984. Calcium and vitamin D metabolism in Guamanian Chamorros with amyotrophic lateral sclerosis and parkinsonism-dementia. Ann. Neurol. **15:** 42–48.

14. PLATO, C. C., R. M. GARRUTO, R. YANAGIHARA, K.-M. CHEN, J. L. WOOD, D. C. GAJDUSEK & A. N. NORRIS. 1982. Cortical bone loss and measurements of the second metacarpal bone. I. Comparisons between adult Guamanian Chamorros and American Caucasians. Am. J. Phys. Anthropol. **59:** 461–465.

15. GARRUTO, R. M., R. FUKATSU, R. YANAGIHARA, D. C. GAJDUSEK, G. HOOK & C. E. FIORI. 1984. Imaging of calcium and aluminum in neurofibrillary tangle-bearing neurons in parkinsonism-dementia of Guam. Proc. Natl. Acad. Sci. USA **81:** 1875–1879.

16. GARRUTO, R. M., S. K. SHANKAR, R. YANAGIHARA, A. M. SALAZAR, H. L. AMYX & D. C. GAJDUSEK. 1989. Low-calcium, high aluminum diet-induced motor neuron pathology in cynomolgus monkeys. Acta. Neuropathol. (Berl). **78:** 210–219.

17. YANO, I., S. YOSHIDA, Y. UEBAYASHI, F. YOSHIMASU & Y. YASE. 1989. Degenerative changes in the central nervous system of Japanese monkeys induced by oral administration of aluminum salt. Biomed. Res. **10:** 33–41.

18. EVANS, D. A., H. H. FUNKENSTEIN, M. S. ALBERT, P. A. SCHERR, N. R. COOK, M. J. CHOWN, L. E. HEBERT, C. H. HENNEKENS & J. O. TAYLOR. 1989. Prevalence of Alzheimer's disease in a community population of older patients. Higher than previously reported. JAMA **262:** 2551–2556.

19. BLESSED, G., B. E. TOMLINSON & M. ROTH. 1968. The association between quantitative measures of dementia and of senile change in the cerebral grey matter of elderly subjects. Br. J. Psychiat. **114:** 797–811.

20. WILCOCK, G. K. & M. M. ESIRI. 1982. Plaques, tangles and dementia: A quantitative study. J. Neurol. Sci. **56:** 343–356.

21. HANSEN, L. A., R. DETEREA, P. DAVIES & R. D. TERRY. 1988. Neocortical morphometry, lesion counts, and choline acetyltransferase levels in the age spectrum of Alzheimer's disease. Neurology **38:** 48–54.

22. MCKEE, A. C., K. S. KOSIK & N. W. KOWALL. 1991. Neuritic pathology and dementia in Alzheimer's Disease. Ann. Neurol. **30:** 156–165.

23. KOSIK, K. S., C. L. JOACHIM & D. J. SELKOE. 1986. Microtubule-associated protein tau (t) is a major antigenic component of paired helical filaments in Alzheimer disease. Proc. Natl. Acad. Sci. USA **83:** 4044–4048.

24. WOOD, J. G., S. S. MIRRA, N. J. POLLOCK & L. I. BINDER. 1986. Neurofibrillary tangles of Alzheimer disease share antigenic determinants with the axonal microtubule-associated protein tau (*t*). Proc. Natl. Acad. Sci. USA **83:** 4040–4043.

25. HYMAN, B. T., G. W. VANHOESE, B. L. WOLOZIN, P. DAVIES, L. J. KROMER & A. R. DAMASIO. 1989. Alzheimer-50 antibody recognizes Alzheimer-related neuronal changes. Ann. Neurol. **23:** 371–379.

26. GRUNDKE-IQBAL, I., K. IQBAL, Y.-C. TUNG, M. QUINLAN, H. M. WISNIEWSKI & L. I. BINDER. 1986. Abnormal phosphorylation of the microtubule-associated protein tau in Alzheimer cytoskeletal pathology. Proc. Natl. Acad. Sci. USA **83:** 4913–4917.

27. BRAAK, H. & E. BRAAK. 1988. Neuropil threads occur in dendrites of tangle-bearing nerve cells. Neuropathol. Appl. Neurobiol. **14:** 39–44.

28. SCHMIDT, M. L., V. M.-Y. LEE & J. Q. TROJANOWSKI. 1991. Comparative epitope analysis of neuronal cytoskeletal proteins in Alzheimer's Disease senile plaque neurites and neuropil threads. Lab. Invest. **64:** 352–357.
29. MUNOZ, D. G. 1991. Chromogranin A-Like immunoreactive neurites are major constituents of senile plaques. Lab. Invest. **64:** 826–832.
30. SHOJI, M., S. HIRAI, H. YAMAGUCHI, Y. HARIGAYA & T. KAWARABAYASHI. 1990. Amyloid B-protein precursor accumulates in dystrophic neurites of senile plaques in Alzheimer-type dementia. Brain Res. **512:** 164–168.
31. STRONG, M. J., R. YANAGIHARA, A. V. WOLFF, S. H. SHANKAR & R. M. GARRUTO. 1990. Experimental neurofilamentous aggregates: Acute and chronic models of aluminum-induced encephalomyelopathy in rabbits. *In* The Etiology of Amyotrophic Lateral Sclerosis: New Advances in Toxicology and Epidemiology. F. C. Rose & F. B. Norris, Eds.: 157–173. Smith-Gordon. London.
32. STRONG, M. J. & R. M. GARRUTO. 1991. Neuron specific thresholds of aluminum toxicity in vitro: A comparative analysis of dissociated fetal rabbit hippocampal and motor neuron-enriched cultures. Lab. Invest. **65(2):** 243–249.
33. STRONG, M. J., A. V. WOLFF, I. WAKAYAMA & R. M. GARRUTO. 1991. Aluminum-induced chronic myelopathy in rabbits. Neurotoxicology **12:** 9–22.
34. WAKAYAMA, I., V. R. NERURKAR, M. J. STRONG & R. M. GARRUTO. 1992. Comparison of progressive motor neuron degeneration in chronic experimental aluminum intoxication and amyotrophic lateral sclerosis. Neurology **42** Suppl. 3: 456.
35. KREKOSKI, C. A., A. MATHEW & I. M. PARHAD. 1988. Neuronal gene transcription is decreased with aluminum treatment. J. Cell. Biol. **9:** 123–138.
36. MUMA, N. A., J. C. TRONCOSO, P. N. HOFFMAN, E. H. KOO & D. L. PRICE. 1988. Aluminum neurotoxicity: Altered expression of cytoskeletal genes. Mol. Brain. Res. **3:** 115–122.
37. BAKER, J. P. & C. L. SCHOFIELD. 1982. Aluminum toxicity to fish in acidic waters. Water, Air and Soil Pollution. **18:** 289–309.
38. GARRUTO, R. M., T. P. FLATEN & I. WAKAYAMA. 1993. Natural and experimental models of environmentally-induced neurodegeneration: Implications for Alzheimer's disease. *In* Alzheimer's Disease: Advances in Clinical and Basic Research. B. Corain, K. Iqbal, M. Nicolini, B. Winblad, H. Wisniewski & P. Zatta, Eds.: 257–266. John Wiley and Sons. London.

Long-term Changes in Glial Fibrillary Acidic Protein and Calcium Levels in Rat Hippocampus after a Single Systemic Dose of Kainic Acid

KORNELIS J. VAN DEN BERG[a,b]
AND JAN BERT P. GRAMSBERGEN[b,c]

[b]Department of Neurotoxicology and Applied Neurosciences
TNO-Medical Biological Laboratory
P.O. B5815
2280HV Rijswijk, the Netherlands

[c]Department of Public Health
Erasmus University
Rotterdam, the Netherlands

INTRODUCTION

Recent neurochemical developments suggest the potential use of glial fibrillary acidic protein (GFAP) and Calcium as biochemical markers of neurotoxicity. GFAP is synthesized and deposited as part of scar tissue during an astrocytic response to insults of the CNS[1] and may, in principle, fulfill the role of a more or less permanent marker of *past* neurotoxic effects.[2] In a variety of pathological conditions, including (excito)toxic exposure, hypertrophy of astrocytes in selectively vulnerable brain areas has been shown using immunocytochemistry with GFAP antibodies.[3,4] Recently, regional changes of GFAP in the brains of animals intracerebrally exposed to excitotoxins[5] or systemically exposed to neurotoxic chemicals such as trimethyl-tin (TMT)[6] or 1-methyl-4-phenyl-1,2,3,6-tetrahydropyridine (MPTP)[7] have also been assessed quantitatively using immunodotblot or ELISA. The time course of changes in GFAP levels in the hippocampus of rats exposed to TMT revealed a maximum response between 2–5 weeks, the levels were still enhanced about 3 months after dosing.[6] In the case of MPTP, a transient increase of GFAP levels in the striatum of exposed mice was found reaching nearly normal levels within a 3 week period.[7]

Calcium overload has been implicated in nerve cell death under a variety of pathological conditions, including cerebral ischemia,[8] status epilepticus[9] or intoxications.[10] Accumulation of $^{45}Ca^{2+}$ in the brain after systemic administration of the radiolabel has been used as an index of experimental brain damage.[11–13] Although those studies report a correlation between the amount of region-specific $^{45}Ca^{2+}$ accumulation and severity of histological damage, the relationship between nerve cell degeneration and cerebral $^{45}Ca^{2+}$ accumulation is still not clear. Therefore, in the present study the early onset and the magnitude of the response as

---

[a] Address correspondence to Kornelis J. van den Berg, Ph.D.

well as persistence of changes in both $^{45}Ca^{2+}$ and GFAP levels were evaluated in target and non-target brain areas of kainate-treated rats. Kainic acid (KA), a potent excitotoxin and convulsant, has been suggested as a model for human temporal lobe epilepsy.[4] KA acts as an agonist at KA- and α-amino-3-hydroxy-5-methyl-4-isoxazole propionic acid (AMPA)-sensitive glutamate receptors. Upon activation of KA receptors, endogenous excitatory amino acids are released, causing increased intracellular calcium levels either indirectly via KA or AMPA receptor mediated depolarization and voltage-dependent Ca-channels or directly via the N-methyl-D-asapartate (NMDA) or AMPA receptor-operated Ca-channels.[14,15]

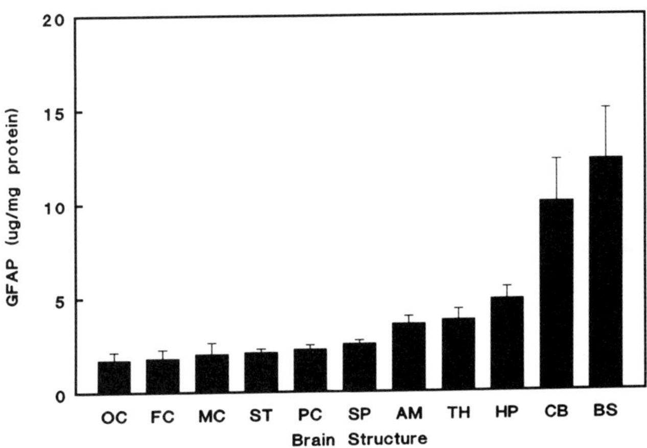

FIGURE 1. GFAP levels in different brain structures of control rats. Brains of untreated rats were dissected and GFAP in the structures was analyzed as described. The data represent mean values ± SEM of 6–11 independent determinations, each comprising a group of 5 animals (*i.e.*, 30–55 animals per structure). **Abbreviations:** OC, occipital cortex; FC, frontal cortex; MC, motor cortex; ST, striatum; PC, piriform cortex; SP, septum; AM, amygdala; TH, thalamus; HP, hippocampus; CB, cerebellum; BS, brain stem.

METHODS

WAG/Rij rats (male, 12 weeks old, 7 animals per group) were treated with a single i.p. dose of 12 mg/kg kainic acid (2 mg KA in 1 ml phosphate-buffered saline) or vehicle. Most of the animals went through a phase of severe convulsions that lasted for a few hours. KA-injected rats without seizures were omitted from the statistical analysis. At selected times, from day 0 (the day of KA administration) up to 6 months after dosing, groups of animals were injected i.p. with 10 μCi (N = 5 for liquid scintilation counting) or 100 μCi $^{45}CaCl_2$ (N = 2 for autoradiography) in 1 ml saline i.p. Twenty-four hours after injection of the radiolabel, the animals were killed by decapitation and their brains were stored at $-70°C$ until use for autoradiography[13] or immediately dissected on dry ice. After weighing, brain tissues of the left hemisphere were dissolved in solubilizer (Soluene, Packard) for measuring radioactivity of $^{45}Ca^{2+}$ in a liquid scintillation counter. Tissues from the other hemisphere were used for quantitative GFAP analysis by a recently

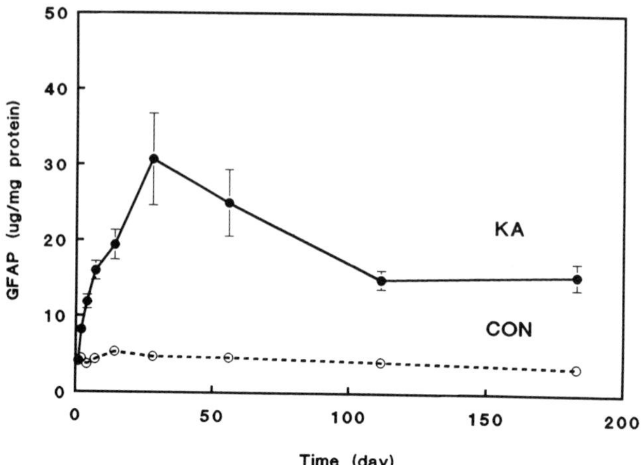

FIGURE 2. Time course of GFAP content in rat hippocampus by kainic acid. Rats were treated with a single dose of kainic acid (12 mg/kg, i.p.). At the times indicated brains were dissected and GFAP in the hippocampus was analyzed as described. Data are means ± SEM of 3–5 rats.

developed ELISA technique,[16] with minor modifications. Protein concentrations of homogenates were determined according to the BCA procedure of Smith *et al.*[17] Mean GFAP levels (μg GFAP/mg protein) ± SEM for each structure were determined. Differences of means between structures of exposed and control animals were evaluated using Students' *t*-test.

RESULTS AND DISCUSSION

Glial Fibrillary Acidic Protein

Various regions of the brain of control animals appeared to differ in levels of GFAP as quantitatively determined by a sandwich ELISA (FIG. 1). The hippocampus, like amygdala and thalamus, generally had GFAP levels somewhat higher than cerebral cortex (frontal, motor, occipital, piriform), striatum, and septum. The highest GFAP levels were encountered in cerebellum and brain stem.

Upon administration of KA, changes in GFAP content in several structures mentioned above were examined over a 6 month time period. The time course with respect to changes in the hippocampus, as an example, is shown in FIG. 2. During the first 24 h after dosing no significant alterations in GFAP levels were noted. Thereafter, GFAP levels started to increase to a maximum level at about 28 days. At this stage GFAP levels in the hippocampus were increased more than 650% compared with control animals. Although GFAP levels declined somewhat during the next 3 months, a permanent increase of 450% over control values remained up to 6 months after a single administration of kainic acid. These permanent changes of GFAP in the hippocampus are consistent with observations on permanent effects, although to a lesser degree, of TMT on GFAP levels in the rat hippocampus.[6] The results are in line with previous findings using other methodologies,[4] indicating that the hippocampus is a highly vulnerable target for KA and that astrocytes in the hippocampus readily respond to insults, thereby leaving a permanent footprint of enhanced levels of GFAP. Both seizure activity and nerve cell death may contribute to this increase.

Long-term alterations of GFAP levels to varying degrees by KA were also encountered in other brain areas, including other limbic structures and striatum, but not in cerebellum and brain stem (details to be published elsewhere).

Calcium

It was of interest to compare the strongly increased reactivity of astrocytes in various brain regions after KA treatment with cerebral calcium accumulation. A time-course of calcium accumulation in the hippocampus is shown in FIGURE 3. In controls a gradually increasing level of $^{45}Ca^{2+}$ was observed with aging. After KA injection, $^{45}Ca^{2+}$ was already increased significantly at day 1, peaked at day 4 and then only gradually declined. By 2 months calcium uptake in the hippocampus of KA rats was still significantly higher than that in controls. Control levels of $^{45}Ca^{2+}$ were reached between 2 and 4 months after dosing.

To study cerebral calcium accumulation in more anatomical detail, *e.g.*, in specific cell layers of the hippocampal formation, and to allow a comparison with histology, autoradiographs were made at each time point after dosing. ^{45}Ca autoradiographs at the level of the dorsal hippocampus at day 7 and day 28 after KA are shown in FIGURE 4. At day 7, heavy labeling is present in the amygdala, some thalamic nuclei, the CA1 area of the hippocampus and the subiculum. Other surrounding brain areas are essentially not labeled above background and have

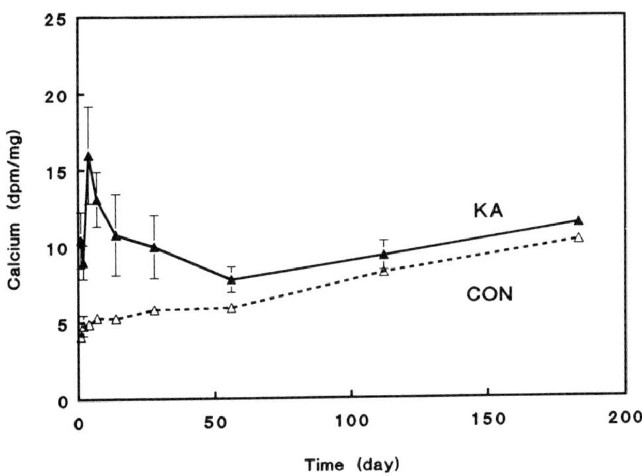

FIGURE 3. Time course of $^{45}Ca^{2+}$ accumulation in rat hippocampus by kainic acid. Rats were treated with a single dose of kainic acid (12 mg/kg, i.p.). One day before sacrifice rats had received 10 μCi $^{45}CaCl_2$ i.p., the hippocampus was dissected and radioactivity was determined as described. Data are means $\pm$ SEM of 3–5 rats.

similar values as control brains. At day 28 less $^{45}Ca^{2+}$ accumulation was observed in most target areas, but in the hippocampus, including both CA1 and CA4 regions substantial labeling was still present. Six months after KA injection autoradiographs of one rat showed a homogenous ^{45}Ca distribution over the brain, identical to those obtained from control brains, whereas autoradiographs of another rat showed still some hot spots in the thalamus (data not shown). In FIGURE 5 thionine stained sections of the dorsal hippocampus of control and KA-treated rats at day

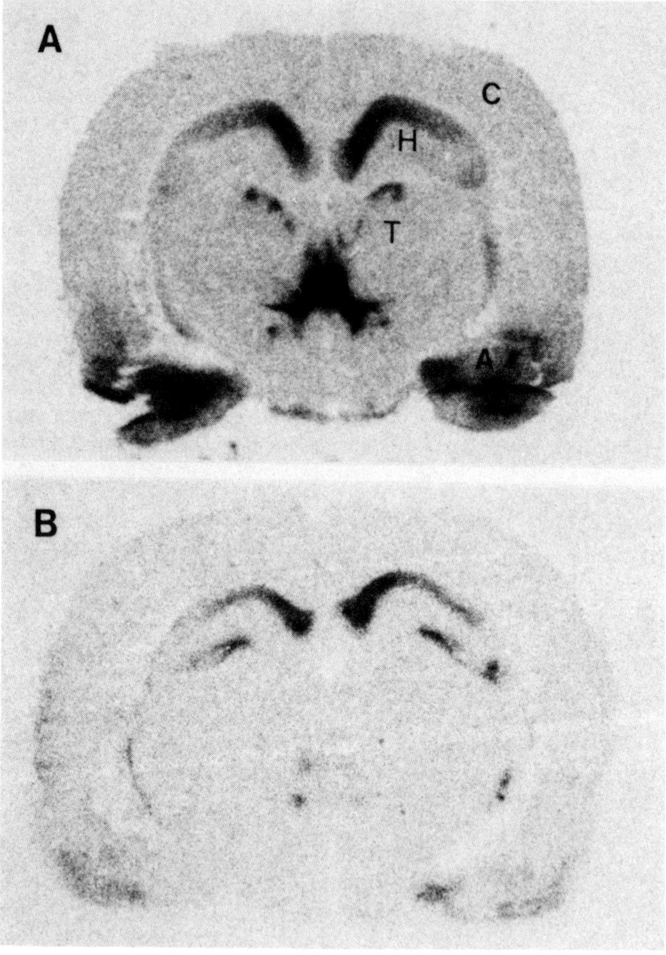

FIGURE 4. ^{45}Ca Autoradiographs of KA-treated rats at day 7 (**A**) and day 28 (**B**) at the level of the dorsal hippocampus. Rats were treated with a single dose of kainic acid (12 mg/kg i.p.). One day before sacrifice rats had received 100 μCi $^{45}CaCl_2$ i.p., frozen brains were cut in a cryostat and 30 μm sections were exposed to hyperfilm β max (Amersham) for one week before being developed in D19 (Kodak). **Abbreviations:** H hippocampus, A amygdala, C cortex; T thalamus.

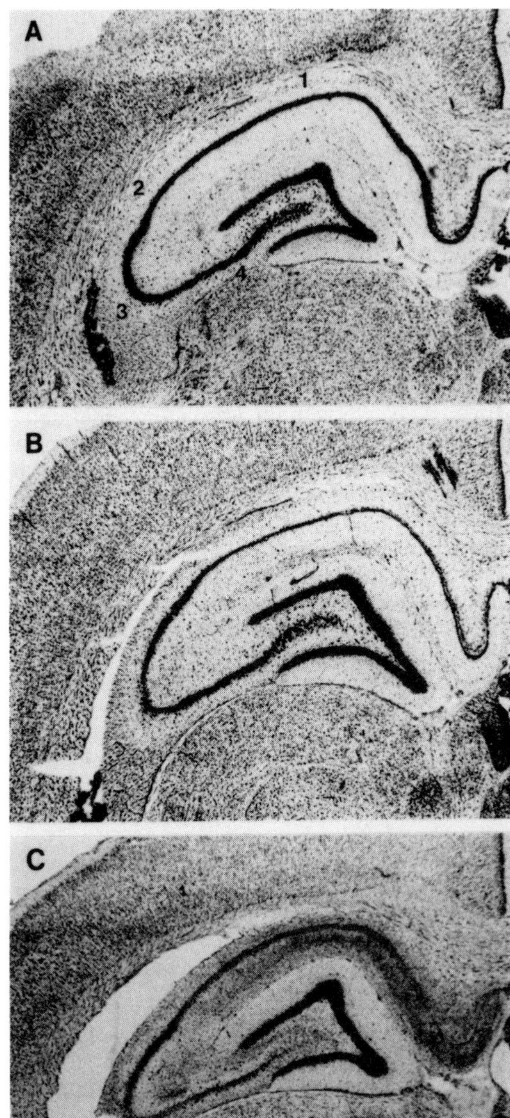

FIGURE 5. Histology of control (**A**) and KA-treated rats at day 7 (**B**) and day 28 (**C**) at the level of the dorsal hippocampus. After exposure to autoradiographic film, brain sections were stained with thionine. For further details see legend to FIGURE 4. 1, 2, 3 and 4 indicate respectively CA1, CA2, CA3 and CA4 area of the hippocampus.

7 and day 28 (same sections were used for autoradiography) show the KA-induced pyramidal cell loss in CA1 and CA3 at day 7 and in CA1, CA3 and CA4 at day 28. The CA2 area is relatively spared at all time points examined. The time course of KA-induced neurodegeneration in CA1 (rich in NMDA receptors) and CA3 (rich in KA receptors) is apparently different, since the CA3 area is only labeled at time points within 48 hours (autoradiographs not shown), whereas CA1 accumulates $^{45}Ca^{2+}$ from day 1 until 4 months after KA. Such a long-term calcium accumulation was also observed in rat striatum lesioned by local injection of quinolinic acid, an endogenous NMDA agonist.[18] In other limbic brain areas examined, but not in cerebellum or brain stem, Ca^{2+} levels were enhanced by KA with a kinetic profile very similar to that observed in the hippocampus (results to be published elsewhere).

A generally consistent pattern was found between brain areas with transiently increased Ca^{2+} and permanently enhanced GFAP levels. Also quantitatively, brain areas with highest Ca^{2+} accumulation were found to have the highest increase of GFAP levels although the absolute magnitude of the effect was larger for GFAP than for Ca^{2+} (results to be published elsewhere). These results indicate a good general correlation between Ca^{2+} accumulation and enhancement of GFAP levels.

It is also of interest to compare the differences in kinetics of Ca^{2+} accumulation and enhancement of GFAP levels which indicate that Ca^{2+} accumulation is a much earlier event, thus preceding alterations in GFAP. One interpretation of the present findings is that the early influx of calcium is associated with the degeneration of neurons, that in turn may provide signals for astrocyte reactivity. In the case of kainic acid, this process appears to proceed for a considerable length of time after only a single dosage.

In conclusion, the results suggest that both GFAP and calcium may be useful as biochemical markers of neurotoxicity. On the basis of differences in kinetics, calcium and GFAP may be utilized on a more prospective or retrospective basis.

ACKNOWLEDGMENTS

We thank Ms. A. van der Sluis and Mr. J. van Vlaardingen for skilled technical assistance, Dr. J. P. O'Callaghan for advice on GFAP analysis and Dr. B. M. Kulig for comments.

REFERENCES

1. ENG, L. F. 1988. The Biochemical Pathology of Astrocytes. Alan R. Liss. New York. Pp. 79–90.
2. O'CALLAGHAN, J. P. 1991. Biomed. Environ. Sci. **4:** 197–206.
3. BJÖRKLUND, H., L. OLSON, D. DAHL & R. SCHWARCZ. 1986. Brain Res. **371:** 267–277.
4. BEN-ARI, Y. 1985. Neuroscience **14:** 375–403.
5. WANG, S., G. J. LEES, L. E. ROSENGREN, J.-E. KARLSSON, T. STIGBRAND, A. HAMBERGER & K. G. HAGLID. 1991. Brain Res. **541:** 334–341.
6. BROCK, T. O. & J. P. O'CALLAGHAN. 1987. J. Neurosci. **7:** 931–942.
7. O'CALLAGHAN, J. P., D. B. MILLER & J. F. REINHARD, JR. 1990. Brain Res. **521:** 73–80.
8. SIESJÖ, B. K. & F. BENGTSSON. 1989. J. Cereb. Blood Flow Metab. **9:** 127–140.
9. GRIFFITHS, T., M. S. EVANS & B. S. MELDRUM. 1984. Neuroscience **12:** 557–567.
10. POUNDS, J. G. 1990. Environ. Health Perspect. **84:** 7–15.
11. DIENEL, G. A. 1984. J. Neurochem. **43:** 913–925.
12. ARAKI, T., H. KATO, K. KOGURE. 1990. Brain Res. **528:** 114–122.

13. GRAMSBERGEN, J. B. P., L. VEENMA-VAN DER DUIN, L. LOOPUIT, A. M. J. PAANS, W. VAALBURG & J. KORF. 1988. J. Neurochem. **50:** 1798–1807.
14. MAYER, M. L. & R. J. MILLER. 1990. TIPS **11:** 254–260.
15. MELDRUM, B. & J. GARTHWAITE. 1990. TIPS **11:** 379–387.
16. O'CALLAGHAN, J. P. 1991. Neurotoxicol. Teratol. **13:** 275–281.
17. SMITH, P. K., R. I. KROHN, G. T. HERMANSON, A. K. MALLIA, F. H. GARTNER, M. D. PROVENZANO, E. K. FUJIMOTO, N. M. GOEKE, B. J. OLSON & D. C. KLENK. 1985. Anal. Biochem. **150:** 76–85.
18. GRAMSBERGEN, J. B. P. & A. J. VAN DER SLUIJS-GELLING, 1991. Soc. Neurosci. Abstr. **17:** 6.6.

Glial Fibrillary Acidic Protein (GFAP) Indicates *in Vivo* Exposure to Environmental Contaminants: PCBs in the Atlantic Tomcod[a]

H. L. EVANS,[b,d] A. R. LITTLE,[b] Z. L. GONG,[b]
J. S. DUFFY,[c] I. WIRGIN,[b] AND H. A. N. EL-FAWAL[b]

[b]*Institute of Environmental Medicine*
New York University Medical Center
Tuxedo, New York 10987

[c]*Texaco Inc.*
Beacon, New York 12508

Reactive gliosis is a common response in the brain's defense against injury,[15] including exposure to toxic chemicals. Glial fibrillary acidic protein (GFAP) is a 50 kilodalton constituent of astrocytic intermediate filaments.[1] Changes in GFAP concentration correlate well with histological evidence of reactive gliosis.[2] Therefore, GFAP may be a practical, quantal marker of *exposure* to potentially neurotoxic chemicals and/or a marker of *toxicity* occurring as a consequence of exposure.[3]

Several studies indicate that GFAP can be a biomarker of neurotoxicity of metals in laboratory rodents.[4,5] It would be desirable to know whether GFAP can indicate exposure to other neurotoxic compounds[6] and whether assays of GFAP can be applied to non-rodent species. Therefore, the studies reported here investigated whether 1) these assays can be used to study GFAP in non-rodent animal species using a mammalian polyclonal antibody, 2) whether GFAP is conserved across many taxa of animals of interest either as lab models of neurotoxicity or as sentinels of environmental contamination, and 3) whether brain GFAP is a marker for *exposure* to polychlorinated biphenyls (PCBs). In addition to indicating GFAP's practical value as a marker of environmental health hazards, this information may also shed light upon the role of astrocytes in the nervous system's response to chemical insult.

METHODS

Animals

Atlantic tomcod of both sexes were captured in the Hudson River and housed in the lab for 60 days to insure freedom from chemical contamination prior to

[a] Supported at New York University in part by a Center Grant ES-00260 and Research Grants ES-04895 and ES-03641, from the United States Dept. Health and Human Services.
[d] Address correspondence to Dr. Evans.

PCB exposure. Other animal species were purchased from commercial suppliers: feral, female *Macaque cynomolgus* monkeys (Hazleton, Port Washington, NY); male white carneau pigeons (Palmetto Pigeon Plant, Sumter, SC) or male F-344 rats (Charles River Corp., Kingston, NY). All animals were adults at time of testing. Care of animals was in accord with NIH guidelines.

Exposure to PCBs

Tomcod were injected i.p. with 1 mg/kg 3,3′,4,4′-tetrachlorobiphenyl (PCB) or an equivalent volume of the corn oil vehicle. All tomcod were sacrificed 4 days later for determination of brain GFAP.

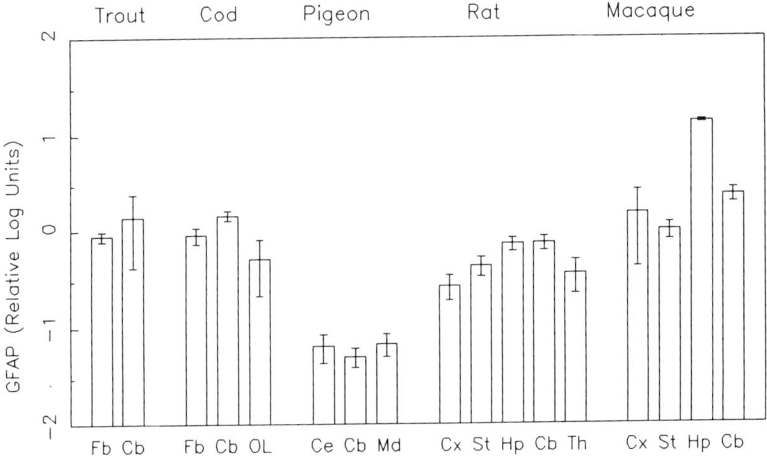

FIGURE 1. Quantification of GFAP immunoreactivity using rabbit anti-cow GFAP, demonstrating the conservation of GFAP across five different vertebrate species. The mammalian antibody can be used with many animals of interest as laboratory models or as environmental sentinels. Y axis shows GFAP immunoreactivity in arbitrary units relative to the standard curve for each species (log scale). Each bar portrays the mean (± SEM) with N ranging from 3 to 6. Abbreviations: cerebellum (Cb), cerebrum (Ce), cortex (Cx), forebrain (Fb), hippocampus (Hp), medulla (Md), optic lobe (OL), striatum (St) and thalamus (Th).

GFAP Determinations

Animals were sacrificed by decapitation (rats), by overdose of sodium pentobarbital (pigeons, macaques) or cervical dislocation (fish). Fresh brains were removed from the skull and snap frozen under liquid nitrogen. Brain regions were dissected, according to standard atlases, on a cold plate. GFAP concentration was determined by an RIA technique.[7,8] The slot-immunobinding assay was based on the propensity of proteins to bind to nitrocellulose. The samples were applied to nitrocellulose sheets through a slotted template. The unbound sites on the sheet were blocked with 0.5% gelatin in Tris buffer followed by exposure to polyclonal anti-GFAP antibodies which bind to the GFAP. The GFAP was then quantified with gamma spectrometry by allowing the bound antibodies to bind with ^{125}I-Protein A. Results are expressed as relative immunoreactivity of each sample to the standard curve.

RESULTS AND DISCUSSION

GFAP in Brains of Normal Animals

The brains of five different animal species show positive immunoreactivity to the GFAP antibody used in the RIA procedure of O'Callaghan.[8] Therefore, one may conclude that GFAP is conserved across many taxa of animals of interest either as lab models of neurotoxicity or as sentinels of environmental contamination (FIG. 1). It may be convenient to be able to use the same procedure to study GFAP in a variety of animal species using a readily available mammalian polyclonal

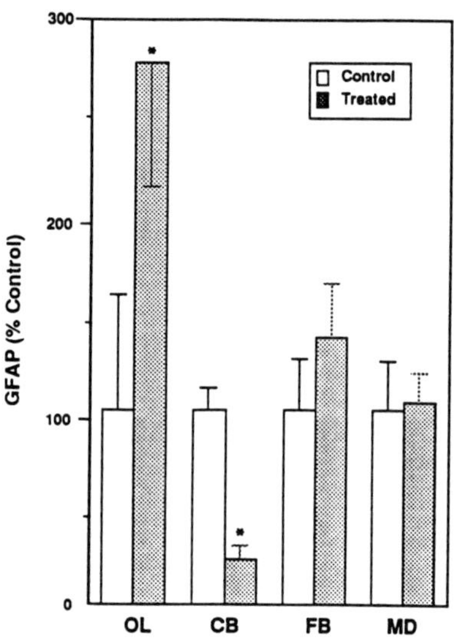

FIGURE 2. GFAP in 4 brain regions of tomcod 4 days after exposure to PCB congener 77 (1 mg/kg, N = 7) as a percentage of vehicle-injected controls (corn oil, N = 6). Significant ($p < .05$, Student's t-test) changes in GFAP concentration were seen as an increase in the optic lobe and a decrease in the cerebellum. No significant changes were measured in forebrain or medulla. Brain regions abbreviated as in FIGURE 1.

antibody. Furthermore, GFAP reactivity varies with brain region *within* a given animal species by as much as GFAP varies *between* the five species shown in FIGURE 1.

Altered GFAP Concentration Tomcod after Exposure to PCBs

FIGURE 2 indicates that the concentration of GFAP in the tomcod's central nervous system changes after sub-lethal exposure to PCBs. The increase in GFAP of treated tomcod relative to control tomcod is compatible with reactive gliosis, which traditionally has been defined by histological evidence. Biochemical changes (GFAP concentration) may be, at least, partially correlated with histological findings of gliosis.[2] The optic lobe is a region of the tomcod's brain which is particularly responsive to PCB exposure. This is particularly significant since the brain region in which GFAP level was most responsive to chemical exposure may not necessarily be the region with the highest baseline GFAP content. Thus, the optic lobe may be a target of PCB neurotoxicity in the fish. Other evidence indicates that GFAP in the fish's optic nerve is especially responsive to injury.[9–12]

Preliminary findings in our lab indicate altered GFAP during *in vivo* exposure to each of several potentially neurotoxic chemicals, *e.g.*, cadmium, methylmercury or trimethyl-lead.[13,14] More data are needed to determine the *sensitivity* of GFAP as a biomarker, *e.g.*, whether changes in GFAP concentration occur very early in chronic exposure to environmental contaminants, at exposure levels below those producing overt signs of toxicity. Very early changes would indicate that GFAP is a sensitive marker of *exposure* to hazardous chemicals. Future research should determine whether GFAP can provide a nearly linear index of acute dose at any given time. Preliminary data with chronic exposures suggest a complex, non-linear relationship of GFAP concentration with dose, exposure duration and tissue sampled.[16] GFAP also may be a marker of *toxicity,* in addition to exposure, but more data are needed to judge the relationship between GFAP concentration and degree of neurotoxicity.

REFERENCES

1. WEINSTEIN, D. E., J. L. SHELANSKI & R. K. H. LIEM. 1991. Suppression by antisense mRNA demonstrates a requirement for the glial fibrillary acidic protein in the formation of stable astrocytic processes in response to neurons. J. Cell. Biol. **112**(6): 1205–1212.
2. BALABAN, C. D., J. P. O'CALLAGHAN & M. L. BILLINGSLEY. 1988. Trimethyltin-induced neuronal damage in the rat: Comparative studies using silver degeneration stains, immunocytochemistry and immunoassay for neuronotypic and gliotypic proteins. Neuroscience **26**: 337–361.
3. O'CALLAGHAN, J. P. 1993. Quantitative features of reactive gliosis following toxicant-induced damage of the CNS. Ann. N.Y. Acad. Sci. **679**. This volume.
4. O'CALLAGHAN, J. P. 1988. Neurotypic and gliotypic proteins as biochemical markers of neurotoxicity. Neurotox. Teratol. **10**: 445–452.
5. O'CALLAGHAN, J. P. & D. B. MILLER. 1984. Neuron-specific phosphoproteins as biochemical indicators of neurotoxicity: Effects of acute administration of trimethyltin to the adult rat. J. Pharmacol. Appl. Therap. **231**: 736–743.
6. MILLER, D. B. & J. P. O'CALLAGHAN. 1993. The Interactions of MK801 with the amphetamine analogues D-METH amphetamine (D-METH) 3,4-methylenedioxy-methamphetamine (D-MDMA) or D-fenfluramine (D-FEN): Neural damage and neural protection. Ann. N.Y. Acad. Sci. **679**. This volume.
7. BROCK, T. O. & J. P. O'CALLAGHAN. 1987. Quantitative changes in the synaptic vesicle proteins Synapsin I and p38 and the astrocyte-specific protein glial fibrillary acidic protein are associated with chemical-induced injury to rat central nervous system. J. Neurosci. **7**: 931–942; 1987.
8. O'CALLAGHAN, J. P. 1991. Quantification of glial fibrillary acidic protein: Comparison of slot-immunobinding assays with a novel sandwich ELISA. Neurotoxicol. Teratol. **13**: 275–281.
9. CARDONNE, B. & B. ROOTS. 1990. Comparative immunohistochemical study of glial filament proteins (glial fibrillary acidic protein and vimentin) in goldfish, octopus, and snail. Glia **3**: 180–192.
10. NONA, S. N., S. A. S. SHEHAB, C. A. STAFFORD & J. R. CONLY-DILLON. 1989. Glial fibrillary acidic protein (GFAP) from goldfish: Its localization in visual pathway. Glia **2**: 189–200.
11. SHEHAB, S. A. S., C. A. STAFFORD, S. N. NONA & J. R. CONLY-DILLON. 1989. Anti-goldfish glial fibrillary acidic protein (GFAP) recognizes astrocytes from rat CNS. Brain Res. **504**: 343–346.

12. STAFFORD, C. A., S. A. S. SHEHAB, S. N. NONA & J. R. CONLY-DILLON. 1990. Expression of glial fibrillary acidic protein (GFAP) in goldfish optic nerve following injury. Glia **3:** 33–42.
13. EL-FAWAL, H. A. N., A. R. LITTLE, Z. GONG & H. L. EVANS. 1992. Glial response to methylmercury in rat brain: Regional-, dose- and time-response. Toxicologist **12:** 312.
14. EVANS, H. L., B. S. JORTNER & H. A. N. EL-FAWAL. 1992. Glial response to trimethyl lead in the macaque monkey. Toxicologist **12:** 317.
15. LINDSAY, R. M. 1986. Reactive gliosis. *In* Astrocytes: Cell Biology and Pathology of Astrocytes. S. Fedoroff & A. Vernadakis, Eds. Vol. 3: 231–262. Academic Press. Orlando, FL.
16. DUFFY, J. S., H. A. N. E. EL-FAWAL, H. L. EVANS, Z. L. GONG & A. S. LITTLE. 1993. Time course evaluation of the glial response to subacute exposure to trimethyltin (TMT) in long-evans rats. Toxicologist **13:** 169.

Growth-associated Protein-43 (GAP-43) Is Expressed by Glial Cells of the Central and Peripheral Nervous System

RORY CURTIS

Regeneron Pharmaceuticals, Inc.
777 Old Saw Mill River Road
Tarrytown, New York 10591

INTRODUCTION

Growth-associated protein-43 (GAP-43) is a developmentally regulated multifunctional phosphoprotein which has been suggested to be restricted to neurons and to subserve a function unique to these cells. Nevertheless, the precise function of GAP-43 is not fully understood. This short review will describe work which has shown that GAP-43 is also expressed by glial cells *in vitro* and *in vivo*. These results have two important considerations. First, the presence of GAP-43 in nonneuronal cells implies that this protein has a role in more generalized cellular processes. Secondly, it necessitates caution in the interpretation of immunohistochemical data, especially in the peripheral nervous system (PNS) where GAP-43 has been used as a marker for regenerating axons.

GAP-43: A NEURON-SPECIFIC PROTEIN?

GAP-43 has been repeatedly discovered in neurons and, in its various guises, has been widely studied in these cells. As p57, it was shown to be a brain-specific calmodulin-binding protein and was subsequently renamed "neuromodulin".[1] As F1, it was identified as a major substrate for protein kinase C, being phosphorylated during hippocampal long-term potentiation.[2] As B50, it was found to be a regulator of inositol phosphate turnover in neurons[3] and subsequently an important component in the neurotransmitter release mechanism.[4] As GAP-43 and GAP-48[5,6] it was identified as a prominent phosphoprotein carried by the fast component of axonal transport in development and during axonal regeneration, which became down-regulated after synaptogenesis.[7] Moreover, it was shown to be a component of growth cone membranes,[8,9] identical to the previously characterized protein pp46,[10] where it may serve a role in guidance by regulating adhesion and/or motility.[11] Studies of neurons *in vivo* and in culture have suggested that GAP-43 is restricted to axons and may indeed help to specify axonal characteristics in developing and regenerating neurites.[12–14]

The involvement of GAP-43 in so many neuronal functions (axonal growth, growth cone guidance, neurotransmitter release, long-term potentiation) led to the suggestion that it is a *neuron-specific* protein. This was supported by biochemical and immunological screens of other organ systems which failed to reveal the presence of GAP-43 in nonneural tissues.[15–17] These studies did not, however, address the issue of GAP-43 expression by non-neuronal cells of the nervous system, *i.e.* glial cells. In the central nervous system (CNS), this question was indirectly answered by immunohistochemical studies which only revealed GAP-43 in neurons during development and in adulthood.[17,18] A direct examination of reactive astrocytes around an electrolytic lesion in adult brain showed that these cells do not express GAP-43.[19] In the PNS, an immunohistochemical study of normal and lesioned adult nerves suggested that this protein was only present in regenerating axons.[20] Furthermore, immunoreactivity was not found in cultured Schwann cells.[21] As a result of these studies, GAP-43 has been widely used as a marker for neurons, and axons in particular.

Glial GAP-43

Evidence that glial cells express GAP-43 first came in 1988 and 1989 from two diverse studies. First, Vitković and colleagues[22] demonstrated GAP-43 immunoreactive astrocytes in CNS mixed glial cultures. However, these cultures contain two types of astrocytes which could be responsible for the observed immunoreactivity and also myelinating glial cells, oligodendrocytes. Secondly, Tetzlaff *et al.*[23] localized GAP-43 in Schwann cells of regenerating peripheral nerves using immuno-electron microscopy but Schwann cells are not a homogeneous cell population and, furthermore, they undergo a change in phenotype when deprived of axonal contact. We therefore set out to determine, using a high-titer antiserum raised against a GAP-43/β-galactosidase fusion protein, which glial populations are capable of GAP-43 expression both *in vivo* and in tissue culture and whether this is modulated by neuronal injury.

Peripheral Glial Cells

In the PNS, Schwann cells are divided into two categories—those that myelinate the axons they ensheath and those that do not. Both types arise from a common Schwann cell precursor and their differentiation is directed by the axons with which they associate (large diameter axons causing Schwann cells to myelinate).[24] When deprived of axons in culture or by nerve transection, Schwann cells revert to a dedifferentiated phenotype similar to the normal non-myelinating phenotype.[25] When we examined Schwann cells in normal nerves and after denervation *in vivo* or dissociation in tissue culture, we found GAP-43 immunoreactivity exclusively in non-myelin-forming Schwann cells and dedifferentiated cells but not in myelinating Schwann cells.[26] Additionally, embryonic Schwann cell precursors isolated from E15 sciatic nerves contained GAP-43 and continued to express immunoreactivity after 24 h in culture. These observations suggest that GAP-43 is expressed early in the Schwann cell lineage and becomes down-regulated in those cells induced to form myelin sheaths by contact with large diameter axons. Furthermore, we utilized metabolic labeling to show that cultured Schwann cells synthesize GAP-43 themselves,[26] rather than acquiring it from neurons as has been suggested.[23]

GAP-43 expression in Schwann cells appears to be controlled differently from other protein markers of the non-myelin-forming Schwann cell lineage, which are down-regulated in myelinating cells by axonal contact and are rapidly re-expressed in dedifferentiating cells (*e.g.*, glial fibrillary acidic protein, N-CAM and the low affinity nerve growth factor receptor).[25] Up-regulation of GAP-43 is delayed relative to these markers, both in transected nerves and in tissue culture. An autocrine mechanism appears to operate in culture as Schwann cells contain more GAP-43 at higher plating densities.[26] The up-regulation of GAP-43 in denervated Schwann cells *in vivo* over a 4-week period may be related to increasing Schwann cell density or accumulation of soluble factor(s) in transected nerves.

The function of GAP-43 in Schwann cells is unclear. By analogy with growth cones, where GAP-43 associates with both the plasmalemma and the sub-membrane cytoskeleton,[11,27] it is conceivable that non-myelin-forming Schwann cells utilize this protein to regulate interactions of the membrane and cytoskeleton which may be related to changes in the diameter of the ensheathed unmyelinated axons, due to axonal transport of organelles.[28]

Central Macroglia

In contrast to the PNS where all Schwann cells are derived from a common pool of precursors, macroglial cell lineages in the CNS are more intricate.[29-31] Myelinating cells (oligodendrocytes) and non-myelinating cells (astrocytes) are distinct from one another and cannot be interconverted. Moreover, two types of astrocytes have been defined in tissue culture according to morphology[32] and expression of cell surface gangliosides.[33,34] Type-1 astrocytes (which show an epithelioid morphology in culture) arise from an as yet unidentified precursor. In culture, type-2 astrocytes (which are stellate and express ganglioside G_{D3}[34]) and oligodendrocytes are derived from a common precursor cell, the so-called O-2A (oligodendrocyte/type-2 astrocyte) progenitor,[35] suggesting that astrocytes and oligodendrocytes do not belong to entirely separate lineages (but see ref. 29). However, type-2 astrocytes have not been detected in developing or adult rat brain,[34,36] and it has been shown *in vitro* and *in vivo* that O-2A progenitors constitutively develop into oligodendrocytes.[37,38]

In culture, we and others have found that O-2A progenitors express GAP-43 and this is maintained as they differentiate into type-2 astrocytes.[39-41] As GAP-43 is an intracellular protein, permeabilization of cultured cells is required for immunohistochemical visualization. GAP-43 is lost as O-2A progenitors differentiate into oligodendrocytes and can not be detected in mature oligodendrocytes, defined by expression of myelin basic protein (MBP).[39] Type-1 astrocytes do not themselves express GAP-43,[41] but in the early stages of primary culture immunoreactivity is seen associated with the outer surface of unpermeabilized cells,[40] possibly due to attached fragments of membranes from growing axons which would be rich in GAP-43. As these cells age in culture, immunoreactivity is lost concomitant with phagocytosis of this axolemmal debris (unpublished observations).

Careful examination of tissue sections from developing rat brain double labeled with oligodendrocyte-specific monoclonal antibodies and anti-GAP-43 antiserum revealed that GAP-43 is expressed by G_{D3} + ve O-2A progenitors and galactocerebroside + ve immature oligodendrocytes but not by MBP + ve mature oligodendrocytes.[39] Thus the developmental progression seen in culture appears to accurately reflect the normal course of events of oligodendrocyte differentiation *in vivo*. In contrast, GAP-43 could not be found in astrocytes in sections of developing or adult brain, nor after the induction of reactive gliosis by mechanical or chemical injuries, confirming earlier studies.[19,39,48] This supports previous suggestions that type-2 astrocytes may not be generated *in vivo*.[29,34]

Speculation on the role of GAP-43 in CNS glia and the differences between *in vivo* and *in vitro* observations have been discussed elsewhere.[39] The function of GAP-43 may be related to the motility of O-2A progenitors[42] or the regulation of differentiation of these cells into oligodendrocytes.[43]

CONCLUSIONS

In the context of this volume, it is important to consider the validity of GAP-43 as a "neuronal" marker. GAP-43 immunostaining has been proposed as a better marker of regenerating axons than neurofilament-based stains (both histological and immunochemical) due to the presence of GAP-43 but not neurofilaments in the growing axon tip.[44] In the PNS, the use of GAP-43 to identify axons is lesioned nerves (or grafts thereof) is complicated by the expression of GAP-43 by non-myelin-forming Schwann cells and dedifferentiated Schwann cells responding to the loss of axonal contact. In the normal adult CNS, GAP-43 is not expressed by mature macroglia and appears to be restricted to neurons, but O-2A progenitor cells persist into adulthood[45] and the potential exists for these cells to express GAP-43. Moreover, it has been proposed that these adult progenitors may initiate a program of oligodendrocyte differentiation in response to demyelinating lesions.[46,47] As oligodendrocytes pass through a GAP-43 + ve stage in their development (see above) both O-2A progenitors and immature oligodendrocytes may represent a non-neuronal source of GAP-43 where demyelination is induced experimentally or pathologically. Thus, GAP-43 should be used with great caution as a marker for neurons and ideally the cellular origin of immunostaining should be confirmed by double labeling with specific markers for neurons and glia.

ACKNOWLEDGMENTS

I would like to thank several people. First and foremost, Graham Wilkin of Imperial College, London, supervised these studies as part of my doctoral thesis. Secondly, I am indebted to my collaborators at Imperial College (Richard Reynolds, Barbara Spruce and Rebecca Hardy) and at University College, London (Helen Stewart, Rhona Mirsky and Kristján Jessen). Finally, I thank my colleagues John Rudge and Peter DiStefano for their critical reading of this manuscript.

REFERENCES

1. LIU, Y. & D. R. STORM. 1990. TIPS **11:** 107–111.
2. NELSON, R. B. & A. ROUTTENBERG. 1985. Exp. Neurol. **89:** 213–224.
3. VAN DONGEN, C. J., H. ZWIERS, P. N. E. DE GRAAN & W. H. GISPEN. 1985. Biochem. Biophys. Res. Commun. **128:** 1219–1227.
4. DEKKER, L. V., P. N. E. DE GRAAN, A. B. OESTREICHER, D. H. G. VERSTEEG & W. H. GISPEN. 1989. Nature **342:** 74–76.
5. SKENE, J. H. P. & M. B. WILLARD. 1981. J. Cell Biol. **89:** 86–95.
6. BENOWITZ, L. I. & E. R. LEWIS. 1983. J. Neurosci. **3:** 2153–2163.
7. JACOBSON, R. D., I. VIRÁG & J. H. P. SKENE. 1986. J. Neurosci. **6:** 1843–1855.
8. MEIRI, K. F., K. H. PFENNINGER & M. B. WILLARD. 1986. Proc. Natl. Acad. Sci. USA **83:** 3537–3541.
9. SKENE, J. H. P., R. D. JACOBSON, G. J. SNIPES, C. B. McGUIRE, J. J. NORDEN & J. A. FREEMAN. 1986. Science **233:** 783–786.
10. HYMAN, C. & K. H. PFENNINGER. 1987. J. Neurosci. **7:** 4076–4083.
11. MEIRI, K. F. & P. R. GORDON-WEEKS. 1990. J. Neurosci. **10:** 256–266.
12. GISPEN, W. H., J. L. M. LEUNISSEN, A. B. OESTREICHER, A. J. VERKLEIJ & H. ZWIERS. 1985. Brain Res. **328:** 381–385.

13. GOSLIN, K., D. J. SCHREYER, J. H. P. SKENE & G. BANKER. 1990. J. Neurosci. **10:** 588–602.
14. VAN LOOKEREN CAMPAGNE, M., A. B. OESTREICHER, P. M. P. VAN BERGEN EN HENEGOUWEN & W. H. GISPEN. 1990. J. Neurocytol. **19:** 948–961.
15. CIMLER, B., T. J. ANDREASEN, K. I. ANDREASEN & D. R. STORM. 1985. J. Biol. Chem. **260:** 10784–10788.
16. BASI, G. S., R. D. JACOBSON, I. VIRÁG, J. SCHILLING & J. H. P. SKENE. 1987. Cell **49:** 785–791.
17. MCGUIRE, C. B., G. J. SNIPES & J. J. NORDEN. 1988. Dev. Brain Res. **41:** 277–291.
18. BENOWITZ, L. I., P. J. APOSTOLIDES, N. PERRONE-BIZZOZERO, S. P. FINKLESTEIN & H. ZWIERS. 1988. J. Neurosci. **8:** 339–352.
19. OESTREICHER, A. B., P. DEVAY, R. L. ISAACSON & W. H. GISPEN. 1988. Brain Res. Bull. **21:** 713–722.
20. VERHAAGEN, J., C. O. M. VAN HOOFF, P. M. EDWARDS, P. N. E. DE GRAAN, A. B. OESTREICHER, P. SCHOTMAN, F. G. I. JENNEKENS & W. H. GISPEN. 1986. Brain Res. Bull. **17:** 737–741.
21. MEIRI, K. F., M. B. WILLARD & M. I. JOHNSON. 1988. J. Neurosci. **8:** 2571–2581.
22. VITKOVIĆ, L., H. W. STEISSLINGER, V. J. ALOYO & M. MERSEL. 1988. Proc. Natl. Acad. Sci. USA **85:** 8296–8300.
23. TETZLAFF, W., H. ZWIERS, K. LEDERIS, L. CASSAR & M. A. BISBY. 1989. J. Neurosci. **9:** 1303–1313.
24. JESSEN, K. R. & R. MIRSKY. 1991. Glia **4:** 185–194.
25. MIRSKY, R. & K. R. JESSEN. 1990. Seminars Neurosci. **2:** 423–439.
26. CURTIS, R., H. J. S. STEWART, S. M. HALL, G. P. WILKIN, R. MIRSKY & K. R. JESSEN. 1992. J. Cell Biol. **116:** 1455–1464.
27. SKENE, J. H. P. & I. VIRÁG. 1989. J. Cell Biol. **108:** 613–624.
28. GREENBERG, M. M., C. LEITAO, J. TROGADIS & J. K. STEVENS. 1990. J. Neurocytol. **20:** 978–988.
29. SKOFF, R. P. & P. E. KNAPP. 1991. Glia **4:** 165–174.
30. NOBLE, M. 1991. Glia **4:** 157–164.
31. CAMERON, R. S. & P. RAKIC. 1991. Glia **4:** 124–137.
32. WILKIN, G. P., G. LEVI, S. R. JOHNSTONE & P. RIDDLE. 1983. Dev. Brain Res. **10:** 265–277.
33. RAFF, M. C., E. R. ABNEY, J. COHEN, R. M. LINDSAY & M. NOBLE. 1983. J. Neurosci. **3:** 1289–1300.
34. CURTIS, R., J. COHEN, J. FOK-SEANG, M. R. HANLEY, N. A. GREGSON, R. REYNOLDS & G. P. WILKIN. 1988. J. Neurocytol. **17:** 43–54.
35. RAFF, M. C., R. H. MILLER & M. NOBLE. 1983. Nature **303:** 390–396.
36. MILLER, R. H., C. FFRENCH-CONSTANT & M. C. RAFF. 1989. Ann. Rev. Neurosci. **12:** 517–534.
37. TEMPLE, S. & M. C. RAFF. 1985. Nature **313:** 223–225.
38. REYNOLDS, R. & G. P. WILKIN. 1991. J. Neurocytol. **20:** 216–224.
39. CURTIS, R., R. HARDY, R. REYNOLDS, B. A. SPRUCE & G. P. WILKIN. 1991. Eur. J. Neurosci. **3:** 876–886.
40. DA CUNHA, A. & L. VITKOVIĆ. 1990. J. Cell Biol. **111:** 209–215.
41. DELOULME, J.-C., T. JANET, D. AU, D. R. STORM, M. SENSENBRENNER & J. BAUDIER. 1990. J. Cell Biol. **111:** 1559–1569.
42. SMALL, R. K., P. RIDDLE & M. NOBLE. 1987. Nature **328:** 155–157.
43. RAFF, M. C., L. E. LILLIEN, W. D. RICHARDSON, J. F. BURNE & M. D. NOBLE. 1988. Nature **333:** 562–565.
44. TETZLAFF, W. & M. A. BISBY. 1989. Neurosci. **29:** 659–666.
45. WOLSWIJK, G. & M. NOBLE. 1989. Development **105:** 387–400.
46. ARMSTRONG, R., V. L. FRIEDRICH, K. V. HOLMES & M. DUBOIS-DALCQ. 1990. J. Cell Biol. **111:** 1183–1195.
47. ARMSTRONG, R. C., H. H. DORN, C. V. KUFTA, E. FRIEDMAN & M. E. DUBOIS-DALCQ. 1992. J. Neurosci. **12:** 1538–1547.
48. CURTIS, R., D. GREEN, R. M. LINDSAY & G. P. WILKIN. 1993. J. Neurocytol. **22:** 51–64.

The Expression of B-50/GAP-43 in Schwann Cells

L. C. PLANTINGA, J. VERHAAGEN, AND W. H. GISPEN

Rudolf Magnus Institute
Department of Pharmacology, Utrecht University
Vondellaan 6
3521 GD Utrecht, the Netherlands

When the axon of a peripheral nerve is crushed, nerve sprouts will grow from the proximal nerve stump to re-form synaptic connections and restore nerve function. During this period of regeneration the pattern of gene expression in the cell bodies of the damaged nerve cells is changed and proteins associated with neuronal outgrowth are induced. One of the proteins of which the expression is substantially enhanced during neuronal outgrowth[1,2] is B-50, also designated GAP 43, pp46, F1 and neuromodulin.[3-7] Following crush lesion of the rat sciatic nerve the expression of B-50 mRNA and B-50 protein increases about 10-fold in rat dorsal root ganglia (DRG), whereas upon reinnervation the expression is downregulated to normal levels.[8-10] B-50 is not only expressed during regeneration but also transiently during the first postnatal weeks in the cortex of the rat, a period in which neurons extend axons.[11] During adult life, B-50 levels are low in most neurons, although restricted subsets of neurons where terminal remodeling is likely to occur continue to express high levels of B-50 throughout life.[12,13] The presence of B-50 in developing and regenerating neurons and the observation that B-50 is greatly enriched in growth cone particles[14,15] indicates that B-50 is implicated in the mechanism of neuronal outgrowth. However, so far no specific function for B-50 in axonal outgrowth has been found.

Although for many years B-50 was considered to be a neuron-specific protein[3,5,16,17] recent data indicate that non-neuronal cells are capable of expressing B-50. The first evidence for the presence of B-50 in non-neuronal cells was obtained by Vitkovic *et al.*[18] who demonstrated B-50 immunoreactivity in the plasma membranes of cultures of neonatal rat cortical astrocytes. More detailed studies[19-21] demonstrated that all three macroglial cell types of the central nervous system, astrocytes type 1, astrocytes type 2, and oligodendrocytes are B-50 immunoreactive in tissue culture although some controversy exists whether type 1 astrocytes express B-50.[20] The expression of B-50 in oligodendrocytes is developmentally regulated as demonstrated both *in vitro* and *in vivo*.[21] Data concerning B-50 immunoreactivity in Schwann cells, the glial cells of the peripheral nervous system, are less extensive. Tetzlaff *et al.*[22] observed B-50 immunoreactivity associated with the bands of Bungner after sciatic nerve injury, but addressed the B-50 positive staining to uptake of B-50 by Schwann cells from degenerating neurons. Besides this observation we detected an unexpected transient increase in B-50 immunoreactivity at the neuromuscular junction 2 days following sciatic nerve injury that could not be explained by reinnervation of the muscle by B-50 positive fibers.[23] Now we have evidence that this increase in B-50 immunoreactivity is due to the expression of B-50 by Schwann cells. Recently B-50 has been localized to S-100 positive cells using double label immunohistochemistry at the neuromuscular junction of the facial nerve of the rat.[24] At the normal intact neuromuscular junction

Schwann cells were virtually devoid of B-50 immunoreactivity although some B-50 positive Schwann cells were detected. Four days following facial nerve crush all Schwann cells were found to express B-50 protein at high levels. In addition to these experiments showing B-50 immunoreactivity in Schwann cells we have demonstrated B-50 mRNA expression in the intact and degenerating sciatic nerves of adult rats, albeit at very low levels if compared to the expression in DRG. This low level of expression may explain the inability to detect B-50 mRNA in the sciatic nerve by others.[16,17] Since the sciatic nerve does not contain neuronal cell bodies, B-50 mRNA present in the nerve segment can only derive from non-neuronal cells, although in the intact sciatic nerve transport of B-50 mRNA from the DRG down to the axon cannot be excluded. However, we believe that the expression of B-50 mRNA demonstrated in the intact sciatic nerve also reflects

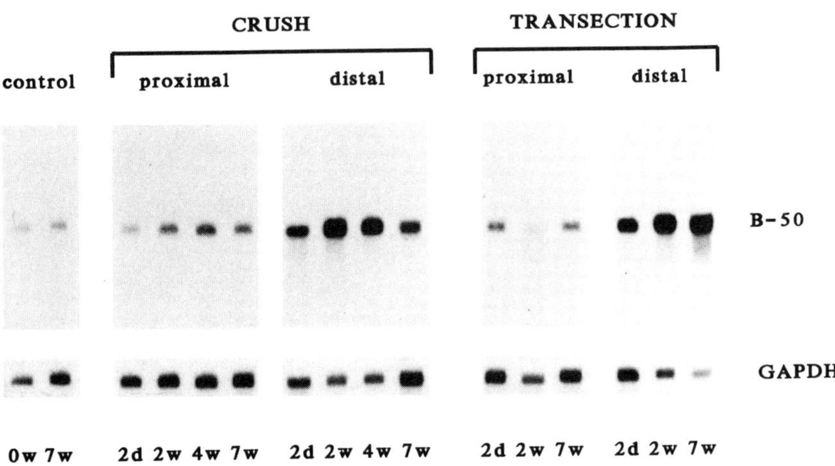

FIGURE 1. Northern blot analysis of the expression of B-50 mRNA in proximal and distal sciaic nerve portions at different timepoints after nerve crush or transection. In the upper panel hybridization with a B-50 CDNA probe is shown, in the lower panel the same blot is hybridized with a glyceraldehyde-3-phosphate dehydrogenase (GAPDH) probe in order to control for variation in sample loading between each lane.

local synthesis by Schwann cells since immunocytochemical data demonstrated B-50 reactivity in some Schwann cells associated with intact axons.[24,25] The observation that Schwann cells are capable of synthesizing B-50 is in line with metabolic labeling studies performed previously by Curtis *et al.*[25]

Since B-50 immunoreactivity in Schwann cells is upregulated following nerve damage, we set out to examine the temporal expression of B-50 mRNA following nerve crush allowing regeneration and following permanent nerve transection (see FIGS. 1 and 2).[26] Following nerve crush we observed a transient increase in B-50 mRNA expression in the distal nerve stump. At day 2 postinjury B-50 mRNA levels were increased and continued to increase till they reached plateau levels after 2 weeks. B-50 mRNA levels remained high at 4 weeks and returned to normal levels at 7 weeks following nerve crush. In contrast, after transection the expression of B-50 mRNA in the distal nerve stump increased at 2 days postinjury but continued to increase up to 7 weeks, the longest timepoint examined. The increase in the expression of B-50 mRNA at day 2 postinjury is in agreement with the observed increase in B-50 protein levels in the sciatic and facial nerves at 2 to 4 days postlesion.[23,24] At variance with our results is the study of Curtis *et al.*[25] who reported an initial increase in immunoreactivity at 4 weeks following nerve transection. At present, we are unable to explain the differences in the initiation of B-50 induction.

It is important to note that in contrast to the increase in B-50 mRNA expression in the distal nerve portion no significant change in B-50 mRNA expression was observed in the proximal nerve portion after crush or transection. Currently we do not know what regulates the expression of B-50 in Schwann cells but it is

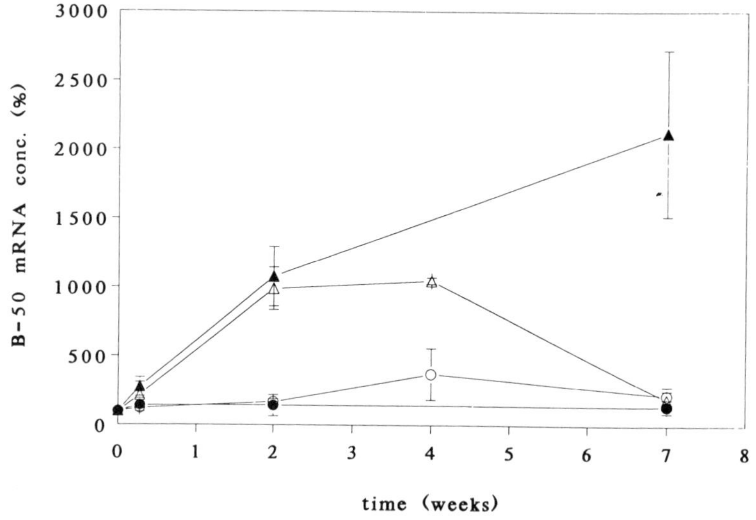

FIGURE 2. Semi-quantitative analysis of the expression of B-50 mRNA in the proximal and distal nerve sciatic stump after crush or transection obtained by densitometric scanning. The signals were normalized to GAPDH hybridization, and the B-50 mRNA expression in control non-injured nerves was set at 100%. In the graph each point represents the two independent observations and is depicted as the mean of which the range is shown. ○ = crush, proximal nerve portion; △ = crush, distal nerve portion; ● = transection, proximal nerve portion; ▲ = transection, distal nerve portion.

tempting to speculate that loss of axonal contact induces B-50 expression directly or indirectly since upon nerve damage the axons distally from the site of injury degenerate and as a consequence Schwann cells lose contact with the axons.[27] Schwann cells respond to the loss of axonal contact by expressing a different set of proteins such as N-CAM[28], nerve growth factor and nerve growth factor receptors,[29] whereas the production of the major myelin genes is sharply reduced.[30] Thus, Schwann cells move from a mature myelin-producing state to an immature proliferating state and produce proteins that are supportive for axonal outgrowth.[31,32] B-50 may be added to the list of proteins expressed by reactive Schwann cells that promote nerve regeneration. In agreement with the hypothesis that Schwann cells produce B-50 upon loss of axonal conact is the observation that B-50 is also expressed in Schwann cell cultures devoid of neurons.[25,26]

However, recent data demonstrated that mature non-myelin forming Schwann cells which are closely associated with intact axons are B-50 immunoreactive.[25] Thus the regulation of B-50 mRNA expression is not likely to depend exclusively on axonal contact. This is in line with the high B-50 mRNA expression we observed at 4 weeks after nerve crush, a time at which nerve sprouts already have innervated their target organs and axon-Schwann cell contact is largely restored. Moreover, B-50 expression in tissue culture is dependent on Schwann cell density suggesting that Schwann cells themselves secrete factors that regulate B-50 expression.[25] Clearly more research is needed to understand how the expression of B-50 in Schwann cells is regulated.

Currently we do not know what the function of B-50 in Schwann cells is. In neurons, B-50 expression is closely associated with nerve fiber extension during axonal development and regeneration. Transfection of non-neuronal cells leads to the formation of membrane extensions.[33] This suggests that B-50 may play a role in the regulation of cell shape. Schwann cells at the neuromuscular junction have been shown to extend numerous processes of considerable length following nerve crush[34] and have been demonstrated to express B-50. Moreover, Schwann cell precursors and nonmyelin-forming Schwann cells which express B-50 have been suggested to be more motile in comparison with intact myelin forming Schwann cells, supporting the suggestion that B-50 is involved in membrane formation and remodeling.

REFERENCES

1. SKENE, J. H. P. & M. WILLARD. 1981. Changes in axonally transported proteins during axonal regeneration in toad retinal ganglion cells. J. Cell. Biol. **89:** 86–95.
2. SKENE, J. H. P. & M. WILLARD. 1981. Axonally transported proteins associated with axon growth in rabbit central and peripheral nervous system. J. Cell. Biol. **89:** 96–103.
3. BENOWITZ, L. I. & A. ROUTENBERG. 1987. A membrane phosphoprotein associated with neural development, axonal regeneration, phospholipid metabolism and synaptic plasticity. Trends Neurosci. **10:** 527–532.
4. GISPEN, W. H., J. BOONSTRA, P. N. E. DE GRAAN, F. G. I. JENNEKENS, A. B. OESTREICHER, P. SCHOTMAN, L. H. SCHRAMA, J. VERHAAGEN & F. L. MARGOLIS. 1990. B-50/GAP-43 in neuronal development and repair. Rest. Neurol. Neurosci. **1:** 237–244.
5. SKENE, J. H. P. 1989. Axonal growth-associated protein. Ann. Rev. Neurosci. **12:** 127–156.
6. PERRONE-BIZZOZERO, N. I., S. P. FINKLESTEIN & L. I. BENOWITZ. 1986. Synthesis of a growth-associated protein by embryonic rat cerebrocortical neurons in vitro. J. Neurosci. **6:** 3721–3730.
7. PFENNINGER, K. H. 1986. Of nerve growth cones, leukocytes and memory: Second messenger systems and growth-related proteins. Trends Neurosci. **9:** 562–565.
8. HOFFMAN, P. N. 1989. Expression of GAP-43, a rapidly transported growth-associated protein, and class 2 beta tubulin, a slowly transported cytoskeletal protein, are coordinated in regenerating neurons. J. Neurosci. **9**(3): 893–897.
9. VAN DER ZEE, C. E. E. M., H. B. NIELANDER, J. P. VOS, S. LOPES DA SILVA, J. VERHAAGEN, A. B. OESTREICHER, L. H. SCHRAMA, P. SCHOTMAN & W. H. GISPEN. 1989. Expression of growth associated protein B-50 (GAP43) in dorsal root ganglia and the sciatic nerve during regenerative sprouting. J. Neurosci. **9**(10): 3505–3512.
10. VERHAAGEN, J., C. O. M. VAN HOOFF, P. M. EDWARDS, P. N. E. DE GRAAN, A. B. OESREICHER, F. G. I. JENNEKENS & W. H. GISPEN. 1986. The kinase C substrate protein B-50 and axonal regeneration. Br. Res. Bull. **17:** 737–741.
11. JACOBSON, R. D., I. VIRAG & J. H. P. SKENE. 1986. A protein associated with axon

growth, GAP-43, is widely distributed and developmentally regulated in rat CNS. J. Neurosci. **6:** 1843–1855.

12. NEVE, R. L., E. A. FINCH, E. D. BIRD & L. I. BENOWITZ. 1988. Growth-associated protein GAP-43 is expressed selectively in associative regions of the adult human brain. Proc. Natl. Acad. Sci. USA **85:** 3638–3642.

13. OESTREICHER, A. B. & W. H. GISPEN. 1986. Comparison of the immunocytochemical distribution of the phosphoprotein B-50 in the cerebellum and hippocampus of immature and adult rat brain. Brain Res. **375:** 267–269.

14. MEIRI, K. F., K. H. PFENNINGER & M. B. WILLARD. 1986. Growth associated protein, GAP 43, a polypeptide that is induced when neurons extended axons, is a component of a neuronal growth cones and corresponds to pp46, a major polypeptide of a subcellular fraction enriched in neuronal growth cones. Proc. Natl. Acad. Sci. USA **83:** 3537–3541.

15. SKENE, J. H. P., R. D. JACOBSON, G. J. SNIPES, C. B. MCGUIRE, J. J. NORDEN & J. A. FREEMAN. 1986. A protein induced during nerve growth (GAP-43) is a major component of growth-cone membranes. Science **233:** 783–786.

16. NEVE, R. L., N. I. PERRONE-BIZZOZERO, S. FINKLESTEIN, H. ZWIERS, E. BIRD, D. M. KURNIT & L. I. BENOWITZ. 1987. The neuronal growth-associated protein GAP 43 (B-50, F1): neuronal specificity, developmental regulation and regional distribution of the human and rat mRNA. Mol. Brain Res. **2:** 177–183.

17. BASI, G. S., R. D. JACOBSON, I. VIRAG, J. SCHILLING & J. H. SKENE. 1987. Primary structure and transcriptional regulation of GAP-43, a protein associated with nerve growth. Cell **49:** 785–791.

18. VITKOVIC, L., H. W. STEISSLINGER, V. J. ALOYO & M. MERSEL. 1988. The 43 kDa neuronal growth-associated protein (GAP-43) is present in plasma membranes of rat astrocytes. Proc. Natl. Acad. Sci. USA **85:** 8296–8300.

19. DA CUNHA, A. & L. VITKOVIC. 1990. Regulation of immunoreactive GAP-43 expression in rat cortical macroglia is cell type specific. J. Cell. Biol. **111:** 209–215.

20. DELOULME, J. C., T. JANET, D. AU, D. R. STORM, M. SENSENBRENNER & J. BAUDIER. 1990. Neuromodulin (GAP-43): A neuronal protein kinase C substrate is also present in O-2A glial cell lineage. Characterization of neuromodulin in secondary cultures of oligodendrocytes and comparison with the neuronal antigen. J. Cell. Biol. **111:** 1559–1569.

21. CURTIS, R., R. HARDLY, R. REYNOLDS, B. A. SPRUCE & G. P. WILKIN. 1991. Down-regulation of GAP-43 during oligodendrocyte development and lack of expression by astrocyes in vivo: Implications for macroglial differentiation. Eur. J. Neurosci. **3:** 876–886.

22. TETZLAFF, W., H. ZWIERS, K. LEDERIS, L. CASSAR & M. A. BISBY. 1989. Axonal transport and localization of B-50/GAP-43-like immunoreactivity in regenerating sciatic and facial nerves of the rat. J. Neurosci. **9:** 1303–1313.

23. VERHAAGEN, J., A. B. OESTREICHER, P. M. EDWARDS, H. VELDMAN, F. G. I. JENNEKENS & W. H. GISPEN. 1988. Light and electronmicroscopical study of the phosphoprotein B-50 following denervation and reinnervation of the rat soleus muscle. J. Neurosci. **8:** 1759–1766.

24. ULENKATE, H. J. L. M., J. VERHAAGEN, L. C. PLANTINGA, M. MERCKEN, H. VELDMAN, F. G. I. JENNEKENS, W. H. GISPEN & A. B. OESTREICHER. 1993. Upregulation of GAP-43/B-50 in Schwann cells at denervated motor endplates and in motoneurons after rat facial nerve crush. Rest. Neurol. Neurosci. In press.

25. CURTIS, R., H. J. S. STEWARD, S. M. HALL, G. P. WILKIN, R. MIRSKY & K. R. JESSEN. 1992. GAP-43 is expressed by nonmyelin-forming Schwann cells of the peripheral nervous system. J. Cell. Biol. **116:** 1455–1464.

26. PLANTINGA, L. C., J. VERHAAGEN, P. M. EDWARDS, E. M. HOL, P. R. BÄR & W. H. GISPEN. 1993. The expression of B-50/GAP-43 in Schwann cells is upregulated in degenerating peripheral nerve stumps following nerve injury. Brain Res. **602:** 69–76.

27. SUTHERLAND, S. 1978. *In* Nerves and Nerve Injuries, 2nd edit. Churchill Livingstone, Edinburgh/London/New York. Pp. 82–88.

28. MARTINI, R. & M. SCHACHNER. 1988. Immunoelectron microscopic localization of neural cell adhesion molecules (L1, N-CAM, and myelin associated glycoprotein) in regenerating adult mouse sciatic nerve. J. Cell. Biol. **100:** 1735–1746.

29. HEUMANN, R., S. KORSCHING, C. BANDTLOW & H. THOENEN. 1987. Changes of nerve growth factor synthesis in nonneuronal cells in response to sciatic nerve transection. J. Cell. Biol. **104:** 1623–1631.

30. TRAPP, B. D., P. HAUER & G. LEMKE. 1988. Axonal regulation of myelin protein levels in actively myelinating Schwann cells. J. Neurosci. **8**(9): 3515–3521.

31. LEMKE, G. & M. CHAO. 1988. Axons regulate Schwann cell expression of the major myelin and NGF recepor genes. Development **102:** 499–504.

32. SALZER, J. L. & R. P. BUNGE. 1980. Studies of Schwann cell proliferation. I. An analysis in tissue culture of proliferation during development, Wallerian degeneration, and direct injury. J. Cell. Biol. **84:** 739–752.

33. ZUBER, M. X., D. W. GOODMAN, L. R. KARNS & M. C. FISHMAN. 1989. The neuronal growth-associated protein GAP 43 induces filopodia in non-neuronal cells. Science **244:** 1193–1195.

34. REYNOLDS, L. M. & C. J. WOOLF. 1992. Terminal Schwann cells elaborate extensive processes following denervation of the motor endplate. J. Neurocytol. **21:** 50–66.

Insulin-like Growth Factors and Cerebral Ischemia

WEI-HUA LEE[a] AND CAROLYN BONDY

Developmental Endocrinology Branch
National Institute of Child Health and Human Development
National Institutes of Health
Bethesda, Maryland 20892

Cerebral ischemia, the sustained interruption of cerebral blood flow, results in an immediate reduction of oxygen and glucose supplies to all cellular elements in the affected area. The sudden shortage of metabolic fuels interrupts oxidative phosphorylation which will eventually lead to cell death.[1] Brain tissue also reacts to the ischemic injury with chronic inflammatory responses as exemplified in middle cerebral artery occlusion (MCAO) which produces a focal cortical infarction.[2] One to two days after the occlusion, the infarct zone is infiltrated by blood-borne phagocytes and by the local proliferation of reactive astrocytes and microglia.[3] Activated macrophages[4,5] and astrocytes[6,7] play central roles in phagocytosis and as producers of mediators that influence the process of healing in ways that may either help or hinder the restoration of neural function. We have investigated patterns of gene expression for insulin-like growth factors (IGFs) and related proteins in brain's response to ischemic injury in the setting of focal cortical ischemia.[8]

Insulin-like growth factors-I and -II (IGF-I and -II) are multifunctional polypeptides that are structurally homologous to each other and to proinsulin. Their biological actions, which include the promotion of both cell proliferation and specific differentiating functions, are mediated by the type-I IGF receptor (IGFR-1), and possibly, the type-II IGF receptor (IGFR-2; IGF-II/Mannose-6-phosphate receptor). In the circulation and interstitial fluids, IGFs are associated with specific, high-affinity binding proteins (IGFBPs) that modulate their action with their receptors. Both IGFs, their receptors and IGFBP2 are synthesized in the normal (non-ischemic) CNS. IGF-I, IGFBP2 and IGFR-1 mRNAs are most abundant in early postnatal development, during which time IGF-I mRNA is contained predominantly in the large, long-axon projection neurons of sensory and cerebellar relay systems,[9] and IGFBP2 is expressed by adjacent astroglia.[10] The synchronized temporo-spatial relationship of the gene expression of IGF-I, its receptor, and IGFBP2 suggests that this IGF 'system' plays a key role in neuronal-glial interaction during brain development. IGF-II mRNA is localized in the mesenchymal support structures of the CNS, including the choroid plexus, meninges, and vascular sheaths, from early embryonic development onward, without apparent developmental regulation.[11,12]

Both IGFs, their receptors and IGFBP2 mRNA levels are increased in the infarct zone as part of the inflammatory response to ischemic injury, but they are

[a] Present address: Riley Research, Room 208, 702 Barnhill Dr., Indianapolis, IN 46202.

418

expressed in different cell populations (FIG. 1).[8] IGF-I mRNA was abundant in reactive astrocytes, which are characterized by thymidine incorporation, high levels of GFAP, active phagocytosis and high metabolic rates.[7,13,14] Astrocytic IGF-I may function in support of the heightened astrocyte metabolism in response

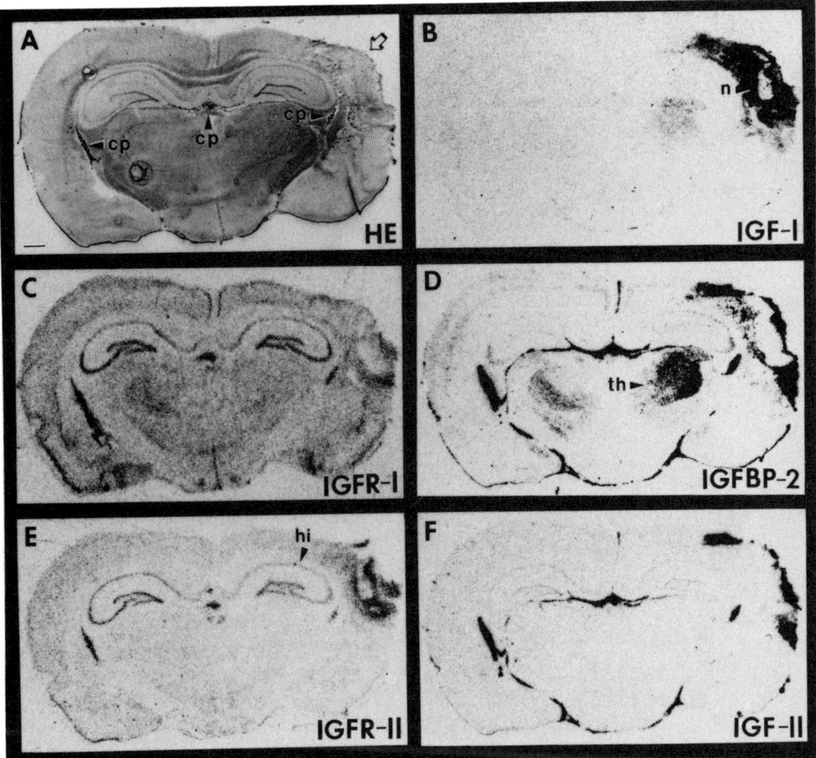

FIGURE 1. Patterns of gene expression for IGFs, receptors, and IGFBP-2 nine days after focal cerebral ischemia, as shown by *in situ* hybridization and film autoradiography. **(A)** A hematoxylin- and eosin-stained (HE) section that is representative of the serial coronal brain sections hybridized to cRNA probes for **(B)** IGF-I, **(C)** IGFR-I, **(D)** IGFBP-2, **(E)** IGFR-II, and **(F)** IGF-II. The infarct is indicated by an open arrow. IGF-I mRNA is abundant throughout the infarct zone except for a small area of necrosis (n). IGFBP-2 and IGF-II mRNAs are also abundant but are localized in the periphery of the infarct. The pattern of gene expression for IGFBP-2 is similar to, but more extensive than, that for IGF-II, IGF-I and, to a greater extent, IGFBP-2 mRNAs were also increased in ipsilateral thalamic nuclei **(B,D).** cp, choroid plexus; th, thalamic nuclei; hi, hippocampus. Bar = 1 mm.

to ischemic injury, for example, by stimulating glucose transporter synthesis, as has been reported *in vitro*.[15] Alternatively, IGF-I released from astrocytes could be directed at other cells in the injured area, *i.e.*, microglia, fibroblasts, and endothelial cells, which are proliferating in the formation of astroglial scar tissue. Activation of IGF-I expression in astrocytes was also reported in a recent study of experimental demyelination, in which high levels of IGF-I mRNA and peptide were found in those reactive astrocytes situated in brain regions selectively affected by demyelination.[16] Astrocytes in this setting are involved in the phagocytosis of degenerating myelin and, possibly, in the stimulation of remyelination by local oligodendrocytes.

IGF-II and IGFBP-2 mRNAs are abundant in activated macrophages congregated around the infarct and in the meninges, vasculature and choroid plexus of the ischemic brain (FIG. 1).[8] As is the case in most tissues, the CNS has its own population of resident macrophages.[17] Brain microglia are macrophages thought to originate from circulating monocytes during early postnatal development, which take up permanent residence throughout the brain parenchyma where they appear as small cells with long, branched processes.[17] On morphological and histochemical grounds these cells are considered to be quiescent tissue macrophages.[17] They are recognized by the ED1 rat macrophage antibody,[8,18] but do not contain detectable IGF-II or IGFBP-2 mRNA under normal conditions. Another group of brain macrophages reside in the brain's mesenchymal support structures—the meninges (mostly between the pia and arachnoid membranes), the choroid plexus and the perivasculature.[17] Macrophages in these strategic sites in the brain's defence perimeter resemble activated macrophages more than glial cells, are ED-1 positive and contain abundant IGF-II and IGFBP-2 mRNA. These cells protect the brain from blood or cerebrospinal fluid–borne threats and scavenge away debris collected by these filtering organs, and thus may be expected to be in a continual state of active phagocytosis. The macrophages congregated around the infarct zone presumably originated from the circulating monocyte pool, although some may have migrated from local meningeal or perivascular sources, or originated from the transformation of local quiescent microglia.[17] IGF-I and IGFBP-2 mRNAs were also increased in the ventrobasal complex of the thalamus ipsilateral to the MCAO.[8] There was histological evidence of neuronal loss and an increase in ED-1 and GFAP immunoreactivity in this region, consistent with a macrophage and astocyte response to localized tissue damage, which may be the result of retrograde degeneration of thalamic neurons that project to the infarcted cortex. It is probable that IGF-I is expressed by astrocytes and IGFBP-2 by macrophages in this site also, although the two cell populations were intermingled such that it was not possible to clearly distinguish the cell of origin of the hybridization signal.

IGF-II and IGFBP-2 mRNAs are co-localized in activated macrophages, both around the infarct site and in the meninges and choroid plexus. How IGFBP-2 is functionally related to IGF-II in this situation is open to speculation. While IGFBPs bind IGFs with high affinity and have been found to inhibit some IGF actions in vitro, in other instances IGFBPs have been shown to enhance IGF effects.[19] In this particular situation, in which local protease activity presumably abounds, IGFBP-2 may function to protect IGF-II from proteolytic digestion. Alternatively, if IGFBP2 is selectively bound (via RGD) to selective cell surfaces or the extracellular matrix protein, it may target the IGFs to particular sites. The fact that both IGFR-1 and IGFR-2 mRNAs are expressed in the infarct zone means that IGF-II could potentially act via both types of receptor in this setting. IGFR-II mRNA was particularly abundant and was found in both astrocytes and macrophages. The type-II IGF receptor has a role in lysosomal enzyme trafficking,[20] and there is evidence that IGF-II promotes this activity.[21] Thus, IGF-II might act via the type II receptor to enhance phagocytic enzyme recycling and via the type-I receptor to enhance metabolic function in support of the activated state.

In summary, we have found that both IGF-I and IGF-II are highly expressed in phagocytic cells during the height of phagocytic activity in the response to brain injury. IGF-I is expressed selectively in reactive astrocytes, and IGF-II and IGFBP-2, in activated macrophages. The function of these peptides in this setting is unknown, but the circumstances suggest that they may be involved in the promotion of phagocytic activity.

REFERENCES

1. CHOI, D. W. 1990. Cerebral hypoxia: Some new approaches and unanswered questions. J. Neurosci. **10:** 2493–2501.
2. BRINT, S., M. JACEWICZ, M. KIESSLING, J. TANABE & W. PULSINELLI. 1988. Focal brain ischemia in the rat: Methods for reproducible neocortical infarction using tendem occlusion of the distal middle cerebral and ipsilateral common carotid arteries. J. Cereb. Blood Flow Metab. **8:** 474–485.
3. HATTEN, M. E., R. K. H. LIEM, M. L. SHELANSKI & C. A. MASON. 1991. Astroglia in CNS injury. Glia **4:** 233–243.
4. GIULIAN, D., J. CHEN, J. E. INGEMAN, J. K. GEORGE & M. NOPONEN. 1989. The role of mononuclear phagocytes in wound healing after traumatic injury to adult mammalian brain. J. Neurosci. **9:** 4416–4429.
5. NATHAN, C. F. 1987. Secretory products of macrophages. J. Clin. Invest. **79:** 319–326.
6. LINDSAY, R. M. 1986. Reactive gliosis. *In* Astrocytes: Cell biology and Pathology of Astrocytes. S. Fedoroff & A. Vernadakis, Eds. Vol. 3: 231–261. Academic Press. New York.
7. RISCHKE, R. & J. KRIEGLSTEIN. 1991. Postischemic neuronal damage causes astroglial activation and increase in local cerebral glucose utilization of rat hippocampus. J. Cereb. Blood Flow. Metab. **11:** 106–113.
8. LEE, W.-H., J. A. CLEMENS & C. A. BONDY. 1992. Insulin-like growth factors in the response to cerebral ischemia. Mol. Cell. Neurosci. **3:** 36–43.
9. BONDY, C. A. 1991. Transient IGF-I gene expression during the maturation of functionally-related central projection neurons. J. Neurosci. **11:** 3442–3455.
10. LEE, W.-H., S. JAVEDAN & C. A. BONDY. 1993. Co-ordinate expression of insulin-like growth factor components by neurons and neuroglia during retinal and cerebellum development. J. Neurosci. **12:** 4737–4744.
11. STYLIANOPOULOU, F., J. HERBERT, M. B. SOARES & A. EFSTRATIADIS. 1988. Expression of the insulin-like growth factor II gene in the choroid plexus and the leptomeninges of the adult rat central nervous system. Proc. Natl. Acad. Sci. USA **85:** 141–145.
12. BONDY, C. A., H. WERNER, C. T. ROBERTS & D. LEROITH. 1990. Cellular pattern of insulin-like growth factor-I (IGF-I) and type I IGF receptor gene expression in early organogenesis: comparison with IGF-II gene expression. Mol. Endocrinol. **4:** 1386–1398.
13. PETITO, C. K., S. MORGELLO, J. C. FELIX & M. L. LESSER. 1990. Two patterns of reactive astrocytosis in postischemic rat brain. J. Cereb. Blood Flow Metab. **10:** 850–859.
14. RICHKE, R. & J. KRIDGLSTEIN. 1991. Postischemic neuronal damage causes astroglial activation and increase in local cerebral glucose utilization of rat hippocampus. J. Cereb. Blood Flow Metab. **11:** 106–113.
15. WERNER, H., M. K. RAIZADA, L. M. MUDD, H. L. FOYT, I. A. SIMPSON, C. T. ROBERTS, JR. & D. LEROITH. 1989. Regulation of rat brain/hepG2 glucose transporter gene expression by insulin and insulin-like growth factor-I in primary cultures and neuronal and glial cells. Endocrinology **125:** 314–320.
16. KOMOLY, S., L. D. HUDSON, H. DEF. WEBSTER & C. A. BONDY. 1991. Insulin-like growth factor I (IGF-I) gene expression is induced in astrocytes during experimental demyelination. Proc. Natl. Acad. Sci. USA. **89:** 1894–1898
17. PERRY, V. H. & S. GORDON. 1988. Macrophages and microglia in the nervous system. Trends Neurosci. **11:** 273–277.
18. SMINIA, T., C. J. A. DE GROOT, C. D. DIJKSTRA, J. C. KOETSIER & C. H. POLMAN. 1987. Macrophages in the central nervous system of the rat. Immunology **174:** 43–50.

19. CLEMMONS, D. R. 1991. Insulin-like growth factor binding proteins. Trends Endocrinol. Metab. **1:** 412–417.
20. ROTH, R. A. 1988. Structure of the receptor for insulin-like growth factor II: The puzzle amplified. Science **239:** 1269–1271.
21. POLYCHRONAKOS, C., H. J. GUYDA, U. JANTHLY & B. I. POSNER. 1990. Effects of mannose-6-phosphate on receptor-mediated endocytosis of insulin-like growth factor-II. Endocrinology **127:** 1861–1866.

Gene Expression in Brain Injury: Identification of a New cDNA Structurally Related to Adhesive and Trophic Agents

TAM THANH QUACH,[a] BRUCE K. SCHRIER,
AND ANNE-MARIE DUCHEMIN

Molecular Neurobiology Unit
Laboratory of Developmental Neurobiology
NICHHD, NIH
Bethesda, Maryland 20892

The brain is a highly complex organ in both structure and function.[1,2] The very large number of neurons and their connections constitute a sophisticated network which transduces and integrates information between the environment and the living organism. Successful functioning of this network is dependent on the maintenance of its physical integrity. When that integrity is interrupted by an injury and its consequent neuronal degeneration, the consequences range from abnormal behaviors to irretrievable loss of one or more functions. The regeneration capacity of injured neurons in mammals is limited. Severed axons in the mammalian peripheral nervous system have been shown to regenerate in response to injury. In contrast, regeneration of the central nervous system neurons remains much less conclusive; however, neurotrophic agents have been shown to aid in the recovery of functional activity in the central nervous system either by early prevention of degeneration, or by the process of regeneration. This response almost certainly requires new patterns of gene expression in the area of the injury, probably involving changes in the level of expression of some genes and induction of new gene expression. To investigate this possibility, we have: 1) examined the production of unique mRNAs by injured tissue using subtractive hybridization of cDNAs from control and injured brain and 2) identified new cDNA clones encoding for trophic, or adhesive factors which may facilitate repair of injured neurons.

MODIFICATION OF GENE EXPRESSION IN INJURED BRAIN TISSUE

In injured brain tissue, while changes in the cytoarchitecture have been clearly established, only a few studies have addressed alterations in the gene expression in surviving neurons, or non-neuronal cells, close to the wound. Elevated levels of RNA synthesis, and an increase in activities of enzymes involved in the metabolism of RNA were observed several days after axonal injury in the fish optic nerve.

[a] Present address: Ohio State University, Biotechnology Center, 1060 Carmack Road, Columbus, OH 43210.

Increases in ^{3}H-uridine incorporation, retinal uridine kinase and uridine mono- and diphosphate kinase were observed in the corresponding retinas, with a peak at day 4 after injury.[3]

It has been shown, that in the rat brain, injury induced clear increase in neurotrophic activity in the area surrounding the damaged region.[4] Extracts from tissue surrounding the wound, and from the gelfoam used to fill the wound cavity, support the survival of a variety of neurons in culture. Some observations also suggest that injury triggers the production of a neurotrophic factor which does not travel far from the injured locus. In the hippocampus, neurotrophic activity is significantly increased within one week after medial septal lesion and can facilitate graft survival. Neurite-promoting activity, different from the neuronal survival activity, is also induced in rat brain following injury and deafferentation.[5] We have previously demonstrated the expression of trophic factors which support the growth of chick sympathetic neurons in Xenopus oocytes injected with mRNA extracted from injured brain.[6,7] These above observations have prompted us to investigate changes in gene expression in injured brain tissue, including the possibility of changes in the gene expression of specific transcripts encoding neuronal survival factors.

For these purposes, we constructed a subtractive cDNA library in a PGEM procaryotic vector. Briefly, total RNA from control and lesioned rat brain tissue[7] was prepared by the guanidium thiocyanate method as described previously.[8] The RNA was then subjected to affinity chromatography on oligo-dT cellulose to obtain substantially purified poly(A+) containing sequences. cDNAs were synthesized from the mRNAs prepared from lesioned brain using AMV reverse transcriptase primed with oligo-dT$_{(20-30)}$. After removal of the template RNA by alkaline hydrolysis, the cDNAs were purified by Sephadex G50, and concentrated with secondary butanol.[9] The single stranded cDNAs from wounded cerebral cortex were hybridized with a 20-fold excess of poly(A+)RNA from control brain cortex to an ER_0t of 4000 at 68°C in order to remove most of the cDNAs which were jointly represented in control and lesioned tissues. Unreacted single stranded cDNAs were then purified by chromatography on hydroxyapatite and used to synthesize double stranded cDNAs with DNA polymerase in the presence of random hexamers. These cDNAs were ligated to the SmaI site of PGEM procaryotic vector, which was then used to transform competent cells E. coli JM109. This library, enriched for lesion-induced sequences, was used in analytical hybridizations. Recombinant bacterial colonies selected at random were grown directly on nitrocellulose filters at low density, and processed for colony hybridization to identify mRNA sequences that are significantly increased during the reactive post-injury period. Nitrocellulose filters were hybridized to ^{32}P-cDNAs prepared from mRNAs from control brain, washed at high stringency and subjected to autoradiography. After stripping off the radioactive probe, the same filters were rehybridized with ^{32}P-cDNAs prepared from mRNAs from lesioned brain. By this technique, we were able to identify 12 colonies, out of 640, which showed a substantial increase in lesioned versus control mRNAs (FIG. 1). This library was 10-fold enriched for lesion-specific cDNAs as judged by the fact that about 90% of the radiolabeled cDNA mass was removed in the subtraction at the hydroxyapatite step. This observation allows a quantitative measurement of the RNA transcripts affected by injury: 0.18% of poly(A+)RNAs showed increased levels of expression in the tissues surrounding the wound. It is of interest that in another model involving an electrolytic lesion in entorhinal cortex, a very similar level of induction of gene expression (0.11%) was observed.[10] Whether these genes are expressed in order to protect cells from post-neurotoxic insults that could lead to cell death, or

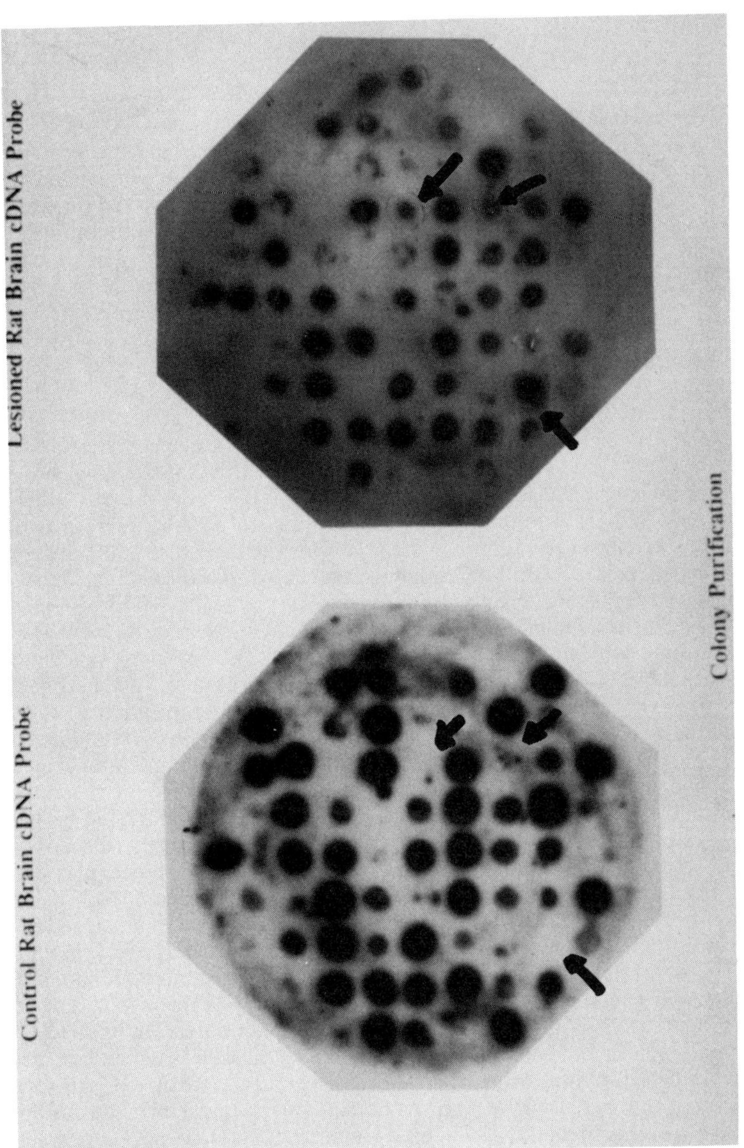

FIGURE 1. Identification of cDNA clones specific to injured brain tissue. Bacterial transformants were grown individually onto nitrocellulose filters, and processed for binding of DNA (see text). Filters were hybridized with ^{32}P-cDNA reverse transcribed from poly(A+)RNAs of control rat brain cortex. After autoradiography and removal of the probe, the same filters were rehybridized with ^{32}P-cDNA from poly(A+)RNAs of lesioned rat brain cortex. Clones with levels of expression increased in lesioned rat brain cortex. Clones with levels of expression increased in lesioned rat brain tissue are marked with arrows.

whether there are actively expressed in neurons as part of a cytocidal death program, is unclear. However, since extracts from lesioned brain tissue present neuronal survival activity, we hypothesize that some of the gene products may serve a beneficial function analogous to a NGF or heat shock-like response which enables deafferented neurons to survive the neurotoxic insult produced by injury.

CLONING AND EXPRESSION OF A NEW cDNA SEQUENCE IN LESIONED CORTEX OF ADULT RAT

After injury to the cerebral cortex, many diffusible substances are released into the tissues which surround the lesion. Some of them affect metabolic activities, neurite extension, survival, and differentiation of the nerve cell. It is likely that these factors keep a maximal number of neurons alive in the area of damage. The substances released by injury may be already known neurotrophic factors, or they may be new molecules specifically induced by the lesion. A number of neurotrophic factors not directly related to injury have been isolated and cloned;[11,12] in the neurotrophin family, NGF is the prototype which has been best characterized.[13,14] BDNF (brain-derivative neurotrophic factor), another representative of this family, was originally discovered in the conditioned medium of a glial cell line.[15,16] Other neurotrophic molecules are neuroleukin and glia-derived-nexin. The above factors are examples of diffusible substances which have been isolated for their neurotrophic activity. Many known growth factors, such as epidermal growth factor, basic fibroblast growth factor, insulin growth factor,[17] or small peptides such as vasoactive intestinal peptide[18] or hydra head activator peptide,[19] also have a neurotrophic activity for specific neuronal types.

In addition to these soluble factors, adhesive molecules also play an important role in the survival and/or differentiation of neurons. The intact extracellular matrix and the availability of some of its components, such as laminin and fibronectin, are important for growth and elongation of nerve fibers both *in vitro* and *in vivo*.[20] In the peripheral nervous system, the existence of an intact basal lamina is prerequisite for nerve regeneration. For example, regeneration in transected sciatic nerve is significantly faster when it is exposed to nerve guide lumen filled with laminin, and *in situ* regeneration of the optic nerve is accompanied by the appearance of laminin immunoreactive sites and of fibrous collagen adjacent to the basal lamina of astrocytes.[21,22] It seems clear that the continuous expression of laminin may be a prerequisite for axonal growth and regeneration. In the peripheral nervous system, the various components of the extracellular matrix, such as collagen and laminin, are produced by Schwann cells. It appears that not only peripheral neurons, but also central nervous neurons, are able to respond to laminin. However, the supportive glial cells in the central nervous system, in contrast to their counterpart Schwann cells in the peripheral nervous system, or the glial cells of central nervous system of fish, are not able to produce laminin. Consequently, further identification of such new molecules—diffusible or extracellular matrix factors—may lead to the understanding of novel mechanisms of neurodegenerative and regenerative processes occurring in injured and aging brain.

For that specific purpose, and on the assumption that a novel neuronal survival factor would contain some common and conservative sequences of neurotrophin family, we have designed a specific 30 mer oligonucleotide common to NGF and BDNF. This oligomer, end-labeled with ^{32}P using T4 nucleotide kinase, was used to screen three different brain cDNA libraries constructed with phage lambda

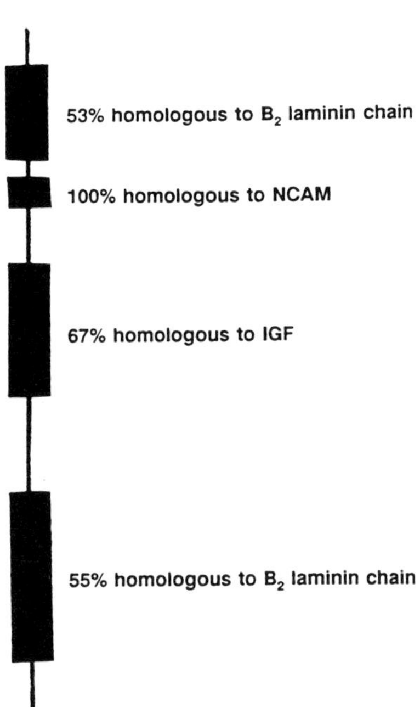

FIGURE 2. Schematic representation of G41 cDNA insert. Sequence comparison of a partially sequenced insert revealed partial homology of G41 with the nucleic acid sequence coding for IGF and B2 chain of laminin. G41 has also a motif presenting 100% homologous to N-CAM.

gt10, gt11, and PGEM procaryotic expression vector. Forty-eight clones which gave positive signals ranging from weak to strong, were partially sequenced. One of the above clones, designated G41, appears to be of special interest in light of the potential trophic or adhesive activity of the gene product(s) (FIG. 2). Partial sequencing of G41 (1200 NT over 1300 NT) has revealed the following nucleotide

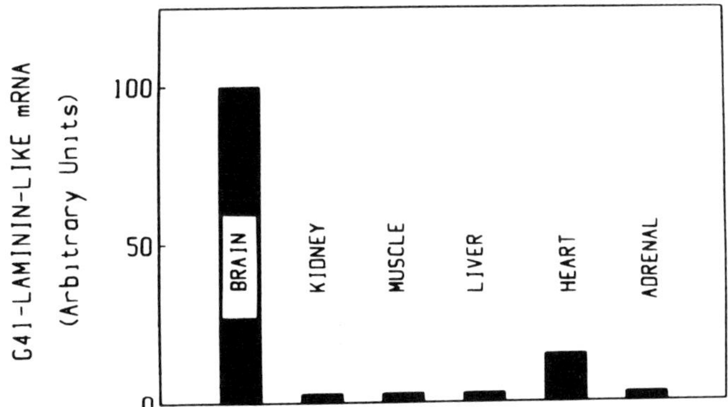

FIGURE 3. Tissue distribution of G41-laminin-like mRNA in the rat. Northern blots of 20 microgram total RNA from different tissues of rat were hybridized with ^{32}P radiolabeled G41 cRNA transcript and autoradiographs scanned with a densitometer. G41mRNA levels are expressed as percent of the levels in the brain.

sequence homologies:

a) from either end of the clone, homologies of 53 and 55% covering 130 and 250 NT, respectively, with the B2 laminin chain;
b) 67% homology with insulin-like growth factor, covering 170 NT in the middle of the insert; and
c) a small motif with 100% homology to N-CAM.

The structural sequence of G41 is interesting in two aspects. Firstly, it raises the possibility that it encodes a novel protein belonging to the laminin gene family that extends beyond the gene coding for three laminin subunits. Secondly, since G41 also has an internal motif representing 67% homology to IGF, over 170 NT, we cannot rule out that G41 presents a new class of active protein, partially similar to IGF, and partially similar to laminin. A similarly complex cDNA structure has been cloned recently.[23] HPSG2 protein core is composed with multiple domains homologous to the low density lipoprotein receptor, laminin, neural cell adhesion molecule, and epidermal growth factor.

We analyzed the expression of G41 mRNA in various tissues, tumors and cell lines using Northern blot analysis. No hybridizing G41mRNA species were

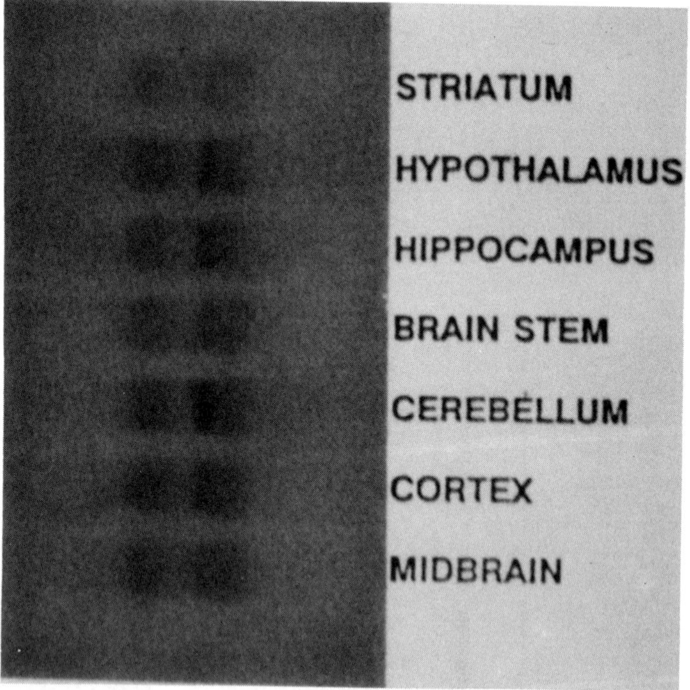

FIGURE 4. Regional distribution of G41mRNA in the rat brain. Brain regions were dissected out as previously described.[25] Total RNA was extracted, electrophoresed and blotted on nylon membranes. Northern blots were hybridized with labeled G41 cRNA transcript and autoradiographed.

FIGURE 5. Expression of G41 mRNA after brain lesion. Lesions of the parieto-occipital cortex of the rat were made by vacuum aspiration. At different times after the lesion, animals were sacrificed and the tissues surrounding the lesion cavity removed. RNA was extracted from these tissues and from similar areas from control animal. Total RNA was blotted and hybridized with a labeled cRNA probe for G41. RNA levels are expressed as percent of the levels in control animals. C: controls; 2,4,6: number of days after lesion.

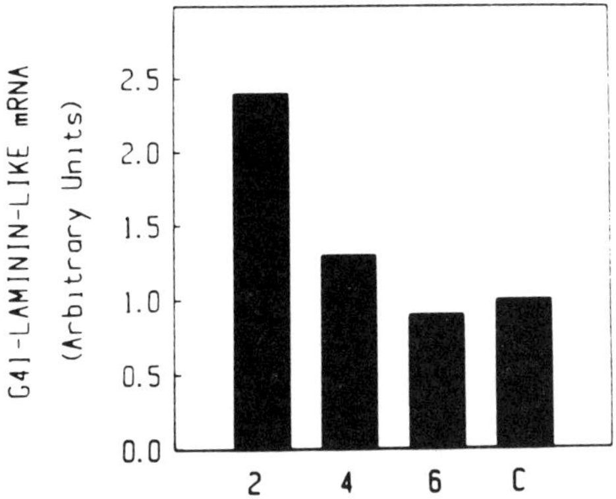

detected from pancreas, intestine, muscle, liver and lung. A low level, relative to brain, was detected in the heart (FIG. 3). The apparently unique 3.8 Kb transcript of G41 was found mostly in brain tissue as expected and in different types of tumor (rat mammary tumor) and cell lines (Neuro 2A and PC12). More detailed analysis of G41 expression in the brain showed that cerebellum, hippocampus, hypothalamus and cortex contain the highest levels of the message. Moderate or low expression was seen in striatum, midbrain and pons (FIG. 4). These observations suggest that the expression of G41 is tissue-specific, and perhaps cell-specific, within the brain.

More interestingly, the levels of G41 mRNA near the wound were increased more than 250% by day 2 and returned to control levels by day 6 post-lesion (FIG. 5). This time-course correlates with the active phenomenon of lesion induced-sprouting and synapse turnover in mammalian brain. In contrast to the temporal increase of G41 gene expression, 3.8 Kb NGF-1A mRNA levels remained unchanged when the same blot was rehybridized with a ^{32}P-radiolabeled pBS-KS plasmid containing a 3.1 Kb NGF-1A insert.[24] Thus, this dynamic change mirrors the specific control of G41 expression by a lesion.

The molecular data presented in this paper unraveled the structural complexity and the potential of G41. The composite of this gene is a result of the assembly of different modular units. Interestingly, these multi-domain units appear to be evolutionarily related to molecules involved in fundamental cellular processes, such as mitogenesis, adhesion, and growth promoting activity. It is tempting to speculate that the G41 gene product(s) would provide several site-specific interactions which collectively or individually affect cellular growth, differentiation, and remodeling following injury.

REFERENCES

1. Molecular Neurobiology. 1983. Cold Spring Harbor Symp. Quant. Biol. Vol. 48. Cold Spring Harbor Laboratory Press.
2. The Brain. 1990. Cold Spring Harbor Symp. Quant. Biol. Vol. 55. Cold Spring Harbor Laboratory Press.
3. KOSHAKA, S., L. A. DOKAS & B. W. AGRANOFF. 1981. Uridine metabolism in the goldfish retina during optical nerve regeneration. J. Neurochem. **36:** 1168–1171.
4. NIETO-SAMPEDRO, M., M. MANTHORPE, G. BARBIN, S. VARON & C. W. COTMAN. 1982. Brain injury causes a time-dependent increase in neurotrophic activity at the lesion site. Science **217:** 860–861.

5. NEEDELS, D. L., M. NIETO-SAMPEDRO & C. W. COTMAN. 1986. Induction of a neurite-promoting factor in rat brain following injury or deafferentation. Neuroscience **18:** 517–526.

6. QUACH, T. T., A. M. DUCHEMIN, B. K. SCHRIER & R. J. WYATT. 1988. Synthesis of neurotrophic factor for sympathetic neurons in Xenopus oocytes by translation of mRNA extracted from rat wounded cerebral cortex. Society for Neuroscience. Toronto.

7. DUCHEMIN, A. M., T. T. QUACH, B. K. SCHRIER, D. M. CHUANG & R. J. WYATT. 1990. Expression of neurotrophic activity in Xenopus oocytes injected with mRNA from wounded rat cerebral cortex. Mol. Brain Res. **8:** 235–241.

8. DUCHEMIN, A. M., T. T. QUACH, M. J. IADAROLA, R. J. DESCHENES, J. P. SCHWARTZ & R. J. WYATT. 1987. Expression of the cholecystokinin gene in rat brain during development. Dev. Neurosci. **9:** 61–67.

9. WALLACE, D. M. 1987. Precipitation of nucleic acid. *In* Methods in Enzymology. J. N. Aberson & M. I. Simon, Eds. **152:** 41–48.

10. POIRIER, J., M. HESS, P. C. MAY & C. L. FINCH. 1991. Cloning of hippocampal poly(A)RNA sequences that increase after entorhinal cortex lesion in adult rat. Mol. Brain Res. **9:** 191–195.

11. SNIDER, W. D. & E. M. JOHNSON. 1989. Neurotrophic molecules. Ann. Neurol. **26:** 490–506.

12. CROSS, M. & T. M. DEXTER. 1991. Growth factors in development, transformation, and tumorigenesis. Cell **64:** 271–280.

13. LEVI-MONTALCINI, R. 1987. The nerve growth factor 35 years later. Science **237:** 1154–1161.

14. MAISONPIERRE, P. C., L. BELLUSCIO, S. SQUINTO, M. E. FURTH, R. M. LINDSAY & G. D. YANCOPOULOS. 1990. Neurotrophin-3: A neurotrophic factor related to NGF and BDNF. Science **247:** 1446–1451.

15. THOENEN, H. 1991. The changing scene of neurotrophic factors. TINS **14:** 165–170.

16. LEIBROCK, J., F. LOTTSPEICH, A. HOHN, M. HOFER, *et al.* 1989. Molecular cloning and expression of brain-derived neurotrophic factor. Nature **341:** 149–151.

17. RECIO-PINTO, E., M. M. RECHLER & D. N. ISHII. 1986. Effects of insulin, insulin-like factor II and nerve growth factor on neurite formation and survival cultured sympathetic and sensory neurons. J. Neurosci. **6:** 1211–1219.

18. PINCUS, D. W., E. M. DICICCO-BLOOM & I. B. BLACK. 1990. Vasoactive intestinal peptide regulates mitosis, differentiation and survival of culture sympathetic neuroblasts. Nature **343:** 564–567.

19. QUACH, T. T., A. M. DUCHEMIN, A. P. OLIVER, B. K. SCHRIER & R. J. WYATT. 1992. Hydra head activator has trophic activity for eucaryotic neurons. Dev. Brain Res. **68:** 97–102.

20. BARON-VAN EVERCOOREN, A., H. K. KLEIMANN, S. OHNO, P. MARANGOS. 1982. Nerve growth factor, laminin, and fibronectin promote neurite outgrowth in human fetal sensory ganglia culture. J. Neurosci. Res. **8:** 179–186.

21. MADISON, R., C. F. DA SILVA, P. DIKKES, T. CHIU & R. L. SILMAN. 1985. Increased rate of peripheral nerve regeneration using bioresorbable nerve guide and laminin-containing gel. Exp. Neurol. **88:** 767–772.

22. REICHARDT, L. F. & K. J. TOMASELLI. 1991. Extracellular matrix molecules and their receptors: Functions in neural development. Ann. Rev. Neurosci. **14:** 531–570.

23. MURDOCH, A. D., G. R. DODGE, I. COHEN, R. S. TUAN & R. V. IOZZO. 1992. Primary structure of the human heparan sulfate proteoglycan from basement membrane (HSPG2/perlecan). J. Biol. Chem. **267**(12): 8544–8557.

24. MILBRANDT, J. 1987. A nerve growth factor-induced gene encodes a possible transcriptional regulatory factor. Science **238:** 797–799.

25. IADAROLA, M., R. J. NARANJO, A. M. DUCHEMIN & T. T. QUACH. 1989. Expression of the cholecystokinin and enkephalin mRNA in discrete brain region. Peptide **10:** 687–692.

Index of Contributors